MW00805575

Central University Libraries
West Coast University
Los Angeles, CA

DISCARDED

The Fundamentals of
ACUPUNCTURE

of related interest

Acupuncture and Chinese Medicine
Roots of Modern Practice
Charles Buck
ISBN 978 1 84819 159 4
eISBN 978 0 85701 133 6

The Acupuncture Points Functions Colouring Book
Rainy Hutchinson
Forewords by Richard Blackwell, and Angela Hicks and John Hicks
ISBN 978 1 84819 266 9
eISBN 978 0 85701 214 2

The Spark in the Machine
How the Science of Acupuncture Explains the Mysteries of Western Medicine
Dr. Daniel Keown MBChB MCEM LicAc
ISBN 978 1 84819 196 9
eISBN 978 0 85701 154 1

Developing Internal Energy for Effective Acupuncture Practice
Zhan Zhuang, Yi Qi Gong and the Art of Painless Needle Insertion
Ioannis Solos
ISBN 978 1 84819 183 9
eISBN 978 0 85701 144 2

Intuitive Acupuncture
John Hamwee
ISBN 978 1 84819 273 7
eISBN 978 0 85701 220 3

The Fundamentals of
ACUPUNCTURE

NIGEL CHING

Foreword by Charles Buck

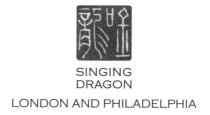

SINGING
DRAGON
LONDON AND PHILADELPHIA

English language edition first published in 2017
by Singing Dragon
an imprint of Jessica Kingsley Publishers
73 Collier Street
London N1 9BE, UK
and
400 Market Street, Suite 400
Philadelphia, PA 19106, USA

www.singingdragon.com

First published in Danish as *Akupunkturens Grundprincipper* by
Klitrose Publishers, Copenhagen, Denmark, 2012

Copyright © Nigel Ching 2017
Foreword copyright © Charles Buck 2017
Illustrations copyright © Klitrose 2017

All rights reserved. No part of this publication may be reproduced in any material form (including
photocopying or storing it in any medium by electronic means and whether or not transiently
or incidentally to some other use of this publication) without the written permission of the
copyright owner except in accordance with the provisions of the Copyright, Designs and Patents
Act 1988 or under the terms of a licence issued by the Copyright Licensing Agency Ltd, Saffron
House, 6–10 Kirby Street, London EC1N 8TS. Applications for the copyright owner's written
permission to reproduce any part of this publication should be addressed to the publisher.

Warning: The doing of an unauthorised act in relation to a copyright work
may result in both a civil claim for damages and criminal prosecution.

Library of Congress Cataloging in Publication Data
Names: Ching, Nigel, 1962- , author.
Title: The fundamentals of acupuncture / Nigel Ching ; foreword by Charles
    Buck.
Other titles: Akupunkturens Grundprincipper. English
Description: English language edition. | London ; Philadelphia : Singing
    Dragon, 2017. | Translation of: Akupunkturens Grundprincipper / Nigel
    Ching. Klitrose Publishers, Copenhagen, Denmark, 2012. | Includes
    bibliographical references and index.
Identifiers: LCCN 2016011560 | ISBN 9781848193130 (alk. paper)
Subjects: | MESH: Acupuncture Therapy | Acupuncture Points | Medicine,
    Chinese Traditional
Classification: LCC RM184.5 | NLM WB 369 | DDC 615.8/92--
dc23 LC record available at http://lccn.loc.gov/2016011560

British Library Cataloguing in Publication Data
A CIP catalogue record for this book is available from the British Library

ISBN 978 1 84819 313 0
eISBN 978 0 85701 266 1

Printed and bound in Great Britain

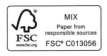

A journey of a thousand miles begins with a single step.

Lao Zi (604 BCE–531 BCE)

CONTENTS

4. The Channel System

5. The Acupuncture Points

FOREWORD

As an educator in acupuncture and Chinese medicine it is tempting to enjoy the reflected glory of past students' achievements. Seeking to resist such empty vanity I instead applaud their accomplishments in the belief that credit properly belongs to those who do the work rather than their teachers. Nevertheless, some pleasure remains in having the opportunity to proudly introduce this textbook and its author Nigel 'Tonto' Ching to the English-speaking acupuncture and Chinese medicine community.

I came to know Nigel in 2000 when he began the three-year training in Chinese herbal medicine on which I was a lead tutor. It quickly became clear that he wished to get his money's worth from this course, as evidenced by the fact that all the assignments I marked of his were close to flawless. Later I came to discover a person who was determined, not only to immerse himself deeply into the wisdom that acupuncture and Chinese medicine offers, but to interpret and share that wisdom with others. Nigel has published three major textbooks in Danish, texts that have become established as standard student resources. His skills as a communicator and dedication to his profession have helped him become a prominent educator in Nordic countries and more widely across the European Union.

What is presented so succinctly in this text is the current *standard model* of acupuncture practice, an understanding that is shared by perhaps a million practitioners worldwide. This is a lucid account of the current interpretation of the extraordinarily diverse scholarly medical tradition of China, a medical system whose literature base extends back almost 2500 years and whose historical literature base runs to many of thousands of volumes. This text provides the foundation that informs modern practice. It provides coherence to a complex historical tradition and sets out the dominant interpretation that is the basis of most acupuncture practice and research worldwide. Before this interpretation was made available to practitioners and students in the West, our learning resources were a confusing mix of fact, fantasy and misapprehension – a mish-mash of Chinese whispers.

In the past, limited scholarship combined with the tendency to romantic orientalism meant that acupuncture study was a frustrating process for those who sought to practice this medicine in a plain, effective and authentic manner. With insufficient information and understanding we coloured this medicine with our own fantasies about what we would expect this medicine to be about, an instance of the human tendency to see things that are *other* in terms of things that are already familiar to us (a trait that was summed up in just six words by the playwright and intellectual Eugene Ionescu as 'the French for London is Paris!'). Fortunately, less than four decades ago, China's new *standard model* for this medicine was delivered to us by scholar-pioneers such as Dan Bensky, John O'Connor, Ted Kaptchuk, Giovanni Macciocia and others. These were exceptional people who had taken the trouble to learn the Chinese language and who had devoted long periods to study extensively in China at a time when travel and life there was difficult. What they brought was a breath of fresh qi for those of us who had previously wallowed in the obscure hinterlands between Chinese philosophy, metaphysics and medicine. The more pragmatic style they brought was appealing because it was congruent with the understanding that we had already learned from exposure to ancient classics such as the *Yijing* (*Classic of Change*) and *Huangdi Nejing* (*Yellow Emperor's Inner Classic*), but the teachings included fewer confusing distractions. The subject was now laid out for us in a coherent, understandable and down-to-earth way. Halleluja! This is the interpretation of China's acupuncture tradition that Nigel offers you here.

In the decades since the introduction of this style of acupuncture practice our profession has continued to mature significantly – we benefit from improved translation resources and ever-greater levels of scholarship. During the same period the *bamboo curtain* almost completely lifted and we gained more direct access to China's classical medical corpus as well as to the generosity of many high-level scholar-practitioners from China. Alongside this, we also gained clearer perspectives on the manner in which this venerable medical tradition was re-interpreted and re-packaged to meet the needs of China's health service in the communist era and to match the political imperatives that dominated the 1960s and 70s. We came to appreciate, too, that ownership of this medicine is not entirely Chinese, that diverse interpretations and styles of practice had emerged over long periods in other East Asian countries, notably Japan, Korea and Vietnam. These countries added their own layers of scholarly interpretation for well over one thousand years and that the styles they have evolved also deserve our attention and respect.

In the 1950s, having made the political decision to include traditional medicine in their healthcare provision, Chinese authorities surveyed the mind-boggling diversity of medically related beliefs and practices that had been acquired over the two previous millennia; essentially an unwieldy mix of sense, half-sense and nonsense, superstition and rationality. Much of what the various medical traditions contained was unworkable in the modern world and so decisions had to be made about what would be included in the medical curriculum and what would be excluded. They will have known, for instance, that the Imperial Medical College of the Song dynasty (960–1278) included extensive study of chanting as a therapeutic modality. It is possible that chanting delivered some useful therapeutic value to people at that time but it did not appear well-matched to the clinical needs in the forward-looking communist world of the 1960s.

Medical practices connect intimately with the cultural beliefs and norms of their time and many of those from old China were no longer congruent with those of today. Belief in the influence of ancestor spirits, astrological notions and the ancient medical practice of writing therapeutic Chinese characters on paper and asking patients to burn this and then swallow the ash were part of the healthcare tradition. The authorities chose to exclude such ideas from the modern scope of practice and so, with this in mind, panels of doctors in the 1950s and 60s were tasked with surveying the formal written tradition. The intention was to reassemble the tradition into a compact practical medicine that was teachable, examinable and a practical means for providing healthcare to millions. As neophytes navigating through the maze of half-understood classical ideas, it was this coherent modern style that my student generation welcomed near the beginning of our journey into this medicine.

Later, as we ourselves gained direct access to the historical literature, we began to understand the way that this sanitisation process had operated and we came to appreciate that this style was only a rough approximation of the tradition. We noticed that thinkers in China had grafted ideas that more properly belonged to the herbal medicine practice onto acupuncture theory, such as the idea of formalised acupoint actions (e.g. *Tai xi – Kidney 3 – Nourishes Kidney Yin*). Whilst not, of itself, an unhelpful innovation, we realised that this was not quite the way things were presented historically. We discovered, too, that some interesting branches of the acupuncture tree had been unceremoniously lopped off in the quest for rationality. The spiritual and emotional content of the tradition had been downplayed and simplified. Now we can see that this was understandable because, after all, communism by definition provides a guarantee of happiness for all. Why would there be any need to include discussions of depression? Further, wishing to see a closer match with modern biomedicine meant that some basic traditional aspects of theory had to be downplayed – chronobiology (the biology of time) and the *wu xing* (five element) model of change, for example.

Having discovered that a wholesale re-styling had taken place, some in the West seized upon this to suggest that modern Traditional Chinese Medicine was not so much a re-interpretation but an invention of the communists. That it was a misleading mutation of the historical medical tradition. It was claimed, for example, that the *Ba Gang* diagnostic framework (八 纲 Eight Principles; Internal-External, Hot-Cold, Excess-Vacuity, Yin-Yang) had been invented in 1947 by a Dr Zhu Wei-ju.

Nigel Ching, myself and many others take the view that the critics overstate the position. The Ba Gang ideas are quite clearly present in the historical medical literature of China, what Dr Zhu did was apply a new label to this fundamental idea, not introduce a new idea. The same applies to the core content in China's *standard model* – that it is practical and substantially accurate. The issue for our profession to consider in the coming years has more to do with what has been excluded than what has been misrepresented. Many consider that the clarity provided by the appraisal of the tradition in the Communist era has, on balance, been a positive thing.

Today, practitioners, translators and scholars in this global profession are better placed to broaden our understanding of the tradition, to evaluate more closely the meaning of the Han dynasty medical classics and to factor in the innovations of medical scholarship from later times. We are better placed now to decide for ourselves what parts of this medicine we believe to be irrational, ineffective, unsuitable or misconstrued and adopt those that make sense to us and that we consider have value for our patients.

Having tracked Nigel Ching's progress towards mastery in acupuncture and Chinese medicine I know that he is familiar with the deeper refinements that lie beyond the scope of this textbook. He knows the territory that lies beyond the TCM *standard model*. Despite this, we both support the notion that the current interpretation of Chinese medicine which dominates in practice today is the most convenient point of entry. It offers a coherent, consensual and substantially accurate overview of the root tradition. It is the starting point to practising this medicine effectively and is one that gives us perspectives that help us interpret other material. What Nigel Ching offers here, in a concise and accurate style, is the interpretation that is understood by perhaps a million practitioners worldwide and it unites this profession together in an agreed common understanding.

Read and study this book well and you will have the opportunity to gain the reliable *standard model* road map that will help you navigate from patient presentation, through interpretation and diagnosis to effective intervention. Later you can journey beyond these roads to find a wonderfully diverse and extensive further landscape of rivers, footpaths and mountains that define a still deeper soul to this medicine.

I have yet to meet anyone who regretted stepping onto this path.

Charles Buck
Chester, UK
July 2016

ACKNOWLEDGEMENTS

If I have been able to see further than others, it is only because I have stood on the shoulders of giants.

Isaac Newton (1642–1727)[1]

In the following chapters you will not read anything new, even though what you are going to read might appear to be new to you. The story that is about to be retold in my words is at least three thousand years old. What you are about to hear is a very faint voice in a huge choir, the sound of whose voices echo way back through the millennia. In this way, I am a single thread, daring to weave itself into a large, intricate and very beautiful tapestry.

For this reason, I will once again use this section of the book to express my sincere gratitude to the learned people whose feet have trodden the path that I have followed the last twenty-five years. It is their knowledge that I have tried to interpret and pass on in this and my other books.

In particular, I owe a huge debt to my teachers, particularly Charles Buck; the authors, whose books I have studied; and the lecturers, whose courses I have participated in. Without these people, this book would not exist.

I have tried, as far as possible, to avoid contributing my own interpretations and ideas to this or my other books, unless these assumptions have been confirmed by wiser and more experienced minds than mine.

I would also like to thank the people who have directly contributed to the making of this book. Books such as this one are dependent on these people, whose efforts are a reflection of their idealism, zeal and a complete lack of economic sense.

A huge thanks to everyone who was involved in the original Danish version of the book, especially Ole Bidsted. His publishing company Klitrose[2] lives up to its name – a tough flower that survives and thrives where other plants do not even attempt to take root. Klitrose is one of the last idealistic publishers left in Denmark, whose faith in the written word outweighs their economic sense.

A big thanks to everyone at Singing Dragon, especially Claire Wilson for convincing me that I should undertake this task, and a special thanks to Jonathan Clogstoun-Willmott for suggesting to Singing Dragon that they should contact me. Thanks also to Jane Evans, Victoria Peters and everyone else who was involved in the production process.

I thank my current and former students, who have been an essential part of the process.

One last thanks goes to my family, my friends and my garden. Thank you for being there.

INTRODUCTION

Chinese medicine's physiological model can be difficult to accept and comprehend for people who have been brought up with a Western scientific view of the body. Western science and Western medicine doctors often perceive Chinese medicine as being superstitious and unscientific. Nevertheless, Chinese medicine is scientific. Chinese medicine is in fact more of a 'natural' science than Western medicine is. It is precisely because Chinese medicine has developed through observation of nature and the cosmos that there is an understanding and that there are fundamental and pervasive principles in the universe and in the world around us. These macrocosmic principles can also be seen in the microcosm of human physiology and in pathology. The human body is not separate or in any way different from the rest of nature or the cosmos in general. The human body and the world around it acts according to the same principles. Chinese medicine can therefore be called a true natural science.

A prerequisite for a system or model to be able to call itself scientific is that a theoretical structure has been defined. In addition, it must be possible to anticipate consequences and results when certain information or stimuli is introduced into this model in specific ways or in certain combinations. In this way, there is no difference between Chinese medicine and Western medicine. What fundamentally separates the two systems is that they have been created around divergent scientific parameters. This is particularly obvious in that Western medicine does not recognise the existence of *qi* and does not have any similar concept. *Qi*, on the other hand, is absolutely essential and fundamental in the theories of Chinese medicine.

Something that is very difficult, when starting to learn Chinese medicine, is that in order to understand a concept, you have to have a simultaneous comprehension of two or three other concepts. This would be fine, apart from the fact that these other concepts in themselves cannot be understood without having a knowledge of either the first concept or of yet another separate concept. This is because knowledge in Chinese medicine is contextual and things can only be seen and understood as a part of this context. Another factor that is a challenge from the outset is the use of many unfamiliar Chinese terms. We often have little idea of how these terms should be pronounced and we do not recognise them from our daily language. Furthermore, it is often a challenge to accommodate an understanding of the body that is different from, and sometimes at odds with, the physiology and pathology that we have learned in school and through previous educations. In some ways it is necessary to empty the glass we are holding before it can be filled with something new. This does not mean that we must reject the Western physiological model, but that we have to put it to one side whilst we encompass a new way of interpreting the body. Nevertheless, as a teacher of Chinese medicine, I have often experienced how Western medical health professionals' scepticism transforms into 'aha' experiences when experiences and situations from their erstwhile profession suddenly begin to make sense, experiences that Western medicine had no explanation of.

Learning Chinese medicine and acupuncture is like learning a new language. In the early stages it is very frustrating, because it is difficult to put all the words into context. In addition, the frustration increases when things you thought that you had understood no longer give meaning – a fog that had started to lift suddenly thickens again. It is important to remember, when this happens, that it is not that we no longer understand what we have already learnt, but that we are in the process of gaining a deeper understanding. This is like a corkscrew. As we turn the corkscrew we return to the same spot with each rotation, but each time at a deeper level. Also, many people have a tendency to focus on what they do not remember and do not understand, rather than what they do comprehend and remember. The concepts you struggle with in the beginning will be simple and obvious facts later on. This is very apparent in my original copy of Giovanni Maciocia's *Foundations of Chinese Medicine* and my early study notes. I can see how my highlights and comments have changed over the years. Things that I highlighted in my first reading of the text seem pointless a few years later, because they are things that I no longer even think about. On the other hand, I can remember how in later readings of the text I highlighted things that I had not even noticed in earlier readings. This was either because I simply did not understand them at the time or because I had not understood the importance of them in previous readings, but that I now comprehend.

Chinese medicine requires great patience in the beginning but, on the other hand, the rewards of this patience are also great. You think that you are going to learn a new way of treating the body and end up discovering a new way of comprehending the world.

The purpose of this book is to give the reader an understanding of Chinese medicine's physiological model. This book explains what the fundamental substances in the body are and how they arise in Chinese medicine. There is a thorough examination of the body's energetic structure and how the organ and channel systems function. To avoid repetition from my other books, I have chosen not to describe pathology, treatment or diagnostic techniques and models. Diagnosis is described in detail in my second book, *The Art of Diagnosis*. Pathology and treatment have been covered in my first book, *Acupuncture and the Treatment of Disease*. This volume therefore completes a trilogy in reverse.

Part 1

BASIC PRINCIPLES

YIN AND YANG

In order to understand Chinese medicine, it is necessary to have at least a superficial understanding of some of the basic principles of Chinese philosophy.

Chinese science, and as a consequence Chinese medicine, is similar to all science in that it is a product of the philosophical climate that it is immersed in. There have historically been three dominant philosophical currents that have had a significant influence on Chinese society – Daoism (Taoism), Confucianism and Buddhism. A relatively recent addition to this list was Maoism, but this has been a very short-term and transient chapter in a very long history.[1] Something that is very typical for East Asian thinking is that these three currents are not necessarily conceived as being contradictory but rather are seen as being complementary. Chinese medicine physiology and pathology is heavily influenced by Daoism, Naturalism (or *Yin Yang* school) and Confucianism. These were the prevailing philosophies during the period of history when much of the Chinese medicine theory was founded. *Yin* and *yang* are a central concept in both Daoist and Naturalistic philosophy, and some of the earliest references to *yin* and *yang* are to be found in books from the Warring States period (475 BCE–221 BCE). It was during this period that the philosophical school, which has laid the foundation for much of today's conception of *yin* and *yang*, had its golden age. The Daoist and Naturalistic philosophers were engaged in understanding nature and the principles of the universe whilst trying to adapt human activity and way of life so that they were in harmony with these principles. It was in the same period that the theory of the Five Phases[2] (Five Elements) was developed. I will discuss Five Phase theory in the next chapter.

Yin and *yang* are the two opposing, yet complementary, forces in the universe. Everything in the universe exists because of the tension between these two poles. It is *yin* and *yang* that create the dynamic of the universe and they are the reason that everything is in a constant process of change. Without *yin* and *yang* the universe would not exist.

In the Daoist understanding of life and the universe, there was no beginning, only an emptiness, a void or *wu ji*.[3] From this void an intention arose. This was *tai ji* (the great wholeness). This wholeness encompassed the first dichotomy – *yin* and *yang*, which is the fundamental tension in the universe. The tension between *yin* and *yang* created *qi*, and from *qi* everything in the universe arose. *Wu ji* is in reality not something that is completely foreign to the Western understanding of the universe. *Wu ji* corresponds to the moment before the 'Big Bang' or the moment before God created light. Chapter forty-two in the seminal Daoist text *Dao De Jing*[4] describes how *yin* and *yang* arose from nothingness and how *qi* is formed from *yin* and *yang*. It is formulated as follows (my interpretation of the text is in brackets):

Dao gave birth to one (tai ji)
One gave birth to two (yin and yang)
Two gave birth to three (qi)
Three gave birth to the ten thousand things (everything in the universe)

Everything from the microcosmic to the macrocosmic is a manifestation of *yin* and *yang*. Everything is subject to, or more correctly is a reflection and a manifestation of, their principles. There is nothing that cannot be understood from a *yin/yang* dynamic. The understanding of *yin* and *yang* is the foundation of everything. In our world there is a fundamental polarity between the sky or Heaven above us (*yang*) and the Earth below us (*yin*). What makes humans unique is that by standing on two legs, we connect the two and link Heaven and Earth.

All physiological and pathological processes in the body can be understood and explained by the principles of *yin* and *yang*.

Yin and *yang* in general

Many of the words and concepts used in Chinese medicine are difficult to translate into English. It is therefore often better to let them remain in Chinese. Instead of translating the term, it is more beneficial to try to gain a comprehension of its meaning. This can be done by looking at the qualities and definitions that these words represent in Chinese and by looking at the structure of the Chinese characters. The Chinese characters for *yin* and *yang* represent the shady side of a mountain and the sunny side respectively.

Already here we can see something that is crucial. Both sides of the mountain are aspects of the same wholeness – the mountain – and both sides are mutually dependent on one another. Each side of the mountain can only exist by virtue of the fact that there is another side.

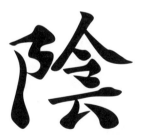
The character for *yin*

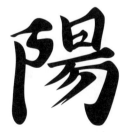
The character for *yang*

Figure 1.1 The Chinese characters for *Yin* and *Yang*

Yin and *yang* determine each other and they are each other's opposites

Yin and *yang* can only exist by virtue of the other. When something is light, it is only because there exists an opposite concept – darkness. Hot and cold, high and low, outside and inside, up and down – these are all expressions of *yang* and *yin* respectively. They are each other's opposites and they are each determined and defined by their counterpart. Something is only *yin* in relation to something that is *yang* and vice versa. A concept only makes sense when there is a counterpart. One can only say that something is high if there exists the concept called low. A front side is determined by, and determines, a reverse side.

Furthermore, even if something is high, it is only high in relation to something else that is lower than itself. This means that you will always be able to further subdivide each of the categories. In the example high and low, we will be able to further differentiate things in the category 'high' between things that are very high and those that are less high. The Empire State Building and a twenty-storey block of flats are both high compared with a bungalow, but the block of flats is low compared with the Empire State Building. That which is less high is *yin* compared with that which is very high. Another example is a glass of water. A glass of water is *yin* compared with a cup of tea. This is because the water is colder than the tea, and thereby it is *yin*. At the same time, the water is *yang* in comparison with an ice cube. This is because the water is warmer than the ice cube and is fluid, whereas the ice cube is colder and is solid. This means that you can never say that something is definitively *yin* or *yang*, only that something is *yin* or *yang* in relation to something else. It is very important to remember that nothing is absolute, only relative.

This is not only a semantic or philosophical concept. It is also seen practically in the world of physics. If you take a magnet, the magnet has a north or a south pole at each end. If you cut the magnet into several pieces, each of these pieces will have a north and a south pole at each end. Even the section that was completely at the tip of the original northern pole will now have a south pole at one end and vice versa. If one again cuts these segments in half, each of the ends will have a north and south pole. You can continuously divide *yin* and *yang* up an infinite number of times and there will still be a *yin* and a *yang* aspect.

Yin and *yang* transform into each other

Yin and *yang* also contain the seeds of one another. As just stated, nothing is absolute, nothing is entirely the one or the other, but will always contain an aspect of its opposite. The north pole contains the potential to be a south pole. This is what makes it possible for *yin* and *yang* to transform and change into each other. *Yin* and *yang* are in a constant cycle where they repeatedly transform and change into each other – high mountains get eroded down and deep river valleys and fathomless lakes silt up. Day turns into night; summer turns into winter. There is a limit to how *yin* or *yang* anything can become. This is what makes the universe dynamic and not static. When something has reached the maximum of its potential, it will not be able to continue and will therefore transform to its opposite. There may be a smooth transition where *yin* or *yang* gradually decreases again whilst the other part increases. This is, for example, seen in the diurnal cycle where the darkest hour (the most *yin* time) is just before dawn (where *yang* starts to grow) or on an annual basis where the length of the day increases until the summer solstice and then decreases again as the nights start to grow longer. If there isn't a gradual transition, then the change will occur suddenly. This can be seen when a balloon is inflated until it explodes. Here, the increasingly *yang* balloon (larger and harder) will become *yin* (small and limp) when it explodes. Nothing in the universe is static; everything is in a process of becoming more or less *yin* or *yang*.

Yin and *yang* consume each other

Because they are each other's opposites, *yin* and *yang* 'consume' each other. This has two main aspects. First, because *yin* and *yang* are opposing aspects, the more there is of the one, the less there is, by definition, of its opposite. The colder it is, the less hot it will be. The lighter it is, the less dark it is. The richer you are, the less poor you are, etc.

Furthermore, because they determine each other, each part will consume its partner. In an oil lamp the flame is *yang* and the oil is *yin*. The flame is bright, dry, warm and constantly moving; the oil is dark, cold, wet and static. Without oil the flame will not be able to exist. The oil is the material potential for the flame. The more you increase the flame, the more the oil is consumed – *yang* consumes *yin*. The opposite can be seen in ice. The more ice there is and the colder the ice is (*yin*), the more heat (*yang*) is required to melt it – *yin* consumes *yang*.

Yin and *yang* control each other

Yin and *yang* control each other. When *yin* and *yang* are equally strong, there is balance and harmony. This mutual control of *yin* and *yang* can be seen in a hot air balloon. *Yang* hot air will cause the balloon to rise upwards. The weight of the *yin* sandbags pulls the balloon towards the ground. If you want to ascend, then there must either be an increase of *yang* (hot air) or a reduction of *yin* (lighter or fewer sandbags). If you want to descend, *yin* must increase (more sandbags) or *yang* must be reduced (let hot air out of the balloon).

These basic principles can be summarised as follows.

- *Yin* and *yang* are each other's opposites – inner/outer, up/down, rich/poor, etc.

- *Yin* and *yang* are mutually dependent. They can only exist because of each other – you cannot have up without down; warm can only exist because there is something called cold.

- *Yin* and *yang* can always be further subdivided into a *yin* and a *yang* aspect – if you divide a line so part of it is to the right and part of it to the left, you will be able to repeat continuously this division infinitely, even on a microscopic scale.

- *Yin* and *yang* control each other – water extinguishes fire; fire evaporates the water.

- *Yin* and *yang* transform each other – day turns into night; night becomes day.

- *Yin* and *yang* consume each other – the hotter it gets, the less cold it feels and vice versa.

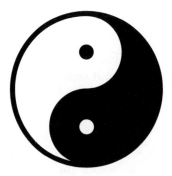

Figure 1.2 The *tai ji* symbol

In the *yin/yang* symbol, more correctly termed the *tai ji* symbol, much of this is represented. The two sides of the symbol are each other's opposite – black and white, but both sides are equally important. The one side of the symbol would not exist without the other. Each contains the seed of the other, and they are in the process of transforming into one another.

It is important to remember that both parts of the symbol are equally important and are equally relevant. Not only can one part not exist without the other, the whole symbol is dependent on both parts being present, otherwise there is imbalance. There is only harmony if both parts are equal.

If there is only heat without any cold or water, everything will be burnt up. Conversely, if there is only water and cold without any heat, there will be no movement and everything will freeze.

In the following table you can see some *yin/yang* relationships.

Yin	Yang
Dark	Light
Moon	Sun
Shade	Sunlight
Rest	Activity
Earth	Sky/heaven
Flat	Round
Space	Time
West	East
North	South
Winter	Summer
Night	Day
Water	Fire
Right	Left
Low	High
Contracting	Expanding
Descending	Ascending
Substance	Energy
Substantial	Non-substantial
Potential	Materialisation

Yin and *yang* are in a process where they are constantly transforming into each other. This is what gives everything in the universe its dynamic. This observation was made at an early stage in history by Chinese thinkers, who realised that nothing in the universe is static and that everything is in a process of change. It is therefore crucial to be conscious of which stage of the transformation process something is in.

When something is as *yin* as it can be, it is called old *yin* and is defined as being *yin* inside *yin*. At this point it cannot become more *yin* and therefore it will soon become *yang* again. During the annual cycle, this is the winter solstice. The days have become shorter and darker. The year cannot become more *yin*. It can only begin to become *yang* again. The cycle never stops. In the spring the heat and light begins to return. This period is called young *yang* or *yang* inside *yin*, because the *yang* aspect is growing within *yin*. The heat and the light continue to gather in strength until mid-summer – old *yang* or *yang* inside *yang*. Now the *yang* has reached its extreme, the day and the light cannot increase further and begin to decline again. The summer turns to autumn, which is *yin* inside *yang* or young *yin*. Now *yin* starts to grow in strength again.

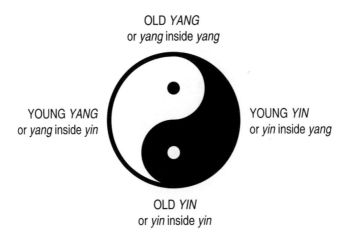

OLD *YANG*
or *yang* inside *yang*

YOUNG *YANG*
or *yang* inside *yin*

YOUNG *YIN*
or *yin* inside *yang*

OLD *YIN*
or *yin* inside *yin*

Figure 1.3 *Yin* and *yang* transform into each other

These processes of change can be seen not only in the seasons and time of day, but everywhere in nature, in the universe and in the body's physiology and pathology.

Winter/midnight	*Yin* inside *yin*	Old *yin*	*Yin* has reached its most extreme stage. *Yang* is at its lowest and weakest point.
Spring/morning	*Yang* inside *yin*	Young *yang*	*Yang* is growing. *Yin* is decreasing.
Summer/noon	*Yang* inside *yang*	Old *yang*	*Yang* has reached its most extreme stage. *Yin* is at its weakest or lowest point.
Autumn/afternoon	*Yin* inside *yang*	Young *yin*	*Yin* is growing. *Yang* is decreasing.

As written earlier, *yin* and *yang* control each other, so there is balance. There are four ways that the relationship between *yin* and *yang* can get out of balance. The four possible imbalances are:

- too much *yin*

- too much *yang*

- too little *yin*

- too little *yang*.

Ostensibly, this might look like the same two scenarios: that there is more *yin* than *yang* and vice versa. However, there is a significant difference between, for example, too little *yin* and too much *yang*, even though in both cases, there is more *yang* than *yin*. When there is too little *yin*, *yin* will not be strong enough to control *yang*. There is only *relatively* too much *yang* and, because *yang* is not controlled or anchored, *yang* can spiral out of control and dominate. Whereas if there is too much *yang*, there is an *absolute* increase in the amount of *yang*. Furthermore, the increased amount of *yang* can in itself injure *yin*. The same is of course true when there is a relative or absolute excess of *yin*.

To get a better understanding of the difference between these conditions, you can again think of the example of the hot air balloon. In this example, *yang* is seen in the hot air and *yin* in the sandbags. If you increase the size of the flame and thereby the heat in the balloon, the balloon will rise upwards. This is a condition of excessive *yang*. If one had instead reduced the amount of sandbags – a state of insufficient *yin* – the balloon would also rise upwards. The result is the same: that there is more *yang* than *yin*, but the cause is different. This is of great importance when diagnosing and treating with Chinese medicine. In Chinese medicine, it is important to be able to distinguish whether a *yang* condition in the body is due to too much *yang* or too little *yin*. If the *yang* is too powerful, then the *yang* should be drained and reduced, whereas if the condition is caused by a deficiency of *yin*, *yin* should be strengthened and increased instead. The same is also true when there is a dominance of *yin*. Here *yin* will be drained or *yang* will be strengthened. This approach will determine which acupuncture points you choose and how these points are stimulated or what herbs are prescribed.

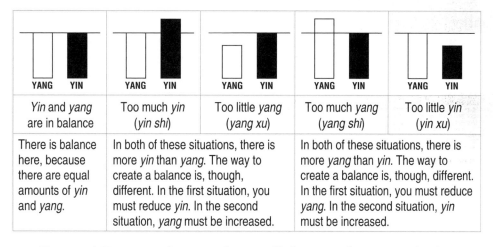

YANG	YIN	YANG	YIN	YANG	YIN	YANG	YIN	YANG	YIN
Yin and *yang* are in balance		Too much *yin* (*yin shi*)		Too little *yang* (*yang xu*)		Too much *yang* (*yang shi*)		Too little *yin* (*yin xu*)	
There is balance here, because there are equal amounts of *yin* and *yang*.		In both of these situations, there is more *yin* than *yang*. The way to create a balance is, though, different. In the first situation, you must reduce *yin*. In the second situation, *yang* must be increased.				In both of these situations, there is more *yang* than *yin*. The way to create a balance is, though, different. In the first situation, you must reduce *yang*. In the second situation, *yin* must be increased.			

Figure 1.4 How *yin* and *yang* can be out of balance in relation to each other

Yin and *yang* in Chinese medicine

Understanding the body through the principles of *yin* and *yang* is the foundation of Chinese medicine. *Yin* and *yang* are used not just as a way of perceiving the body's anatomy, but also to analyse the body's physiological processes in relation to pathology and treatment with needles and herbs. Everything in Chinese medicine is only a refinement and further development of the basic principles described in this chapter. The principles of *yin* and *yang* are used to draw a rough sketch. Later you learn how to paint a more detailed picture. You will, though, always be able to take a step back and use this rough sketch to look at the body and understand its physiology and pathology. This is especially important to remember when things start to seem overwhelming.

Yin and yang are each other's opposites and are mutually dependent, and they can be further differentiated with regards to each other

Anatomically the body can be divided into *yin* and *yang* aspects. As previously written, it is important to remember that these aspects are not absolute but are relative. This means that something can only be defined as being *yin* because you can compare and relate it to something that is *yang* and vice versa. Furthermore, every aspect of the body can further be divided into *yin* and *yang*. For example, the internal organs are *yin* in relation to the skin and muscles, but of these organs, the so-called hollow organs are *yang* relative to the solid organs, which are defined as being *yin* organs.

At the same time, the skin is *yang* in relation to the muscles, even though the muscles are *yang* in relation to the internal organs. Nevertheless, taken as a whole, all physical aspects of the body, including the skin and muscles, are *yin* because they have physical form. Whereas all the body's physiological processes are *yang*, because they do not have form, but are defined by their activity.

The upper parts of the body, that is to say the head and the thorax, are *yang* in relation to the lower parts of the body. The anterior aspect of the body is considered to be *yin* and posterior aspects of the body *yang*. This is because the front of the body is softer and more vulnerable than the back, which is harder and more protective. These are, respectively, *yin* and *yang* qualities. In addition, if a person stands on all fours, like an animal, the posterior aspect will be the area that is illuminated by the sun. The anterior aspect of the body will be shaded; again these are respectively *yang* and *yin* qualities. Furthermore, when standing on all fours, the posterior aspect of the body will be the area that is the highest up, furthest away from the *yin* earth and thus closest to heaven, which is *yang*. It is on the anterior aspect of the body that the *yin* channels traverse,[5] while *yang* channels traverse the posterior aspects of the body.

As stated, the body's anatomical structures as a whole are *yin* compared with the physiological processes, because they have the physical form, while the physiological processes are energetic activity. Of these anatomical structures, the most superficial, exterior aspects such as the skin, the channels, the sense organs and the muscles are *yang*, compared with the deeper, inner structures such as the organs and bones.

The right side of the body is considered to be *yin* and the left side *yang*. This classification is based on the fact that when the Emperor sat on his throne, he faced southwards. This meant that the sun rose (*yang*) on the left-hand side of his body and sank (*yin*) on the right side.

The body consists of the so-called vital substances *jing, shen, qi, xue* and *jinye*. These concepts cannot be translated satisfactorily into European languages, because we do not have the same physiological understanding of the body. A common translation of these concepts though is: *jing* – essence; *shen* – psyche/spirit/soul/ mind/consciousness; *qi* – bodily energy; *xue* – blood; and *jinye* – body fluids. These vital substances, which will be explained in detail in the following sections, can be understood as being *yin* and *yang* in relation to each other. *Jing*-essence, *xue*-blood and *jinye*-body fluid are *yin* compared with *qi*-bodily energy and *shen*-mind/spirit, because *jing*, *xue* and *jinye* are condensed and have form. Of these, the most *yin* substance is *jing*, whereas *shen* is the most *yang* form of *qi*.

Jing is a substantial form of *qi* that is inherited from one's parents. *Jing* is the potential that creates life and creates the body. It is like an acorn that has the potential to become a giant oak tree. *Jing* is defined as *yin* because it has potential and it is the foundation of everything else in the body, as well as being the most concentrated form of *qi* in the body.

Shen, which can be translated as mind, spirit, consciousness or psyche, is extremely *yang*. Unlike *jing*, *xue* and *jinye*, *shen* is ethereal and without form. *Shen* is created by *jing* and nourished and rooted in the body by *yin* and *xue*. Here you can see some of the other *yin/yang* principles: *yin* and *yang* transform into each other – *jing* is the material basis that creates *shen*, and *shen* is nourished by *yin* and *xue*; *yin* and *yang* control each other – *yin* and *xue* anchor and hold *shen* inside the body. Due to its *yang* nature, *shen* can be affected from one moment to the next. *Yin* substances on the other hand are slower in their movements. *Jing*, for example, operates in seven- and eight-year cycles and only changes gradually over months and years. *Shen* on the other hand can change instantaneously. One moment you can be happy and serene listening to music, and within a split second on seeing a masked intruder in the room, you would be frightened and terrified.

Qi is relatively *yin* compared with *shen*, but *qi* is relatively *yang* compared with *xue*. *Qi* is *yang* compared with *xue* because *xue* is slower in its movement and *xue* has physical form. In this way one can again see that nothing is *yin* or *yang*, only *yin* or *yang* in relation to something else.[6]

Yin	*Yang*
Anterior aspects of the body	Posterior aspects of the body
Lower part of the body	Head and the upper portion of body
Interior aspects of the body	Exterior aspects of the body
Right side of the body	Left side of the body
Structure	Function
Internal organs	Skin and muscles, channels
Solid organs	Hollow organs
Ying qi (nourishing *qi*)	*Wei qi* (protective or defensive *qi*)
Xue (blood)	*Qi* (body energy)
Jing (essence)	*Shen* (mind/spirit)

Yin and yang are transformed into each other and yin and yang consume each other

There are countless examples of how *yin* and *yang* substances transform into each other and how the one consumes the other. This is in reality much of what this book is going to be about. Overall, one can say that when the body is functioning and is active, the liquids and food that have been consumed are transformed into *qi* and *xue*[7] – thus *yang* (*qi* and *xue*) is created and *yin* (the nutrients in the food) is consumed. *Qi* and *xue* are used to nourish the muscles and organs in the body, thereby creating *yin* (the body's muscles and organs), and *yang* (*qi* and *xue*) is consumed.

In the body, we need *yang* to activate, transport, transform and warm *yin* substances. We need *yin* substances to nourish, moisten, cool and anchor *yang* aspects of the body.

We will later see how in each of these *yin* and *yang* processes we can see further *yin* and *yang* aspects.

In practice this means that the more active and *yang* we are, the more we consume our *yin*, because *yang qi* is created from *yin*. Conversely, the more *yin* we are exposed to or consume, the more *yang* is needed to heat, transform and transport *yin*. For example, the more physically active a person is, the more food (*yin*) they need to consume so that it can be transformed into *yang*. If they do not ingest enough food, the body's *yin* structure – fat and muscles – is instead transformed into *yang qi* and the person will lose weight or they will lack energy.

At the same time *yang qi* is used to transform *yin* food. If too much food is consumed, especially food that is very nutritious and rich (very *yin* foodstuffs), extra *yang qi* will be required to transform this. This can be seen when you eat a big meal or rich food, like pasta with cream sauce for example, and you feel tired afterwards. Furthermore, if the person's *yang* is weak, or they excessively consume too much *yin,* especially *yin* foods such as sugar, dairy products, etc., they will be less able to transform it into *qi*. This untransformed *yin* will deposit itself around the body in what Chinese medicine calls Dampness and Phlegm, and thus the person will become more *yin* in appearance (fat, soft, round) and they will feel heavy and sluggish.

Another example is cold and heat. The more cold we are exposed to, the more *yang* heat will be used to maintain the body temperature and the physiological processes in the body. A person exposed to excessive cold temperatures or who consumes large amounts of cooling food and liquids will eventually have a condition of either too little *yang* or too much *yin* in their body. Conversely, if a person has a state of pathological 'Heat' in their body, this will injure their *yin* aspects. This is because *yin* substances will be used to cool the body, but also because Heat over-activates the body's physiological processes. This over-activity will consume more *qi* than the body is able to produce from the food consumed, so the body has to draw on its *yin* reserves.

Yin	*Yang*
Nourishes	Activates
Moistens	Transports
Cools	Transforms
Anchors	Warms

Yin and yang control each other

Yin and *yang* control each other, thereby maintaining the body's homoeostatic balance. If there is too much or too little of one or the other, there will be imbalance and ultimately disease. The balance of *yin* and *yang* is a general principle and it is also seen in all the relationships between the organs and vital substances and in relation to pathological *qi*. A very simple example is when the body gets too hot. Here the body becomes too *yang*. This excess of *yang* is controlled by, amongst other things, sweating. Sweat droplets are *yin* – these cool the body and thereby control *yang*. Conversely, if you freeze, the body has become too *yin*. This will result in the body's muscles starting to shiver and the teeth chattering. This activity creates heat, which is *yang*, and thereby controls the *yin*.

Yin and yang in pathology

In Chinese medicine diseases develop when there are imbalances in the body's *qi*. These imbalances can be diverse and complex, but generally they can be differentiated as being *yin* or *yang* conditions. In a *yin* condition there will be a relative or absolute excess of *yin*. That is, there is more *yin qi* in the body than *yang qi*. Conversely, there will be a relative or absolute excess of *yang qi* in a *yang* condition.

When there is a *yang* condition, *yang* qualities will be dominant and generally the excess of *yang* will over-stimulate, heat up and dry out the body. On the other hand, if *yin qi* dominates, the body's physiology will be characterised by a lack of heat and the body's physiological and mental activities will be reduced.

Many of the symptoms and signs[8] attributed to a *yang* condition can reflect the presence in the body of Heat.[9] The presence of Heat will mean that a person's subjective sense of their body temperature will be hotter. It may also mean that a person's skin and especially their head feels hot on palpation. The head in particular becomes red and hot because the *yang* nature of Heat causes it to rise upwards. The *yang* nature of Heat will over-activate the blood and force it outwards to the surface of the body, making a person's skin feel hot and become more red in colour. This corresponds to the physiological explanation in Western medicine; here the redness of the skin is explained by the fact that there will be an increased circulation of blood in the superficial blood vessels under the skin when the body temperature rises and the body tries to dissipate the heat. Conversely, a lower body temperature will result in blood being drawn inwards away from the surface and down into the interior to reduce heat loss. This will make the person's skin, especially at the extremities, feel cold and they will look pale, which is typical in a person who has too little *yang* or a condition of Cold in the body. These colours will be also be evident on the tongue. The presence of Heat usually manifests with a tongue body that is more red in colour, whereas a lack of Heat will mean that the tongue body is pale.

As mentioned above, Heat causes physiological processes to accelerate. This means, for example, that the heart will beat faster. The pulse will therefore be more rapid than normal. Conversely, a lack of *yang* or too much *yin* will mean that the heart beats more slowly and therefore the pulse will be correspondingly slower.

In Chinese medicine *shen* has its residence in the Heart. If the Heart becomes agitated by Heat, it usually manifests with mental restlessness. The person's thoughts are over-activated. They will find it difficult to find mental calm. It can also be seen by the fact that the person has difficulty falling asleep or that they often wake at night.

If there is an absence of Heat, as in a *yin* condition, the mind will not be activated enough. This can mean that a person's thoughts are slower and duller than usual. Generally, the body will be characterised by inactivity and the person will have a greater need for sleep. When they sleep, they sleep with nightclothes on and they will lie curled up, in a subconscious attempt to reduce their surface area and thereby preserve body heat. A *yang* person will on the other hand tend to sleep naked or throw off the bedclothes, to reduce the heat.

In the presence of *yang* Heat the bodily fluids begin to dry out. The skin will become dry and the person will be thirstier than normal. Their urine will be darker and more sparse. A person with a *yin* condition will in turn lack *yang*'s transforming power. This will mean that body fluids do not get transformed and transported. The body fluids start to accumulate and the person can therefore lack thirst and may have a tendency to oedema. A person with a *yin* condition will typically have a tongue that is wet, whereas a *yang* person's tongue will more typically be dry. Furthermore, the untransformed fluids will seep downwards in the body and result in increased urination. The urine will be clear and voluminous, due to the amount of untransformed water in it. A lack of *yang* can also mean that a person finds it difficult to keep the urine inside the body and they may have problems with frequent urination and incontinence.

The stools are difficult to differentiate in the same way. Generally, constipation is seen in *yang* conditions, because Heat dries out the stools, but Heat can also over-activate the intestinal tract, causing the stool to move so quickly through the system that the body does not have time to draw fluids out of them. This will give rise to explosive diarrhoea. Cold and a lack of *yang* will result in the food and liquids not being transformed as they should, with loose stools or diarrhoea as a consequence. A lack of *yang* or Cold can though also result in constipation when there is not enough *yang* or *yang* is blocked, so the stools do not move through the intestines.

Yang has an expansive energy. This will mean that a particular area of the body will be distended and feel physically harder on palpation when there is a *yang* condition. It may be a larger area, such as the abdomen, but it can also be smaller areas such as an abscess. A *yang* boil will be hard, red and swollen, whereas *yin* sores will be sunken and weeping.

It is important to remember that these are general guidelines and that there will be many situations where other factors also have an influence. For example, *yang* conditions are usually acute. This is because *yang* is fast and active. *Yang* results in rapid changes, and this means that acute conditions will often be *yang*. Nevertheless, the body can be invaded by exogenous Cold, which is a *yin* pathogen. This will be an acute condition, but it will be an acute condition of *yin* symptoms and signs. Often an acute Cold condition will quickly transform into a *yang* condition. In such a case, the person will often subsequently develop a fever.

Similarly, you can have chronic *yang* conditions or conditions where there is a mixture of both *yin* and *yang* symptoms.

Yin and yang pathological conditions

Yin	Yang
Cold	Heat
Inactivity, lethargy	Restlessness
Wet	Dry
Soft	Hard
Reduced or blocked activity	Increased or accelerated activity
Chronic	Acute
Slow changes	Rapid changes
Hypersomnia	Insomnia
Sleeps curled up	Casts off the bedclothes
Pale face	Red face
Slow pulse	Rapid pulse
No thirst	Thirsty
Weak voice	Powerful voice
Clear, voluminous urine	Dark, scanty urine
Pale tongue body	Red tongue body

As written in the introduction to the principles of *yin* and *yang*, there are only four possible imbalances of *yin* and *yang*:

- too little *yin*
- too much *yang*
- too much *yin*
- too little *yang*.

This means that the two pathological *yin* and *yang* states described above can be further refined. In Chinese medicine there is talk of the following four imbalances between *yin* and *yang*.

- **Too little *yin* not controlling *yang*.** This is called *yin xu*[10] – also called *yin* deficiency or 'empty' *yin*. This is a state of deficiency. There is too little *yin* and it results in a *relative* excess of *yang*. There will both be symptoms and signs indicating a lack of *yin*, whilst at the same time there will be symptoms and signs that relate to an excess of *yang*. The *yang* signs will not be as dominant and extreme as those seen in an *absolute* excess of *yang* – which is called *yang shi* (*yang* excess or 'full' *yang*). This is because *yin xu* symptoms and signs arise when *yin* is not able to control *yang*. Examples of *yin xu* signs for instance could be hot flushes and a dry mouth.[11] The difference between this person and a person who has too much Heat (*yang shi*) is that when there is *yin xu*, the Heat will come in waves and the Heat will manifest mainly in the evenings and at night. The thirst will not be excessive, but rather there will be a dryness in the mouth and throat. This is because the person lacks *yin*'s moistening qualities, rather than it being Heat damaging fluids and drying out the body. It's a bit like the difference between water gradually evaporating from a bowl because no additional water is added to the bowl and a kettle boiling dry because the flames under the kettle are too hot. In general, the symptoms and signs of *xu* (deficiency) conditions are not as severe as those seen in a *shi* (excess) condition. Furthermore, it is important to note that there is a difference between physiological and pathological *yin* and *yang*. For example, *yang* heat (physiological heat) is a fundamental necessity for all the body's physiological processes. Pathological Heat though has no positive effect on the body's physiological processes. On the contrary, pathological Heat only has a negative effect on the body. This is also the reason that I use a capital H when writing about pathological Heat. The same rule applies for other pathological forms of *qi*, such as Dampness, Dryness, Wind, etc.

- **Too little *yang* not activating *yin*.** This is called *yang xu* – *yang* deficiency/ empty *yang*. When there is *yang xu*, the body lacks the necessary *yang qi* to carry out the functions and activities that are attributed to *yang*. This will mean that many of the body's physiological processes will be slower and there will be a reduced efficiency. The body will also be characterised by so-called 'Cold' symptoms such as sensitivity to cold, a pale face or a lack of thirst. Again, because it is a *xu* (deficiency) condition, these signs and symptoms will be less intense than that of a *shi* (excess) condition.

- **Too much *yang* over-activating the body and injuring *yin*.** This is called *yang shi*[12] – *yang* excess or 'full' *yang*. When there is *yang shi*, it is not because the body has too little *yin* to control *yang*, as in a *yin xu* condition, but because the body actually does have too much *yang*. This means that the symptoms and signs are more aggressive and more powerful than in a *yin xu* state. It could mean, for example, that where there were hot flushes in the evening in a *yin xu* condition, there will be a persistent fever or constant feeling of heat in the body in a *yang shi* condition. Where the face in a *yin xu* condition was only red on the cheekbones, the whole head will be red when there is a *yang shi* condition. Instead of a dryness of the mouth and throat, there will in a *yang shi* condition be a strong thirst with the desire to drink large gulps of cold water.

- **Too much *yin*, which restricts and inhibits the body's activity and damages *yang*.** This is called *yin shi* – *yin* excess/full *yin*. This is again an *absolute* excess condition. This time the body is affected by an excess of a so-called *yin* pathogen. This will most probably be Cold or Dampness. *Yin* pathogens will inhibit and restrict the body's physiological processes. Unlike in a *yang xu* condition, this condition is not characterised by a lack of the energy that is necessary so that physiological processes can take place optimally. Instead, in a *yin shi* condition the *yang qi* is not depleted, but it is blocked and cannot perform its functions. Symptoms and signs will resemble those seen in *yang xu*, but again *yin shi* symptoms will be stronger and more pronounced. Moreover, *yin shi* will manifest not only with signs that there is a lack of activity but also that there is an actual stagnation and blockage. For example, urination in a *yang xu* state can be frequent with copious amounts of clear urine. In a *yin shi* condition the urination can be blocked or impeded. This is because a *yin* pathogen will block the *yang qi*, so it cannot expel the urine out of the body.

If *yin* and *yang* become so imbalanced that they completely separate from each other, death will occur.

Yin and *yang* in treatment

In all simplicity, all treatment is an attempt to recreate balance and harmony between *yin* and *yang* in the body.

This means that there are therapeutically four main treatment strategies.

- Nourishing *yin* in *yin xu* conditions.

- Tonifying *yang* in *yang xu* conditions.

- Draining *yang* in *yang shi* conditions.

- Draining *yin* in *yin shi* conditions.

These four strategies will determine which combinations of acupuncture points, needle techniques, herbal prescriptions, dietary and lifestyle changes, etc. are used in the treatment of disorders and diseases.

THE FIVE PHASES

Wu xing or the 'Five Phase' theories are almost as fundamental and seminal in Chinese medicine as *yin* and *yang* theories are. *Wu xing* is often incorrectly translated as the 'Five Elements'. In Chinese *wu* means five, and *xing* means movement or process. Five Phases infers a more dynamic understanding of the concept, than translating *wu xing* as Five Elements. The word 'element' has a more static connotation. By translating *xing* as phase, there is more of a sense that things are in a state of change and have a dynamic relationship, rather than a world split up into five fixed categories. The Chinese character *xing* represents a man who places one foot in front of the other. It is the same character as 'to walk' or a crossroad. In both of these images, the understanding is: 'as things move'. *Xing* is also used as the term for planets' trajectories.

The theory of the Five Phases was developed around the same time in Chinese history as the theories of *Yin Yang*, i.e. in the Warring States period (475 BCE–221 BCE). The philosophy of the Five Phases is attributed to the semi-legendary figure Zhou Yan, but should more be seen as a synthesis of many philosophers' and theoreticians' work.

Five Phase theory is based on the premise that everything in the universe is created by *qi* or is a manifestation of *qi*. *Qi* as a concept will be discussed in detail in the next section, which deals with the vital substances in the body. As we have seen in the chapter on *yin* and *yang* (page 20), *qi* is created by the interaction of *yin* and *yang*. *Qi* is something other and more than just pure energy. Everything in the universe consists of *qi*. The theory of the Five Phases has as its founding premise that there are five fundamental resonances of *qi* in the universe. This means that things that have the same resonance will be related to each other. They are manifestations of the same energy.[13] The universe is conceived as having five basic energies or resonances. These are known as the Five Phases, which are: Water, Wood, Fire, Earth and Metal.

It is important to remember that things are not arbitrarily divided into different phases. Objects, processes, colours, climates, etc. are just manifestations of *qi*, which have similar energetic qualities. This is the reason that these things are classified as being of the same phase. They resonate with each other. The Wood Phase is not the green colour, but the green colour resonates with other things around us and in the universe, which can be classified as being an aspect of the Wood Phase.

The Five Phases are not static. They are in a state of constant change, as, for example, the seasons are. Spring follows winter, which is succeeded by summer. The phases also have a dynamic relationship with each other. This is not dissimilar to the relationship between *yin* and *yang*. The Five Phases are mutually dependent on each other; they control each other and they create each other. Water creates or is followed by Wood, which creates or is followed by Fire and so on. At the same time, Water extinguishes Fire, Fire burns Wood, etc.

The Five Phases can be understood as being a refinement or development of *Yin Yang* theory. The Five Phases can be viewed as an explanation of the way in which *yin* and *yang* transform into and control each other.

The *sheng* cycle

The cycle in which the Five Phases follow or create each other is called the *sheng* cycle.

It can be translated into English as the generating or creative cycle. Some call the *sheng* cycle the nourishing cycle. The relationship between the two phases that follow each other in the *sheng* cycle is described as a mother-and-son relationship. The first phase is mother to the phase that follows it in the *sheng* cycle. For example, Water is mother of Wood. The generating cycle can be seen everywhere, not only in seasons as described above, but also in all aspects of life. Night follows the evening and then is itself followed by the morning. We also see it in a lifecycle, where a plant sprouts from a seed and then blossoms, and this then turns to fruit and finally to seed. People start their lives as helpless individuals, unable to walk, fed by others and incapable of controlling their urination, only to end up in the same condition again eighty years later. The *sheng* cycle as described here is nothing other than the principle of *yin* and *yang* transforming into each other. The *sheng* cycle is the process of *yang* growing until it reaches its zenith and then fading again as *yin* grows in strength.

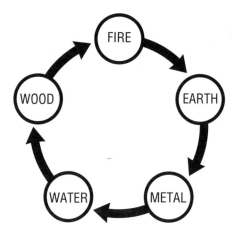

Figure 1.5 The *sheng* cycle

The *ke* cycle

The *sheng* cycle is not the only cycle or dynamic relationship between the phases. All of the principles of *yin* and *yang* can be seen in the relationships of the Five Phases.

Water and Fire, for example, are each other's opposites and they control each other, but at the same time they are mutually dependent on each other. The Metal Phase's energetic dynamic is inward or centripetal, whilst the Wood Phase is expanding or centrifugal. Phases can only exist by virtue of each other, whilst simultaneously balancing and controlling each other. The way in which the phases control each other is known as the controlling cycle or *ke* cycle. In this cycle the different phases keep each other in check or, more correctly, in balance. Fire controls Metal, which in turn controls Wood. Wood controls Earth and Earth controls Water, which again controls Fire.

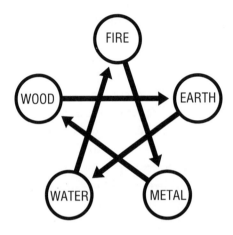

Figure 1.6 The *ke* cycle

The combination of *sheng* and *ke* cycles results in a finely tuned and balanced system, where one phase nourishes the next phase, but the phase that it nourishes controls a third phase, which for its part controls the first phase.

Imbalance can, however, arise. A phase may be too dominant and can oppress another phase. Instead of keeping the second phase in check and having a balancing effect, it oppresses and thereby weakens the following phase in the *ke* cycle.

A phase may also be too weak, so that it is no longer capable of controlling the next phase in the *ke* cycle or the phase that it should be controlling has become too strong. The end result of both situations is a phase that no longer controls the next phase in the *ke* cycle, but instead is 'insulted' by a phase that should be subservient to it. There is a reversal of the relationships in the *ke* cycle. An example could be that if Water is weak, instead of controlling Fire, Fire starts to dominate Water instead.

These relationships can be used to diagnose and treat the body when the body has become energetically imbalanced resulting in physical and emotional symptoms.

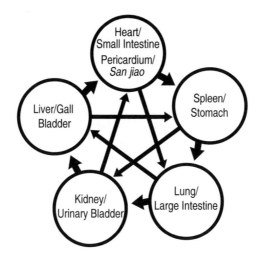

Figure 1.7 The Five Phases and the organ relationships

The Cosmological sequence

The relationship between the Five Phases can be presented in another way. The oldest model is the Cosmological cycle. In this model the Earth Phase is not positioned between Fire and Metal. Instead all the phases pass through Earth, which is in the centre, before proceeding to the next phase in the cycle. The Earth Phase is the beginning and the end of all the phases. In the annual cycle, the Earth Phase is no longer late summer, but is instead the last nine days of each season and the first nine days of the following season. Earth is the central position that is passed through each time there is a change of direction.

In the Cosmological sequence there is a central, vertical axis, consisting of Water, Earth and Fire. This axis reflects the relationship between the planet Earth, Man and Heaven.[14] The Cosmological cycle is less well known than the *sheng* and *ke* cycles, but nonetheless it reflects several aspects of the Five Phases and the universe. In the Cosmological cycle the compass directions of the phases are more correctly represented with the Earth Phase being the centre and having no direction. The Cosmological model is also more representative of the physical and physiological relationships between the internal organs in the body. The central axis represents the relationship between the so-called three treasures – *jing*, *qi* and *shen* – and their relationship to the Kidneys, Spleen and Heart and their respective positions in the body.

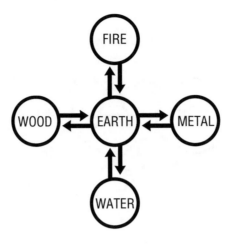

Figure 1.8 The Cosmological sequence

The theory of the Five Phases is not unique to Chinese medicine. These theories were the prevailing philosophy in Chinese society during the Warring States period. This way of observing and understanding the universe was used for virtually everything. Whether it was agriculture, astrology, medicine or politics, or even military strategies, everything was subjected to a Five Phase analysis of the situation. It is not by coincidence that the Yellow Emperor is called the Yellow Emperor. Emperors and their dynasties viewed themselves as being or having qualities reflecting the various phases. Initially dynasties replaced each other in relation to the *ke* cycle (the controlling cycle), i.e. the new dynasty overpowered the preceding dynasty in the *ke* cycle. As society developed in a more peaceful direction, the *sheng* cycle (or the creative cycle) was used to explain or interpret the succession of the dynasties.[15]

Everything being equal, the philosophy of the Five Phases was a quantum leap forward in the development of Chinese medicine. It was in this period that Chinese medicine advanced away from superstition and into scientific analysis. Chinese medicine is not scientific when defined from a Western scientific viewpoint. Nevertheless, it is still scientific. It is just based on different parameters to Western science. Up until this point in time, Chinese medicine had viewed disease as being caused by evil spirits and ghosts. Now the understanding developed that a person was an integral part of the world that they were surrounded by and of the universe as a whole. Through observation of the world around them, the Chinese recognised universal, governing principles. It is these principles that determined that everything has certain characteristics and behaves in a certain way. The Chinese observed that everything in the universe is affected by, and affects, everything else. Therefore, when disease occurs in a person, it will have arisen due to influences from the world around them.

The theory of the Five Phases has had both high and low periods in Chinese medical history. In Chinese medicine today in China, the Five Phase theories are still very relevant in relation to the understanding of the body and what it is affected by, but they are of less importance with respect to actual treatment.[16] In China, Five Phase theory is deemed by many as being too rigid and inflexible to be used as a treatment system. As stated above, the Five Phases though are used to understand the body and its relation to the universe. Five Phase dynamics underpin the physiological and pathological relationships in the body.

Each of the Five Phases has certain energetic directions, which are characterised by their *yin* and *yang* qualities.

- Water is old *yin* or *yin* in *yin* and thus has a descending energy.

- Wood is young *yang* or *yang* in *yin*. It has a centrifugal energy.

- Fire is old *yang* or *yang* in *yang* and thus has an ascending energy.

- Metal is young *yin* or *yin* in *yang*. It has a centripetal energy.

- Earth is in the centre of everything. It has no energetic direction.

The Five Phases

The Water Phase

The Water Phase is ultimate *yin* or old *yin*. This is the lowest point in a circle. It is both the beginning and the end. It is here that one cycle ends and the next begins.

Water as a physical substance has extreme *yin* qualities and therefore it is not by chance that the most *yin* phase in the cycle of transformation is called the Water Phase.

Water is cold unless it has been exposed to *yang* heat. In fact, water will freeze and be immobile without *yang* heat. Water is soft and passive and seeps downwards. This is reflected in the fact that the Water Phase *qi* dynamic is descendent.

The Water Phase is winter. The Sun has sunk in the west and is now in the north, from where its rays cannot reach us. It is night; it is cold. It is the deepest and darkest point in a cycle. The warm and bright *yang* has faded, so much as it possibly can. *Yang* cannot decrease any more and therefore it will soon begin to grow again. The days grow shorter and shorter until the winter solstice, only to lengthen again the day after. The darkest hour is just before dawn.

Night time and winter are the time for regeneration. *Qi* is stored and activity is reduced. It is *yin* qualities that are dominant. *Qi* is drawn inwards, so it can be used again in the spring. *Yang qi* must be preserved and *yin qi* nurtured. Humans sleep at night, a bear will sleep throughout the winter and bushes and trees draw their sap down into their roots in the winter. It is not death; the cycle of life continues again in the morning and in the spring. The Water Phase is both the beginning and the end of the cycle of life. It is here that life has its origin and here that life ends. It is in winter that the seed lays buried in the ground waiting for the spring, waiting for heat and light, so that it can begin to grow.

In the same way that farmers in winter store their surplus corn for next year's crops, the body stores *qi* as *jing* in the Kidneys. This is something that we must be aware of in our lifestyle. It is in the Water Phase organ, the Kidneys, that we have our reserves, our energetic warehouse. It is from here that energy is drawn when we overexert ourselves and use more *qi* than we are able to produce.

Jing is unmanifested potential. It is the potential for growth and change. *Jing* can be seen in plants as seeds or as semen and eggs in humans. This stored *qi* is used to enable the growth of the next generation in the lifecycle. We as individuals age and die, but new life grows and develops from our *jing*.

In winter, and especially in the evening and at night, we should think about how peasant farmers traditionally behaved during the winter. Like many animals, they were extremely active, getting up early and going to bed late in the summer time. They toiled all day long. In the wintertime they would sleep longer and go to bed earlier than they did in the summer. In the winter they did not toil in the same way as during harvest time. The work on the farm consisted more of carrying out small repairs and maintenance. If we are to follow a natural cycle, we should therefore be calm and tranquil in the evening and sleep when it gets dark. The invention of the electric light, and electricity in general, has had a crucial effect on our ability to disrupt the natural balance between day and night and in our bodies. It is now possible and even regarded as normal to be active and *yang*, when we in reality should be tranquil and *yin*.

The Wood Phase

The Wood Phase is *yang* in *yin* or young *yang*. It is morning, it is spring and it is youth. This is where the potential of the Water Phase will be transformed into growth. The seed that lay dormant in the soil germinates and emerges into the light. The tree's branches grow upwards and outwards. There is a plethora of green growth everywhere. Spring is characterised by abundance, rapid change and a green hue. The Wood Phase has a very dynamic energy that is characterised by growth and development. But it is also precisely because of the powerful dynamic that is inherent in the Wood Phase that you can see the risk of imbalance. When there is so much momentum, dynamic and resoluteness, it can easily be at the expense of others.

Wood energy, when it is in balance, is characterised by flexibility. A tree will bend when it comes under pressure, but when the pressure is released, the tree will rise up again and continue its growth upwards. On the other hand, when Wood is imbalanced, it does not yield, but stiffly refuses to bend until the pressure is too great and it snaps. The tree though can also be too limp and feeble and thus not be capable of growing upwards and bending too easily when put under pressure.

The sun rises in the east, which is the direction of the Wood Phase. It is in the morning and in the spring that the light and warmth return after the dark and cold of the winter and the night. Out in nature and on the farm life is characterised by activity. After a period of rest there is renewed energy. This energy is used to initiate the preparations made during the winter. The seed, which has been lying dormant in the ground all winter, breaks through the surface of the soil and grows upwards into the light. The sap, which had been drawn down into the roots, rises upwards through the stem and out into the new green leaves. When a plant is growing, we can see the dynamic of the Wood Phase; things grow upwards and outwards.

The Fire Phase

Fire is the most *yang* of all the phases. It is termed *yang* in *yang* or old *yang*, because *yang* has reached its most extreme point. From here there is only one way, and that is that *yin* will begin to increase and *yang* will decrease again. This is seen when the sun is highest in the sky at noon or when the summer sun is hottest. After the summer solstice the days grow shorter and the nights grow longer. It is in the summer that flowers bloom most beautifully, before they start to wither and fade.

On the farm and in nature life is almost hectic. The farmers and wild animals get up early and go to sleep late. Plants are blossoming and manifesting their full potential. Everything is characterised by *yang* activity.

Fire is the diametric opposite of Water. Where the water itself is extremely *yin*, cold and wet and descends downwards, fire is hot and dry and has an ascending energy. In the same way that water always seeps downwards, the heat from fire always floats upwards. In Chinese medicine physiology the relationship between Water and Fire is extremely important. The activating *yang* energy of Fire is needed to invigorate and transform the *yin* potential of Water. At the same time the *yin* cooling energy of Water is needed to control Fire and make sure that it does not get out of hand.

Fire, due to its extreme *yang* nature, is extremely transformative. It is the catalyst that enables things to transform themselves. However, it is also a force that must be controlled so that it does not cause damage. This is not just poetic Chinese philosophy. You can see these relations in Western physiology. For example, the stomach needs acid (Fire) so that the digestion of food can take place, but if there is too much acid, the lining of the stomach wall (*yin*) gets damaged, resulting in stomach ulcers.

The Earth Phase

The Earth Phase is characterised by maturity, fertility and nutrition. It is in the soil that seeds are planted and from where crops are harvested. The Earth Phase is slightly more difficult to understand and explain in the annual and diurnal cycles. Some sources classify the Earth Phase as being late summer and the harvest time in the annual cycle and as the afternoon in the diurnal cycle. This is because the Earth Phase is, amongst other things, characterised by the fact that the summer flowers have now matured to fruit and are ready to be harvested. The Earth Phase is in reality much more than this. It is the last nine days of each of the other phases and the first nine days of the following phase in the cycle. This is because the Earth Phase is neither north, south, east nor west. It is the centre. This is the place from which all directions originate and where all directions meet. This is the axle that all the other phases rotate around. This is the place that all the other phases have to pass through on their way to the next phase. This relationship is apparent in the Cosmological cycle. Nevertheless, the Earth Phase is placed between the Fire and Metal Phases in the *sheng* cycle, whilst simultaneously controlling the Water Phase and being controlled by the Wood Phase in the *ke* cycle.

The Earth Phase has no dynamic direction. Whilst the other phases' *qi* is characterised by being ascendant, descendent, centrifugal and centripetal, the Earth phase is static. This is because it is in the middle; it is the centre. This lack of dynamic in the Earth Phase is a strength – it provides stability, trust and loyalty – but it also can result in a tendency to stagnation, lethargy and sluggishness, unless activated by others.

The Metal Phase

We have reached autumn in the cycle of transformation. *Yang* is waning and *yin* is growing in strength. This is called *yin* in *yang* or young *yin*. The sun is sinking in the west. It is evening, the light is fading and darkness is on the increase. After the summer's intense heat and light comes the autumn, where the evenings start to grow longer and the days shorter. There is less noise and activity. Calm and tranquillity start to settle, but there is also a slight sense of melancholy. The air is sharper and colder and the first night frosts are on their way. Even though the length of day is the same at the autumn equinox, there is a very different dynamic than at the spring equinox. The energetic dynamic has changed direction and the movement is now inwards and contracting. Plants and the trees draw their sap into the stem and down into the roots. The leaves lose their nutrition and fall to the ground together with the seeds and nuts. The nuts and the seeds will lie in the ground the whole winter and will sprout and grow upwards, when *yang* warmth returns in the spring.

In the greater picture the individual person, animal or plant comes and goes, but the cycle itself is eternal.

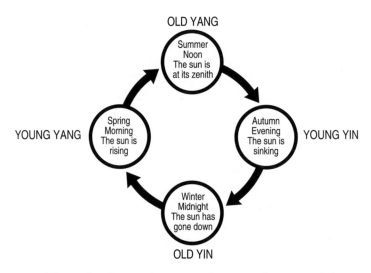

Figure 1.9 The cycle of *yin* and *yang* in relation to the sun and the seasons

Five Phase relationships

In the Five Phase way of thinking, everything in the universe, everything in the world and everything in our body is conceived of as being resonances of the Five Phases. In the table below, you can see some of these Five Phase relations. The classifications of the categories into the various phases is not arbitrary. The physical functions and manifestations listed below often relate to the *zang* organ that is itself a resonance of that phase. Other manifestations relate to seasons, astrology, numerology and energetic directions. These depend on the *yin* and *yang* dynamic of the phase and whereabouts in the cycle of transformation that the phase is located.

Observation of changes in the aspects and functions that relate to the human body are used when diagnosing with Chinese medicine.

It is important to bear in mind that the descriptions of the physical aspects of the Five Phases are based on functional relationships and not on inherited truths that have been written in stone. These relationships are dependent on the individual organs' physiological functions. This means that more than one of the internal organs, as well as various forms of *xie qi* (pathological *qi*), can have an influence on a particular aspect of the body or its physiology. For instance, urine is an aspect of the Water Phase. This is because the Urinary Bladder stores and expels urine and Kidney *yang* transforms fluids, thereby creating urine. Also, Kidney *yang* both keeps the urine in the Urinary Bladder and expels the urine out of the Urinary Bladder, when a person urinates. That said, Damp-Cold and Damp-Heat can often result in urinary difficulties, as can Heart Fire and Liver *qi* stagnation. In Chinese medicine, it is important not just to look at the manifestation. Things should always be seen in relation to a larger context and it is important to try and identify the root cause.

This means that the Five Phase relations can be used as a starting point for further investigation. Chinese medicine, and its associated physiological model, is therefore much more complex than the immediate impression one gets when looking at the table below.

An explanation and description of the internal organs' functions and physiology is to be found in the relevant chapters on the internal organs, also called *zangfu* organs. This section nevertheless provides an overview of some of the various Five Phase relationships that relate to the *zangfu* organs.

	Water	Wood	Fire	Soil	Metal
Season	Winter	Spring	Summer	Either late summer or no season[17]	Autumn
Compass direction	North	East	South	Centre	West
Energetic dynamic	Descending	Expanding or centrifugal	Ascending	None/static	Contracting or centripetal
Colour	Black or dark blue	Green	Red	Yellow	White
Flavour	Salt	Sour	Bitter	Sweet	Spicy
Climate	Cold	Wind	Heat	Dampness	Dryness
Developmental stage	Dormancy	Sprouting	Blooming	Fruiting or ripening	Withering
Number	6	8	7	5	9
Planet	Mercury	Jupiter	Mars	Saturn	Venus
Yin Yang	Old *yin*	Young *yang*	Old *yang*	The centre	Young *yin*
Animals	Shellfish	Fish	Bird	Man	Mammal
Cattle/livestock	Pig	Goat or cockerel[18]	Goose	Oxen	Dog or goat
Cereal	Millet	Wheat	Beans	Rice	Hemp
Yin or *zang* organ	Kidneys	Liver	Heart and Pericardium	Spleen	Lung
Yang or *fu* organ	Urinary Bladder	Gall Bladder	Small Intestine and *san jiao*	Stomach	Large Intestine
Sensory organ	Ear	Eyes	Tongue	Mouth	Nose
Body tissue	Bones	Tendons	Blood vessels	Muscles	Skin
Emotion	Fear	Anger	Joy	Worry	Sorrow
Sound	Groaning	Shouting	Laughing	Singing	Crying
Body fluid	Urine	Tears	Sweat	Saliva	Phlegm
Odour	Putrid	Rancid	Burnt	Fragrant aromatic	Rotten
Sense	Hearing	Vision	Speech	Taste	Smell
Shen aspect	*Zhi*	*Hun*	*Shen*	*Yi*	*Po*

I have already explained some of the Five Phase relations such as the seasons, times of day, energetic directions, etc. in the introduction. In the following subsections I will try to expand on some of the other Five Phase relations.

Colours

Colours are of great importance in relation to the Five Phases. Most of the colours are quite logical when you take into account the other qualities of the respective phases. The black or midnight blue colour is seen in both the colour of deep water and the colour of the sky when the night is at its darkest. The green colour is to be seen everywhere in the spring when there is a verdurous explosion. The fire's flames are red, etc.

In addition, the colour of foodstuffs can sometimes give an indication of the organs that they have a beneficial effect on. Green-leafed vegetables, for example, have a highly nourishing effect on the Liver's *xue* or Blood aspect.

It is especially in relation to diagnosis that the observation of how colours have changed is utilised. It is most often the skin on the face that is observed for changes, but the skin in various parts of the body can also alter its hue when there is an imbalance. These changes can be related to certain organs or types of *xie qi* (pathogenic *qi*). For example, the skin turns red when there are Heat conditions in the body; Dampness and especially Damp-Heat can give the skin a yellow tinge; a person with a deficiency of Lung *qi* (also called Lung *qi xu*) will have a pale, white face; a greenish tinge around the mouth or in the temporal area can be a sign of Liver *qi* stagnation.

The Five Phase interpretation of these colours means that there are sometimes big cultural differences between how and when these colours are used in the East compared with the West. White is used for wedding dresses in Europe because it represents innocence and purity. In China white is used at funerals, because it symbolises sadness by virtue of its relationship to the Metal Phase. On the other hand, red is used for weddings in China, because it is the Heart's colour.

Colour	
Water	Midnight blue or Black
Wood	Green
Fire	Red
Earth	Yellow
Metal	White

Flavours

In Chinese herbal medicine and Chinese medicine dietary therapy, the flavour of food and herbs has a determining influence on their physiological effect. The flavour of some foodstuffs may at times seem strange and not founded in reality. This is because the flavour is not necessarily defined by how the herb or the foodstuff is perceived by the taste buds on the tongue, but by the way it affects the body's *qi*. This dynamic determines how its flavour is defined. Each flavour has an energetic direction and dynamic, which determine how it affects *qi*. The flavour will also resonate specifically with one of the internal organs. This can be used to direct the desired effect towards a specific organ. The spicy flavour is used, for example, to expel invasions of external Wind-Cold and to disseminate Lung *qi*. An example of this is when ginger, garlic or a hot whisky toddy is used to get rid of a cold. The bitter taste can drain Damp-Heat and activate the Heart, something that is clearly seen in the impact coffee can have on the speed of the heartbeat.

Flavour can also be used diagnostically. A bitter taste in the mouth is usually a sign that there is a condition of Fire in the body, i.e. an excess of Heat in one or more of the internal organs. People with a deficiency condition of their Spleen, i.e. Spleen *qi xu*, will often have an urge to consume things that have a sweet taste.

Flavour	
Water	Salt
Wood	Sour
Fire	Bitter
Earth	Sweet
Metal	Spicy

Climates

The five climates are the prevailing climates of the respective seasons. They are also the climatic effects that have a negative effect on the organs of the corresponding phase. Cold is the prevailing climate in the winter and, at the same time, cold has a damaging effect on the Kidneys. This is because the Kidneys are the root of all *yang* and thereby the root of physiological heat in the body. At the same time, a deficiency of Kidney *yang* (Kidney *yang xu*) will cause a person to be sensitive to cold and have difficulty keeping warm. Wind is characteristic of the Wood Phase's dynamic. Wind is a very *yang* form of *qi*. Wind is a necessity to prevent stagnation. Wind clears the air, but too much wind can be catastrophic. If the wind is too strong, it can be devastating for everything in the vicinity. This can be seen all around us in nature and inside the body. In the body, the Liver makes sure that there is constantly a well-regulated movement of *qi*. If so-called Liver Wind arises, *qi* can ascend in an uncontrolled manner up to the head, resulting in a headache or in the worst case a stroke.

Summer is characterised by sunshine and heat. Heat has an ascending *yang* energy. The Heart, due to its relationship to the Fire Phase, has difficulty controlling heat and can therefore easily overheat, both when there is too little Kidney *yin* – cool water that controls the heat – or when there is a surplus of Heat in the body. Due to its *yang* nature, heat in the body will rise upwards. Therefore, Heat will almost always affect the Heart at some point (because the Heart is located in the upper part of the body).

Dampness is particularly burdensome for the Spleen, which is the primary organ of the Earth Phase. Dampness is heavy, sticky and stagnant. This reflects the same lack of dynamic that can be seen in the Earth Phase. This means that it is difficult to disperse and spread Dampness when it has accumulated. The Spleen creates Dampness internally in the body when it is imbalanced, and at the same time the Spleen is weakened by food that creates Dampness.

In the autumn the air is extremely dry in large parts of China; much dryer than it can ever be in Denmark or the British Isles, because these have a maritime climate. This is one of the reasons that the climate that is attributed to the Metal Phase is dryness. A second reason that dryness is attributed to the Metal Phase is that the Metal Phase's direction is West. The Gobi Desert, which is extremely dry, is located in western China. The Lung,[19] which is the Metal Phase's *yin* organ (or *zang* organ), is easily damaged by dryness. This can be seen when people who live in buildings with a dry climate, such as concrete flats, develop respiratory problems, such as dry mucous membranes and a dry cough.

Climate	
Water	Cold
Wood	Wind
Fire	Heat
Earth	Dampness
Metal	Dryness

Numerology

Numerology or numerical dynamics has always been of great importance in China. Each of the phases has a number that resonates with this particular phase. The numbers ascribed to the phases can appear confusing, not only because they start at five and run to nine, but also because the numbers do not follow the sequence of the more well-known *sheng* cycle.

In the older Cosmological arrangement of the phases, where the phases are located on a north/south and an east/west axis, with Earth in the centre, the phases have the following sequence: Water, Fire, Metal, Wood and Earth. The phases in this arrangement are then assigned the numbers one to five.[20] All phases are necessary in the creation of life. This is a creative or *sheng* cycle, and the phases pass through this cycle in order to create a complete whole cycle so that something can be manifested physically. When something manifests, it contains the whole (all five phases) plus its own unique *qi*. The Water Phase is therefore five plus one and thereby six; Fire is five plus two and thereby seven; Wood is eight; and Metal is nine. Earth can in fact be defined as being both five and ten. This is because when something has reached the number five, there is already a completion and therefore it is already whole.

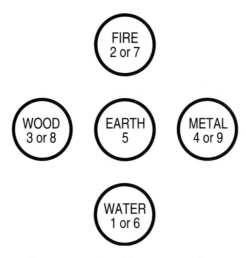

Figure 1.10 Five Phase numerology

Planets

The foundation of the Five Phases approach is that everything from the microcosmic to the macrocosmic is determined by the same natural principles. This is because everything is a manifestation of *qi* and of the interplay between *yin* and *yang*. That is why the various planets in our solar system are represented in presentations of the Five Phases. At the time that the theory of the Five Phases was created, only five planets in our solar system could be observed with the naked eye. These planets have a fundamental resonance with the other aspects of their phase.

Planet	
Water	Mercury
Wood	Jupiter
Fire	Mars
Earth	Saturn
Metal	Venus

Internal organs

Each of the phases is associated with a so-called *yin* organ and a so-called *yang* organ. *Yin* organs have a solid structure and store pure and refined forms of *qi*. These organs are called *zang* organs in Chinese. *Yang* organs have a hollow structure. They are constantly filled and emptied. Their task is to receive coarse and impure substances, which they help to transform and to excrete waste products. These hollow organs are called *fu* organs. There will be a detailed examination of each of these organs' functions in the section about *zangfu* organs. The relationship between a phase's *yin* and *yang* organs or its channels is called a husband/wife relationship.

The *zang* organ of the Water Phase is the Kidneys. One of the primary functions of the Kidneys is to store *jing*, which is the most *yin* form of *qi* in the body. *Jing* is the *qi* that is received from the parents at conception. It is the *qi* that can create new life in the form of sperm and eggs. This is an example of how *qi* is drawn inwards in the Water Phase to create new life and how the start of a new *sheng* cycle begins. *Jing* is involved in creating life itself. At the same time the consumption and decrease of *jing* is one of the causes of ageing. This decrease of *jing* in old age can be seen by the fact that many of the things *jing* has an influence on, such as bones, hair, potency, fertility and hearing, all become weaker the older we get.

Jing has a major influence on many of the aspects that are seen as being aspects of the Water Phase. *Jing* is the foundation of our life and existence.

The Kidneys' partner *fu* organ is the Urinary Bladder. The Kidneys and the Urinary Bladder have a close relationship, both physically and functionally. They have a fundamental influence on fluid physiology, particularly the storage and excretion of urine.

The Wood Phase's *zang* organ is the Liver and its *fu* organ is the Gall Bladder. These also have a very close physical and physiological relationship to each other. One of the Liver's most important functions is to ensure that *qi* flows freely and without hindrance. The Gall Bladder is dependent on this free flow of *qi* to carry out its functions. The Liver and Gall Bladder work closely together with regards to making decisions and planning. All *zang* organs have a spiritual or psychological aspect called the organ's *shen* aspect. The *shen* aspect of the Liver is called the *hun*. It is the *hun* that gives us the ability to have visions, ideas and dreams. This enables us to create strategies, lay plans and thereby take decisions. The Gall Bladder gives us the resolution and courage to carry out these decisions. The Liver is also a reservoir that stores Blood or *xue* and constantly ensures that there is an appropriate amount of *xue* circulating in the body.

The Fire Phase is special in that two *zang* and two *fu* organs are ascribed to this phase. There was originally only one *zang* organ in the Fire Phase – the Heart. The Pericardium was added later as a separate organ, and it is also for this reason that some books speak of five *zang* organs and six *fu* organs. The Pericardium's main function is to protect the Heart, because the Heart is considered to be the most important organ in the body. The Heart is where *shen* has its residence. *Shen*, which will be discussed in greater detail in the next section of this book, can be translated as mind, consciousness, spirit and intelligence. Where *jing* is the most *yin* form of *qi* in the body, *shen* is the most *yang* form of *qi*. This is a reflection of the Water and Fire Phases' *yin/yang* polarity. *Jing* is the material foundation for *shen*, and *shen* is the *yang* manifestation of *jing*. The relationship between the Fire Phase *zang* organs and their partner *fu* organs is not as close as with the other phases. The Heart's partner is the Small Intestine, whose main functions are related to the separation of pure and impure substances. *San jiao*, whose partner is the Pericardium, is a strange organ seen with Western eyes, as it has no physical structure. In some ways this is an advantage, as it is important to remember that when an organ is discussed in

Chinese medicine, it is more a sum of different physiological and mental-emotional processes than it is a physical structure that is being discussed. Furthermore, many of the functions attributed to the various organs can be quite different in the two medical systems.

The Earth Phase's organs are the Spleen and the Stomach. Their functional relationship is so close that they can almost be viewed as being the same organ. Nevertheless, they do have their own separate functions and each is more typically affected by different forms of pathological *qi*. The Stomach and the Spleen are located in the middle of the body. This is consistent with the Earth Phase, which is characterised as being in the centre. All upward and downward movement of *qi* must pass through the centre and the Spleen and Stomach have an important *qi* dynamic (called *qi ji* in Chinese). The Spleen and Stomach respectively send *qi* upwards and downwards. The Earth Phase's organs are the root of post-heavenly *qi*. This is the *qi* that is created daily from the food and liquid that has been consumed.

Internal organs	
Water	Kidneys and Urinary Bladder
Wood	Liver and Gall Bladder
Fire	Heart, Small Intestine, Pericardium and *san jiao*
Earth	Spleen and Stomach
Metal	Lung and Large Intestine

The organs of the Metal Phase are the Lung and the Large Intestines. The Lung is also involved in the production of the post-heavenly *qi*. This is seen by the fact that it is the Lung that draws the pure air into the body, which is then combined with the *qi* that the Spleen has extracted from the ingested food. When the *qi* from the food is combined with the pure air that the Lung has inhaled, *zong qi* is created. *Zong qi* is the foundation of post-heavenly *qi*. The Large Intestine's most important functions relate to fluid physiology and the expulsion of the unused residue from the digestive process.

Sensory organs

Each phase and each *zang* organ has a sensory organ that it has a close relationship to. It is important to remember that these relationships are not exclusive and that other organs may also have a very close relationship to the sensory organ.

The sensory organ of the Water Phase is the ears. The ears consist primarily of cartilage, which is also an aspect of the Water Phase. Cartilage is created by *jing*, and it is *jing* that nourishes the inner ear, enabling us to hear. The older we get, the greater the decline in the quality and quantity of our *jing*. This is reflected in the fact that many of the things that have been created and nourished by *jing*, such as our auditory sense, diminish in strength and quality the older we become. In daily practice, problems with the ears such as tinnitus, earache, etc. will just as often relate to imbalances in the Liver, Gall Bladder and *san jiao*, or to invasions of external pathological *qi* (exogenous *xie qi*).

The eyes are nourished by Liver *xue* (Liver Blood). In addition, the *shen* aspect of the Liver, *hun*, travels to the eyes during the day. Tang Zong Hai wrote in the *Xue Zheng Lun*: 'When *hun* wanders to the eyes, they can see.' The *hun*, which can be translated as the ethereal spirit, provides us with vision, both on the physical level as sight, but also vision as in dreams and goals in life. The *Treatise of the Golden Flower* (*Taiyi Jinhua Zongzhi*) in chapter two says: 'In the daytime *hun* is in the eyes and at night in the Liver. When it is in the eyes we can see. When it is in the Liver we dream.' It is therefore logical that the eyes are an aspect of the Wood Phase. When there is a deficiency of the Liver's *xue* or Blood aspect, called Liver *xue xu* in Chinese medicine, there can be floaters in the visual field and there can be difficulty in focussing and a lack of visual acuity. In a similar way to the ears, it is important in the diagnosis of eye and visual problems to also pay attention to the channel connections to the eyes, as well as invasions of *xie qi*. The eyes are particularly sensitive to conditions of Heat in the body. This can be both external invasions of Heat and internally generated Heat.

The sensory organ of the Heart is the tongue. The Heart is in general a very special organ that in many ways differentiates itself from the other organs due to its unique nature. The Heart and *shen* are our connection to the universe. That is why the Heart should preferably be empty, so that there is space for the *dao*, or the universal *shen*, to be able to flow freely. The other sensory organs are hollow and the body uses them to absorb impressions. The tongue though is different. Unlike the other sensory organs, the tongue has a solid structure. Furthermore, the tongue is used to empty the mind and thereby the Heart of feelings and thoughts via speech. The sense of taste, which is associated with the tongue, is something that can be related to the Heart in Chinese medicine, but is also a function of the mouth and thereby the Spleen, as the Spleen and Stomach control the mouth and oral cavity. Often, changes and problems with the lips, gums and oral cavity will be due to Stomach or Spleen imbalances.

The nose and the rest of the respiratory tract is controlled by the Lung and thereby they are an aspect of the Metal Phase. The Lung is the only *zang* organ that directly opens to its sense organ. The Lung is also the only *zang* organ that is in direct contact with the world that is outside of the body. The Lung is in direct contact with the external world through the nose and respiratory passages and through the skin, which is controlled by the Lung. All the other *zang* organs connect to their sensory organs and to the outer world via the channel system. This means that the Lung is easily affected by exogenous *xie qi*. When the Lung has been disturbed by exogenous *xie qi*, it will often manifest itself with symptoms in its sense organ such as sneezing, snivelling, nasal drip or a blocked nose and sinuses.

Sense organ	
Water	Ear
Wood	Eye
Fire	Tongue
Earth	Mouth
Metal	Nose

Senses

The senses that are attributed to the various phases relate to their sensory organs.

Hearing is an aspect of the Water Phase. The ears are nourished by Kidney *jing*, and the acuity of the hearing decreases over the years as *jing* becomes weaker. Similarly, tinnitus can be a sign of a Kidney imbalance.

As described in the section above, the eyes are nourished by Liver *xue*, which is of great importance for the quality of our vision. Liver *xue xu* can manifest with symptoms such as floaters, difficulty focussing and poor visual acuity. The *hun* of the Liver gives us vision, also metaphorically. The *hun* gives us our dreams in life, as well as the dreams we have whilst we are sleeping.

Communication is an important aspect of the Heart. It is through our Heart that we open ourselves to others. We talk to people when we communicate with them and when we want to make contact. When the Heart is imbalanced, the person will often talk too much, too fast or too little. When people are anxious and their *shen* is unsettled, they will often stammer.

The sense of taste is an aspect of the Spleen. The Spleen enables a person to distinguish the five flavours. If the Spleen is imbalanced, a person can lose their sense of taste.

The nose is controlled by the Lung. When the Lung is in balance, the nose can smell and distinguish the different scents and odours. On the other hand, the sense of smell can be greatly reduced if the nose is blocked, such as when a person has a cold for example.

Sense	
Water	Hearing
Wood	Vision
Fire	Speech
Earth	Taste
Metal	Smell

Body tissues

As was the case with the sensory organs, it is important to remember that an organ and thereby a phase's relationship to specific types of body tissue is far from exclusive. There will often be more than one organ that has a close relationship to a particular type of tissue in the body. Nonetheless, we can see that various organs have a close relationship with specific types of tissue.

Jing, which is stored in the Kidneys, creates physical structures in the body, such as bones, cartilage, teeth and the hair on the head. Bones also contain, and are dependent on, the mineral salts, which are also an aspect of the Water Phase. When Kidney *jing* is decreasing, these structures will be physically weaker, bones become fragile, the teeth fall out and the hair loses its colour and rooting.

Liver *xue* nourishes the sinews and tendons in the body and together with Liver *qi* maintains the flexibility and strength of the sinews and tendons. The fingernails are also seen as being an extension of the sinews in Chinese medicine physiology. A weakening of Liver *xue* can therefore manifest with fingernails that are weak and break easily or that are dry and ridged.

The blood vessels can in some ways be seen as a direct extension of the Heart. The Heart organ is in direct physical connection with the blood vessels, and it is the muscles of the Heart that pump *xue* through the blood vessels.

The Spleen is the post-heaven root of *qi* and *xue*. *Qi* and *xue* are used to create and nourish the muscles. Some modern authors' interpretation of the Five Phase relationships is that the Spleen controls the muscles in the arms and legs and the Liver controls muscles in the rest of the body. In my view this is a misunderstanding and a simplification. The Spleen has a significant influence on muscle volume and size by virtue of the fact that it is *qi* and *xue* that nourish the muscles. As stated, it is the Spleen that is the post-heaven root of these substances. The free flow of Liver *qi* ensures that the muscles are flexible and supple. The Liver thereby influences their functionality. When Spleen *qi* is weak, the person often experiences fatigue and weakness in their limbs, whereas they will feel heaviness in their arms and legs if there is Dampness in the body. Liver *qi* stagnation will often result in muscles that are stiff and tense.

Even though the skin and body hair are an aspect of the Metal Phase, and thereby the tissue of the Lung, it is by no means true that all skin diseases are related to the Lung. On the contrary, many skin diseases are caused by Damp-Heat or *xue* imbalances. This is because it is *xue* that nourishes the skin. The skin is the body's largest respiratory organ. In the same way that air can pass through the tissue of the Lung, air can enter and leave the body through the pores in the skin, which are controlled by *wei qi* (defensive *qi*). It is through the skin that pathogens such as Wind and Cold enter the body and disturb the Lung in its functioning.

Body tissue	
Water	Bones and cartilage
Wood	Tendons and sinews
Fire	Blood vessels
Earth	Muscles
Metal	Skin

Body fluids

The urine's relationship to the Water Phase can be clearly seen in the key role played by the Kidneys and the Urinary Bladder in the production, storage and expulsion of urine. The Wood Phase's relationship to tears can at first seem to be more tenuous. Nevertheless, wind, which is the climatic aspect of the Wood Phase, often causes people's eyes to water. People whose eyes start to tear when they are outdoors often have Liver *xue xu*.

On first sight one might assume that sweat would be more relevant as an aspect of the Lung in the Five Phases, as it is the Lung that controls the pores. It is important to bear in mind that many people spontaneously sweat when they are nervous or when they are emotionally uncomfortable. When we are nervous, our *shen* is not being anchored by the *yin* aspects of the Heart. Furthermore, the areas people sweat from when they are nervous are under the arms and in the palms of the hands. These places are at the start and the end of the Heart channel. At the same time as they are spontaneously sweating due to nervousness, a person will typically also experience palpitations and their cheeks will redden. The cheeks are the area of the face that relates to the Heart.

In Western physiology saliva is something that is used in the digestive process. Furthermore, saliva is produced in the mouth. Both of these facts are consistent with Chinese medicine physiology, as the oral cavity is controlled by the Stomach and Spleen, which are the two most important digestive organs. The Stomach and Spleen have saliva as their body fluid, and Stomach and Spleen imbalances can manifest with disturbances in the production of saliva.

The body fluid that is usually ascribed to the Lung is Phlegm. One of the aphorisms of Chinese medicine is that 'Phlegm is produced in the Spleen and stored in the Lung'. This is because the Phlegm that accumulates in the Lung is often the result of Spleen *qi xu* or poor diet. Nevertheless, a disruption of the Lung's function of spreading fluids throughout the body can result in the accumulation of thin, watery Phlegm in the Lung itself.

Body fluid	
Water	Urine
Wood	Tears
Fire	Sweat
Earth	Saliva
Metal	Phlegm

As previously stated, the application of Five Phase theories marked a significant shift in Chinese medicine. Chinese medicine changed from being a shamanistic medicine to being an analytical and knowledge-based medicine. Disease was now seen as arising due to imbalance in the dynamic of a phase and its components. One of the phases was seen as being weaker or more dominant in relation to the other phases. The phases could be dominant or weak due to the dynamics of the internal organs or due to aetiological factors that resonated with a particular phase. Cold could, for example, have a detrimental effect on the Water Phase; eating too much sweet food could have created Dampness and thereby weakened the Spleen of the Earth Phase. Unexpressed anger could have created an imbalance in the Wood Phase.

People are a mixture of all five phases, but often one or two of the phases will be dominant in that person's constitution. Furthermore, the influences that a person is exposed to throughout their life affect the balance between the phases. The relative dominance or weakness of the various phases is ascertained through observation of the person. Observation of changes in how the Five Phases manifest themselves in a person was used, and is still used today, to diagnose physical, emotional and mental imbalances. It is both through the observation of changes in the physiological functions that are carried out by the *zang* and *fu* organs and through changes in other aspects of the person that conclusions are drawn. These changes can both be physical and emotional. I will not venture here into describing how to diagnose using the parameters of the Five Phases. The reader is instead referred to *The Art of Diagnosis in Chinese Medicine* (Ching 2009)[21] or *Five Element Constitutional Acupuncture* (Hicks, Hicks and Mole 2004). I will however discuss a couple of the relations that are included in the overview table at the beginning of the chapter.

Sounds

The sound qualities attributed to the Five Phases are: a shouting voice in the Wood Phase; laughter or a voice that has a jovial quality in the Fire Phase; a complaining or moaning voice in the Water Phase; a singing voice in the Earth phase; and a crying voice in the Metal Phase.

The sound of a person's voice should contain qualities of all the Five Phases when there is harmony. If a phase is deficient or is *xu*, the voice will lack the sound quality that resonates with that phase. Conversely, if the phase is excess or is *shi*, the voice will be dominated by the associated sound quality. The sound in a person's voice will of course change in relation to their emotions and what they are talking about. This reflects the emotions relating to the various phases. When there is an imbalance the dominance or lack of a quality can also be heard when the sound of the voice does not match with what they are talking about or to the situation.

The Water Phase has a voice that has a moaning or groaning quality. The voice is very flat and lacks variation in the tone. The voice can also sound as if it is on the point of breaking. This will be particularly noticeable if the *qi* of the Water Phase is deficient.

The Wood Phase is characterised by a shouting voice. This a hard and clear-cut voice. The voice has a harsh quality and it has power, volume and direction. The voice travels clearly through the air and can often be heard through doors and walls. The voice of a person with Liver *xue xu* will lack these qualities and they will often have a weak voice that lacks sonority. A person with what is known as Liver Fire on the other hand will have a loud voice that sounds as if they are on the verge of shouting – a voice that can often be heard through doors and walls. This is the tone that is heard in the voice of someone who is angry.

Fire imbalances manifest with either a voice that is flat and sad, lacking a joyful quality, or the opposite, the voice being excessively jovial. The joviality in their voice can sound exaggerated or even false. It could also be that the person either does not laugh or laughs excessively or inappropriately. People who are Heart *yin xu* often punctuate their sentences with a nervous laugh.

When the Heart is in balance, we can hear the quality of joy in that person's voice. This is the voice you expect to hear when a person tells you of a happy event. The voice will have vitality. The Heart is nurtured by, and manifests with, joy. In conditions where there are Heart *xu* imbalances or where there is a stagnation of Heart *qi*, the voice will generally lack this quality. There will be a flatness and sadness in the voice. Conversely, when there is Heat in the Heart, the voice can be exaggeratedly happy. This may be a constant nervous giggle whilst they are talking. It can also be a 'life and soul of the party' type voice, a person who is constantly laughing and trying to be funny. As mentioned earlier, the voice should be appropriate to what the person is saying. A person whose voice is glad and full of vitality, or who laughs whilst talking about something sad or tragic, will most probably have a Fire imbalance. On the other hand, a voice that is flat and sad, lacking variation in tone when they are talking of a happy event, will also be a sign of a Fire imbalance.

The Earth Phase manifests with a voice that is singing. It is a voice whose tone varies up and down whilst the person is speaking. It is the voice you would use when reading a story out loud.

As in the case of the Fire Phase, the voice that is a manifestation of the Metal Phase characterises the emotion that is associated with this phase. The emotion of the Metal Phase is sadness, and the voice of the Metal Phase has a quality that makes it sound as if the person is close to tears. There can be a slight choking of the words. An extreme version of this voice is heard in children when they are trying to tell you something just after they have burst into tears. The voice can lack strength and the person's sentences can have a tendency to fade out before they are completed. This is because the Lung *qi* is affected and there is therefore not enough *zong qi* to complete the sentences.

Sound	
Water	Groaning or moaning
Wood	Shouting
Fire	Laughing
Earth	Singing
Metal	Crying

Odours

Each of the phases has a specific odour, which can be noticeable when there is imbalance in that phase. Often it can be difficult to smell anything relevant. This is mainly because most people bathe frequently and regularly wash their clothes, and use fabric softeners, perfumes, aftershave, creams, deodorants, etc., all of which make it difficult to smell the person's natural odours.

The following description of the Five Phase odours is mainly based on the descriptions that Hicks *et al.* use in their book *Five Element Constitutional Acupuncture* (2004) and J. R. Worsley uses in his book *Traditional Acupuncture: Volume II* (1990).

- Water Phase – Rotten and putrid: The Chinese character *fu* can be translated into English as putrid. The character is built up of two components. The first has the meaning of a building or shed, and the second component means to dry meat that is tied together. This gives the character a sense of the odour you would expect to smell in a shed that is used to dry meat. The difference between this odour and the odour of the Metal Phase is that the *fu* odour is more tart and caustic.

- Wood Phase – Rancid: *Sao*, as this smell is called in Chinese, is the smell that animals or urine can have. This is rancid, as in rancid butter or rancid fats, but even sharper. Hicks *et al.* (2004) describe this smell as newly mown grass, but without that smell being pleasant.

- Fire Phase – Burnt: This odour is called *zhuo* in Chinese. The smell can be described as being similar to toast that has been burnt, clothes that have just come out of a tumble dryer, a shirt that has been burnt with an iron or vegetables burning dry in a saucepan. In the same way that the smell varies depending on what it is that is burning, the burnt smell can vary from person to person. The aroma may be noticed when a person has a high fever.

- Earth Phase – Sweet and aromatic: The Chinese word *xiang* means aromatic. It is a word that is used in the name of many aromatic herbs for example.

This though can be misleading, as the odour referred to here has a heavy, sticky, almost nauseating aroma.

- Metal Phase – Rotten: Rotten is called *lan* in Chinese. This is the rotten odour that is smelt when meat, fish or vegetables rot. This odour can be smelt in old dustbins or garbage trucks.

Odour	
Water	Putrid
Wood	Rancid
Fire	Burnt
Earth	Sweet and aromatic
Metal	Rotten

Emotions

All the organs have both physical functions and mental-emotional aspects. This means that they can be negatively affected by the excessive long-term presence of certain feelings and emotions. Conversely, people often manifest an excessive tendency towards certain emotions when an organ is imbalanced.

It is important to remember that all emotions have both a positive and negative aspect. This is the same as *yin* and *yang*. A certain portion of every emotion is necessary to function normally, but too much or too little of any emotion or an excessive manifestation of this emotion in inappropriate situations is pathological and problematical. This can be clearly seen in fear, which is the emotion of the Water Phase. Fear gives a person the necessary respect in situations that can be dangerous or risky. If a person is completely fearless, they will sooner or later end up in a situation that is life-threatening. Conversely, a person who suffers from acute anxiety and whose life is totally controlled by fear is often not able to act, because they are paralysed by fear and often see signs of danger all around them.

Anger in a Chinese medicine context is understood as being more encompassing than just anger – it is also frustration, irritation and aggressiveness. Anger is very characteristic of *qi* in the Wood Phase and the Liver in particular. Anger is a very focussed and dynamic form of *qi*. It is sometimes also needed to set and assert boundaries. Similar to wind, which is the climatic aspect of the Wood Phase, anger can be the necessary force needed to bring about change. Anger has a powerful dynamic. On the other hand, if anger is excessive and uncontrolled it can, like wind, be very destructive and devastating. A pathological lack of anger can be seen in some people, such as people who fail to react to injustices or who have difficulty asserting their boundaries in relation to other people.

Joy is a spontaneous manifestation of the Heart. When the Heart and thereby the *shen* is in balance, there is a harmonious sense of calm and happiness in a person. If the Heart *qi* is stagnant or weak, there will often be sadness and lack of joy.

Conversely, if the Heart and *shen* is agitated by Heat, the person will often be too ecstatic and easily excited.

The Spleen has the task of transforming the food and drink consumed into pure *qi* that can be used by the body, whilst at the same time separating out the impure *qi* that cannot be used. The process also occurs on a mental level. Thoughts and impressions must also be digested. The emotion that is attributed to the Spleen is contemplativeness and worry. If there is Spleen *qi xu* or a condition of Dampness that hampers and obstructs the Spleen, a person can have a tendency to be too contemplative and to worry a lot. They have a tendency to get lost in their thoughts and their thoughts do not lead to a constructive conclusion where the relevant information is extracted and the irrelevant information discarded. Rather than reaching a conclusion, they start the process again and again.

The Metal Phase is attributed the emotion of grief and sadness. The Lung has, like the other *zang* organs, a *shen* aspect. This aspect of the Lung is the *po*. Unlike the *hun* of the Liver, the *po* does not survive the physical body at death but dies with the body. Some people therefore mean that the mortality of the *po* characterises the Metal Phase and gives the Metal Phase an aspect of melancholy and grief.

Many people associate the autumn with melancholia. Life is waning and nature is moving towards winter's dormancy and death. Nature is in a process where the individual life is let go of, but life itself continues. As we approach old age, we must relate to the fact that we must let go of life and that those around us, who we care for, die.

Throughout life, we must be able to grieve. Only by giving space to grief can we let go of it. It is important to let go of grief to be able to move forward. Chinese culture has traditionally provided allotted time periods for grief after a person dies. It is important that a person grieves in this period, but it is also important that they also can let go of the grief afterwards. By letting go of the sorrow and loss of the one that you loved, you are able to love again. Only in this way is it possible to move on.

It is not only on the emotional level in the Metal Phase that the necessity of letting go of the old, to create the space so something new and nourishing can enter, is seen. The Lung and the Large Intestine both have the job of releasing from the body things that are no longer nourishing in the form of impure air and faeces. Only by releasing these from the body is it possible to take in new nourishment. A person with Lung imbalances can have a tendency to sadness and they may have difficulty releasing their grief.

Emotion	
Water	Fear
Wood	Anger
Fire	Joy
Earth	Worry
Metal	Sorrow

Shen aspects

In addition to having physical and emotional aspects, each organ has a so-called *shen* aspect. These aspects will be discussed in greater depth in the next section on the vital substances, as well as in the individual chapters about the *zangfu* organs.

It is possible to talk about both an overall *shen* and about specific aspects of *shen* that relate to the five *zang* organs. *Shen* can be translated amongst other things as spirit, consciousness and mind. *Shen* is a much broader concept than all three of these words.

Prior to the foundation of Five Phase philosophy, there was in Chinese physiology more a concept of three *shen* aspects – *hun*, *po* and *shen*. These three have their residence in, and have a close relationship to, the Liver, the Lung and the Heart respectively. *Shen* is the universal *qi* that permeates everything, but it is also our own individual refraction of this *qi*. *Shen* is all embracing and omnipresent; therefore *shen* is infinite and timeless.

Hun is the ethereal spirit; though bearing some similarities to the Western concept of soul, it is nevertheless not the same. *Hun* survives the body after death and rises up out of the body and returns to the universe. *Hun* enables a person to have visions and dreams, both in the sense of goals in life, but also dreams at night and sight.

Po is the animal or physical spirit. *Po* is responsible for the automatic physical functioning and reflexes in the body. It is *po* that responds when the body is physically stimulated, such as when the skin is touched. *Po* is the aspect of a person that ensures that the lungs inhale and exhale, that the stomach empties and the muscles of the intestines send the food downwards and the body heals after a physical trauma. It is all the things that the body does without a person consciously thinking about it. It is our instincts, reflexes and responses to physical stimuli.

Two other aspects of the *shen* were added around the time that the theories of the Five Phases were founded. These two aspects are *yi* and *zhi*. *Yi* and *zhi* appear to be less spiritual than *shen*, *hun* and *po* and ostensibly are more mental or psychological. In Chinese medicine it is difficult to be so categoric, as there is no clear division between the psyche and the spirit in the same way that there is no clear division between the psyche and soma. They are all just refractions of the same *qi*.

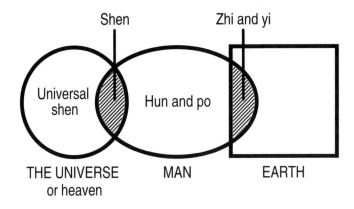

Figure 1.11 The relationships between the various *shen* aspects

Zhi is our willpower. It is the perseverance that allows us to complete our projects. Without *zhi*, *hun* would just create a lot of empty ideas that never amounted to anything. *Zhi* is an aspect of us that gives us stability. It keeps us on the path and stops us from running after each and every new idea. *Zhi* has also a relationship to our fundamental animal drives and instincts, for example our sexual urges. It is the will to live and the will to continue life in the next generation.

Yi can be defined as our mental faculties, our intellectual focus. *Yi* ensures that we can digest information and that we can reflect on our experiences and impressions. *Yi* relates to the sorting, mental recording and digestion of information. That is why it is so closely connected to our intellectual capacities. *Yi* can also be translated as intention. It is that which focuses our *qi*.

Heart	Liver	Lung	Spleen	Kidneys
Shen	*Hun*	*Po*	*Yi*	*Zhi*
Individual refraction or aspect of *dao* or the universal *shen* or *qi*	Ethereal soul that rises up and out of the body at death to return to the universe	Corporeal spirit dies together with physical body and returns to the ground below us	Mental faculties, intellectual focus	Willpower, stamina
Consciousness	Dreams and visions	Instincts and reflexes	Thoughts and reflections Intention, mental focus	The fundamental will to live, determination and perseverance
Fully awake and conscious	Dream world, REM sleep	Reflexes and responses	Thoughts and reflection	Deep sleep
Propriety	Benevolence and compassion	Reverence, righteousness	Trust, sincerity	Wisdom

Five Element body types

Within J.R. Worsley-style Five Element acupuncture, people are diagnosed, amongst other things, by their constitutional type. The physical body and the character are observed to assess which phase or phases the person is a manifestation of. The analysis of body type is also used to assess the relative severity of an imbalance. It is better to have an imbalance that 'matches' the constitutional phase, rather than an imbalance that matches the controlling phase.

The theory is that all humans are born with a constitutional body type. It is their starting point in life. There are therefore five main body types, which correspond to the Five Phases, but it is rare that a person is only one type. We are all mixtures of all five phases simultaneously. One or two of the phases, however, will often be dominant in relation to the others. Furthermore, your life experiences, the food you have eaten, your long-term environmental influences, lifestyle and diseases you have suffered will also have had a fundamental influence on the body and its physiology.

Huang Di Nei Jing – Ling Shu, chapter sixty-four, lists the following characteristics of the five constitutional types.

Wood type

- Sinewy
- Greenish skin colour
- Small head
- Long face
- Broad back and shoulders
- Straight back
- Small torso
- Tall
- Small hands and feet
- Intelligent
- Not physically strong
- Persistent when they work
- Tendency to worry

Fire type

- Ruddy skin colour
- Small head
- Thin face
- Wide back
- Well-developed muscles in the shoulders, back, abdomen and buttocks
- Small hands and feet
- Curly hair
- Quick tempered
- Quick thinking
- Quick body movements
- Firm gait and the body moves whilst they walk
- Can have a tendency to be anxious

Earth type

- Yellowish skin colour
- Rotund body shape
- Large head
- Round face
- Broad jaws
- Large abdomen
- Large thighs and calf muscles, strong legs
- Relatively small hands and feet
- Well-proportioned body
- Steady gait
- Raises feet slightly whilst walking
- Solid muscles
- Quiet and generous
- Not overambitious
- Easy to get on with

Metal type

- Pale skin colour
- Square face
- Small head
- Narrow shoulders and upper back
- Small abdomen
- Lean
- Small hands and feet
- Fine bone structure
- Powerful voice
- Thinks quickly
- Honest and reliable
- Quiet and calm, but solid

- Determined
- Good leader
- Quick, swift movements

Water type

- Dark complexion
- Wrinkled face
- Large head
- Angular jaw and chin
- Round and narrow shoulders
- Large abdomen
- Moves the whole body when they walk
- Long spine
- Relaxed
- Loyal
- Attentive and sensitive

Part 2

THE VITAL
SUBSTANCES

INTRODUCTION TO THE
VITAL SUBSTANCES

The very foundation of Chinese medicine physiology are the so-called vital substances. The vital substances are even more important than the internal organs themselves. This is not only because the vital substances are the foundation of the internal organs, but also because all diagnosis and all treatment in the final end is based on the quality and condition of these substances.

In Chinese medicine physiology there are substances that do not exist at all in Western medicine physiology. For example, *qi*, *shen* and *jing* have no counterpart in Western medicine physiology, yet they are three of the most important aspects of the body in Chinese medicine. The importance of these substances that are 'non-existent' in Western medicine is seen in their common title – the Three Treasures. This means in practice that Chinese medicine is based on a fundamentally different physiological model than Western medicine. It is necessary that you accept and understand this model if you want to work with acupuncture and Chinese medicine. It can be difficult in the beginning to let go of an ingrown conception of how the body works and what it is comprised of. It is often initially difficult to accept that there can be another way of understanding the body's physiology and pathology. This is partly due to the Western, Cartesian way of thinking, where there is a tendency always to view things as being either/or, i.e. if there exists a truth, then it excludes alternative or parallel truths. East Asian thought is different. Here there is more of a both/and view. This means that just because a truth is correct, it does not mean that there may not be other truths simultaneously. This is perhaps an over-simplification, but one does not have to go back much more than one hundred years in the history of Western medicine before meeting the opinion that the psyche did not exist and that the emotions did not influence the physical body. At this time Western medicine only conceived of the body as having physical form. Now it is commonly accepted knowledge in Western medicine that the body consists of both physical and mental-emotional aspects and that they have an influence on each other.

Apart from having to accept the fact that the Chinese medicine physiological model operates with the concepts of *qi*, *shen* and *jing* that do not exist in Western medicine physiology, one also has to cope with the fact that even though the organs and many of the bodily substances bear the same names in Chinese medicine, they are attributed very different functions than those that they have in Western medicine.

Furthermore, where Western medicine primarily focuses on the physical structure and form of the organs and bodily substances, Chinese medicine focuses more on the functions of an organ and the relationship and cooperation between the various organs and substances, as well as how these are affected by the world around them.

This can create difficulty for a Western novice when trying to understand Chinese medicine. Not only must they comprehend Chinese medicine and its associated physiological and pathological model, they must also comprehend the fundamental concepts and philosophy that this model is based upon.

This becomes very obvious when defining what *qi* is.

Qi as an overall concept

Qi, which is the most fundamental aspect of Chinese medicine, is a substance and a concept that does not exist in the Western world, neither linguistically nor philosophically and certainly not in the Western medicine physiological model. This means that it is not possible to directly translate *qi* into English, Danish, Dutch or any other European language. There is no concept that embraces all the various connotations of *qi*. A student from China, Japan, Vietnam and Korea who is about to learn acupuncture or Chinese herbal medicine will already be familiar with the word *qi*. It will be a concept that is already a part of their vocabulary and their way of thinking. An East Asian acupuncture student will only have to learn the physiological functions that *qi* has in the body, how *qi* behaves, how it is produced and how it is brought out of balance. *Qi* as a concept is something that they have grown up with.

As described above, *qi* is not just a word, but also a concept that does not exist in European languages and philosophies or Western medicine physiology. In a Chinese dictionary, there are twenty-three definitions of the word *qi* (Rose and Zhang 2001, p.9). This in itself makes it very difficult to translate the word *qi* into a singular word in a European language.

Qi is often translated as energy or bodily energy, but this is a very narrow definition of something that is so comprehensive. In East Asian philosophies, and thereby also in East Asian traditional science, the universe is created from, and consists of, *qi*. At the same time *qi* is the energy or the potential that creates all movement and change in the universe, but *qi* is also the result of this change and dynamic. In Chinese philosophy there is no clear distinction between energy and matter – they are part of a continuum. *Qi* manifests both as solid, physical structures and as immaterial energies. But even this does not give a complete understanding of *qi*. Whatever word we choose to translate *qi* as, it will be too unequivocal in its definition to be able to embrace *qi*.

Something that is difficult for the Western way of thinking is that *qi* is not something that is definitive and constant. We are accustomed to thinking of things as being solid and unchanging and that things are defined by their form, especially when they have a physical structure. We find it more difficult to comprehend that everything is in a constant process, where it is not only being broken down and built up, but also things can change form and are defined by their function. The key to comprehending *qi* is perhaps to think of *qi* as being something that is in a constant process of change, both in terms of its form and function and as being something that is defined by its activity and function.

Qi is one of the oldest words or characters in the Chinese language. The character is to be found in some of the oldest texts that are in existence. The character has gone through a number of changes over time, not only with regard to the definition of the word but also how the character is written. Originally, the ideogram for *qi* consisted of three horizontal lines. These lines represented vapours that were rising upwards to form a cloud. This creates an image of something that cannot necessarily be seen but that can be sensed, experienced and understood through the changes it creates. In this way, *qi* is similar to wind. You cannot see wind, but you can see the consequences of its existence. The leaves and branches of the trees sway, a flag flutters, etc. but we cannot actually see the wind itself.

Over the course of time *qi* assumed additional definitions. One of these was that *qi* is something that can be inhaled and exhaled from the body. This definition was particularly relevant for Daoists, who developed various respiratory techniques to enhance the production and conservation of *qi*, in their attempt to achieve a longer lifespan. A second development of the word was the addition of the radical for rice, giving the character a characteristic of nourishment. Roughly translated, the character could be interpreted as being steam or vapours that rise up and nourish or the steam or vapour that rises up from the rice.

So what is *qi*? How can we briefly summarise and comprehend *qi* in a Chinese medicine context? An attempt could be: '*Qi* is that which makes us alive, whilst at the same time all matter is *qi*, i.e. everything that we are, both our minds and our physical body, are *qi*.' In Chinese medicine physiology, everything in the body consists of *qi*, whilst all of the body's physiological processes are created and controlled by *qi*. All the body's structures and all the vital substances in the body are forms of *qi*. To make it more practical, all the various forms of *qi* are of course defined as being independent substances, structures and processes. In the following chapters I will try to define the various bodily substances and what their functions in the body are. Some forms of *qi* are more *yin*, such as *jing* (essence), *xue* (blood), *jinye* (fluids), bones, etc. Some forms of *qi* are more *yang*, such as *shen* (mind/spirit/consciousness), *wei qi* (protective or defensive *qi*) and *yuan qi* (original *qi*). All of them though are *qi*, in the same way that icebergs, glaciers, waterfalls, rivers, lakes, oceans, mist, steam, clouds, rain, hail, snow, sleet and frost are all water.

Furthermore, apart from the various forms of *qi* that the body consists of and that are essential for the body's physiology, the body can also be negatively affected by *qi*. This means that *qi* can be conceived, not just as being something physiological, but also as being pathological. *Xie qi* – 'evil' or 'perverted' *qi* – is *qi* that has a negative effect and disturbs the body's physiology. *Xie qi* can be exogenous and invade the body from the environment, or it can be internally generated, arising from poor diet, emotions, imbalances in the organs, etc. This can lead to disease in Chinese medicine.

The vital substances in the body are:

- *jing* or essence
- *qi*
- blood or *xue*
- fluids or *jinye*
- mind/spirit/consciousness or *shen.*

These five substances are broad categories and there are various sub-categories and different forms of most of these substances.

JING OR ESSENCE

Jing is one of the most *yin* manifestations of *qi* in the body. *Jing* is often translated as 'essence'. As the word essence indicates, *jing* is one of the most fundamental forms of *qi* and is the basis for all other forms of *qi* in the body. *Jing* is the fundamental potential for life and growth in the body. *Jing* has the overall responsibility for the body's physiological growth and development and the body's structure, as well as fertility and reproduction. *Jing* is used to create the bones, the teeth and the hair on the head. *Jing* is also that which creates semen and eggs and is thereby the basis for reproduction and fertility. *Jing* is bone marrow, which in Chinese physiology is the root of the brain. This means that *jing* not only has a determining influence on the body's physical structure, but also that it has an impact on a person's mental capabilities. This is also confirmed by the fact that *jing* is considered to be the material root of *shen* (awareness/mind/mental-emotional aspects).

There are three types of *jing*: pre-heaven *jing* (*xian tian zhi jing*), post-heaven *jing* (*hou tian zhi jing*) and Kidney *jing* (*shen jing*). These three forms of *jing* are not separate, but they are aspects of each other and in part create each other. Pre-heaven *jing* is something that you are born with, hence the name pre-heaven, which means that it is pre-natal. Post-heaven or post-natal *jing* is created throughout life from the surplus of the body's physiological processes. Kidney *jing* is a specific form of *jing*, which is created by the interaction of pre- and post-heaven *jing* and is stored in the Kidneys. *Jing* and the Kidneys have in general a very close relationship, and their respective conditions are often a reflection of each other.

In the following chapters we will see how *jing*, when it is transformed to *yuan qi* (original *qi*), is involved in the production of all the vital substances in the body. On the other hand, *jing* is nourished throughout life by *qi* and *xue* (blood). *Jing*, though, is something that decreases over the years. The weakening of *jing* helps to explain many of the changes that take place in the body in old age such as poor hearing, infertility, weak teeth, hair loss, weak bones, impotence, etc., because all of these (and many other things) are aspects of *jing* and reflect its functions in the body.

Pre-heaven *jing*

Pre-heaven *jing* is something that is inherited from one's parents and something that is passed on to the next generation. The nearest concept we have in Western medicine physiology is DNA. However, we must be careful when making direct correlations between the two disparate ways of seeing the body, and DNA is only one aspect of *jing*.

Pre-heaven *jing* arises when the *jing* of the two parents unites at the moment of conception. It is this *jing*, together with the maternal Kidney *jing*, *xue* and *qi*, which nourishes the foetus during pregnancy. It is not only in humans that we can see this *jing* aspect, but also in all living creatures. For example, it is pre-heaven *jing* that enables a seed to sprout and grow into a new plant. Pre-heaven *jing* is the energy that enables things to grow. It is pre-heaven *jing* that provides the seed with the energy that is necessary to sprout and push upwards through the soil until it is able to produce energy itself from the soil and the sun. The nourishment that the plant subsequently gets from the sun and the soil is equivalent to post-heaven *jing* in humans. In humans, post-heaven *jing* is created from the food and drink that is consumed and the air that is inhaled.

Pre-heaven *jing* determines a person's basic constitution, strength and vitality. As described above, pre-heaven *jing* is created from the parents' *jing*. From this it can be concluded that a person's constitution, and their basic vitality, is dependent upon the quality of their parents' *jing*. A person's pre-heaven *jing* can be negatively affected if the parents were old, sick or weak or if their *jing* was in other ways affected at the moment of conception and during pregnancy (in the case of the mother). If the parents were drunk or under the influence of drugs at the moment of conception, this will also have a negative effect on a person's *jing*.[1] If they were old or weak, if their own *jing* was weak, this will also mean that a person's *jing* will probably be weak.

Because pre-heaven *jing* is inherited from the parents, some call it 'hereditary *qi*'. Furthermore, because it is hereditary, this means that it is difficult to affect *jing* beneficially. *Jing* is something that can be cultivated and preserved so as not to further consume it, but it is difficult to renew *jing*. It is not possible to create new pre-heaven *jing*. In some ways, pre-heaven *jing* can be seen as a car that you are given to drive in your journey through life with. Some people have been given a sparkling new BMW; others a rusty old Toyota. If you have a rusty old Toyota, you have to be more careful how you use it. It needs to be looked after and regularly serviced and the oil should be checked and changed more frequently. You will not be able to drive as fast, and you will have to take more frequent breaks if you are going to travel a long distance, but the car will be able to get you there if you take care of it. However, even if you have a brand new BMW, you cannot just put your foot down and constantly travel at one hundred and fifty mph. If you never stop for a rest or service the car, even a new BMW will end up breaking down. The new BMW can handle more, but it is not invulnerable. A person with a weak pre-heaven *jing* is more fragile and delicate, but a person with strong *jing* can also 'burn out' and fundamentally weaken themselves if they live life too long in the fast lane.

You can see how a strong and a weak *jing* manifests itself when you look at a litter of puppies. There are usually a few robust and healthy individuals (strong *jing*), which we recognise as strong and healthy dogs. At the same time there will typically be a small, delicate puppy (weak *jing*). Quite often this puppy does not survive. If it is to have a hope of surviving, it must be nurtured more than the other puppies. If you were to purchase one of these puppies to use as a working dog, it would not be the one you would select. It would simply not be robust enough.

Post-heaven *jing*

Post-heaven *jing* is the aspect of *jing* that is created after birth. Post-heaven *jing* is therefore also called post-natal *jing*. *Qi* and *xue* (blood) is produced from the food and liquids that we consume and the air that we breathe. These are used throughout the day, to carry out all the activities of the body, both physical and mental. If there is any *qi* and *xue* left at the end of the day, this surplus is transformed into post-heaven *jing* during the night and will be stored in the Kidneys. The Kidneys are called the root of pre-heaven *jing*, because it is here that *jing* is stored. The Spleen and Stomach are called the root of post-heaven *jing*, because they are responsible for the transformation of the food and liquids we consume that can be transformed into *jing*.

There is a mutual relationship between pre- and post-heaven *jing*. Post-heaven *jing* nourishes and supports pre-heaven *jing*. Pre-heaven *jing*, on the other hand, is the foundation for all *qi* and *xue* production in the body. This is because all production of *qi* and *xue* is dependent on *yuan qi* (original *qi*). *Yuan qi* is a form of *qi* that is created by the transformation of Kidney *jing*.

In a way you can see *jing* as a savings account in the bank and *qi* production as a person's wages. A person should preferably not spend more than they earn. When they consume more *qi* than they create, they have to draw on their reserves and thereby weaken their *jing*. Conversely, if a person who has a good production of *qi* does not overstrain their *qi* and *xue*, then they will be able to replenish their *jing*.

Kidney *jing*

Often when *jing* is discussed, both in physiology and pathology, it is the aspect of *jing* known as Kidney *jing* that is being discussed. Kidney *jing* is a specific form of *jing*. Kidney *jing* is a very functional form of *jing*. Kidney *jing* is created by the interaction between pre- and post-heaven *jing*. In general, there is a very close relationship between the Kidneys and *jing*. This also means in practice that the weakening of *jing*, among other things, will manifest itself with a weakening of the Kidneys. Many of the functions that are attributed to *jing* are also considered to be functions of the Kidneys.

Jing is stored in the Kidneys and circulates mainly through the part of the channel system that is called the eight extraordinary vessels.[2] The fact that *jing* circulates through the eight extraordinary vessels confirms that *jing* is something that is fundamental to the body's physiology and development. This is because the extraordinary vessels are one of the first structures that are formed in the body whilst it is an embryo. Furthermore, the eight extraordinary vessels are involved in shaping the body throughout life and are responsible for relevant transformations taking place at different ages.

It may well be appropriate to compare *qi* and *jing* here. Despite the fact that all of the vital substances can in reality be considered to be *qi*, in practice it is practical to differentiate between them. *Qi* is more *yang* than *jing*. *Qi* circulates in the body in daily cycles. *Jing* is *yin* in nature, and this can be seen amongst other things in that it has cycles that are seven or eight years in length, depending on a person's gender. Furthermore, because *qi* is relatively *yang*, it can be affected negatively and positively relatively quickly. *Jing* however takes much longer to be weakened and to be replenished. Where *jing* is difficult to replenish once it has been weakened, *qi* is relatively quick to recover.

Jing is used by the body for both physiological processes and in the formation of physical structures. Bone Marrow, which is considered to be an organ[3] in Chinese medicine, is created by *jing*.

Bone marrow is something other and more than bone marrow is in Western anatomy. In Chinese medicine Bone Marrow produces the bones themselves and cartilage. Bone Marrow is also seen as filling the spinal cord. The Brain is also seen as being created by the spinal cord. The Brain is described as a flower at the top of the spinal cord. The Brain is also known as the 'Sea of Marrow'. Problems that are related to the Brain not being 'nourished' by Bone Marrow include symptoms such as poor concentration, poor memory, dizziness and an empty feeling in the head.

Congenitally weak *jing* can manifest as weak bones or delayed development. There may be problems of delayed closure of the fontanelle, lack of growth, etc. The child will be fragile and have a weak immune system. Weak *jing* can manifest mentally with a child being mentally handicapped.

Jing decreases with age, and the older we become, the weaker our *jing* is. This can be seen in old age when the bones become porous, weak and brittle.

The teeth are considered to be a surplus of the bones. This means that the teeth are also an aspect of *jing*. *Jing*'s progressive weakening over the years means that the teeth will loosen and start to fall out in old age. *Jing xu* (deficiency of *jing*) can also be seen when teeth do not develop as they should in children, when their teeth are very weak or when the milk teeth do not fall out and get replaced with permanent teeth or the wisdom teeth do not develop.

The hair on the head is created and nourished by the Kidney *jing* and is nourished by *xue*. This means that the hair can lose its lustre, turn grey or there can be premature balding or hair loss when the Kidney *jing* is weak.

The ear's physical structure is made of cartilage, which in itself is an aspect of the bones and thereby Kidney *jing*. Furthermore, its functionality is dependent on Kidney *jing*. Congenital Kidney *jing xu* or weakening of the Kidney *jing*, such as in old age, can give rise to symptoms such as tinnitus and deafness.

Jing, which is the most *yin* aspect of *qi*, is the foundation and the root of *shen*, which is the most *yang* aspect of *qi*. *Jing* is transformed to form *shen*. This means that a person's *shen* reflects and is dependent on their *jing*. *Jing xu* can manifest itself already at birth, with some children being born mentally handicapped or having learning difficulties. It can also be seen in old age, when some people lose their mind or their memory.

Where Kidney *jing* is an aspect of Kidney *yin*, *mingmen* (the Gate of Fire) is considered to be an aspect of Kidney *yang*. *Mingmen* will be described in the next chapter. Kidney *jing* and *mingmen* have a close and mutual relationship. Kidney *jing* is dependent on *mingmen*'s transformative power to be able to realise and manifest its potential. *Mingmen*'s transformation of *jing* creates one of the most vital forms of *qi* in the body – *yuan qi* (original *qi*). *Yuan qi* is used for all transformations in the body and is therefore the foundation of all post-heaven *qi*.

Kidney *yang*'s transformation of Kidney *yin* also creates Kidney *qi*, which is used by the Kidneys to perform all its physiological activities. For this reason, *jing* is considered to be the root of Kidney *qi*. Kidney *qi*'s features will be discussed in a later chapter (page 122).

Jing cycles

Jing's control of growth and development is not only seen in the formation of bones, teeth, cartilage, etc., but *jing* also determines the developmental changes that occur in the body at various ages. These changes in the body occur in cycles that are several years long. In women these cycles are seven yearly, whilst in men they are of eight years. These cycles are described in the *Huang Di Nei Jing – Su Wen* (*The Yellow Emperor's Classic – Simple Questions*), chapter one. Qi Bo, the Yellow Emperor's advisor, explains to the Yellow Emperor how the body ages:

> When a girl is seven, her *jing* is rich, her hair grows and the milk teeth are replaced with permanent teeth.
>
> When she is fourteen, the extraordinary vessels *ren mai* and *chong mai* fill up and begin to overflow, so that menstruation starts and conception is possible.
>
> When she is twenty-one, *jing* peaks, growth is complete, the wisdom teeth emerge.
>
> When she is twenty-eight, her tendons and bones are strong, the hair is long and the body is strong and in full vigour.
>
> When she is thirty-five, the *jing* begins to decline, the skin starts to wrinkle, the muscles become weaker, the teeth loosen and the hair starts to fall out.
>
> When she is forty-two, her face darkens and the hair turns grey.
>
> When she is forty-nine, *chong mai* and *ren mai* have dried up, menstruation ceases and fertilisation is no longer possible.
>
> When a boy is eight, his *jing* is rich, the hair grows and the milk teeth are replaced with permanent teeth.
>
> When he is sixteen, his *jing* is even stronger, the semen arrives and conception is possible.
>
> When he is twenty-four, his *jing* peaks, his bones and teeth are strong, the wisdom teeth arrive and his growth is complete.

When he is thirty-two, his bones and tendons are at their strongest, his muscles are strong and solid.

When he is forty, the *jing* starts to decline, his teeth loosen and the hair thins.

When he is forty-eight, his face darkens and the hair turns grey.

When he is fifty-six, the tendons become stiff and he loses his fertility.

When he is sixty-four, his teeth and his hair fall out.

This difference between girls' and boys' cycles can help to explain why girls develop faster, physically and mentally, than boys of the same age.

These cycles also show the influence that *jing* has on fertility. It is in adolescence that boys and girls become fertile. As the strength and quality of *jing* declines over the years, the ability to reproduce diminishes. *Jing* is that which creates the next generation. *Jing* is the pre-heavenly *qi*. *Jing* manifests as semen in men and eggs and menstrual blood in women. The sperm and menstrual blood are called *tian gui* or in English 'Heavenly Water', and this is created from *jing*. Weak *jing* can therefore manifest as infertility, poor quality semen or eggs and in some hereditary diseases.

In addition, *jing* is weakened through ovulation, menstrual bleeding, pregnancy, births and abortions in women, and through ejaculation in men. Some are also of the belief that women also lose *jing* when orgasming.

Jing is also weakened when more *qi* is used than is produced. This can be a consequence of weakness in one or more of the *qi*-producing organs, chronic illness, stress or malnutrition. Due to the close relationship between some of the aspects of *jing* in Chinese medicine physiology and DNA in Western medicine physiology, one could be tempted to conclude that things that have a negative effect on DNA will also have a negative influence on *jing*.

It can also be discussed whether *jing* can be strengthened at all when it is weak. This is because *jing* is essentially something that is hereditary. *Jing* can only be weakened and it is not possible to add new pre-heaven *jing* to the body. It is, though, possible to increase the production of post-heaven *jing* and thereby improve the quality of the *jing* that there is. Furthermore, the remaining *jing* can be preserved and its quality improved through an appropriate lifestyle, i.e. adequate rest, not overdoing things, avoiding stress and through celibacy. Some people think that the quality of *jing* can be strengthened by practising Daoist and tantra sex.

Foods that are attributed *jing*-nourishing qualities are royal jelly, eggs, roe/caviar, seeds, nuts, propolis/pollen, bone marrow, brain, kidney, oysters, seaweed and algae, artichokes, raw milk, nettles and oats.

Meditation, *qi gong* and yoga are considered to be *jing* nourishing.

Acupuncture points considered to have a direct influence on *jing* and *mingmen* are Ren 4 and Du 4. The Kidneys are the root of the pre-heaven *jing*. Therefore, the treatment of Kidney channel points, especially Kid 3, will have a beneficial effect on *jing*.

The properties of Kidney *jing* can be summarised as follows:

Jing

- is created by the interaction of pre- and post-heaven *jing*
- is stored in the Kidneys, but circulates throughout the body, particularly in the eight extraordinary vessels
- has a close relationship to *mingmen*
- is responsible for growth, development and reproduction
- is the foundation for the production of *qi*, *xue* and *jinye*
- manifests in the bones, head hair and teeth
- is the basis for Kidney *qi*
- creates the bone marrow
- creates the ears and hearing
- is the foundation of the constitutional strength
- is the basis for, and is a part of, the Three Treasures – *jing*, *qi* and *shen*
- is weakened by: chronic weakness of one or more of the *qi*-producing organs; using more *qi* than is produced; births; chronic disease; old age; and too much sex
- can be strengthened through lifestyle and diet and by the use of acupuncture points such as Kid 3, Ren 4 and Du 4

MINGMEN

As was seen in the last chapter, *jing* can be seen as the most fundamental *yin* aspect of the body. The most fundamental *yang* aspect of the body is *mingmen* or 'the Gate of Fire'. In reality, *jing* and *mingmen* are just each other's *yin* and *yang* aspects and they are mutually dependent on each other. They can be understood as the oil and the flame in a lamp. The flame is the manifestation of the energetic potential of the oil. Without the oil there will be no flame. At the same time though, the oil would be just an inert and inactive substance without the transformative power of the flame. It is exactly the same with *jing* and *mingmen*. *Jing*, the most fundamental *yin* aspect of the body, is the potential for life, development, reproduction, *shen* and much more. *Jing* though is dependent on *mingmen*, the most fundamental form for *yang* in the body. *Mingmen* transforms and activates *jing*. Without *mingmen*, *jing* would just be an inert substance, solid, sticky and full of potential, but without the possibility to manifest this potential. This is also seen in the seed lying in the ground, which was mentioned in the previous chapter. An acorn has the potential to develop into an eighty-foot tall oak tree, but it is dependent on the warmth of the Sun to activate this potential. Without the Sun's *yang qi*, the acorn would just lie in the ground and end up rotting away.

In the same way that the acorn lying in the soil has to be transformed so it can develop and manifest its potential, *jing* is transformed so that a foetus can develop. This means that both *jing* and *mingmen* are present just after the moment of conception.

Mingmen's close relationship to *jing* is also seen in its physical location in the body. Whereas *jing* is conceived of as being stored in the Kidneys, *mingmen* is seen as being located between the two Kidneys. It is therefore found that acupuncture points such as Ren 4, Ren 6 and especially Du 4 have a tonifying effect on *mingmen*.[4] In early Chinese medical texts, such as the *Nanjing*, the left Kidney was considered to be the Kidney organ itself, whilst the right Kidney was *mingmen*. This is also reflected in the *chi* pulse position (proximal pulse position) on the left-hand side being seen as reflecting Kidney *yin*, whilst the right *chi* position reflects Kidney *yang*.

Functions

Mingmen is closely linked to Kidney *yang*. Kidney *yang* is dependent on the *mingmen's* fire to be able to carry out its activities. *Mingmen* is the foundation of Kidney *yang* in the same way that *jing* is the foundation of Kidney *yin*. *Mingmen's* transformation of *jing* is used to create *yuan qi* or original *qi*. *Yuan qi* is used in all transformations in the body and is the basis for all post-heaven *qi*. *Yuan qi* is supported in its functions by *mingmen's* fire.

Mingmen is the root of all *yang* in the body, and many organs are dependent on the *mingmen's* fire to able to carry out their processes and activities. The Kidneys and the Urinary Bladder are supported by *mingmen* in their functions with regards to the transformation of fluids. The Stomach and Spleen use the heat of the *mingmen* to transform the food that has been consumed. *Mingmen* also aids the Kidneys in grasping the *qi* that the Lung has sent downwards.

Whereas *jing* is fundamentally important in fertility and reproduction, *mingmen*'s role is more related to sexual function and desire. *Mingmen* is used to transform *jing* after fertilisation, but it also plays a significant role before then. Sexual function and arousal are dependent on the fire from *mingmen*. This can be seen for instance when the cheeks and the lips become red and the temperature of the skin feels warmer during sexual arousal. If *mingmen* is weak, there may be impotence and a lack of libido. If *mingmen* fire is overactive, there may be an exaggerated sexual appetite. The Uterus, or *bao* in Chinese, is warmed by *mingmen*. If *mingmen* is weak and does not warm the *bao*, there can be problems with fertility. *Bao* is not only found in women; in men *bao* is the place where semen is created and stored. Once again we can see the close relationship between *jing* and *mingmen*.

As we saw in the last chapter, *jing* is the root of *shen*. Once again, it is *mingmen* that transforms this *yin* potential, so it can express itself as a *yang* manifestation. *Mingmen* also warms the Heart, where *shen* has its residence. In practice, this means that a person whose *mingmen* is weak will have a tendency to be apathetic, mentally dull or perhaps depressed. An overactive *mingmen*, on the other hand, can agitate the Heart and result in manic behaviour.

Mingmen is weakened by too much sex, physical overwork, cold and old age. On the other hand, *mingmen* can be strengthened by keeping the lumbar and lower abdomen warm; through *qi gong*; by eating a diet that is rich in foods that are energetically hot, such as ginger and cinnamon; and by using acupuncture and moxa on acupuncture points such as Ren 4, Ren 6 and especially Du 4.

Mingmen's properties can be summarised as follows:

Mingmen

- is physically located between the Kidneys
- is the source of all *yang* in the body
- is the root of *yuan qi*. Yuan qi is motivated *jing* – *jing* that has been transformed by *mingmen*
- supports *yuan qi* in its functions
- has a close relationship to Kidney *yang*
- heats the lower *jiao*
- supports all organs in their physiological activities
- harmonises sexual functions
- warms *jing* and *bao*
- transforms *jing* to *shen*
- warms Kidney *yang*, so that it can grasp *qi*

QI

As we have already seen in the 'Introduction to the Vital Substances', *qi* is a concept that is difficult to translate into English. *Qi* is, as previously described, an overarching concept, something that everything in the universe consists of. All of the various vital substances and all of the organs' physiological activity are therefore *qi*. Although all the vital substances are in reality *qi*, *qi* is at the same time also defined as being something specific, something that is different from the other vital substances. *Qi*, as a specific vital substance, is *yang* in relation to three of the other vital substances – *jing* (Essence), *xue* (Blood) and *jinye* (Fluids) – because it is lighter and less condensed, moves faster and is less substantial. On the other hand, *qi* is *yin* compared with *shen* (consciousness, mind, spirit).

Further distinction is made between the different forms of *qi* in the body. Although these forms of *qi* are all '*qi*', it is relevant to further differentiate them from each other. Differentiating the various types of *qi* is important both in relation to understanding the body's physiological processes and in the diagnosis and treatment of disease.

In this chapter I will discuss:

- *qi*'s general functions

- the various forms of *qi*, their functions and how they are produced.

Functions

Qi has six main functions in the body.

Qi:

- transforms

- transports

- warms

- holds

- raises

- protects.

That *qi* is an aspect of *yang* can be seen in all of these functions being active processes. As a rule, it is *yin* substances that are transformed, transported and kept in place by *qi*, and it is *yin* structures that are raised upwards and held up by *qi*. Warming and protecting are also *yang* activities.

Transforms

Post-heaven *qi* is made from the food and liquids that we consume and from the air that we breathe. For these foods and liquids to become usable *qi*, *xue* and *jinye*, they need to be transformed from their crude form to more refined and subtle forms of *qi*. This is no different than Western medicine physiology, where the food we eat is broken down into nutrients that can be absorbed and utilised by the body. In addition, different substances in the body can transform into each other. *Jing* is transformed into *yuan qi*, *qi* is transformed into *xue*, *xue* and *qi* to *jing*, etc. Transformation is an active process that requires *qi*. *Yuan qi* (original *qi*) is the form of *qi* that is primarily responsible for the majority of transformations in the body.

Transports

All transportation in the body is carried out by *qi*. *Qi* is used to transport vital substances around the body from their production sites to where they are to be used or stored. Waste products are transported by *qi* and expelled from the body.

All movement in the body is dependent on *qi*. This includes the physical activity of muscles, but also what is referred to as *qi ji* or 'qi mechanism'. Each organ sends its *qi* in specific directions and *qi* moves in and out of the body's tissues. This movement of *qi* can be upwards, downwards, inwards or outwards. It is this dynamic movement of *qi* that is called *qi ji*. When there are *qi* imbalances, this dynamic can be disturbed. It can come to a standstill (stagnation of *qi*) or *qi* can move in the wrong direction (rebellious *qi*).

Warms

This is a specific function of *yang qi*. *Yang qi* warms, amongst other things, the body. Without heat, all physiological processes would grind to a halt. *Yang* heat is needed to transform and transport *yin* substances. Therefore, if a person's *yang qi* is weakened, they will not only be sensitive to the cold, but also many of their physiological processes will be weakened or sluggish. A weak Spleen *yang qi* can, for example, mean that the food that has been consumed is not transformed to *gu qi* (food *qi*).

Holds

Yang qi keeps *yin* substances such as *xue* and *jinye* in place and inside the body. Examples of this are Spleen *qi*, which keeps *xue* inside the blood vessels; *wei qi* (defensive *qi*), which keeps sweat inside the body; and Kidney *qi*, which keeps the urine inside the Urinary Bladder.

Raises

Qi is used to counteract gravity and keep organs, etc. in their place. It is mainly Spleen *yang qi* which performs the task of lifting and holding organs and blood vessels in place. The Kidneys also lift the Uterus and keep the foetus in place.

Protects

Wei qi circulates in the space between the muscles and the skin, protecting the body against exogenous *xie qi*, which will have a detrimental effect on the body's *qi*.

The various forms of *qi* and their functions

Qi is defined as a specific substance, which is separate from *xue*, *jing*, *shen* and *jinye*. *Qi* can be further differentiated into various forms of *qi*. These forms of *qi* are defined by their function, origin or location in the body. The various forms of *qi* are not definitive and they can transform into each other.

Yuan qi

Yuan qi, or original *qi*, is closely linked to *jing*. *Yuan qi* can be understood as *jing* in a more mobile or lighter form, or as *jing's yang* aspect. In fact, *yuan qi* and *jing* are respectively referred to as *yuan yang* and *yuan yin*, because they are the two fundamental or original forms of *yin* and *yang qi* in the body and because they have the same root. *Yuan qi* is generated when *jing* is transformed by *mingmen*.

Functionally, *yuan qi* is closely connected to *mingmen*, and its place of origin is the same place as *mingmen*, i.e. between the Kidneys.

Yuan qi is nourished on a daily basis by post-heaven *jing*.

Yuan qi is distributed throughout the body, from its place of origin between the Kidneys, via the *san jiao*.[5] *San jiao* can be understood as a complex passageway where, among other things, fluids and *yuan qi* circulate in various directions. *San jiao* is also said to differentiate and separate *yuan qi* into its various forms so it can perform its relevant functions around the body. *Yuan qi* is sent to the organs, where it is the motivating force that enables organs to carry out their functions. *Yuan qi* is also sent through *san jiao* and into the individual channels via their *yuan* source points. This is why the use of *yuan*-source points can have a strong, tonifying effect on the body.

Yuan qi's functions can be summarised as follows.

Yuan qi

- is a motivating force
- is a transformative force
- is the basis for Kidney *qi*

Motivating force

Yuan qi is the motivating *qi*, which is the driving force behind all functional activity in the organs. Without *yuan qi*, all activity in the organs would come to a halt.

Yuan qi is the foundation of vigour and stamina in the body. This is because *yuan qi* is created by *jing* and is therefore a manifestation of *jing*. *Yuan qi* can be understood as being the link between the *yin* substance *jing*, which is denser, more fluid-like and slower in its cycles, and the *yang* substance *qi*, which is lighter, more rapid in its cycles and without form. That *yuan qi* is the link between *jing* and *qi* can also be seen by the fact that *yuan qi*, which is created by *jing*, is the catalyst that is needed in the production of *qi* and *xue*. As so often in Chinese medicine, there is a reciprocal relationship between *qi* and *yuan qi*. *Yuan qi* is the foundation for the production of *qi* in the body, but the *qi* that is produced nourishes *jing* and thereby *yuan qi*.

Transformation

Yuan qi is the transforming force that is the catalyst in the production of the three vital substances, *qi*, *xue* and *jinye*. It is *yuan qi* that transforms *zong qi* (gathering or pectoral *qi*) in the chest to the more refined *zhen qi* (true *qi*), which flows inside and outside the channels and is used by the organs. *Gu qi* (food *qi*) is transformed into *xue* by *yuan qi* in the Heart. *Yuan qi* is the foundation of Kidney *qi* and is used in the transformation of the fluids consumed into *jinye*.

Basis for Kidney *qi*

Yuan qi is the basis of Kidney *qi* and it is involved in all of the Kidneys' activities. *Yuan qi* can therefore be interpreted as being an aspect of Kidney *yang*. *Yuan qi* is, together with *mingmen*, the root of the physiological heat that is necessary for all physiological processes in the body.

Yuan qi can be tonified by the use of points such as Ren 4, Ren 6 and Du 4. These acupuncture points are located in the area of the body where *yuan qi* has its origin. By stimulating these points, especially with moxa, you can tonify and activate *yuan qi*. *Yuan qi* can also be stimulated by activating the various channels' *yuan*-source points. This approach is especially used on the *yin* channels.

Gu qi

Gu qi, which is translated as food *qi*, or basis *qi*, is the *qi* that is made from the food and liquids that have been ingested through the mouth. The food and liquid is passed from the mouth down to the Stomach, which is responsible for receiving food and liquids. It is said that the Stomach 'ripens and rots' the food. The Stomach prepares the food so that it can be transformed by Spleen *qi*. *Gu qi* is a coarse and unrefined form of *qi*, which the body cannot use until it has been further transformed and refined.

When the Spleen transforms food, it separates the pure and usable *qi* from the impure or unusable *qi* (as previously stated, the same process is also seen in the transformation of fluids). The pure *qi* that has been extracted is sent upwards to the Lung by the Spleen, whilst the impure residue is sent downwards to the Small Intestine by the Stomach.

If the Spleen is weak, this process of separation and transformation will not function optimally. This can have a significant effect on a person's energy level.

As stated above, *gu qi* is too coarse to be used in its current form and must therefore be further refined. *Gu qi* is sent upwards from its place of production in the middle *jiao* to the upper *jiao*. Here a portion of the *gu qi* is mixed with air (*da qi*) from the Lung to create *zong qi* (see below) and the rest is sent to the Heart, where *yuan qi* transforms it into *xue*.

Gu qi is tonified by eating a diet that is beneficial for the Spleen and by the use of acupuncture points such as Sp 3, Sp 6, St 36, UB 20, UB 21 and Ren 12.

Zong qi

Zong qi is translated very differently from author to author. Giovanni Maciocia translates it into English as 'gathering' *qi* (Maciocia 2005). Others translate it as 'ancestral' *qi*. Maciocia writes that it can be confusing to use the direct translation, which is inherited or ancestral *qi*, as this term creates associations to *jing*, which *zong qi* is not an aspect of. Other Chinese terms for this type of *qi* are *da qi* (big *qi*) and *xiong qi* (chest *qi*), which in some books is translated as 'pectoral' *qi*.

Zong qi is generated when the air (also called *da qi*) that we breathe is mixed with *gu qi*, which the Spleen has sent up to the Lung. *Zong qi* is a more refined form of *qi* than *gu qi*. Unlike *gu qi*, *zong qi* can be used by the body without being further transformed. *Zong qi* is used, for example, by the Lung and the Heart to perform some of their functions. *Zong qi* is also very important when it is further transformed to create *zhen qi* (see below).

Zong qi is used by the Lung and the Heart to circulate *qi* and *xue* rhythmically around the body and to regulate the breathing and the heartbeat. *Zong qi* does not itself circulate through the channels and blood vessels, but it is the driving force behind the movement of *qi* and *xue* in these. Without *zong qi*, *xue* and *qi* would not circulate in the extremities, and this can be seen when a person with *zong qi xu* has cold fingers and toes or has a tingling sensation or numbness in the extremities. It is not only *zong qi*'s driving force that has an influence on the movement of *qi* and *xue* in the vessels and channels – Liver *qi*, for example, ensures the free movement of *qi* throughout the body; stagnations of *qi*, *xue* and Phlegm can block the flow in the channel, etc.

Zong qi is also the *qi* that gives the voice its strength. The relative strength of a person's *zong qi* can therefore be assessed from how powerful or weak their voice is.

There is a reciprocal relationship between *yuan qi* and *zong qi*. *Yuan qi* ascends to the chest where it transforms *zong qi* to *zhen qi* and assists the respiration. *Zong qi* is sent down to the lower *jiao*,[6] where it nourishes *yuan qi* and assists the Kidneys.

Zong qi gathers in the chest, where it creates the 'Sea of *qi*'. This means that acupuncture points in the thorax can be used to stimulate *zong qi*. One of the most important acupuncture points that stimulates *zong qi* is Ren 17, which is a so-called *hui*-gathering point for *qi*. Lu 9, which is the *yuan*-source point of the Lung, is another acupuncture point that is often used to tonify *zong qi*.

Zong qi can also be tonified through breathing exercises.

Zhen qi

Zhen qi (genuine *qi* or true *qi*) is created when *zong qi* is transformed by *yuan qi* in the upper *jiao*.[7] *Zhen qi* is therefore a more refined form of *qi* than both *zong qi* and *gu qi*. *Zhen qi* is *qi* that is in a form that can be used by the body without the need for any further transformation. *Zhen qi* is the *qi* that circulates inside and outside of the channels. It is used to nourish all the organs and tissues in the body and to protect the body against invasions of exogenous *xie qi* (pathogen *qi*).

Zhen qi has two aspects – *ying qi* and *wei qi*. *Ying qi* is relatively *yin* compared with *wei qi*, which is relatively *yang*.

Ying qi

Ying qi (nutritious *qi*) is the *yin* aspect of *zhen qi*. The main function of *ying qi* is to nourish all the tissues and all the organs of the body. *Ying qi* is conceived of as being more *yin* than *wei qi* for several reasons. *Ying qi* is nutritious, whereas *wei qi* is protective and warming. *Ying qi* circulates deeper in the body inside the channel system, whereas *wei qi* circulates in the space between the muscles and skin.[8]

Ying qi has a very close relationship to *xue*. *Ying qi* and *xue* circulate together in the channel system and the vessels, where they mutually nourish all the tissues and organs of the body. *Zhen qi* can be observed in a person's energy level and in how their organs function. *Zhen qi* can be tonified by tonifying the *qi*-producing organs: the Kidneys, Spleen and Lung. This can be achieved through the use of acupuncture points such as Sp 3, St 36, Lu 9, Kid 3, UB 13, UB 20, UB 21 and UB 23.

Wei qi

Wei qi (protective or defensive *qi*) is the *qi* that circulates in the space between the muscles and skin and in the thorax and abdominal cavity. Its primary task is to protect the body against invasions of exogenous *xie qi* (pathogen *qi*). In addition to protecting the body, *wei qi* warms and moistens the skin.

Wei qi helps to control the body temperature. It does this by controlling the opening and closing of the pores.

There is a close relationship between *wei qi* and *jin*, which is the thin, lighter aspect of the body fluids. *Jin* circulates together with *wei qi* and moistens the skin. If *wei qi* is blocked, the thin fluids will accumulate. This can be seen, for example, in a person who has a cold. The invasion of *xie qi* will have blocked the *wei qi*, and the resulting disturbance of the distribution of *jin* under the skin can be seen in a puffiness around the eyes.

Wei qi controls the pores, thereby influencing how much a person sweats. If *wei qi* is weak (*wei qi xu*) and cannot control the pores, the person will sweat spontaneously and *jinye* will be weakened.

Wei qi circulates throughout the body fifty times a day – twenty-five times a day, whilst the person is awake, in the exterior aspect of the body (between the muscles and skin), and twenty-five times during the night in the interior, flowing down to and through the *zangfu* organs, where it helps to nourish them.

Wei qi xu can manifest with a person often being ill and catching frequent colds (due to invasions of *xie qi*), having difficulty keeping warm (because *wei qi* is not heating the skin) and spontaneous sweating (*wei qi* not controlling the pores). The organs that have the greatest influence on *wei qi* are the Lung, the Kidneys and the Spleen, all of which are involved in the production of *wei qi*. It is these organs that are treated in a condition of *wei qi xu*. The Lung has in general a very close relationship with *wei qi*, both because they are involved in the creation of *zong qi*, which is an antecedent to *zhen qi*, and also because it is the Lung that spreads *wei qi* throughout the body. *Wei qi* can be activated by activating the Lung's spreading function. The *taiyang* (Urinary Bladder/Small Intestine) channel, which is the most *yang* channel and thereby the body's most exterior and protective channel, also has a close relationship to *wei qi*. For this reason, *wei qi* can also be activated by activating the *taiyang* channel.

Zheng qi

Zheng qi (correct or upright *qi*) is not an independent form of *qi*, but it is the sum of the body's anti-pathogenic *qi*. In some aspects, *zheng qi* can be seen as the immune system in Western terminology. *Zheng qi* is not the same as *wei qi*. *Wei qi* is an aspect of *zheng qi*, but other forms of *qi*, such as *ying qi*, *yuan qi* and organ *qi*, are also involved in combating *xie qi* when it has invaded the body. *Zheng qi* is usually only used as a term in the context of *xie qi* when discussing their relative strengths.

Zhong qi

Zhong qi (central *qi*) is just another name for Stomach and Spleen *qi* or the *qi* of the middle *jiao*. It is sometimes used to describe the Spleen's function of transforming, transporting and raising *qi*.

Zang fu zhi qi

Something that is crucially important when trying to understand Chinese medicine physiology is that things are usually defined by their function and not their form. *Zang fu zhi qi* (internal organ *qi*) is not an independent form of *qi* that is different from the above-mentioned forms of *qi*, it is just the sum of an organ's physiological activity.

Jing luo zhi qi

Jing luo zhi qi (channel *qi*) is the *qi* that flows through the channel system, hence the name *jing luo*. Again, this is not an independent form of *qi*, but the sum of the various forms of *qi* that are flowing through the channels.

Xie qi

Although *xie qi* is not one of the vital substances, I have chosen to discuss it in this section. This is because *xie qi* is something that will be mentioned many times throughout the book. Furthermore, *xie qi* can be seen in contrast to *zheng qi*.

Xie qi can be translated directly as perverse or evil *qi*. Instead of translating *xie qi* as perverse or evil *qi*, many books use the terms pathogen, pathological *qi* and pathological factor, because *xie qi* is a form of *qi* that causes disease. As stated above, *xie qi* can be regarded as the opposite of the body's *zheng qi*. *Zheng qi*, or the correct *qi*, is the body's anti-pathogenic *qi*. One could be tempted to call *zheng qi* the body's immune response, but *zheng qi* is also the sum of the body's *qi*. Even though it is *zheng qi* that combats *xie qi* in the body, *zheng qi* is something other and more than *wei qi*. *Zheng qi* encompasses *wei qi*, but *wei qi* is only one aspect of *zheng qi*. *Wei qi* is the body's first line of defence, which protects the body's exterior. It is here that the first reactions occur if exogenous *xie qi* invades the body, but if exogenous *xie qi* in the form of climatic factors penetrates deeper, it is combated by other forms of *qi* in the body.

The body is also disturbed by other forms of *xie qi* than just external pathogens. All forms of *qi* that have a negative effect on the body are classified as *xie qi*. Many internal imbalances in the body can lead to the creation of *xie qi*. Spleen *qi xu* can, for example, result in Dampness,[9] stagnations of *qi* can generate Heat, and Heat and Dampness can both result in the formation of the Phlegm.

Exogenous *xie qi* invades the body when the body is exposed to climatic influences, bacteria, viruses, allergens, etc. Internally generated *xie qi*, on the other hand, will usually arise when there are internal imbalances in the body, especially *zangfu* organ imbalances. It is important to remember that *xie qi* is defined both in terms of its origin and in the way it manifests itself. This means that when an internal imbalance leads to a person having an excessive thirst, a red face, physical and mental restlessness, a rapid pulse and a red tongue, then this will be defined as *xie* Heat. The difference between this and an external invasion of Heat is that the cause here is an internal imbalance and is not due to contact with an external pathogen. When *xie qi* is internally generated, the aetiology, the signs and symptoms that are manifesting and the treatment itself will be different from if it were an invasion of the external aspect of the body by exogenous *xie qi*.

It can be confusing that some of the various forms of *xie qi* have the same names as some of the body's physiological aspects. It is important to understand that *xie qi* only has negative properties. Although these pathogenic forms of *qi* have the same names as aspects of *zheng qi*, there is still talk about two different kinds of *qi*. For example, all transformations in the body are dependent on physiological heat. Without *yang* heat, *yin* substances would only be inactive potential. There is a need for physiological heat to release this potential. On the other hand, pathological Heat has no properties that enable it to transform *yin*. On the contrary, *xie* Heat injures *yin*. Furthermore, *xie* Dampness has no moistening or lubricating properties. Pathological Dampness will only block the movement of *qi* and other vital substances. In fact, Dampness can block *jinye*, so that it cannot perform its function of moistening and lubricating parts of the body. For its part, physiological heat and *jinye* only have positive physiological properties and they will not damage the *yin* or block the movement of *qi* or fluids in the body.

This means that *xie qi* is any form of *qi* that has a negative or disruptive effect on the physiology of the body.

In Part 6 on the causes of imbalance (page 691), there is a more detailed description of the various types of *xie qi*.

Chinese name	English name	Definition and function
Yuan qi	Original *qi*	Circulates in the regular channels and extraordinary vessels and in *san jiao* Gathers in *yuan*-source points Motivating force that is the foundation for all physiological activities Basis for Kidney *qi* and is closely related to Kidney *yang*'s functions and activity Transforms *zong qi* into *zhen qi* Transforms *gu qi* into *xue*
Gu qi	Food or basis *qi*	Food that has been transformed into unrefined, coarse *qi* Is combined with *da qi* to create *zong qi* Transformed by *yuan qi* into *xue*
Da qi	Air	Combined with *gu qi* to create *zong qi*
Zong qi	Gathering, ancestral or pectoral *qi*	Combination of *gu qi* and *da qi* The driving force behind respiration and the heartbeat Propels *xue* and *qi* through the channel system Creates the voice Nourishes *yuan qi* and assists the Kidneys

Chinese name	English name	Definition and function
Zhen qi	True or genuine qi	Created when zong qi is transformed by yuan qi Has a yin and a yang aspect – ying qi and wei qi Nourishes the organs and tissues of the body Protects the body Circulates inside and outside the channel system
Ying qi	Nourishing qi	Circulates together with xue in the channels and vessels Nourishes the organs and tissues of the body
Wei qi	Protective or defensive qi	Circulates in the space between the muscles and skin and in the thorax and abdominal cavities Protects the body against exogenous xie qi Warms the skin Circulates together with jin and moisturises the skin Controls the pores Circulates twenty-five times in the exterior during the day and twenty-five times in the interior at night
Zheng qi	Correct or upright qi	The sum of the body's anti-pathogenic qi
Zhong qi	Central qi	The qi of the middle jiao The Stomach and Spleen's physiological functions
Zang fu zhi qi	Zangfu or organ qi	The various organs' physiological activity
Jing luo zhi qi	Channel qi	Qi that circulates through the channel system
Xie qi	Pathogenic qi	Qi that has a negative or pathological effect on the body Does not have any beneficial physiological properties

Qi production and transformation

Qi production starts in the lower *jiao* (the lower part of the abdominal cavity), when *jing*, which is stored in the Kidneys, is transformed by *mingmen*. This produces *yuan qi*. For this reason, the Kidneys are called the pre-heaven root of *qi*.

This means that *jing*, which in part has been inherited from one's parents, is of fundamental importance in all *qi* production throughout life. *Yuan qi* is needed to transform *zong qi* to *zhen qi*, so that it can be used by the whole body. At the same time, *yuan qi* is the motivating force necessary for all the *qi*-producing organs' physiological activity. Furthermore, *mingmen* is the fundamental *yang*, which is necessary to transform the food that has been ingested and received by the Stomach. There is, however, as there usually is in Chinese medicine, a reciprocal relationship. *Jing*, *mingmen* and *yuan qi* are the pre-heaven root of *qi*, but *qi* is the post-heaven nourishment that is used to replenish *jing*.

The post-heaven aspect of *qi* production starts in the middle *jiao* with the creation of *gu qi*. *Gu qi* arises when Spleen *yang qi* transforms the food and drink consumed through the mouth. Food and liquid passes from the mouth down to the

Stomach, whose task it is to 'rotten and ripen' the food. To rotten and ripen means that the Stomach prepares the food so that it can be transformed by the Spleen. This is in some ways similar to Western medicine physiology, where the muscles of the stomach, the stomach acid and enzymes released in the stomach start to break down the food as one of the first of the digestive processes.

Spleen *yang qi*, which is supported by the fire of *mingmen*, transforms the food in the Stomach and separates the pure and usable *qi* from the impure residue. Spleen *yang qi* then sends the pure *gu qi* up to the upper *jiao*, where a part of it is combined with *da qi* from the Lung to create *zong qi*. Some of the *gu qi* is sent to the Heart, where it is transformed into *xue* by *yuan qi*. The impure dregs are sent down from the Stomach to the Small Intestine, where there is a further separation of the pure and the impure.

Gu qi is a form of *qi* that is too unrefined to be able to be used by the body in its current form. To be usable by the body, *gu qi* needs to be refined and further transformed. This transformation takes place in the upper *jiao*.

The Spleen is one of two organs that are termed the post-heavenly root of *qi*. The other is the Lung, which is located in the upper *jiao*. The Lung draws *da qi* into the body from the world outside of the body. *Da qi* is mixed with the *gu qi* that the Spleen has sent up to the upper *jiao* from the middle *jiao*. This creates *zong qi*. *Zong qi* is, as described earlier, a form of *qi* that can be used in its present form to perform certain functions. However, it is also necessary to further refine *zong qi* so that it can be used by the rest of the body. This process takes place when *yuan qi* is sent up through the *san jiao* from the Kidneys to the upper *jiao*, where *yuan qi* transforms *zong qi* into *zhen qi*.

Zhen qi has two aspects. *Ying qi* is the *yin* aspect of *zhen qi*, and it is *ying qi* that flows through the channel system, helping to nourish all tissue in the body. *Wei qi* is the *yang* aspect of *zhen qi* and flows outside of the channels themselves in the space between the skin and muscles.

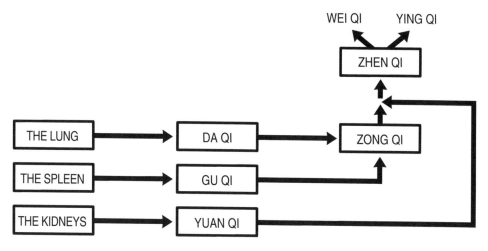

Figure 2.1 The production of *qi*

Qi production and transformation in summary

Kidneys

- Store *jing*.
- *Mingmen* is located between the two Kidneys.

Jing

- Pre-heavenly root of *qi*.
- *Yuan qi* is generated when *jing* is transformed by *mingmen*.

Mingmen

- Transforms *jing* to *yuan qi*.
- The fundamental *yang* heat, which supports Spleen *yang*, when it transforms the food in the Stomach to *gu qi*.

Yuan qi

- Transforms *zong qi* into *zhen qi*.
- Motivating force for all the *qi*-producing organs' physiological processes.

Stomach

- Receives food and drink.
- Rots and ripens the food.
- Sends the dirty residue down to the Small Intestine.

Spleen

- Transforms food and liquids to *gu qi*.
- Sends the pure *gu qi* up from the Stomach to the upper *jiao*.

Gu qi

- Unrefined *qi* that has been extracted from the food and drink that has been consumed through the mouth and has been prepared by the Stomach.
- Sent up to the upper *jiao* to be further transformed.

Lung

- Inhales *da qi* from the world outside of the body.

Da qi

- Air from the world outside of the body.
- Combines with *gu qi* to create *zong qi*.

Zong qi

- Combination of *gu qi* and *da qi*.
- A form of *qi* that can be utilised for some purposes in its current form.
- Transformed by *yuan qi* to create *zhen qi*.

Zhen qi

- *Zong qi* that has been transformed by *yuan qi*.
- Refined *qi*, which can be used by the body in its present form.
- Has two aspects – *ying qi* and *wei qi*.

Ying qi

- Nourishing *qi*.
- *Yin* aspect of *zhen qi*.

Wei qi

- Defensive *qi*.
- *Yang* aspect of *zhen qi*.

San jiao

- Ensures that *yuan qi* comes from the lower *jiao* to the upper *jiao*.

Strengthening the production of *qi*

The pre-heavenly root of *qi* is *jing* that in part has been inherited from the parents. This aspect is therefore difficult to improve. However, it can be preserved and replenished by having a sufficient production of post-heaven *qi* and by tonifying the Kidneys. Tonifying the Kidneys is important, because the Kidneys store *jing*, which is the pre-heavenly root of *qi*, but also because of the Kidneys' relationship to *mingmen* and *yuan qi*.

When there is *jing xu*, it is imperative that a person gets adequate rest and does not overexert themselves mentally or physically. Men with *jing xu* should avoid having too many ejaculations. Pregnancy and childbirth will further weaken a woman who is *jing xu*. With regard to diet, the person will benefit from eating eggs, seeds, nuts, bone marrow and foods that are rich in vitamins and minerals. People with *jing xu* should avoid stimulants, in particular coffee and caffeine-rich substances. Many *qi gong* and yoga techniques have a restorative effect on *yuan qi*, *mingmen* and *jing*.

Acupuncture and moxa on points such as Kid 3, Ren 4, Du 4 and UB 23 is recommended.

The Spleen is dependent on three things if it is going to be able to create a sufficient production of *gu qi*: that the food that is consumed is sufficient in quality and quantity; that the Spleen itself is strong enough to transform the food that has been consumed; and that the *mingmen*'s fire is powerful enough to support Spleen *yang*.

The food that is consumed must, of course, be commensurate with the energy that is being used by the body. Furthermore, in Chinese medicine it is not enough just to eat sufficient food and eat food that is rich in nutrients and calories. The Spleen is strengthened by consuming food that is easily digestible and that is cold neither in temperature nor energy. The Spleen benefits from eating food that has been cooked, i.e. soups and stews, boiled or steamed vegetables and stir-fried dishes, where the physical heat from the stove has already started the transformation process. The Spleen is burdened not only by cold food, but also by very rich food, coarse food and food that creates 'Dampness'. Examples of foods that create Dampness are dairy products, sugar, bananas, orange juice and wheat.

The Spleen can be tonified by the use of acupuncture points such as Sp 3, Sp 6, St 36, Ren 12, UB 20 and UB 21.

The Lung, which helps to create *zong qi*, is dependent on its own *qi* being strong enough and that the *da qi* that is inhaled is of good quality. This means that the Lung can be tonified by being in places where the air is pure and fresh and through breathing exercises. Treatment of acupuncture points such as Lu 7, Lu 9, Ren 17, UB 13 and UB 42 can tonify the Lung and *zong qi*.

XUE

Xue means 'blood', but *xue* is something other and more than blood in Western medicine physiology and anatomy. *Xue* is both the red fluid that circulates in the blood vessels and a *yin* form of *qi*. The Western concept of blood encompasses only the physical aspect of *xue*, its visible form. *Xue* is that which can, for example, be seen when a blood vessel is cut, but *xue* is also an energetic aspect of the body, i.e. a form of *qi*. We can perhaps say that the word blood only encompasses the quantitative aspect of blood, that which can be measured, whereas *xue* also includes its *qi* qualities. This means that when a person is diagnosed as being *xue xu*, i.e. that their Blood, as defined in Chinese medicine, is deficient, it may well not be possible to measure anything negative in a Western medicine blood analysis. On the other hand, it will almost always be possible to diagnose a condition of *xue xu*, if a client has been told by a Western physician that they are anaemic, have low blood pressure or their blood values are low.

In this chapter I will discuss:

- *xue*'s overall functions

- how *xue* is produced

- *xue*'s relationship to *jing*, *qi*, *jinye* and *shen*.

Xue functions

The main functions that *xue* is responsible for are:

- to nourish

- to moisten

- to anchor *shen*.

Xue flows through the channel system and blood vessels together with *ying qi*. They support each other in nourishing all the tissues and organs of the body. Through their nourishment, *xue* and *qi* enable the body to grow, repair and regenerate itself. There is, however, a difference between *ying qi* and *xue*. Although they are both nourishing, *xue* is also moistening, something that *qi* is not. This is a significant difference between the two and is important when it comes to diagnosis. When there is a condition of *xue xu*, dry skin, dry hair and dry lips will be important diagnostic characteristics. *Xue* is moistening due to its close relationship with *jinye* and *xue*. *Jinye* thins *xue* and keeps it fluid. *Jinye* for its part benefits from the nutritional qualities of *xue*, because *xue* helps *jinye* to moisten and nourish the body.

Xue has a very close relationship to *shen*. *Shen*, which has its residence in the Heart, is nourished by Heart *xue*. *Shen*, which is *yang* in its nature, needs to be anchored and 'held down'. This function is in part performed by the *yin xue*. If a person is *xue xu*, they can be forgetful, have poor concentration and have a tendency to be absent minded. This is because *shen* is undernourished. They may also have difficulty sleeping, because their *shen* is not anchored at night by the *yin xue* and therefore the *yang shen* floats upwards.

It is also *xue* that, by anchoring *shen*, leads to *shen* throughout the body and its tissue. This allows *shen*, which is the Emperor in the body, to be aware of all that is happening in its realm. This means there can be a sensation of numbness or a tingling sensation in certain parts of the body where *xue* is not circulating. This is typically experienced in areas where there is scar tissue or when the supply of blood to an area is restricted.

Production of *xue*

Like *qi*, *xue* has a pre-heaven and a post-heaven root. The pre-heavenly root of *xue* is *yuan qi*. *Yuan qi*, which is transformed *jing*, is the catalyst in the transformation of *gu qi* to *xue*. The production of *xue* would grind to a halt without the presence of *yuan qi*. The post-heavenly root of *xue* is *gu qi*. *Gu qi* is produced by the Spleen from the food that has been ingested. *Gu qi* is sent upwards from the middle *jiao* by the Spleen to the upper *jiao*. In the upper *jiao*, the Lung pushes the *gu qi* across to the Heart, where it is transformed by *yuan qi*, which has ascended from the Kidneys, via the *san jiao*. The Heart then pumps *xue* out into the rest of the body. The Heart gets the strength to do this from *zong qi*.

Giovanni Maciocia is of the opinion that *xue* can also be created by the bone marrow. In *The Foundations of Chinese Medicine* (Maciocia 2005) he refers to a text from 1695, where Zhang Lu in his book *Medical Transmission of Zhang Family* writes 'that if *qi* is not exhausted, it returns essences to the Kidneys, where it creates *jing*; if *jing* is not depleted, it returns *jing* to the Liver to be transformed into *xue*'. This is not something that is confirmed by the classic texts. Elisabeth Rochat de la Vallee (Larre and Rochat de la Vallee 2003) writes that this originates from a passage in *Huang Di Nei Jing – Su Wen*, chapter five. Here it says that it is the Marrow that creates the Liver and it does this through Kidney *jing*. This refers to the *shen* cycle of the Five Phases, where Water creates Wood. In any case, Kidney *jing* is essential in the production of *xue*, because *jing* is the foundation of *yuan qi*, which is the catalyst that is needed to transform *gu qi* to *xue*. Therefore, Kidney *jing* is the pre-heavenly root of *xue*.

The production of *xue* is dependent on the organs that are involved in its production, i.e. the Spleen and the Kidneys, as well as the quality and quantity of the food consumed. It is the food that has been consumed that gets transformed to *gu qi* and subsequently to *xue*. Examples of foods that directly nourish *xue* are red meat, liver, green-leafed vegetables, beetroot, black sesame seeds, black beans, kidney beans and nettles. Acupuncture points that can help to strengthen the production of *xue* are points that tonify the Spleen and the Kidneys such as Sp 3, Sp 6, St 36, Kid 3, Ren 4, UB 20, UB 21 and UB 23, as well as UB 17, which is an acupuncture point that specifically nourishes *xue*.

Relationship to *zangfu* organs

There is a mutual relationship between *xue* and the internal or *zangfu* organs. *Xue* nourishes and moistens the whole of the body and thereby also the *zangfu* organs. On the other hand, *zangfu* organs produce *xue*, as well as storing, controlling and circulating *xue*. The role played by the *zangfu* organs in the production of *xue* is described above. I will therefore now describe the roles *zangfu* organs play in relation to *xue* that do not relate to the production of *xue*.

The Spleen, apart from creating *gu qi*, the raw material for the production of *xue*, also has the task of keeping *xue* inside the blood vessels. This means that Spleen *qi xu* can directly result in *xue xu* (*xue* deficiency) if it is not capable of transforming food into *gu qi*. Spleen *qi xu* can also indirectly be a cause of *xue xu*, if Spleen *qi xu* has resulted in spontaneous bleeding, heavy menstrual bleeding, irregular menstrual bleeding, etc. by not being able to hold *xue* in the vessels. Spleen *qi xu* can also manifest as a tendency to being easily bruised.

The Liver has an important role to play in relation to *xue*. The Liver is not involved in the production of *xue*, but it is the Liver that stores *xue*. It is said that the Liver is a reservoir for *xue*. The Liver is responsible for making sure that there is a sufficient quantity of *xue* out in the channel and vessel system at any given time. The amount of *xue* circulating in the body must always be appropriate to the level of activity and the body's needs. This means that when we sleep or when we are at rest, *xue* flows back to the Liver where it is stored. When we are physically active, the Liver sends *xue* out into the system again, so it can be used by the muscles and by the rest of the body. The Liver also has another important role to play in relation to *xue*. *Xue* is moved by *qi*, and the Liver is responsible for the free flow of *qi* in the whole body and thereby also the free flow of *xue*. This means that a stagnation of Liver *qi* can lead to a stagnation of *xue*. *Xue* for its part is important for the Liver, as *xue* nourishes, moistens and keeps the Liver supple. This is because the Liver is a reservoir that stores *xue* and the stored *xue* moistens the Liver, so it does not become stiff and inflexible. A consequence of this relationship can be seen in practice, when a condition of *xue xu* in the Liver can result in the Liver becoming 'dry' and 'rigid'. This can then result in Liver *qi* stagnation. This dynamic is in fact a very typical cause of Liver *qi* stagnation in women, because women lose *xue* each month during their menstrual bleeding.

The Heart governs *xue*. The Heart has the overall responsibility for governing *xue*, because it is the Heart that pumps *xue* through the blood vessels.

Summary of these relationships

- The Spleen produces *xue*.
- The Spleen controls *xue*.
- The Heart governs *xue*.
- The Liver stores *xue*.

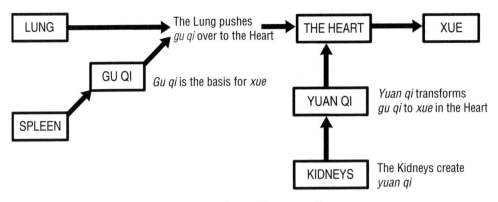

Figure 2.2 The production of *xue*

Xue's relationships

Jing

- The root of *yuan qi*, which transforms *gu qi* to *xue*.

- The root of Bone Marrow, which some sources say can create *xue*.

- Nourished and supplemented by *xue*.

Kidneys

- Send *yuan qi* up to the Heart to transform *gu qi* to *xue*.

Yuan qi

- Pre-heaven root of *xue*.

- Is sent up to the Heart to transform *gu qi* to *xue*.

Spleen

- Creates *gu qi* from the food consumed.

- Sends *gu qi* from the middle *jiao* up to the upper *jiao*.

- Spleen *qi* holds *xue* in the blood vessels.

Gu qi

- The basis for *xue*. Created by the Spleen and transformed into *xue* by *yuan qi* in the Heart.

Lung

- Pushes *gu qi* to the Heart, where it is transformed by *yuan qi* to *xue*.
- *Zong qi* pumps *xue* rhythmically around the body.

Heart

- The place where *xue* is created.
- Pumps *xue* around the body.

Shen

- *Xue* nourishes and anchors *shen*.
- *Shen* travels around the body with *xue*.

Ying qi

- Flows with *xue* in channels and vessels.
- Nourishes the body together with *xue*.
- Activates *xue*.

Jinye

- Is a part of *xue* and ensures that *xue* is fluid.
- Moistens the body together with *xue*.

Bone Marrow

- Can be transformed into *xue*.

San jiao

- Ensures that *yuan qi* and *gu qi* travel to where they are needed.

Liver

- Stores *xue*.
- Ensures that *qi* and thereby also *xue* flow freely and unhindered.
- *Xue* moistens and thereby ensures that the Liver is supple and flexible.

The relationship between *xue* and the other vital substances

The relationship between *qi* and *xue*

The relationship between *qi* and *xue* has four aspects:

- *qi* creates *xue*

- *qi* moves *xue*

- *qi* holds *xue* in place

- *xue* nourishes *qi*.

Xue is created when *yuan qi* transforms *gu qi*. Therefore, it is said that *qi* creates *xue*.

Xue is *yin* in nature. This means that *xue* is heavy, sticky and motionless. *Xue* is dependent on *qi's* activating force to be able to circulate around the body. It is *zong qi* that is the driving force behind the Heart's pumping of *xue* around the body, and it is *ying qi* that flows with *xue* through channels and vessels. This can be seen when blood leaves the body. The *qi* floats away from *xue*, which then stagnates without the *qi's* moving force. Furthermore, Liver *qi* ensures that *xue* moves freely and unhindered throughout the body.

Spleen *qi* has the important function that it keeps *xue* inside the blood vessels. If there is Spleen *qi xu*, a person can have a tendency towards spontaneous bleeding, bruising and menstrual disturbances.

Although it is *qi* that creates *xue*, *qi* is itself dependent on *xue*. *Xue*, which is very nourishing, nourishes the organs that produce *qi*. Therefore, there is a mutual relationship where the organs that produce the *qi* that is used in the production of *xue* are themselves dependent on being nourished by *xue* in order to function. *Xue*, by being much more nourishing than *qi*, enhances *ying qi* in its function of nourishing the body's tissues and organs.

Furthermore, *xue* is more *yin* than *qi*. *Qi* is anchored by *xue*, as they flow together through the channels and vessels. Without *xue*, *qi* would have a tendency to float upwards. Without *qi*, *xue* would stagnate.

These four relationships are summarised in a single sentence: *Qi* is the commander of *xue*; *xue* is the mother of *qi*.

Relationship to jing

If there is any nourishment left when *xue* has performed its various tasks around the body, the remaining nourishment will be used to nourish and supplement *jing*. *Jing* is the root of *yuan qi* and thereby the root of both the production of *qi* and the transformation of *gu qi* to *xue*. Some authors are of the opinion that *jing* can be directly transformed to *xue*.

Relationship to shen

Shen has its residence in the Heart. Heart *xue* anchors and nourishes *shen*.

Shen travels with *xue* through channels and vessels.

The relationship between xue and jinye

- *Jinye* thins *xue*.

- *Xue* nourishes *jinye*.

Xue and *jinye* have a close relationship to each other, both in their form and in their function. They are both *yin* substances and their roles in the body are partially overlapping.

However, there are also significant differences between the two. *Jinye* dilutes and thins *xue* and keeps *xue* fluid. On the other hand, *xue* is much more nutritious than *jinye*. *Xue* can therefore nourish and supplement *jinye*. Their close relationship can be seen by the fact that excessive or persistent sweating can lead to *xue xu*, while a heavy or persistent blood loss can weaken *jinye*.

As well as being more nutritious than *jinye*, *xue* also has the characteristic that it can anchor *shen*. This is not something that *jinye* can do. *Jinye* is more moistening and lubricating than *xue* is.

JINYE

Jinye is a general term for all the normal fluids in the body. *Jinye* includes saliva, sweat, tears, synovial fluids and the mucosa of all the mucous membranes in the body. *Jinye* has the task of moistening, lubricating and nourishing the skin, muscles, joints and the body's orifices. *Jinye* has a close relationship to *xue*; in particular it is *jinye* that thins *xue* and ensures that *xue* is fluid.

Jinye is manufactured from the food and liquids that are consumed. *Jinye* is created through a complex process, involving several organs. The body fluids are differentiated into two different types of fluid: *jin* and *ye*. *Jin* is lighter, less dense and has more of the character of a mist. *Jin* is conceived as being the more *yang* of the two types of body fluid. *Ye* is denser, stickier and is therefore more *yin*.[10]

In this chapter I will discuss:

- *jinye's* overall functions
- how *jinye* is produced
- the relationship between *jinye* and the other vital substances.

Functions of *jinye*

Jin

As stated above, *jin* is the most *yang* of the two types of body fluid. *Jin* is conceived of as being mist-like. *Jin* is clear, thin and watery. *Jin* flows easily and moves quickly. *Jin* circulates primarily in the space between the skin and muscles together with *wei qi* and in the channels and vessels together with *ying qi* and *xue*. The image that is sometimes used is that *jin* flows together with the channel *qi* and *xue* in the same way that a mist flows together with the water in a stream in the early morning. This circulation and distribution of *jin* is controlled by the Lung. *Jin* primarily has the function of moistening the skin and muscles and partly also of nourishing them. *Jin* is not as nutritious as *xue*, but it is more moistening. *Jinye* has in general a close relationship to *xue*, diluting *xue* and keeping it fluid. *Jin* can be directly observed in sweat, in tears and to a certain degree in saliva.

Ye

Ye is more turbid, thick and oily than *jin*. *Ye* is slower in its movement. *Ye* is used by the body to lubricate the joints, and *ye* is also the mucus that lubricates the body's orifices, such as the eyes, nose, mouth, ears and vagina. *Ye* also supplements *jing* and it strengthens the Brain and Bone Marrow.

Production of *jinye*

The entire production of *jinye* is a very complex process, with a repeated separation of the pure and impure fluids. There is a constant recycling process, where pure fluids are extracted from the remaining impure liquids, so no pure fluids go to waste. This is similar to a gold mine, where the gold ore that is extracted in the mine is separated from the rock. This gold is very impure and needs to be processed, as there are still remnants of worthless rock mixed in with the gold. There will then be a repeated process, where the valuable gold is constantly refined. The rock and dust that is separated from the pure gold is not discarded though. It still contains traces of valuable gold. This means that the impure dust and rock will be worked on again to extract the pure gold that is still present in the dust. Finally, when there is no gold remaining in the dust and rock, the debris will be discarded on the slag heap.

The process of fluid physiology starts with the pure fluids being separated out from the food and liquids that have been consumed. Afterwards there is a constant refinement and preservation of fluids where the pure fluids is sent upwards in the body and the impure fluids are sent down to be further processed. At each stage of the process, the pure fluids are separated out of the remaining impure fluids and the impure fluids are sent downwards to be further processed. The process continues until the last remaining impure fluids are separated and expelled from the body in the form of urine.

The first stage in the process is when the food and liquids that have been consumed are received by the Stomach. Spleen *qi* separates the pure fluids out of these liquids. The Spleen sends the pure fluids up to the Lung, where there is a further separation of the pure and impure parts. The pure part of these fluids is spread with channel *qi* through the body as a fine mist. Some of the pure fluids exit the body as sweat. The impure part that was separated by the Lung is sent down to the Urinary Bladder. The Urinary Bladder retains the fluids until they can be evaporated by Kidney *yang*. This evaporation separates the pure aspect of the fluids. These pure fluids are sent upwards through the lower and middle *jiao* to the upper *jiao*. The impure residue that is left remains in the Urinary Bladder. Now there is nothing remaining that can be recovered and utilised. The last impure fluids are expelled from the body as urine. Some of the fluids that the Lung sent down to the Urinary Bladder are evaporated by the Kidney *yang* and are sent back up to the Lung again to keep the Lung moist.

The impure fluids that were not transformed by the Spleen will be sent down from the Stomach to the Small Intestine. In the Small Intestine there is a further separation of the pure and impure fluids. The impure part that has been separated in the Small Intestine is sent to the Urinary Bladder to be processed.[11] The pure part of the fluid is sent upwards through the body via *san jiao*.

From the Small Intestine the remaining solids or dross is sent down into the Large Intestine, which then absorbs the remaining pure liquid. The remaining untransformed solids are expelled from the body as faeces.

The impure fluids that were separated in the Small Intestine and were sent downwards are received by the Urinary Bladder. These, and the impure fluids that the Lung sent down, are once again transformed under the influence of Kidney *yang*. After this transformation the usable pure residues are sent upwards through *san jiao* to create sweat. The Urinary Bladder sends the remaining impure fluid out of the body (again under the influence of Kidney *yang*) as urine.

All of the transport of pure and impure fluids takes place through *san jiao*. Similarly, it is also through *san jiao* that the passage of the *yuan qi*, which is to be used by all of these transformation processes, takes place.

San jiao controls the water passages

Most organs' roles in fluid physiology have been described above. I will go into more depth below with regards to the role played by *san jiao* in relation to fluid physiology. *San jiao* is an organ that 'has function, but does not have form'. That is, *san jiao* is an organ that cannot be seen, but that manifests through its functionality. This is in reality no different to the other organs in Chinese medicine. The difference between *san jiao* and the other organs is that they are also specific physical organs in Western anatomy. Nevertheless, they can still have completely different and variant properties in Chinese medicine physiology. As we will see later in the book, *san jiao* can be defined in several ways. At this stage, it is enough to know that *san jiao* can be understood both as all cavities and spaces in the tissue of the body and as a threefold division of the torso, the division being in an upper, middle and lower part.

San jiao is the organ that has the overall responsibility for the body fluids being transformed, transported and discharged properly.

San jiao's official title in the hierarchy of the body, as described in the *Huang Di Nei Jing – Su Wen*, is the 'official with responsibility for the drains and irrigation'. This is, of course, not quite such a fine title as the Emperor or the Ambassador, but it is crucial that someone performs these vital functions and looks after the more practical aspects of the realm.

When we refer to *san jiao* and fluids, there are several conditions that apply. *San jiao* is responsible for *yuan qi* arriving at the appropriate places and in the form that it is to be used. *Jinye* production and physiology is completely dependent on *yuan qi*. The Spleen, Small Intestine, Lung, Kidneys and Urinary Bladder all utilise *yuan qi* to transform and transport the body fluids. In addition, *san jiao* maintains the passages and directs the fluids up and down and in and out of the body. *San jiao* ensures that *jinye* arrives where and when it should and that the pure and impure parts will be sent to where they should be afterwards.

The classical texts describe the three *jiao* as having different roles in relation to *jinye* physiology.

In the upper *jiao*, *jinye* is described as being like a mist. In the upper *jiao*, *jin* is dispersed as a fine mist out into the rest of the body in the spaces between the skin and muscles. The middle *jiao* is characterised as a fermentation chamber or a bubbling cauldron. The fluids are initially 'rotted and ripened' here. They are then transformed and the pure aspect is sent up to the upper *jiao*. The lower *jiao* is seen as a drain or a ditch. It is here that the impure, turbid fluids are sent down to and subsequently expelled from the body.

San jiao is, as described, all spaces in the body, including the spaces in the tissue and the inside of the joints. *San jiao* also controls the movement of body fluids here. *San jiao* ensures for instance that the joints are constantly lubricated.

Jinye's relationships

Stomach

- Receives the food and liquids consumed and retains them until the Spleen has transformed them. The Stomach is therefore called the root of *jinye*.

- Sends the impure fluids down to the Small Intestine.

Spleen

- Transforms food and liquids in the Stomach.

- Separates the pure from the impure.

- Sends the pure fluids up to the Lung.

San jiao

- The passage through which all *jinye* is transported.

- Ensures that *yuan qi* arrives where it is needed to assist in the transformation of *jinye*.

Lung

- Receives the pure fluids from the Spleen and further refines and separates the pure and impure aspects.

- The pure fluids are spread as a fine mist throughout the body together with *ying qi* and *wei qi*.

- The impure fluids are sent downwards to the Urinary Bladder for further processing.

Small Intestine

- Further separates the pure and impure fluids.

- Impure fluids are sent down to the Urinary Bladder and the pure aspects are sent up through the body via *san jiao*.

- Sends the remaining solids down to the Large Intestine.

Urinary Bladder

- Receives the impure fluids from the Small Intestine, Lung and *san jiao*.

- Sends pure fluids up through *san jiao* to the exterior to form sweat.

- Expels the impure fluids from the body as urine.

Kidneys

- Kidney *yang* evaporates and transforms the fluids in the Urinary Bladder.

- Sends some of the pure fluid up to the Lung to moisten it.

- Kidney *yang* holds the urine inside the Urinary Bladder, and it expels the urine out of the Urinary Bladder upon urination.

Large Intestine

- Receives the remaining food residues and liquids that have not already been transformed.

- Extracts the remaining fluid aspect of these dregs and sends it upwards through *san jiao*.

Yuan qi

- Is used in all transformation processes where the pure and the impure are separated from each other.

Wei qi

- Spreads *jin* fluids in the space between the skin and the muscles.

Ying qi

- Spreads the *ye* aspect to the joints and orifices.

The relationship between *jinye* and the other vital substances

The relationship between *qi* and *jinye*

- *Qi* transforms and transports *jinye*.

- *Qi* holds *jinye* in place.

- *Jinye* plays a minor role in relation to the production of *qi*.

- *Qi* is lost through sweating.

Qi and *jinye* have a *yin/yang* relationship. *Qi* is *yang* and *jinye* is *yin*. *Qi* is both lighter and less substantial than *jinye*. Furthermore, the *yang qi* transforms and transports the *yin jinye*.

Qi is involved in all the stages of *jinye* production. Without *qi*, there would be no transformation of fluids to *jinye*. It is both the *qi* of the individual organs and *yuan qi* that are involved in these processes. In addition, it is *qi* that transports *jinye* around the body. Without *qi*, *jinye* would accumulate and become a pathological substance (*xie qi*): Water, Dampness or Phlegm. The three organs that are primarily responsible for transporting *jinye* are the Lung, the Spleen and the Kidneys. There can be visible oedema and accumulations of fluids if these organs are in imbalance.

The Lung is primarily responsible for transporting *jinye* in the upper *jiao*. If the Lung is disturbed in this process, there can be a tangible puffiness to the face and arms and fluids can accumulate in the Lung and in its sensory organ, the nose. This is seen, for instance, when a person has a cold and the Lung's ability to spread *wei qi* and *jinye* is blocked by *xie qi*. This will result in the above-mentioned puffiness around the eyes and thin watery mucus in the nose and possibly also in the lungs themselves.

The Spleen and the Kidneys are primarily responsible for transporting *jinye* in the middle and lower *jiao* respectively. Imbalances in this function can result in abdominal oedema or oedema of the legs. It is important to remember that *jinye* is a form of liquid and thus *yin* in nature. When *jinye* is not moved by *qi*, it will always seep downwards. Oedema is therefore most often seen in the legs.

As well as keeping *xue* inside the blood vessels, *qi* also has the task of keeping *jinye* inside the body. It does this by keeping the pores in the skin closed, holding the urine in the Urinary Bladder and keeping *jinye* inside of the body's orifices. If there is a condition of *qi xu*, the body may not be able to perform these functions, resulting in symptoms and signs such as incontinence, spontaneous sweating and vaginal discharge.

Jinye plays a very limited role in *qi* production. The Stomach, which 'ripens and rots' the food and liquids before the Spleen *qi* transforms them, is damaged by Dryness. It is therefore important that the Stomach does not dry out. *Jinye* helps to moisten the Stomach.

When a person sweats, they lose not only *jinye*, but also *qi*. *Qi* escapes from the body together with *jinye*. This is why night sweats are known in Chinese medicine as the 'thief who comes in the night'.

The relationship between xue and jinye

- *Jinye* thins *xue*.

- *Xue* nourishes *jinye*.

Xue and *jinye* have a close relationship to each other, both in form and function. They are both *yin* substances and their role in the body is partially overlapping. At the same time there are also significant differences between the two.

Jinye dilutes *xue* and maintains the fluidity of *xue*. *Xue*, on the other hand, is much more nourishing than *jinye*, so *xue* can nourish and supplement *jinye*. Their close relationship can be seen in the fact that excessive or persistent sweating can lead to *xue xu*, while a heavy or persistent blood loss can weaken *jinye*.

Xue is not only more nutritious than *jinye*, but it also anchors *shen*. This is not something that *jinye* can do. *Jinye*, on the other hand, is more moistening and lubricating than *xue*.

The relationship between jing and jinye

Yuan qi, which is created from *jing* in the Kidneys, is used in all transformations of fluids to *jinye* and to transport of *jinye* via *san jiao*.

Ye, which is lubricating and moistening, supplements *jing* and its aspects: the Bone Marrow and the Brain.

The relationship between shen and jinye

Shen is created from *jing*, but is also dependent on nourishment from all of the post-heaven *qi*, which *jinye* is also a part of.

When *shen* is in balance, it ensures that all the physiological processes in the body are harmonious, including the transformation and transport of *jinye*.

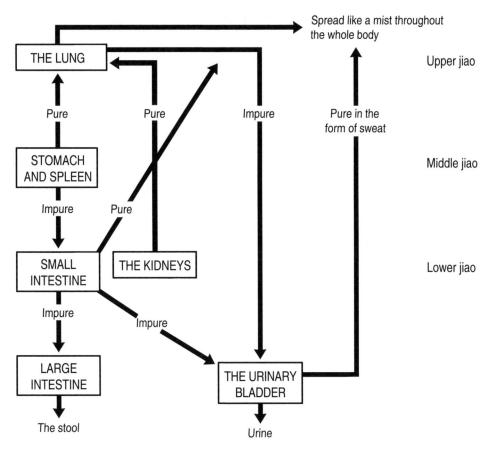

Figure 2.3 The production of *jinye*

SHEN

Shen is a difficult concept to translate into English. This is the same problem that was seen with regards to *qi*. *Shen* is more than a single word or term. In the same way that there are no English or European words that directly correspond to *qi*, there is no word or concept that directly corresponds to *shen*. Furthermore, the relationship that *shen* has to the body's physiology is quite alien and differs significantly from the existing concepts in modern, Western medicine.

Shen is translated differently by different authors. This reflects that there are different definitions, or more correctly aspects, of *shen*, but also the importance that various authors attach to these aspects. In modern TCM,[12] which has been developed and practised in China over the last fifty years, there is a very 'material' understanding of *shen*. In TCM *shen* can be translated as mind, as the sum of our mental capacities and our psyche. This reflects the Maoist society that TCM is a child of. In the more doctrinaire TCM, the more spiritual aspects of *shen* that are described in classic Daoist, Buddhist and Confucian texts are not easily reconciled with a materialistic, Western, scientific understanding of the body and the universe. The classical conception of *shen* was therefore downplayed or even ignored. To only understand *shen* as mind is a very narrow and deceptive definition of what *shen* is. This is because, as a concept, *shen* is much more comprehensive than just the mind. *Shen* is more than the sum of our mental activities. It is the sum of our mental, emotional and not least spiritual aspects. TCM had to appease and be accepted by the Maoists and their purely materialistic view of the world. This meant that everything that had to do with the spirit or soul needed to be hidden away as much as possible.

In this chapter, I will try to highlight some of the aspects of *shen* that are of relevance in Chinese medicine. The aspects I will describe are as follows.

- *Shen* as a part of the universal *shen*.

- *Shen* as the sum of the body's mental, emotional and spiritual aspects.

- *Shen* as an aspect of the Heart.

- *Shen* and its relationship to Heart *yin* and Heart *xue*.

- *Shen* as one of the Three Treasures.

- *Shen* and its relationship to *xue*.

- *Shen* as vitality and radiance.

Shen as a part of the universal *shen*

In the ancient philosophical texts there is a more esoteric description of *shen*. Here *shen* is described as being something that is transcendental – something that is greater than humans and their physical organs. In fact, *shen* transcends even *yin* and *yang*. It is the universal *yuan qi*. In *The Great Commentary to the Yi Jing* (*Yi Dazhuan*) it says, 'that which is beyond *yin* and *yang* is called *shen*'. In this context *shen* has the same sense as *dao*. That is, that which everything is a part of. It is that which is beyond time and space. It is that which is without form. This aspect of *shen* is not used directly in Chinese medicine, but it still has relevance. This is because our own *shen* is a refraction or an individual manifestation of this universal *shen*.

Shen as, the sum of the body's mental, emotional and spiritual aspects

Shen is the overall consciousness in the body, and at the same time it is the sum of the five *shen* or, in Chinese, *wu shen*. Each of the *zang* organs has a *shen* aspect. These are called *shen*, *hun*, *po*, *yi* and *zhi* and these relate respectively to the Heart, Liver, Lung, Spleen and Kidneys. Each of these *shen* has specific and unique characteristics. In the chapters on the *zang* organs, the functions and characteristics of the individual *shen* are discussed in detail. Observation of how these five *shen* manifest themselves can be used to diagnose both the psycho-emotional imbalances and physical disorders. This is because the five *shen* are each aspects of the organs that they are related to. Changes in the body's *qi* will manifest itself with changes in the organ's *shen* aspect.

As can be seen, *shen* is the sum of the five *shen* and at the same time it is also one of them. This is because when Heart *shen* is referred to there is talk of an aspect of *shen* that is specific to the Heart.

Shen as an aspect of the Heart

It is this *shen* that is usually referred to when *shen* is mentioned in Chinese medicine.

Heart *shen* has several aspects, which I will try to explain here. Some of the most important aspects of the Heart *shen* are:

- consciousness
- mental capacities
- wisdom
- fellowship.

Consciousness

It is *shen* that is our consciousness. It is *shen* that enables us to know who we are. It is our cognitive sense. *Shen* is also awareness of the stimuli and impressions we experience. It is *shen* that makes us aware of what it is we experience. It is *po* that senses the skin being touched or when we touch something. It is the Spleen that distinguishes the five tastes from each other when we eat. It is the Liver that is affected by anger. It is the ear that hears the five sounds, but it is *shen* that makes us conscious of all these experiences. Without our *shen* all of these things would just be physical and energetic reactions in the body, but we would not be aware of the fact that something had happened. This is the same as when the nerves in the fingers register the fingers touching something, but it is the Brain that receives the signal and makes the person aware that something is being touched. We can see that many of the Brain's functions in Western anatomy are similar to those of *shen*. In Chinese medicine the Brain is one of the so-called extraordinary *fu* organs (see the chapter on the extraordinary *fu* organs, page 216, for more detail). The Brain is created from *jing* and is seen as a flower that grows out of the spinal cord. The Brain is nourished by Heart *xue*. From this we can see that there are similarities with *shen*. They are both created and nourished by *jing* and Heart *xue*. In fact, some older Daoist traditions in Chinese medicine view *shen* as having its residence in the Brain. The relationship between the Brain and *shen* can be seen in the fact that many *du mai* acupuncture points can be used to influence *shen* when it is agitated or blocked. This is because *du mai* connects directly to the brain and *du mai* transverses the head. In reality, it is not of great importance whether the residence of *shen* is in the Brain or the Heart, as *du mai* connects both to the Heart and the Brain, and the treatment will largely be the same.

A second aspect of consciousness is that *shen* makes us aware of what is appropriate or normal behaviour. *Shen* enables a person to conform to their surroundings. People whose *shen* is disturbed often lack this ability. They say and do things that to them are normal but to others seem strange. They often dress and act strangely.

Mental capacities

Shen encompasses the intellect, i.e. our ability to think and our intelligence. This is both academic capabilities and intelligence, as well as the ability to learn things and to remember. We will see later in the book that other organs, particularly the Kidneys and the Spleen, are also involved in the processes of learning and memory. The Heart and thereby *shen* also have a close relationship to long-term memory. When *shen* is not nourished or when *shen* is blocked by Phlegm, the abilities to think and to learn things can be impeded. *Shen* is that which enables a person to think rationally. If *shen* is blocked by Phlegm or agitated by Heat, this capacity is compromised.

Wisdom

Shen is not only an intellectual intelligence. It is also wisdom and insight. *Shen* enables a person to comprehend the world around them and themselves.

It is *shen* consciousness that is cultivated in meditation and esoteric exercises.[13]

Fellowship

Shen is an aspect of the Heart and, at the same time, it is an aspect of the universal *shen* or *dao*, which everything in the universe is a part of. *Shen* is a refraction of this *qi.* When a person's *shen* is in contact with the universal *qi*, they will feel at ease, tranquil and safe and have a sense of belonging. The universal *shen* is beyond time and space and thus immortal and infinite. When a person's *shen* is in contact with this, they will feel at ease. When *shen* is not in contact with this, because it is either undernourished, agitated or blocked, they will experience loneliness, desolation, mortal fear, panic and despair.

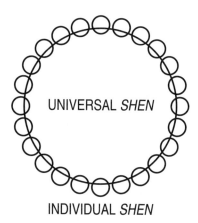

Figure 2.4 The relationship between the individual and universal *shen*

Shen and its relationship to Heart *yin* and Heart *xue*

Heart *shen* has a very close relationship to Heart *yin* and Heart *xue*. Once again, there is a *yin/yang* relationship. *Shen* is the most *yang* aspect of the Heart and it is nourished and also controlled by the Heart's *yin* aspects, which are Heart *yin* and Heart *xue*. If there is a condition of the Heart *yin xu* or Heart *xue xu*, *shen* will not be nourished as it should, nor will it be anchored. When *shen* lacks nourishment, there can be problems with the memory and concentration, and there can be a tendency to anxiety, nervousness or being easily startled. When *shen* is not being anchored, there can be insomnia. This is because *shen* should rest in the Heart during the night, and it is the Heart's *yin* aspects that hold *shen* down and within the Heart. *Shen* not being anchored can also manifest with signs such as anxiety, nervousness and being easily startled.

Shen as one of the Three Treasures

Shen is a part of the continuum – *jing*, *qi* and *shen*. In this we can see that in Chinese medicine there can be no separation of body and mind. They do not just influence each other, as they are conceived as doing in Western holistic medicine. They are each other. They are just different manifestations of the same *qi*. *Jing*, *qi* and *shen* affect, and are affected by, each other, because they are manifestations of the same *qi*. The difference lies in their density. *Shen* is the most *yang* and least material of the various manifestations of *qi* in the body. *Jing*, which is the most *yin* form of *qi* in the body, is the most dense. *Jing* is the material foundation for *shen*, which is the most *yang* and ethereal form of *qi*. *Shen* is a manifestation of the pre-heavenly *jing* and is nourished by the post-heaven *qi* and *xue*. An imbalance in one of the Three Treasures will create an imbalance in the other two. They are mutually dependent on each other. If *jing* is weak, *shen* will also be weak. *Shen* for its part activates and motivates *jing*.

The Three Treasures reflect the perpetual division into the number three that is seen not only in Chinese medicine, but also in Chinese philosophy in general. This division reflects a *yin/yang* continuum, where *yang* Heaven and *yin* Earth are connected by Man. In the body this is reflected in the Three Treasures – *jing*, *qi* and *shen*, but also in the three *jiao* and the organs that are situated in these. Each of the Three Treasures has an affinity to one of the *jiao*. *Jing*, which is the ultimate *yin*, is stored in the lower *jiao*, which is the most *yin*. The Water Phase, which is an aspect of the Kidneys, is also the most *yin* phase. The root of the post-heaven production of *qi* is the Spleen and the Stomach, which are situated in the middle *jiao*. The middle *jiao* reflects Man, who connects Heaven and Earth in the same way that the middle *jiao* connects the lower and the upper *jiao*. *Shen* resides in the Heart, which is a Fire organ. The Heart and the Fire Phase are the most *yang* aspects of the body. The Three Treasures' *yin/yang* qualities can be seen in their functions and cycles (see table below).

Whereas *jing*, which is very material, is stored in the Kidneys and moves through the body via the eight extraordinary vessels, *shen* is immaterial and ethereal and has its residence in the Heart. *Shen* is anchored by and moves through the body together with *xue*, but because *shen* is ethereal, it is in a certain sense also outside the body. That *shen* is also something that is outside the body can sometimes be experienced; for example, sensing that there is a person behind you staring at you or the sensation you can have that a person sitting in a seat on the train is deranged without them having said a word. There is something about the person's *shen* that our own *shen* registers and that makes it uneasy. The two *shen* affect each other without there being any direct contact.

Jing	*Qi*	*Shen*
Relatively *yin*	Relatively *yang* in relation to *jing* Relatively *yin* in relation to *shen*	Relatively *yang*
Dependent on the parents' *jing*	Dependent on the diet consumed and on the quality of *jing*	Dependent on *jing*, *qi* and especially *xue* (which is created by *jing* and *qi*)
Difficult to influence and restore	Recreated from hour to hour	Extremely easily affected
Circulates in seven- and eight-year cycles	Circulates in shorter cycles, some on a daily basis	Daily cycles
Circulates mainly in the eight extraordinary vessels	Circulates in the whole body	Is both inside and outside the body
Changes very slowly	Changes relatively quickly	Changes immediately
Mainly treated via the Kidneys	Mainly treated via the Spleen, Lung and Kidneys	Mainly treated via the Heart, Pericardium and *du mai*

Shen and its relationship to *xue*

Shen has a very close relationship to *xue* and in particular Heart *xue*.

Xue and *shen* have three overall relationships.

- *Shen* is nurtured by *xue*.

- *Shen* is anchored by *xue*.

- *Shen* moves around the body with *xue*.

Shen has its residence in the Heart, and it is Heart *yin* and Heart *xue* that nourish *shen*. *Shen* is created by *jing*, but is nourished constantly by Heart *xue*. This means that in a *xue xu* condition, *shen* will not receive the nourishment it needs to carry out its functions and activities. This can manifest with a person being absent minded, having difficulty concentrating and having difficulty remembering things. In addition to being nourished by Heart *xue*, *shen* is also anchored by it. It is the *yin xue* that anchors and keeps the *yang shen* in place. If there is Heart *xue xu*, *shen* will not be anchored. This will primarily be seen by the *shen* not being held down and at rest at night. The person will have difficulty sleeping. *Shen* not being anchored can also manifest with nervousness, anxiety and being easily startled.

If Heart *xue* becomes too hot, it can result in *shen* being agitated. This can manifest with insomnia, manic behaviour, restlessness and difficulty concentrating.

The anchoring of *shen* by *xue* allows *shen* to travel through the body to all of the places that *xue* permeates. This enables *shen* to be conscious of everything that is going on in the body. This is not dissimilar to the Western concept of the brain and nervous system, although it is not possible to make direct parallels between the two physiological models.

Shen as vitality and radiance

The term *shen* is used in diagnostic contexts to describe a quality that should be present in the skin, the eyes, the face, the tongue, the pulse, etc. When *shen* is present, there will be a glow and radiance. There will be vitality. The presence of *shen* will show that *xue* and *ying qi* are strong and that there is a good prognosis even in serious conditions.

Part 3

THE INTERNAL ORGANS

ZANGFU ORGANS

A prerequisite for understanding Chinese medicine is acceptance of the fact that when organs are referred to, it is the Chinese medicine concept of organs that is inferred. Often there is significant divergence between the Western and Chinese medicine perception of the internal organs. It is not only the fact that Western medicine operates with a biochemical physiological model, whereas Chinese medicine uses a *qi-* or energetic model, it is also because in Western medicine it is the organ's physical anatomy that is definitive. In the Chinese medical model, the physical structure of the body is of limited importance. Here it is the organ's function and not form that is most important. This is the hallmark of Chinese medicine, where function and context are the defining qualities. This can be enormously frustrating and appear to be unscientific and superstitious when you are brought up with the Western scientific, analytical model. Nonetheless, the Chinese medicine model is also analytical and it is constructed around the observation of the body's physiology and pathology and how these relate to natural principles.[1] Common to both systems is that you can anticipate the consequences of actions and influences that affect the physiology of the body. In practice, this means that it is necessary to let go of the Western medicine perception of the body whilst reading about the body in a Chinese medicine context. A very clear example of this is the Spleen. In Chinese medicine the Spleen is the most important digestive organ – a function that this organ has no relation to in Western medicine. Furthermore, the internal organs are attributed mental and emotional characteristics and properties in Chinese medicine, which is not the case in Western medicine physiology. It is due to these differences in the perception of organs that the initial letter of the names of the organs are capitalised throughout this book when it is the Chinese medical understanding of the organ that is being referred to.

In the Chinese medicine model, there are twelve internal organs. These are called *zangfu* organs. Six of these organs are defined as being *yin* organs.[2] These organs are solid in their structure and are called *zang* organs. The other six organs have a hollow structure and are called *fu* organs. *Fu* organs are defined as being *yang* organs. In addition to the structural differences, there is also a difference between *zang* and *fu* organs' overall functionality, energetic level and importance.

Each of the six *zang* organs has a *yin/yang* relationship to one of the six *fu* organs and they are regarded as each other's partner organ.

As well as the twelve *zangfu* organs, there are six so-called extraordinary *fu* organs. These are organs that have the structure of a *fu* organ but the functions of a *zang* organ. These extraordinary *fu* organs will be discussed in a separate chapter (page 216).

Zang organs' solid structure should be understood as being relative to the *fu* organs. The Lung and the Heart have hollow spaces, but in comparison to the

Stomach, the Intestines and Bladders, their structure is still relatively solid. *Fu* organs' hollow structure reflects their function. *Fu* organs receive, transmit and excrete. For example, the Stomach receives the food and liquids that are ingested through the mouth. After the Spleen has transformed the food, the Stomach sends the remaining residue to the Small Intestine. Furthermore, *fu* organs are in contact with impure and untransformed substances, where *zang* organs are only involved in processing and storing pure and refined substances. *Zang* organs do not receive or transmit in the same way as *fu* organs do. *Zang* organs' primary task is to store the vital substances *qi*, *xue*, *jing* and *shen*. The Kidneys, for example, store *jing*.

Fu organs receive food and liquids and excrete urine and faeces from the body. They are therefore in direct contact with the exterior. *Zang* organs are energetically located deeper inside the body and, with the exception of the Lung, they are not in direct contact with the exterior. By lying deeper inside the body and not being in contact with the exterior, *zang* organs are more protected. *Zang* organs store vital substances and it is therefore important that they are protected against climatic *xie qi*.

Zang organs' general functions can be summarised as follows.

Zang organs

- store vital substances
- store pure and refined substances that they have received from *fu* organs
- are located deeper inside the body and are viewed as being of greater importance than *fu* organs
- with the exception of the Lung, are not in direct contact with the outside world
- have a solid structure

Fu organs' general functions can be summarised as follows.

Fu organs

- do not store pure or vital substances
- constantly fill and empty
- transform and refine food and liquids to vital substances
- have the function of receiving, transmitting, digesting and excreting
- expel waste products
- are hollow in structure
- with the exception of the Gall Bladder, are in direct contact with the exterior

---

The concepts relating to *zangfu* organs are central to Chinese medicine and most treatments of physiological problems are based on a so-called *zangfu* diagnosis. This is because the whole channel system, and thereby acupuncture points, is directly connected to the *zangfu* organs, but also particularly because of the role played by *zang* organs in the production, transport and storage of the vital substances *qi*, *xue*, *jinye*, *jing* and *shen*.

The internal organs are an integrated part of an energetic context, and these organs are not only physical but also energetic structures. *Zang* organs are considered more important than *fu* organs. This is not only based on the functions that they perform – it is also due to the relationships they have with other aspects of the body. The various relationships that are attributed to the Five Phases, i.e. tissue, sensory organ, smell, sound, etc., refer mainly to the *zang* organs. *Fu* organs are in reality subordinate to the *zang* organs. For example, the majority of the processes that take place in the Small Intestine are governed by the Spleen and the Kidneys, and the Small Intestine's *qi* is regulated by the Liver and the Stomach. The majority of *zangfu* imbalances are also *zang* organ imbalances. In relation to the channel system, however, *yang* and *yin* organs' channels are equally important.

In *Huang Di Nei Jing – Su Wen*, chapter eight, the various organs are allocated positions in the imperial court or in society. This reflects Confucian philosophy, where everyone has a specific position and responsibility in society. It also reflects the various organs' functions and how important these are viewed as being. For example, in the same way that the Emperor was not physically involved in the daily tasks of the realm, the Heart is not directly involved in any of the transformation processes of *qi*, *xue* or *jinye*. Nevertheless, the Heart's role is considered to be of crucial importance. This is because the Heart, like the Emperor, has the overall responsibility for the well-being of everyone and everything, and is at the same time responsible for all processes being carried out in harmony with the universal laws.

Organ	Court position	Task it is responsible for the realm
Heart	Emperor	Governs *shen*, residence for *shen*
Pericardium	Ambassador	Joy and delight
Lung	Prime Minister	Regulation
Spleen and Stomach	Civil servants	Responsible for the storage and granaries
San jiao	Civil servant	Irrigation and the ditches
Gall Bladder	Upright civil servant	Responsible for decisions
Liver	General	Planning and strategies
Kidney	Strong official	Ingenuity and skill
Urinary Bladder	Province capital	Storage of liquids until they are expelled by *qi*
Small Intestine	Civil servant	Receiving, to be filled and to transform
Large Intestine	Civil servant	Passage and transportation

Each *zang* organ will, in addition to influencing the vital substances, manifest itself in various other ways. Furthermore, organs can be affected by certain emotions, climatic factors, etc. Many of these correspondences – things that affect these organs and things that are affected by these organs – are the same as the Five Phase correspondences. This is the explanation of many of the relationships that are seen in the Five Phase system.

Each *zang* organ has a relationship to a specific:

- vital substance

- body tissue

- sensory organ

- emotion

- external manifestation of the body

- fluid

- climatic factor

- odour

- colour

- flavour

- posture

- sound

- virtue

- *shen.*

These relationships will be discussed separately for each of the individual organs in the following chapters. It is important to remember when you read about these relationships that they are not exclusive. The Liver, for example, manifests in the eyes because, amongst other things, Liver *xue* nourishes the eyes. Other organs though also influence the eyes. Kidney *yin* helps to moisten and nourish the eyes. Furthermore, there are several channels that either start or terminate in the eyes. This means that imbalances in these organs, especially if there is Heat, will possibly manifest in the eyes.

ZANG ORGANS

THE KIDNEYS

Deep down in the dark, moist soil nestles the roots of a flower. It was in these dark depths that a seed once germinated. It was from here that the seedling forced its way upwards and broke through the surface of the soil, reaching up into the light. It was in the dark soil that the seed, formed from the union of the *jing* of two other plants, was to be found. It was in this seed that the resources needed by the seed to germinate and grow upwards were activated, providing the energy that was necessary for the plant to germinate and grow upwards until it could generate its own energy from the sunlight. From these depths came the will to live and the willpower needed to enable the seedling to force its way up and past obstacles in its pursuit of light. Without the willpower and without the inherited potential that the seed contained, the flower would never have been able to blossom, manifesting the full potential of its beauty.

But even after the plant has matured and grown to its maximum height, the roots are still the foundation of its life. Though the leaves absorb and photosynthesise the sunlight, whilst inhaling carbon dioxide and expelling oxygen, the whole plant is still completely dependent on the minerals and the water that rise up from the roots. Without the roots, the leaves and the flowers would fade and wither. This in reality is no different from a human body. In the human body, the Kidneys are the root. The Kidneys, which are to be found deep in the lower *jiao*, store *jing*. *Jing* is the potential for life that arose from the union of the two parents' *jing*. It was *jing* that determined the development of the foetus, and it was *jing* that created the fundamental growth of the body until the post-heaven *qi* was created and could assist in the body's development and growth. Although the Lung and the Spleen create *qi* on a daily basis in the form of *gu qi* and *zong qi*, they are still reliant on the fundamental nourishment that the Kidneys' pre-heaven *jing* provides. As we saw in the previous section, the physiological processes that are centred on the production of *qi*, *xue* and *jinye* are all processes that are dependent on *yuan qi*. *Yuan qi* is *qi* that is formed when the body's fundamental *yang* aspect, *mingmen*, transforms the body's fundamental *yin* aspect, *jing*. Without *yuan qi*, *gu qi* would remain an untransformed potential and there would be no production of *qi* and *xue*; neither would there be a transformation or distribution of *jinye*. Without the pre-heaven *jing* and post-heaven production of *qi* and *xue*, the Heart's *shen* could not manifest itself like a beautiful flower blossoming in the sun.

The functions of the Kidneys

As we can see in the above, the Kidneys' primary function is to store *jing*. Through *mingmen*'s transformation of *jing*, *yuan qi* is created. The Kidneys are thereby the root of all *yin* and *yang* in the body. Kidney *yin* and *yang* are therefore termed, respectively, the primary *yin* and the primary *yang* in the body. This means that the Kidneys influence all organs and all physiological processes in the body. A weakening of one of the Kidneys' aspects will have a decisive influence on the rest of the body. Conversely, due to the fact that the Kidneys are nourished by the post-heaven *qi*, a chronic *xu* (deficiency) condition in another organ will end up having a debilitating effect on the Kidneys.

The Kidneys are also unique amongst the internal organs. This is because the Kidneys are the only organ that have no *shi* (excess) patterns of imbalance and can only have *xu* states. Most of the Kidneys' functions relate to *jing*, *mingmen* and *yuan qi*. The condition of these and the condition of the Kidneys are therefore inextricably linked. This means that the treatment of these aspects and the treatment of the Kidneys will be more or less identical. The Kidneys have a determining influence on our reproductive abilities – not only fertility, but also potency and libido. The Kidney *jing* aspect is also reflected in the body's physical development and ageing processes. Another major area of influence is fluid physiology, where the Kidneys' *yang yuan qi* has a determining influence on most of the processes. Furthermore, it is the Kidney *yang* aspect that has the task of not only holding the urine in the bladder, but also expelling the urine out of the bladder. The functions and relationships of the Kidneys can be summarised as follows.

The Kidneys

- store *jing*
- are located in the same area of the body as *mingmen*
- are the root of the post-heaven *qi*
- produce marrow and control bones
- manifest in the teeth and hair
- control water
- control the lower orifices
- control the receiving of *qi*
- open to the ears
- control hearing
- control saliva
- are affected by Cold

- hate Dryness
- are affected by the salty flavour
- manifest with a putrid odour
- manifest with a complaining, moaning voice
- are affected by, and manifest with, the black-blue colour
- are weakened by standing too much
- are weakened by lifting
- are the residence for *zhi*
- have wisdom as their virtue
- are influenced by, and manifest with, fear

The Kidneys store jing

The Kidneys are the place in the body where *jing* is stored. As we saw earlier, Kidney *jing* has two aspects: a pre-heaven *jing* aspect, which is created at conception from the union of both parents' *jing*, and a post-heaven *jing* aspect, which is created from the surplus of the daily production of *qi* and *xue*. Kidney *jing* is created by the interaction of these two aspects. Like the pre-heaven *jing*, Kidney *jing* is stored in the Kidneys, but Kidney *jing* also circulates around the body, especially in the eight extraordinary channels.

Kidney *jing* can be seen manifesting in the bones, the ears, the hair on the head and in the teeth. A person with Kidney *jing xu* can therefore have weak teeth, brittle or poorly developed bones, a balding head or thin hair and small ears. In general, *jing* has a determining influence on a person's fundamental strength and constitution. A person with strong *jing* will have a solid constitution. They will be generally healthy and strong. On the other hand, a person who is *jing xu* will often have a more fragile health. Physically, they will not have the same strength and endurance as other people have. *Jing* is also the foundation of *shen*. A person with a weak *jing* can have problems with their memory, concentration and intellectual abilities in general. Due to the fact that *jing* has a fundamental influence on our physical strength and mental abilities, it is said that 'the Kidneys control strength and skill'. *Jing* determines an individual's growth from the fertilised egg through childhood and adolescence and in adulthood. This means that the condition of Kidney *jing* has a decisive influence on our basic constitution, our ability to reproduce and our development throughout life. It is through the cycles of Kidney *jing* that our bodies develop and change. *Jing* has seven- and eight-year cycles for women and men respectively. These cycles have been described earlier in the chapter on *jing* (page 72). While Kidney *jing* is the foundation of our lives and the basis for our development throughout life, *jing* is also the foundation for the continuation of life in the next generation. When *jing* is transformed by Heart Fire, *tian gui* (Heavenly Water) is created. *Tian gui* manifests as sperm in men and eggs in women. This means that a person who is Kidney *jing xu* may well have problems with their fertility. *Jing* is waning throughout our lives and it is one of the factors that determines the ageing process and impairment in old age. When *jing* declines, the hair starts to grey and begins to fall out, the teeth become loose, the bones weaken, the hearing fades, the memory weakens and we lose our potency and fertility. This is experienced by everyone. It is not a question of whether our *jing* becomes weaker. It is a question of how quickly and how much it weakens. The quantity and quality of the *jing* that has been present from the beginning is of great importance, but one's lifestyle is of equal importance. *Jing* is consumed by living beyond one's means, by using more *qi* than can be produced, by burning the candle at both ends. The Chinese also believe that, when men ejaculate, they lose *jing*, as semen is *jing*. Daoists therefore developed various sexual practices to withhold the sperm. This is also why sexual abstinence is recommended for men with Kidney *xu* conditions. The general opinion is that *jing* cannot be replaced when it is lost, as it is something you inherit from your parents. However, a person can make sure that they do not consume more of their *jing* than necessary through their lifestyle and by making sure that they get enough rest, as well as peace and quiet. A person can also optimise and improve the quality of the *jing* they have by optimising the production of the post-heaven *jing* and by practising *tai ji*, yoga and *qi gong*.

The Kidneys are located in the same area of the body as mingmen

In addition to storing *jing*, which is the fundamental aspect of *yin* in the body, the Kidneys are also the place where *mingmen*, the fundamental *yang*, is to be found. In older Chinese medical texts, the two individual Kidneys were regarded as two separate organs. The right Kidney was considered to be *mingmen*, whilst the left Kidney was the actual Kidney itself. This conception is still apparent in the pulse positions. The right *chi* (proximal) pulse position is used in some pulse systems to assess the condition of the Kidney *yang* aspect, whilst the left *chi* pulse position is used to assess the quality of the Kidney *yin*.

Mingmen is the source of physiological fire in the body. Without *mingmen* fire, no transformation could take place in the body and all of the body's physiological processes would grind to a halt. *Mingmen*'s transformation of *jing* creates *yuan qi*, which is the motivating *qi* that all the organs in the body depend upon to carry out their functions. At the same time, *yuan qi* is the catalyst that is essential in the production of *qi* and *xue*, as well as being used in all the processes related to the production of *jinye*. *Mingmen* warms the lower *jiao* and the Urinary Bladder. Without *mingmen* heat all activity in the lower *jiao* would stop. This is particularly important for the Kidneys' and Urinary Bladder's transformation of *jinye* and in the production, storage and excretion of urine. *Mingmen* warms the Spleen and Stomach, so the Stomach can 'rot and ripen' the ingested food and the Spleen can transform and transport it. Spleen *yang* is particularly dependent on support from the *mingmen* when it transforms the food in the Stomach. *Mingmen* has a crucial influence on our sexual functions and on our ability to reproduce. The *bao* must be warm enough for fertilisation to take place. *Yang* heat is required to transform *jing*. This has implications for both men's and women's fertility. Without *yang* heat, *jing* would not be transformed into sperm and the sperm would not have the necessary movement and activity that it should have. This means that men whose sperm has poor motility will often be Kidney *yang xu* and have a weak *mingmen*. Women need the heat from *mingmen* fire to mature eggs and to release the ovum at ovulation. *Yang* heat is also used when the released egg travels through the fallopian tubes. The heat is necessary to dilute or dissolve the mucus within the fallopian tubes so that the egg can pass freely through them. Heat from *mingmen* is also used to keep pathological Cold out of the *bao*. This is necessary, as Cold would otherwise create stagnation, blocking the two *jing* from connecting and merging in the woman's *bao*. If fertilisation does take place, the Cold can block *qi* and *xue* from circulating freely, preventing the egg from getting the nutrition that is necessary to be able to develop.

It is not just the ability to reproduce that is affected by the *mingmen*. Sexuality in general is influenced by *mingmen*. When a person is sexually aroused, *mingmen* fire flares up. This is seen in the increase in body temperature during sexual arousal, which manifests with an increase in colour in the cheeks, lips, nails, etc. There is an increased circulation of blood in the genitals. If *mingmen* is weak, the person's libido may also be weak. Furthermore, a man is physically dependent on heat from the *mingmen* to force *xue* out into his penis to create an erection. Consequently, a condition of pathological Heat can mean that some people have an exaggerated sex drive. Because Kidney *yang* is dependent on *mingmen*, the relationship between the lower and upper *jiao* can be affected by a weak *mingmen*. Kidney *yang* must grasp the *qi* that is sent down from the Lung. If this function is impaired, the person could have difficulty breathing, especially on inhalation. The Heart and *shen* are also dependent on the heat of *mingmen* fire. A weak *mingmen* can result in a person being apathetic, mentally lethargic or depressed. Pathological Fire on the other hand could mean that a person is manic.

The Kidneys are the root of the post-heaven qi

As described above, *yuan qi* is created when *mingmen* transforms *jing*. *Yuan qi* is indispensable in all the physiological processes involved in the creation of *qi*, *xue* and *jinye*. The Kidneys are therefore the pre-heavenly root of the post-heaven *qi*. A weakening of either *mingmen* or *jing* will have a decisive impact on the production of *qi* and *xue* in particular.

The Kidneys produce marrow and control bones

Both the Bones and Bone Marrow are classified as extraordinary *fu* organs. These organs have the structure of a *fu* organ, but at the same time store 'treasured substances'. They both have a very close relationship to *jing* and thereby also to the Kidneys. Bone Marrow is directly created by *jing*, and in Chinese medicine it is the Marrow that creates the Bones. This is because the Bone Marrow, like so many other organs and body substances, is something different from and greater than it is in Western physiology. A person with Kidney *jing xu* may have weak bones. This can be seen, for example, in elderly people who are Kidney *jing xu*. They often have osteoporosis and their bones are generally more fragile than the bones of younger people.

The Bone Marrow – and thereby Kidney *jing* – also has a profound influence on another of the extraordinary *fu* organs, the Brain. The Brain is considered to be a flower on top of the stem that is the spinal cord. This means that the Brain is created by Kidney *jing*. Again we can see the influence *jing* has on our mental capacities and abilities. In old age *jing xu* can manifest as conditions such as dementia and Alzheimer's or just a poor memory. *Jing xu* can also be congenital, such as in Down's Syndrome.

The Kidneys manifest in the teeth and hair

Each internal organ manifests in an aspect of the body's external structure. This means that by observing these structures, one can assess the condition of the various internal organs. The Liver manifests in the fingernails, the Spleen in the lips, etc. The state of the Kidneys can be observed in a person's hair and in their teeth. The hair on the scalp is created by *jing*. This can be seen in younger people generally having a stronger growth of hair on their heads than older people do. That's because the older we get, the less *jing* there is to create the hair on the head. However, it is important to remember that *xue* also nourishes the hair and that pathogenic Heat can scorch the roots of the hair. Therefore, these can also be factors in hair loss.

The teeth are also created by *jing*. As a consequence, the condition of *jing* can be observed in a person's teeth. On entering the second *jing* cycle, seven- or eight-year-olds lose their milk teeth and the permanent teeth emerge. At the transition from the third to the fourth *jing* cycle, the wisdom teeth emerge. When *jing* weakens and a person grows old, their teeth become loose and start to fall out. The fact that a person's fundamental constitution can be gauged through the teeth and bones is something that slave traders utilised in their time (and horse traders still do) when determining which individual to buy. Strong teeth and thick bones are a sign of a strong constitution.

The Kidneys control water

The Kidneys have a very close relationship to water and body fluids in general. *Yuan qi*, which is created in the Kidneys, is involved in all the various processes involved in the production of *jinye*. The transportation of *jinye* through the *san jiao* is also dependent on *yuan qi* and thereby Kidney *yang*.

The Urinary Bladder is especially dependent on Kidney *yang* to carry out its functions. The impure fluids sent to the Urinary Bladder from the Lung and the Small Intestine are transformed by Kidney *yang* in the Urinary Bladder, and the pure fluids are sent up through the body again. The impure residue that remains is stored in the Urinary Bladder as urine. The urine is held within the Urinary Bladder by Kidney *yang*. Kidney *yang xu* can therefore manifest with incontinence. When the urine is to be expelled from the body, Kidney *yang* is again the active force that drives the urine out. A weak stream of urine and difficulty emptying the bladder may be a sign of Kidney *yang xu*.

The Kidneys also have a significant influence on sweat. The production of sweat is dependent on Kidney *yang*. *Yuan qi* and Kidney *yang* are directly involved in the transformation of the impure and untransformed fluids that sweat is an aspect of. *Wei qi*, which has its roots in the Kidneys, is also used to control the sweat pores. If the Kidneys and *wei qi* are *xu*, a person can have difficulty keeping the sweat pores closed and the person will experience spontaneous sweating and perspiration even during light activity.

The Kidneys control the lower orifices

It is said that the Kidneys control the lower orifices in the body. A similar statement is: 'The Kidneys control opening and closing.' The orifices in the lower part of the body that these statements refer to are the urinary tract, the anus and the vagina. This controlling of the lower orifices is an aspect of Kidney *yang*. It is an active process in which the Kidneys ensure that there is no involuntary leakage out of the body. As seen above, Kidney *yang* is used to keep the urine in the Urinary Bladder, and Kidney *yang xu* may lead to involuntary urination and incontinence. The Kidneys' failure to control the anus can be seen in older people who are very Kidney *yang xu* and can no longer control their bowel movements and suffer from faecal incontinence. Furthermore, one can see that fear, which weakens the Kidneys and has a powerful downward dynamic, can cause involuntary urination and defecation.

The vagina is also under the influence of Kidney *yang*. Kidney *yang xu* can therefore lead to excessive vaginal discharge.

Kidney *yang* is also necessary to keep the *bao* closed. Kidney *yang xu* can be the cause of menstrual bleeding irregularities and involuntary abortions. In men, Kidney imbalances lead to involuntary or premature ejaculation from the *bao*.

The Kidneys control the receiving of qi

Kidney *yang* grasps the *qi* that is sent down from the Lung. Kidney *yang xu* can therefore result in the *qi* that is sent down from the upper *jiao* not being grasped and anchored. This will result in breathing difficulties where the person has problems on inhalation.

The Kidneys open to the ears

The ears' outer structure consists of cartilage, which is created from Kidney *jing*. This in turn means that you can assess the condition of Kidney *jing* from the ears' structure. Strong Kidney *jing* will be seen in the ears not being too small and in the cartilage feeling firm when squeezed. It is not only the ears' structure, but also especially the ears' function, that is influenced by the Kidneys. Problems such as deafness and tinnitus can often result from Kidney *yin xu* or Kidney *jing xu*. However, it is important to remember that other organs such as the Liver and other channels, especially the *san jiao* and Gall Bladder channels, also affect the ears.

The Kidneys control hearing

As we have just seen, it is not only the ears' structure, but also their function, that is under the influence of Kidney *jing*. This means that the sense of hearing is attributed to the Water Phase in Chinese medicine. Conditions of Kidney *yin xu* and Kidney *jing xu* can manifest with disorders such as deafness, poor hearing and tinnitus. This is typically seen in old age, when *jing* has diminished and poor hearing and deafness are therefore more common.

The Kidneys control saliva

The Kidneys control the thick saliva (*tuo*). Thick saliva is differentiated from the thin saliva (*xian*) created by the Spleen. *Tuo* is used to support digestion. It is said that *tuo* is produced under the tongue, where the inner branch of the Kidney channel terminates.

The Kidneys are affected by Cold

The Water Phase is the most extreme *yin* aspect of the transformation cycle. It is winter in the seasonal cycle and it is the darkest and coldest time of day. This means that the various aspects of the Water Phase will have a special resonance with coldness. When the Kidneys are in balance, their *yin* aspect has a cooling effect on the rest of the body, especially the Heart's Fire aspect.

On the other hand, pathological Cold has a detrimental effect on Kidney *yang*, which is the fundamental warming aspect of the body. If a person experiences repeated invasions of Cold, this will have a debilitating effect on Kidney *yang*. It is especially important to keep the lumbar region warm and protected from the cold and draughts.

Food and beverages that are cold in their temperature or energy will primarily weaken Spleen *yang*, but in the long term this will also have a negative effect on *mingmen* and Kidney *yang*.

The Kidneys hate Dryness

Dryness is the climatic influence that resonates with the Metal Phase. Even so, it is said that the Kidneys hate Dryness. This is because Dryness damages *yin* and *yin*'s ability to moisten the body. The Kidneys are the fundamental *yin* organ in the body, and they will therefore be strained when *yin* in the body is damaged.

The Kidneys are affected by the salty flavour

The salty flavour is related to the Kidneys and to the Water Phase in general. The sea, which is representative of the Water Phase, has a salty taste. Urine created by the Water Phase's internal organs also tastes of salt. Food with a salty flavour has an affinity with the Kidneys, and the salty flavour can be used to affect the Kidneys.

The Kidneys manifest with a putrid odour

The smell the body can have if the Kidneys are imbalanced is called *fu* in Chinese. This translates into English as 'putrid'. The Chinese character is composed of two components. The first character represents a building or shed and the second component meat hanging to dry. This gives the ideogram the characteristic of the smell that will be in a shed that is used to dry meat. The odour will characteristically be quite sharp. Ammonia and chlorine have this characteristic.

The Kidneys manifest with a complaining, moaning voice

This voice, which is heard when the Kidneys are out of balance, is a very flat voice, lacking in tonal variation. The voice also sounds like it is about to break into tears. It is the opposite of the Fire Phase voice, which is full of joy and laughter.

The Kidneys are affected by, and manifest with, the black-blue colour

Black, dark blue or midnight blue are the colours that are attributed to the Water Phase. The colour of the Water Phase is dark and cool. This colour is the same as is seen in the oceans and in the night sky. By virtue of its resonance with the Water Phase, dark blue and black have a tonifying effect on the Kidneys. Conversely, this colour is sometimes seen manifesting in the skin when there are Kidney imbalances. For example, dark circles under the eyes are often indicative of a Kidney *xu* condition. If the skin here is moist, it is more likely that the condition is one of Kidney *yang xu*. In Kidney *yin xu* the skin under the eyes will also be dark, but this time it will be more dryish.

Cold, which is an aspect of the Water Phase, can also cause the skin of the body to become bluish.

The Kidneys are weakened by standing too much

The body position that is most detrimental for the Kidneys is standing upright. This is typically seen in people who are Kidney *xu*, when they stand for long periods of time. These people will often report that they easily get tired in the lower back and in their knees. The lumbar region and the knees are both areas where the Kidneys have a special influence. People with Kidney *xu* conditions often suffer from aches and fatigue in the lower back and knees. This is partly due to a branch of the Kidney channel running through the lumbar vertebrae. Furthermore, the extraordinary channels *du mai*, *ren mai* and *chong mai* have their origin between the Kidneys. All these channels also pass through the lumbar vertebrae. Furthermore, the Kidneys' partner channel, the Urinary Bladder, also passes through the lumbar muscles. People whose work consists of having to stand up all day will therefore have an increased tendency to be Kidney *xu*.

The Kidneys are weakened by lifting

Lifting heavy objects has a draining effect on the Kidneys' *yang* aspect. This means that people whose work involves a lot of lifting and carrying heavy loads will have an increased tendency to be Kidney *yang xu* and Kidney *qi xu*.

The Kidneys are the residence for zhi

Willpower, or *zhi* in Chinese, has its residence in the Kidneys. If the Kidneys are strong, we have the will to implement the projects we create in our minds, i.e. the projects that the Liver and the *hun* have visualised and planned. Without *zhi*, *hun* would just be a creator of empty ideas that never come to fruition. *Zhi* gives us stability so that we keep to our path and do not start to run after each new idea. It anchors us.

There is also a close relationship between the Spleen *yi* and the Kidneys' *zhi*. *Yi* is intention, which is used to focus *qi*, but in order to complete a project this requires persistence.

Zhi can also be seen in the will to live. It is the desire to grow that is seen in germination. The seedling is determined in its growth up towards the light. It is also the determination to continue life and to procreate that is manifested in sexual desire.

The Chinese character *zhi* also has an aspect of memory. This makes sense when we take into account the fact that the Brain is nurtured and created by *jing*. As stated earlier, one can see problems with memory, particularly short-term memory, when *jing* is weakened.

The Kidneys have wisdom as their virtue

The Kidneys' virtue is wisdom and insight. This is both because *zhi* has a relationship to the storage of information and because *jing* is the material foundation for *shen*. There is a direct correlation throughout life between *jing* and *shen*. Furthermore, the Kidneys are regarded as the gate between life and death. This is because the Water Phase is both the start and the end of a lifecycle. When we see ourselves as part of a larger cycle, we will be able to escape the fear of death. By transforming our fear of death, we become wise.

The Kidneys are influenced by, and manifest with, fear

Fear, or *kong* in Chinese, affects Kidney *qi*. The energetic dynamic of fear causes *qi* in the body to sink downwards. This is seen clearly when people, especially children, are afraid and temporarily lose control of their bladder or in extreme cases their bowels. Here, the downward movement of *qi* caused by fear, together with fear's weakening of the Kidneys, results in the Kidneys no longer being able to keep the 'lower orifices' closed.

On the other hand, Kidney *xu* conditions can result in a person being overly fearful. It can manifest as conditions such as anxiety, OCD, paranoia, etc. or in a person just being extremely cautious and having a tendency to see signs of danger all around them.

The Kidneys' relationship to other organs

The Kidneys and the Heart

This is the fundamental relationship between Fire and Water, between the upper and lower *jiao* and between *yin* and *yang* in the body. The Kidneys and *jing* in the lower *jiao* are corporeal aspects of the Water Phase. They thereby constitute the ultimate *yin* in the body. The Heart and *shen* in the upper *jiao* are the corporeal aspects of the Fire Phase and thus the ultimate *yang* in the body. The *yin* aspects of the Kidneys are both an anchor for, but also the basis of, *shen*. *Shen* manifests the potential that *jing* contains. *Jing* is the material foundation that roots and nurtures the ethereal *shen*. A strong *jing* is a necessity for a strong and stable *shen*. In turn, a weak or disturbed *shen* will not control *jing* and the person will feel exhausted and lack motivation.

It is said that 'Fire and Water engender each other'. By this it is meant that Kidney *yin* rises to the upper *jiao* to nourish Heart *yin*. Kidney *yin* also helps to control and cool the Heart's *yang* aspects. Fire from the Heart descends to the lower *jiao*, where it warms and activates Kidney *yin*.

The menstrual cycle is also dependent on communication between Heart Fire and Kidney Water. This cooperation influences the transformations from *yang* to *yin* and *yin* to *yang* that occur throughout the menstrual cycle. There is a direct connection from the Heart to the Uterus (*bao*) via the internal channel called *bao mai*. A second internal channel, *bao luo*, connects the Kidney and the *bao*. The Heart ensures that the *bao* opens at the correct moments during the cycle, whilst the Kidneys ensure that *bao* closes at other times during the cycle.

Kidney *yang* plays a pivotal role in most of the aspects of fluid physiology. The Heart can be negatively affected by the accumulations of fluids, which can be the result of Kidney *yang xu*.

The Heart and Kidneys are also connected to each other via the *shaoyin* channel, which they both form a part of.

The Kidneys and the Lung

The Lung and the Kidneys cooperate with each other, both with regards to respiration and with fluid physiology.

When we breathe in, the Lung sends *qi* downwards through the body to the Kidneys, which grasp the *qi*. For this cooperation to function optimally, both organs' *qi* must be strong enough. At the same time, the *qi* of the Lung must not be blocked by exogenous *xie qi*, Phlegm or other stagnations. If the Kidneys or the Lung are disturbed in this cooperation, dyspnoea can result.

The Kidneys and the Lung's collaboration in fluid physiology consists of the Lung sending impure fluids down from the upper *jiao* to the Urinary

Bladder, where they are transformed by Kidney *yang*. In return the Kidney *yang* sends clear fluids up to the Lung, keeping the Lung moist so it does not dry out. Lung imbalances can lead to oedema and to urinary problems. Kidney imbalances can result in the Lung drying out and thus becoming *yin xu*. *Zong qi* and *yuan qi*, which have a close relationship to the Lung and Kidneys respectively, also have a relationship with each other. *Yuan qi* ascends to the upper *jiao* to transform *zong qi* to *zhen qi*. *Zong qi* descends to the lower *jiao*, where it helps to nourish *yuan qi* and assist the Kidneys in their functions.

The Kidneys and the Spleen

The Spleen and Kidneys' relationship is a reflection of the relationship between pre- and post-heaven *qi*. The Kidneys and Spleen are mutually dependent on each other and help to strengthen and nurture one another. Kidney *yang*, *mingmen* and *yuan qi* are all involved in the production of *qi* and *xue*, as is Spleen *qi*. Spleen *yang* is supported by Kidney *yang* and *mingmen*. Without these the Spleen's physiological fire would peter out, and the transformation and transport of *qi* and *jinye* would break down. The Spleen's production of *gu qi* is, for its part, the beginning of the post-heaven *qi* production cycle. Post-heaven *qi* nourishes and replenishes the pre-heaven *jing*. Kidney *jing* is therefore dependent on the Spleen's *qi* production.

The Spleen and the Kidneys are both involved in the transformation and transportation of *jinye*. A *xu* condition in one or the other can lead to oedema, diarrhoea or urinary imbalances.

The Kidneys and the Liver

The relationship between the Kidneys and the Liver is a reflection of the relationship between *jing* and *xue*, which mutually nourish each other. It is said that Liver and Kidney *yin* have a common root. This can be seen in a *yin xu* condition in one of these organs, which is usually accompanied by a *yin xu* condition in the other. Similarly, Liver *xue xu* can often lead to Kidney *yin xu*, as Liver *xue* is an aspect of the Liver *yin* and because Liver *xue* should nourish Kidney *jing*.

The Kidneys and the Urinary Bladder

The Urinary Bladder and the Kidneys have a close functional relationship with regard to fluid physiology. Kidney *yang* is responsible for several of the processes that the Urinary Bladder is involved in.

The Urinary Bladder is, for example, responsible for storing and expelling urine from the body. Kidney *yang* actively holds the urine in the Urinary Bladder so that there is not involuntary or uncontrolled urination. This is one of the ways in which 'the Kidneys control the lower orifices'. Kidney *yang* is also used by the Urinary Bladder to expel the urine out of the Urinary Bladder upon urination.

Furthermore, the final transformation of the fluids in the body is a process that takes place in the Urinary Bladder but is carried out by Kidney *yang*. It is also Kidney *yang* that sends the pure fluids from this transformation up from the Urinary Bladder to form sweat.

The Kidneys and the Stomach

The Stomach is the root of *jinye* in the body. This is because it is in the Stomach that the initial and greatest transformation of the ingested liquids takes place. Kidney *yin* will be negatively affected if the Stomach does not perform this role properly. Chronic Stomach *yin xu* can lead to Kidney *yin xu*. Stomach *yin* for its part is dependent on Kidney *yin*.

The Kidneys and the Small Intestine and the Large Intestine

The Small Intestine and the Large Intestine are dependent on *yuan qi* to carry out their functions with regard to fluid physiology.

THE SPLEEN

The Spleen is a problematical organ when discussing Chinese medicine with people who are brought up with Western medicine's conception of anatomy and physiology. In Western medicine the Spleen has nothing to do with the digestive process. In Western medicine physiology the Spleen is mainly responsible for the filtering of blood and is a part of the immune system. In Chinese medicine, on the other hand, the Spleen is considered to be one of the most important organs with regard to transforming the food that has been consumed into *qi* and *xue*.

The Spleen's role in extracting nutrients from the food has led some Western writers to be of the opinion that when the Chinese refer to the Spleen, they are in reality referring to the pancreas. Some books even go so far as to term the Spleen the Spleen/pancreas. I personally believe this is a mistake. In Chinese medicine the physical form and structure of an organ is of limited importance. The organ's functions and activities, its relationships to other organs and its relationship to the vital substances are what is weighted in Chinese medicine. An organ is defined more by its functions and activities and less on the basis of its structure and form.

I do not dispute that many of the functions of the pancreas can be related to the Spleen in Chinese medicine. The pancreas plays a central role in the digestion of food, and the pancreas has a special relationship to the sweet taste through the secretion of insulin and the regulation of sugar levels in the blood. But there are also other organs and substances in Western medicine that are involved in the transformation of food to nutrients and the subsequent absorption of these. You could therefore say that the Chinese medicine Spleen also encompasses the gastric enzymes, the enzymes that are in the saliva, the hormones that are excreted in the duodenum and which stimulate the pancreas's release of digestive enzymes, the wall of the small intestine and not least the intestinal flora.

Furthermore, the Spleen is responsible for many other functions that are not related to digestion. The Spleen holds *xue* within the blood vessels, it prevents the prolapse of the inner organs, it contributes to mental abilities such as learning and memory, it influences emotional states such as worrying and pensiveness, it is involved in fluid physiology and it has a significant influence on the mouth and lips. All of these are things that the pancreas has nothing to do with in Western physiology.

In reality, it does not matter what names are used in our own model, as long as the model itself is consistent and logical. It only becomes a problem when we have to communicate with others whose terminology is based on another system. We have already seen that terminology in general is a problem when discussing Chinese medicine in a Western medicine context, as we operate with concepts such as *qi, shen* and *jing*, which have no counterparts in the Western model. That does not mean that it is not possible to see parallels between models. On the contrary, a great many of the processes in the Western medicine model can in fact be understood from a

Chinese medicine perspective. Initially though, it is usually an advantage to let go of the Western medicine model entirely for a while whilst learning Chinese medicine. Later it is no problem at all to understand the one system when viewing it through the prism of the other.

The functions of the Spleen

The Spleen and the Stomach are the crankshaft in the centre of the body. They are the engine room. It is here that energy for the rest of the system is produced. The Spleen does not have as fine a title as many of the other *zang* organs. It even has to share its court title with its partner organ, the Stomach. Together they have the title of 'officials with responsibility for storage and granaries'. Even though their title is not that fine, their work is of great importance. Without them, the population would starve to death and the Empire would collapse.

The Spleen and the Stomach are the central organs in the middle of the body. They are the axle in the centre of the body's wheel. Their mutual *qi ji* is of crucial importance for the movement of all *qi* in the body. The Spleen sends its *qi* upwards and the Stomach sends its *qi* downwards. Just like the edges of a wheel, both sides are dependent on the movement of the other.

By virtue of their location in the middle *jiao*, the Earth Phase organs have considerable influence on the body's vertical Fire-Water axis. The relationship and link between the fundamental *yin*, which is Water, and Fire, which is the most extreme *yang*, is of great importance. There are countless examples of how Fire and Water control and activate each other, of how *jing* and *shen* are mutually dependent on each other and how Kidney *yin* must nourish Heart *yin* so that Heart *yang* is controlled. All of this cooperation and communication has to pass through the middle *jiao*. If the Spleen is in imbalance and there arises Dampness or if the Spleen and the Liver relationship becomes pathological, this communication up and down through the body will be disturbed. This relationship between the three *jiao* and the Three Treasures (*jing*, *qi* and *shen*) is a reflection of the relationship between Heaven, Earth and Man, where Heaven and Earth are connected through Man.

In the same way that the Kidneys in the lower *jiao* and the Heart in the upper *jiao* have a close relationship to *jing* and *shen*, the Spleen has a close relationship to the third of the Three Treasures, *qi*. The Spleen is the post-heavenly root of *qi*. The Spleen creates *gu qi* from the food that has been consumed. This is why the Spleen has the title of the 'official responsible for storage and granaries'. The granaries are the place where grain is stored, but also the place from which the grain is distributed to the rest of the realm. The Spleen ensures that the fruit of the spring and summer's growth is utilised optimally.

It is not only on the physical level that the Spleen transforms. In the same way that food is transformed into *qi*, impressions and information are transformed into knowledge and understanding. *Shen* is nourished by *xue*, which is the fruit of the Spleen's efforts, and *shen* consciousness is supplied with the knowledge that the Spleen has transformed from the information that the body has received.

The functions and relationships of the Spleen can be summarised as follows.

The Spleen

- is the root of post-heaven *qi*
- transforms and transports *qi*
- transforms and transports *jinye*
- keeps *xue* inside the blood vessels
- raises clear *yang* upwards
- holds the organs up
- controls the muscles and the four limbs
- manifests in the lips
- opens to the mouth
- controls the sense of taste
- controls saliva

- relates to Dampness
- is affected by the sweet flavour
- manifests with the aromatic odour
- manifests with a singing voice
- is affected by, and manifests with, the yellow colour
- is overburdened by sitting too much
- has trust as its virtue
- is the residence of *yi*
- is affected by, and manifests with, worry, speculation and overthinking

---

The Spleen is the root of post-heaven qi

The Spleen's absolute most important function on the physical level is that, together with the Stomach, it transforms the coarse, unprocessed substances that have been ingested through the mouth into usable *qi*. This is the daily production of *qi*, which is used in the day-to-day functioning of the body and which supplements and nourishes the *jing* that has been inherited from the parents.[3] Furthermore, *shen* and *hun* are nourished and anchored by *xue*. This is why the Spleen's role in the body is so important. The Spleen's production of post-heaven *qi* affects all the organs and substances in the body. A key sign that the Spleen is not functioning optimally is therefore tiredness and a lack of energy.

The Spleen transforms and transports qi

The Stomach receives and temporarily stores the food and liquid that have been consumed. The Stomach 'ripens and rots' the food, thereby preparing it for the Spleen to transform it to *gu qi*. It is the Spleen's *yang* aspect, supported by *mingmen*, that transforms the coarse, unrefined food and liquids to this 'basis' *qi*, which is the root of *zhen qi* and *xue*. Because it is *yang* heat that transforms the food, Chinese medicine views raw fruit and vegetables (particularly salads), food that comes straight from the refrigerator and cold drinks as having a detrimental effect on the Spleen and the production of *qi*.[4] It is much more demanding for Spleen's *qi* and *yang* to transform food that has not been prepared and that is difficult to digest than it is to transform something that has been cooked and is easily digestible, such as porridge, soups and stews. Furthermore, things that are cold, both energetically and in their temperature, weaken the Spleen's *yang qi* and thus weaken the transformation of food to *qi*.

The Spleen has the task of separating the pure and usable *qi* from the impure residue. The pure *qi* is sent upwards to the upper *jiao* by the Spleen, where further transformation will take place, until it becomes *zhen qi* and *xue*. Some of the pure, refined essences from the ingested food will be transported by the Spleen to the other *zang* organs. These essences, called *jing wei*, are the five flavours. The essence from the sour flavour goes to the Liver, the essence from the bitter flavour to the Heart, etc. The impure residue that is left is sent down by the Stomach to the Small Intestine, where there is a further separation of the pure and the impure. The Spleen's functions of transporting and transforming is called *yunhua* in Chinese. This function is of crucial importance for the energy levels, for the production of *xue* and thereby for all the body's physiological processes. Apart from resulting in a lack of *qi* and *xue*, a weakening or disruption of the Spleen will often also result in the production of Dampness and Phlegm, which will have a further disruptive effect on the Spleen because it will block its *qi ji*.

The Spleen transforms and transports jinye

It is not only the solid food that the Spleen transforms to usable *qi*. The Spleen also has the task of separating the pure from the impure fluids and transforming these to *jinye*. It is also the Spleen that transports these pure fluids up to the Lung, from where they are spread throughout the body.

The Spleen keeps xue inside the blood vessels

The Spleen has a very close relationship with *xue*. As well as being the fundamental *xue*-producing organ, the Spleen is also responsible for keeping *xue* inside the blood vessels. That is why it is said that 'the Spleen controls *xue*'. This sounds almost identical to the Heart's function of 'governing *xue*'. The difference lies in the fact that the Spleen's controlling function is to keep *xue* inside the blood vessels, whereas the Heart's governing function is to maintain a regular, harmonic and rhythmic movement of *xue* through the vessels. If the Spleen is weak and does not carry out its function, there can be spontaneous bleeding and a tendency to bruising. An imbalance of the Heart will more probably manifest with an irregular pulse, a weak pulse or a pounding pulse.

The Spleen raises clear yang upwards

The Spleen raises and sends *qi* upwards from the middle *jiao*. It is the pure essences from that which has been ingested that is sent up through the body. If the Spleen is weak or if there is impure *yin*, i.e. Dampness mixed in with the pure *yang*, then the pure *yang* will not be able to ascend to the head. This can result in a person feeling that their sensory organs are dull or blocked, their vision is blurred, their sense of smell is reduced, their hearing is poor or everything tastes bland. A lack of pure *yang* in the head can result in an empty feeling in the head or dizziness. If impure *yin* travels up to the head with the pure *yang*, there can be a heavy headache and a fuzzy feeling in the head and difficulty thinking.

The Spleen holds the organs up

The ascending dynamic of the Spleen's *qi* enables the Spleen to keep organs and structures in place in the body. This means that when there is Spleen *qi xu* and Spleen *yang xu*, a person can experience a heavy, dragging sensation in the body, especially during menstruation. There can also be a slumped posture or haemorrhoids. If the Spleen is very weak, there may be prolapse of organs or hernias.

The Spleen controls the muscles and the four limbs

The Spleen has an influence on the muscles in general and the muscles of the arms and legs in particular. By being the root of the post-heaven *qi*, the Spleen creates the *qi* and *xue* that develop and maintain the muscles. Spleen *qi xu* can therefore manifest as underdeveloped and weak muscles. This will first and foremost be seen in the limbs. As well as this being visually observable from the outside, the person will also have a sense of weakness and fatigue in their limbs.

Spleen imbalances can also affect limbs in other ways. Spleen *qi xu* can result in Dampness or Damp-Heat. In these situations, a person can feel that their arms and legs are very heavy and, when there is Damp-Heat, there can also be soreness.

The Spleen manifests in the lips

The lips are a part of the mouth and therefore in the Spleen's sphere of influence. The condition of the Spleen can be observed here. The lips can, therefore, in the same way as the tongue, be used as a fairly precise diagnostic tool. Pale lips are often interpreted as being a sign of Spleen *qi xu*. The pale colour of the lips displays that there is not enough *xue* in the lips to give them their characteristic redness. This lack of *xue* is often a consequence of Spleen *qi xu*. The lack of *qi* will also mean that *qi* is not powerful enough to propel *xue* out to the extremities, also resulting in a lack of *xue* in the lips. *Xue xu* itself manifests with pale and dry lips, whereas other *xue* imbalances, such as *xue* stagnation and *xue* Heat, manifest with blue/purple lips and red lips respectively.

The Spleen opens to the mouth

The Stomach and Spleen open to the mouth. This is logical when one considers that the mouth is the start of the digestive canal. Food is macerated in the mouth as the first stage in the process of transformation.

The sense that is attributed to the Spleen is the sense of taste, and in Chinese medicine the mouth is involved in tasting the food. A manifestation of Spleen *qi xu* can be that a person lacks the ability to differentiate the various flavours. The pattern of imbalance known as Dampness, which is often related to Spleen *qi xu*, can manifest with a sticky sensation in the mouth.

The Spleen controls the sense of taste

In Western medicine, the sense of taste is mainly related to the tongue, which is the Heart's sense organ. Nevertheless, the sense of taste is attributed to the Spleen in Chinese medicine. This is because the Spleen controls the mouth and the oral cavity. The Heart has a determining influence on our sense of taste. This is because it is Heart *shen* that makes us aware of what we are tasting in the same way that *shen* makes us conscious of other sensations. Our sense of taste is also dependent on the nose, because the aromatic flavours are perceived in the nose. This means that some people who have a chronically impaired sense of taste will often have Phlegm-Dampness blocking their nose. Phlegm-Dampness is usually the result of Spleen imbalances, even though Phlegm-Dampness often manifests in the Lung. This has led to the following adage in Chinese medicine: 'Phlegm has its root in the Spleen, but is stored in the Lung.'

The Spleen controls saliva

The Spleen has a direct influence on the production of saliva, which is used to moisten the food and thereby make the food easier to transform. In Western medicine physiology, the saliva contains enzymes that initiate the digestive process. Chinese medicine physiology differentiates between watery saliva (*xian*), which is controlled by the Spleen, and the more thick and sticky saliva (*tuo*), which is an aspect of the Kidneys.

The Spleen relates to Dampness

There is a direct and negative relationship between the Spleen and Dampness. It is said that 'the Spleen loathes Dampness'. This is because conditions of Dampness in the body and an excessive intake of Damp-producing foods will burden the Spleen. The intrinsic nature of Dampness means that it will block the free movement of *qi*. This thereby impairs the Spleen's ability to send its *qi* upwards. In addition, rich, heavy foods with a Damp nature will be difficult for the Spleen to transform, thereby exhausting Spleen *qi* over time.

The Spleen also has a tendency to create Dampness when it is *qi xu*. This is because one of the Spleen's primary tasks is to separate the pure from the impure. The Spleen is like a sharp knife that cuts clean through, separating the two parts from each other. If the knife is blunt, there is not a clean cut and there is a lot of sludge where the two parts are mixed together. This means that a portion of the pure *qi* gets sent downwards along with the impure dregs, resulting in poor production of *qi* and *xue*. At the same time that some of the pure *qi* is being sent downwards and out of the body, murky Dampness that should have been sent downwards is getting sent upwards together with the pure *qi*. Dampness, due to its *yin* nature, will have a tendency to stagnate in the vicinity of where it is created. This means that Dampness from Spleen *qi xu* will initially collect in the middle *jiao*. Later on the Dampness will have a tendency to seep downwards to the lower *jiao*, due to its *yin* nature.

Invasions of exogenous Dampness can rapidly affect the Spleen and Stomach *qi ji*, resulting in nausea, vomiting or diarrhoea. Damp weather and humid conditions will often have a negative effect on people who have conditions of internal Dampness or Phlegm.

The Spleen is affected by the sweet flavour

The sweet flavour resonates with the Earth Phase and thereby with the Spleen. Most foods that we eat have a slightly sweet flavour. This can be difficult to discern for many people, because their taste buds have been overburdened by an excessive intake of sweets, cake, sugar, etc. Nevertheless, if a person chews a mouthful of rice, for example, for a couple of minutes they will often be able to taste how sweet it actually is.

The sweet flavour is necessary to produce *qi*, but as with everything in Chinese philosophy, a small amount of something is beneficial, while too much of the same thing has a negative effect. The Spleen is strengthened by the sweet flavour, but too much of the sweet flavour has a damaging effect on the Spleen.

A classic sign of Spleen *qi xu* is that a person has a craving for the sweet taste, which in some cases can be completely uncontrollable. That the body desires the sweet flavour is logical enough; it is the flavour that tonifies the Spleen. The problem lies in the intensity of the sweet flavour of the food. Whilst things such as rice, millet and root vegetables all have a sweet flavour and will thereby tonify the Spleen, many people consume sweets, chocolate, cake, etc. when the craving for something sweet arises. These very sweet substances are a strain on the Spleen, as they are difficult to transform due to their rich, cloying nature. They are even more difficult to transform if the Spleen is already weak. A vicious circle can soon arise in which a weak Spleen tries to recover by craving the consumption of something sweet but becomes overloaded, and thereby even weaker, when the person consumes foods that have a very concentrated sweet flavour.

It is also a problem for the Spleen that the sweet flavour has no directional dynamic. Whilst the spicy flavour sends *qi* upwards and outwards and the sour flavour causes *qi* to contract inwards, there is no movement or *qi* dynamic in the sweet flavour. This means that an excessive consumption of sweet-tasting food, or the consumption of food that has an extremely sweet flavour, will lead to a stagnation of *qi* in the middle *jiao.*

The Spleen manifests with the aromatic odour

The Chinese word *xiang* means 'aromatic'. This word is seen in the name of many aromatic herbs, for example *mu xiang* and *huo xiang.* Aromatic is in some ways a bit of a misnomer, as the odour that relates to the Spleen is a sticky, almost nauseating aroma. Lilies and hyacinths have this aroma. People with Phlegm-Dampness can report that they have an aversion to these flowers, as the fragrance of them compounds their Phlegm-Dampness and thereby aggravates some of their symptoms, such as nausea or heaviness in the head.

Skin diseases caused by Dampness can sometimes also have a sweet, sticky smell.

The Spleen manifests with a singing voice

The Spleen manifests with a singing voice. This is a voice that is varied in its tone. The tone fluctuates up and down. It is the voice that you would use when reading a story out loud. A voice that has either too much or too little of this quality will indicate a Spleen imbalance.

The Spleen is affected by, and manifests with, the yellow colour

The yellow colour resonates with the Earth Phase. Yellow is the dominant colour in the late summer, when corn matures. The yellow colour in general will have a beneficial effect on the Spleen. This can be seen, for example, in the way that many foods that are yellowish are viewed as Spleen tonics.

The yellow colour can also be a pathological sign and can sometimes be seen as a manifestation of certain Spleen imbalances, in particular patterns of Dampness and especially Damp-Heat. These patterns that often have their root in conditions of Spleen *qi xu* will often result in the skin of the face and the eyes turning yellowish.

The Spleen is overburdened by sitting too much

According to the relationships of the Five Phases, the posture that has a negative influence on the organs of the Earth Phase is the sitting position. This is mainly because when sitting still for long periods of time the lack of movement in the abdominal muscles will mean that the Spleen and Stomach are not physically supported in sending *qi* upwards and downwards. Even worse is when a person sits bent forwards or with a twisted midriff; this will physically impede the free passage of *qi* up and down in the middle *jiao.* This is one of the reasons that Spleen *qi xu* and its accompanying imbalances are so prevalent in our culture. Add to this the excessive consumption of wheat, dairy products and sugar, as well as people's tendency to worry, speculate and ruminate, all of which burden the Spleen. This is made worse again by the fact that many people not only have a sedentary job, but they also sit in a car to and from work. When they get home they then sit in front of the television or the computer.

The famous Chinese doctor Sun Si Miao (581–682 CE) placed great emphasis on the importance of lifestyle changes when treating diseases and disorders. Sun Si Miao recommended that you should take a walk of one hundred steps after a meal. He also said that you should not pedantically count the steps, as this in itself can lead to imbalance. The idea was that a light stroll would support the Spleen and the Stomach by creating a rhythmic movement of *qi* in the middle *jiao* through gentle physical activity. Heavy exertion, such as jogging or cycling, is not recommended after you have eaten, as it will consume *qi*, so there is less available for the Spleen's transformation processes. If it is not possible to take a light walk after eating, it can be a good idea to stand up and do some light stretching or just walk back and forth across the floor for a while.

The Spleen has trust as its virtue

The potential of the Spleen is trust, loyalty and reliability. When the Spleen is in balance, a person has confidence in themselves and the world around them. When the Spleen is weak, they can lose this basic trust and begin to worry and speculate too much about things. They no longer trust life itself.

The Spleen is the residence of yi

The Spleen's *shen* aspect is called *yi*. *Yi* can be defined as our mental faculties – our ntellectual focus. *Yi* enables us to digest information and helps us to integrate our experiences and impressions. This reflects, to a certain degree, the Spleen's functions on the physical level with regard to the transformation of the coarse food and liquids into refined and usable *qi* and *jinye*. *Yi* absorbs, sorts and digests the information we receive intellectually. In addition, *yi* is closely related to our ability to learn and store information. It is for this reason that it is so intimately associated with our intellectual capabilities.

Yi is also the aspect of us that can be translated as intention – the way in which we can focus our thoughts and our desires. For example, it is *yi* that is utilised when an acupuncturist performs various needling techniques. It is not so much the physical effects of the technique – whether the needle is rotated clockwise or anticlockwise a certain number of times, for example – it is more that by carrying out these instructions, the practitioner's *yi* is focussed and it is *yi* that then focuses and directs the practitioner's *qi*.

As well as reflection and pensiveness being a characteristic that *yi* has a significant influence on, there is also an aspect of spontaneity in *yi*. It is the spontaneity that arises upon comprehending a situation. When the mind is clear, focussed and without worry, we can then act with spontaneity.

The Spleen is affected by, and manifests with, worry, speculation and overthinking

When the Spleen is weak or burdened, it can be difficult to separate the pure from the impure, the usable from that which can't be used. This can mean that, on the physical level, the pure *qi* and the murky residue are not separated completely, creating Dampness. On the mental level, it can mean that relevant information and thoughts are not separated from irrelevant ones. This can result in worry, speculation and thinking in circles.

Conversely, constantly speculating, worrying, thinking in rings or studying for long periods, reading too much or being constantly intellectually active can be a strain on the *yi*. The Spleen will constantly be working overtime. It is also for this reason that it is not recommended that people watch television, read or work on the computer while they are eating or immediately afterwards. This is because the Spleen should use its *qi* to transform the food that has been consumed and not sort and transform information.

Summary of the functions of *yi*

- mental and intellectual focus
- intention
- thoughts and reflection
- informative learning

The Spleen's relationship to other organs

The Spleen and the Lung

The Spleen and the Lung have a close relationship. This is particularly evident in their roles in the production of post-heavenly *qi*. The Spleen separates the pure from the impure, both in the production of *gu qi* and in the production of *jinye*. These pure aspects are sent upwards by the Spleen to the Lung for further transformation. *Gu qi* is combined with *da qi* from the Lung to create *zong qi*, whilst the pure fluids that have been sent up from the Spleen are further transformed and subsequently distributed by the Lung. Because they are both directly involved in the production of *qi*, a *qi xu* condition in one of these organs will often lead to a *qi xu* condition in the other.

The Spleen and the Lung are both dependent on each other's *qi ji* in order to be able to send their *qi* upwards and downwards respectively. If the Lung is not capable of sending its *qi* downwards or the Spleen its *qi* upwards, this will have a negative effect on the other's ability to send its *qi* in the opposite direction. There will not be enough space for it, and so the *qi* will stagnate in either the middle or upper *jiao*.

Another example of how the two organs can affect each other negatively is seen in that Damp-Phlegm, which can be a consequence of Spleen *qi xu*, will often accumulate in the Lung. That is why it is said in Chinese that the 'Phlegm is produced in the Spleen, but stored in the Lung' and 'to treat Phlegm in the Lung, you must treat the Spleen'.

The Lung and Spleen relationship is also seen in their channel relationship. Both are part of the *taiyin* channel.

The Spleen and the Heart

The Spleen and the Heart cooperate in relation to *xue*. The Heart is the organ that governs *xue*, and Heart *shen* is anchored and nourished by *xue*. The Spleen is the organ that creates *gu qi*, which is the foundation of *xue*. This means that Spleen *qi xu* can lead to Heart *xue xu* with a resultant influence on the person's *shen*. This is something that is often seen in the clinic, especially in women. One of the major Chinese herbal prescriptions *Gui Pi Tang* focuses precisely on treating this combination of imbalances.

The Spleen and the Stomach

The relationships between some organ pairs can appear to be rather tenuous, whilst other pairs have a very close relationship. The Stomach and Spleen are almost inseparable in their functions – they are completely dependent on each other when performing their functions. The Stomach receives the food and liquids that have been consumed. The food 'rots and ripens' in the Stomach in preparation for the Spleen's transformation of it. If the Spleen does not transform the food, it will stagnate in the Stomach and create a pattern of imbalance known as food stagnation. The Stomach can be understood as being a cauldron that contains the ingredients of a soup. The Spleen is the flames below the pot. *Gu qi* are the vapours that rise up from the pot when the soup boils. Without the flames, the ingredients would remain raw and uncooked and there would not be any vapours rising up from the pot.

The Spleen and the Stomach are the first stage in the production of *jinye*. It is said that the Stomach is the root of *jinye*, because it is here that the initial and the greatest transformation of fluids takes place. The Spleen is the organ that is responsible for this transformation, and it is the Spleen that transports the pure fluids up and away from the Stomach.

The Spleen and the Stomach send *qi* in opposite directions. The Spleen sends the pure *qi* up and the Stomach sends the impure residue down. Both movements are partly dependent on the other organ sending its *qi* in the opposite direction. If the upward and downward movement of *qi* in the middle *jiao* is disturbed, there can be a loss of appetite, nausea, vomiting, abdominal pain and bloating of the upper abdomen.

In spite of their close relationship, and the fact they are inseparable in their functionality, there are some essential and fundamental differences between what they are affected by and how they thrive. It is said that the Spleen loathes Dampness. This is because Dampness will block the Spleen's *qi ji*. Dampness in this context includes food that has a Damp nature, which is often difficult to transform to *gu qi* and Dampness, as in a humid climate. The Spleen can also be 'drowned' by drinking too much liquid, especially at mealtimes. Too much liquid intake will extinguish the flames of the Spleen *yang*, so that the food is not transformed. The Stomach on the other hand is damaged by Dryness. This is because the Stomach has a tendency to overheat and dry out. This is reflected by Stomach Fire and Stomach *yin xu* being the two most common patterns of imbalance in the Stomach. Both of these conditions are characterised by the Stomach being too hot and either lacking *yin* moisture or Stomach *yin* being injured by the Heat. Because of its tendency to overheat and because of its need for *yin*, the Stomach is damaged by substances that are hot in their energy, such as chilli, pepper, alcohol, lamb, etc., or by foods that are drying, such as baked foods, crispbread, ricecakes, crackers, dry food, etc. The Spleen is harmed, however, by food that is cold, either in its temperature or its energy. Whereas lettuce, cucumber, melon, tomato and milk are cooling and thereby beneficial for the Stomach, especially when there is Stomach Fire or Stomach *yin xu*, they will have a detrimental effect on Spleen *yang*. Harmony between the two organs can be maintained by eating a predominantly neutral diet or a diet where the food is prepared and boiled, such as soups and stews. This food will be warm and already partly transformed. This will help the Spleen in its processes and at the same time it will nourish Stomach *yin*, because it is moist.

The Spleen and the Liver

The Spleen dynamic of sending *qi* upwards is supported by the Liver, which ensures that *qi* flows freely and without hindrance in the body and that *qi* flows in the right direction. When Liver *qi* stagnates, it often becomes rebellious and 'invades' the Spleen. This means that instead of supporting Spleen *qi*, the stagnated Liver *qi* disrupts and blocks Spleen *qi*. Therefore symptoms and signs relating to a disturbance of Spleen *qi* are so often seen when there is Liver *qi* stagnation. These could be symptoms and signs such as nausea, bloated stomach, abdominal pain, alternating diarrhoea and constipation, and oedema.

On the other hand, a stagnation of *qi* or Dampness in the middle *jiao* will disturb the Liver in its task of ensuring the free flow of *qi* throughout the body.

The Liver is dependent on the Spleen's production of *gu qi*, which is the raw material for *xue*. The Liver is a reservoir for *xue*. *Xue* is stored in the Liver when it is not being used by the body. The stored *xue* moistens and nourishes the Liver, ensuring the Liver does not become rigid and inflexible. If the Liver does become stiff, this will result in Liver *qi* stagnation. A vicious circle can quickly develop, where a stagnation of Liver *qi* disturbs the Spleen in its production of *gu qi*. This results in *xue xu*, which can lead to the Liver becoming rigid and inflexible, thereby creating Liver *qi* stagnation, which then invades the Spleen.

The Spleen and the Kidneys

The Spleen and the Kidneys' relationship is a reflection of the relationship between pre-heaven and post-heaven *qi*. Both are mutually dependent on the other, and each strengthens and nourishes the other. Kidney *yang*, *mingmen* and *yuan qi* are all involved in the production of *qi* and *xue*, as is Spleen *qi*. Spleen *yang* is supported by Kidney *yang* and *mingmen*. Without these the Spleen's fire would die out and the transformation and transportation of *qi* and *jinye* would grind to a halt. The Spleen's production of *gu qi* on the other hand is the start of the post-heavenly production of *qi*. Post-heaven *qi* nourishes and replenishes pre-heaven *jing*. This means that Kidney *jing* is dependent on the Spleen's production of *qi*.

The Spleen and Kidneys are both involved in the transformation and transportation of *jinye*. A *xu* condition in one or the other can lead to oedema in the body, diarrhoea and urinary imbalances.

THE LUNG

The Lung[5] is described as being a canopy in the top of the thorax. From this position in the upper *jiao*, the Lung rhythmically sends *qi* down through the whole body and through the channels and vessels. The Lung governs *qi* and respiration.

The Lung is also the boundary between the interior and the exterior. The skin and *wei qi*, which are under the influence of the Lung, protect the body against external influences and against exogenous *xie qi*. The Lung is the only *zang* organ that is in direct contact with the exterior. This is because the air from outside of the body passes directly into the Lung. It is through this interface that there is a constant exchange between the interior and the exterior. Pure air is absorbed, and the old, used air is eliminated from the body.

From its position at the top of the body the Lung receives the pure essences from other organs and it helps to send the impure residue downwards. The Lung has a particularly close cooperation with its partner organ, the Large Intestine, in relation to the excretion of the dross that is left behind after the separation processes involved in the production of *qi* and *jinye*.

As we will see later, it is not only on the physical level that the Lung helps the body to get rid of the old and used.

The position that the Lung has been assigned in the hierarchy of the internal organs is that of the 'Prime Minister with responsibility for regulation'. This is a reflection of the close relationship between the Lung and the Heart, both physically and functionally. In the governing of a realm, there is a close cooperation and coordination between the Emperor and his Prime Minister. The Lung governs *qi* and the Heart governs *xue*. The regular, rhythmic movement of *qi* from the Lung is used by the Heart to send *xue* out through the body and it will be used to send *qi* via the channel system to all parts of the body. In this way, the Lung has a determining influence on all physiological activity in the body. The Lung being 'responsible for regulation' also relates to the function of the Lung's *shen* aspect, which is *po*. *Po* is responsible for the overall management of all the physiological activities, movement and reflexes that take place in the body without the person consciously thinking about them. This includes things like breathing, reflexes, perception of stimuli, touch, etc.

Functions of the Lung

As written in the introduction, the primary function of the Lung is the constant, rhythmic exchange of pure and impure air in and out of the body, as well as the rhythmic movement of *qi* downwards and throughout the body. The Lung inhales *da qi* (big *qi* or air) into the body. *Da qi* is blended with the *gu qi* (basis, food or grain *qi*) that the Spleen sends up from the middle *jiao* to create *zong qi*. A major difference between *zong qi* and *gu qi* is that *zong qi* is a form of *qi* that can be used by the body without the need for further transformation. *Zong qi* is used by both the Lung and the Heart to carry out their functions, particularly to support their rhythmic circulation of *qi* and *xue* around the body. The quality of a person's *zong qi* and thereby also the Lung can be heard in a person's voice, which is created by *zong qi*. A strong voice is a sign that *zong qi* is strong. However, it is important to remember that other factors will also have an influence on the voice, such as *xie qi*, the Heart and the Liver.[6]

Zong qi is also transformed. *Yuan qi* transforms *zong qi* to create *zhen qi*, which is a form of *qi* that can be used by the whole body. This means that the Lung is of great importance and influences not only the spreading of *qi* and *xue* throughout the whole body, but also the production of *qi* itself. If the Lung is weak, as it is for example when it is disrupted by *xie qi*, this will have an immediate impact on the production of *qi*. This can be seen clearly when a person catches a cold or gets a cough. Not only is their breathing affected, but they also experience fatigue and low energy levels.

The role played by the Lung in the production of *qi* is another example of how Heaven and Earth meet in Man, which is a recurring theme in Chinese medicine. Another name for *da qi* or air is *tian qi* or Heavenly *qi*. This is the *qi* that is above and around us. *Gu qi* is also known as *di qi* or earth *qi*, because it is created from the food that grows in the ground. These two *qi* are combined in man to create *zong qi*, which is then further transformed to *zhen qi*.

The relationship of the Lung to the production and distribution of *jinye* is very similar to the relationship of the Lung to the production and distribution of *qi*. The pure fluids are sent up to the Lung from the middle *jiao* by the Spleen. The Lung carries out a further transformation before the pure *jin* is spread as a fine mist around the body and the heavier *ye* is sent to the joints and orifices, whilst the impure fluids that are left over are sent down through the body to the Urinary Bladder.

The functions and relationships of the Lung can be summarised as follows.

The Lung

- controls *qi* and breathing
- controls the channels and vessels
- descends and spreads *qi* through the body
- spreads *jin* through the whole body
- regulates the water passages
- is the upper source of *jinye*
- controls *wei qi*
- controls the skin and the space between the skin and the muscles
- manifests in the body hair
- opens to the nose
- controls the sense of smell
- controls the nose

- is the delicate or vulnerable organ
- is damaged by Dryness
- hates Cold
- is affected by lying down
- is affected by, and manifests with, the white colour
- is affected by the spicy flavour
- manifests with a rotten odour
- controls the voice
- manifests with a crying or weeping voice
- is affected by grief, sorrow, worry and melancholy
- has reverence as its virtue
- is the residence of *po*

The Lung controls qi and breathing

The Lung draws pure *qi* into the body and exhales impure *qi*. This is consistent with the Western understanding of the lungs' relationship to the inhalation and exhalation of oxygen and carbon dioxide.

The Lung inhales *da qi* from the environment into the body, where it is combined with *gu qi* to create *zong qi*. In this way, the Lung is one of the fundamental *qi*-producing organs and has a huge influence on the quantity and quality of *qi* in the body.

The Lung has a specific relationship to *zong qi*, which it both creates and uses to support its own functionality. *Zong qi* is the driving force behind the movement of *qi* in the channel system. That is why it is said that the Lung controls *qi*. *Zong qi* is used by the Lung to carry out its function of regulating the breathing so it is rhythmic and harmonious.

The Lung controls the channels and vessels

It is said that the Lung controls the channels and vessels. The Lung does this by creating *zong qi* and spreading *qi*. *Zong qi* is the driving force behind *qi* in the channels and it assists the Lung in spreading *qi* through the channel network. Lung *qi* and *zong qi* assist the Heart in pumping *xue* through the channels and vessels.[7] It is therefore said that the Lung 'controls the hundred vessels'.

The relationship between the Lung and the Heart is in general a reflection of the relationship between *qi* and *xue*. This is summarised in the adage that '*qi* is the commander of *xue*; *xue* is the mother of *qi*'. *Zong qi* is used by the Heart to pump *xue* through the channels, whilst Heart *xue* nourishes the Lung so it is capable of performing its tasks. This relationship between the Lung, *zong qi* and the Heart can be seen, in practice, when shortness of breath, heart palpitations, breathing difficulty and chest oppression are often seen together. Furthermore, when a person suffers acute cardiac problems or asthma, they often have difficulty speaking because *zong qi* is blocked.

The Lung's relationship to the blood vessels is also seen in the fact that the *hui*-gathering point for the blood vessels is Lu 9, which is also the *yuan*-source point of the Lung. By stimulating one of the most tonifying acupuncture points of the Lung, *zong qi* will be tonified, and this will have a significant influence on the movement of *xue* in the blood vessels.

The Lung descends and spreads qi through the body

The Lung, which is like a canopy or a roof over the other organs, sends *qi* downwards through the body. The Lung creates a constant, rhythmic movement, where *qi* is sent down to the lower *jiao*. The *qi* is grasped by the Kidneys. This means that the condition of both the Lung and the Kidneys has a significant influence on respiration. An imbalance in one or both of these organs will mean either that *qi* is not sent down from the upper *jiao* or that it is not grasped by the Kidneys. This will result in *qi* accumulating in the chest, with subsequent breathing difficulties, coughing or chest oppression.

The ability of the Lung to send *qi* downwards is of great importance to its partner organ, the Large Intestine. The Large Intestine uses the *qi* that the Lung sends down to drive the stools down and out of the body.

This downward movement of *qi* is also of significance for the Spleen. When the Lung sends *qi* downwards, this creates space for the *qi* that the Spleen sends upwards. Apart from sending *qi* downwards, the Lung spreads *qi* throughout the body. *Zong qi* supplies the power and the rhythmic movement to circulate *qi* through the channel system.

The Lung spreads jin through the whole body

It is not only *qi* that is spread throughout the body by the Lung. The Lung also has several other important tasks; in particular, the Lung plays an important role in fluid physiology. One of these tasks is to spread *jin* through the body like a fine mist. *Jin* is the light *yang* aspect of the body fluids. *Jin* is spread by Lung *qi* together with *wei qi* in the space between the skin and the muscles. This space is called *cou li* in Chinese medicine. *Jin* then moistens and, to a certain extent, nourishes the skin. It also circulates through the channel system with *ying qi* and *xue*. A pictorial description of the relationship between *jin* and channel *qi* is that *jin* flows with channel *qi* and *xue* in the same way that mist flows above the water of a river in the early morning.

When there is a disruption of this function, there can either be a puffiness to the skin, because of oedema, or the skin will be dry, because it has not been moistened by *jin*. The heavier and more sticky *ye* flows together with *ying qi* and *xue* in the channels.

The Lung regulates the water passages

It is said that the Lung regulates the water passages. This is because:

- the Lung spreads *jin* through the space in between the skin and muscles

- *wei qi*, which is controlled by the Lung, controls the opening and closing of the pores

- the Lung sends impure fluids down to the Urinary Bladder for further transformation.

The Lung spreads *jin* together with *wei qi* through what is called *cou li*. *Cou li* is conceived of as being the space that is between the skin and muscles, as well as the small spaces in all the tissues of the body. As *wei qi* circulates below the skin, it also controls the pores in the skin. This is of great importance in the balance of fluids in the body. If *wei qi* is blocked by exogenous *xie* Cold, the Cold will block both the circulation of *jin* and the pores in the skin so that they cannot open. This will result in a person not being able to sweat. If the Lung is *qi xu*, *wei qi* will also be *xu*. This will mean that *wei qi* no longer controls the pores in the skin and the person will sweat spontaneously or during light exertion.

The Lung is also involved in regulating the movement of fluids upwards and downwards in the body. The Lung sends impure fluids down to the Urinary Bladder and receives pure fluids from the Spleen, as well as being moistened by pure *jinye* from the Kidneys.

The consequence of these relationships can be seen when *wei qi* is blocked by exogenous *xie qi* or if the Lung is in a state of imbalance. These situations can result in oedema. The oedema will manifest in the upper part of the body, especially the face. When the Lung can no longer spread *jinye*, it will accumulate in the Lung, resulting in thin, watery Phlegm collecting in the Lung and the respiratory passages. Disturbance of the Lung's ability to send fluids down to the Urinary Bladder can lead to urinary disturbances. Here there will be a lack of urination and an acute oedema due to the impure fluids that should have been expelled as urine accumulating in the upper *jiao*.

The Lung is the upper source of *jinye*

The production and distribution of *jinye* is a complex process involving many organs and takes place in all three *jiao*. The Lung is called the upper source of *jinye*, because it is the Lung that receives the pure fluids that the Spleen has sent upwards from the middle *jiao*. The pure fluids that the Spleen sends up to the Lung are the result of the transformation of liquids that have been ingested via the mouth and received by the Stomach. The Lung carries out a further transformation and sends the pure *jinye* out into the body, and the unclean remains are sent down to the Urinary Bladder, where they will be further transformed.

The Lung controls *wei qi*

The Lung relates to *wei qi* in two ways. The Lung and the Spleen are the post-heavenly root of *zhen qi* and thereby *wei qi*. The Lung is also responsible for spreading *wei qi* throughout the body. This means that the Lung is inextricably involved in the body's ability to protect itself against exogenous *xie qi*. A person who frequently falls ill or is sensitive to draughts will often be Lung *qi xu*. We also see that when *wei qi* is blocked or disrupted by *xie qi* there will often be signs and symptoms that the Lung's functionality is disturbed. As well as there being chills and aches in the muscles and skin, which in themselves are signs that circulation of *wei qi* is blocked, there can be sneezing, coughing and clear watery mucus in the nose. There can also be a puffiness in the face and around the eyes.

The influence that the Lung has on *wei qi* can be seen in the acupuncture points that often are used to treat an invasion of exogenous *xie qi*. Acupuncture points such as Lu 7, LI 4 and UB 12 are often chosen, precisely because these acupuncture points activate and regulate the Lung. The use of these points activate and spread *wei qi*, which opens the pores in the skin and thereby expels *xie qi* through the skin.

The Lung controls the skin and the space between the skin and the muscles

The Lung controls *wei qi*, which is the *qi* that mainly circulates in the space between the skin and the muscles, the area that is called the *cou li* in Chinese. By circulating here, *wei qi* is able to protect the exterior part of the body against invasions of exogenous *xie qi*, whilst simultaneously keeping the skin warm. *Jin*, which circulates together with *wei qi* in this space, helps to moisten and to some extent nourish the skin.

Wei qi controls the opening and closing of pores in the skin. If Lung *qi* or *wei qi* are *xu*, and are not strong enough to keep the pores closed, there can be spontaneous perspiration or sweating, even if there is only light exertion.

The Lung manifests in the body hair

The hair on the head is under the influence of the Kidneys, whilst the body hair is under the influence of the Lung. This relates to the fact that the skin in general is an aspect of the Lung. It also relates to the Lung's relationship to *wei qi*. When the body is exposed to cold weather and draughts, one of the first physical reactions is that the hairs on the body rise up and the pores in the skin close. This is a sign that *wei qi* is activated and is protecting the body against the external Cold and Wind.

The Lung opens to the nose

The sensory organ that is an aspect of the Metal Phase, and thereby the Lung, is the nose. This is logical, because the Lung is directly physically connected to the whole of the respiratory tract. When there are imbalances in the Lung, there will often be visible symptoms and signs that manifest in the nose. This could, for example, be a runny or blocked nose, or there could be sneezing. Furthermore, it is not only the nose but all parts of the upper airways, such as the sinuses, that are an aspect of the Lung and that can therefore manifest imbalances of the Lung. The throat, however, is both a part of the upper airways and a part of the alimentary canal and connects to the Stomach. This means that problems in the throat can relate to both Lung and Stomach imbalances.

The Lung controls the sense of smell

By controlling the nose, the Lung has an important influence on the sense of smell. This is seen clearly when a person has a cold with a blocked nose. Their sense of smell will often be greatly reduced. Even though the sense of smell is attributed to the Metal Phase and the Lung, it is in reality not only the ability to discern odours and fragrances that is affected by a blocked nose or by Phlegm-Dampness – our ability to taste flavours is also dependent on the nose. The tongue distinguishes the flavours of salt, sour, bitter and sweet, but the aromatic flavours are perceived in the nose. This means that some people who complain that they have lost the ability to taste often have Phlegm-Dampness blocking the nose.

The Lung controls the nose

Each organ has an impact on a specific form of *ye* or bodily fluid. The *ye* of the Lung is the mucus that is formed in the membrane lining the nose. This mucus moistens and lubricates the interior of the nose. When there is *yin xu* or *shi* Heat, the mucous membrane of the nose can become dry. *Shi* Heat can congeal *ye* in the nose so that it becomes thick, sticky and yellowish Phlegm. Wind-Cold can also disrupt the Lung's function of spreading *jin*, which then accumulates and stagnates, turning into Phlegm. The Phlegm can then be carried up to the nose by the rebellious Lung *qi*, so that there will be an increased amount of mucus in the nose. The mucus will be thin and watery in this case.

The Lung is the delicate or vulnerable organ

The Lung is unique amongst the *zang* organs. The Lung is the only *zang* organ that is in direct contact with the exterior. The Lung is directly connected to the external environment through the upper airways and the skin, which is an aspect of the Lung. The Lung also controls *wei qi*, which is the *qi* that keeps exogenous *xie qi* out of the body.

It is this direct contact to the exterior that makes the Lung so vulnerable. The Lung is therefore often the first organ that is affected when exogenous *xie qi* invades the body. For this reason the Lung is called the 'delicate or sensitive organ'.

Being in direct contact with the climate outside of the body means that the *yin* aspect of the Lung is particularly vulnerable to Dryness.

The Lung is damaged by Dryness

Dryness in general has a negative influence on the organs of the Metal Phase. The Lung is easily desiccated because it is a *zang* organ that is in direct contact with the environment. This is the reason that the Kidneys must constantly send *jinye* up to the Lung to keep it moist. Lung *yin* is easily damaged if the air is very dry. This should not be a problem for people in north-western Europe, where there is a maritime climate. Lung *yin* can however be damaged by living or working in buildings that have a very dry indoor climate. The effect of a dry indoor climate on the Lung will be the same as when the Lung is invaded by exogenous *xie* Dryness. Lung *yin* is also damaged by *shi* and *xu* Heat.

The Lung hates Cold

As we have seen, the Lung is highly vulnerable to exogenous *xie qi*. This applies to all kinds of exogenous *xie qi*. It is said, however, that 'the Lung hates Cold'. This is due to the Lung's relationship to *wei qi*. Cold is the *xie qi* that has the most detrimental effect on *wei qi*. Cold blocks the circulation of *wei qi* and it blocks the pores in the skin, thus preventing *wei qi* from expelling the Cold from below the skin. Cold will also, by virtue of its contracting nature, block the Lung's ability to sink and spread *qi*. This is why sneezing is such a common symptom of Wind-Cold. Sneezing arises because the blocked Lung *qi* becomes rebellious. In addition, the Lung is prevented from spreading *jin* throughout the body. This can result in puffiness of the face. There will also typically be watery exudation from the nose and eyes that tear.

The Lung is affected by lying down

The posture that has a negative effect on the Lung is lying down. This is because Damp-Phlegm can collect in the Lungs in the recumbent position. The Lung will also have greater difficulty spreading and descending the *qi* when a person is lying flat. Sitting slumped or bent forwards will also hinder the Lung in spreading and descending the *qi* from the upper *jiao*. Poor posture can be one of the underlying causes of Lung imbalances, such as asthma.

The Lung is affected by, and manifests with, the white colour

The white colour resonates with the Metal Phase. This is apparent when the Lung is *qi xu* and the person has a pale face, the cheeks in particular being pale. It is important to remember, however, that other forms of *qi xu* and *yang xu* can also manifest with paleness of the face.

The Lung's resonance with the white colour can also be seen in the white colour of many of the foods that affect the Lung. Onions, garlic, radishes, mushrooms, pears and milk all have an effect on the Lung. It is not possible to say whether this effect is positive or negative – that depends on which type of imbalance there is and the amount of these foods that is consumed. If a person is extremely Lung *yin xu*, milk will have a beneficial effect, because it is highly nutritious for Lung *yin*. Conversely, milk will have a decidedly negative effect if the person has a tendency to Phlegm-Dampness in the Lung.

The Lung is affected by the spicy flavour

Just as the white colour resonates with the Metal Phase, so does the spicy flavour. Food and spices with a spicy flavour will therefore often affect the Lung.

The spicy flavour has an intrinsic dynamic that is very *yang*. Its dynamic is centrifugal, i.e. it moves upwards and outwards from the centre. This dynamic can have a beneficial effect on the Lung if there has been an invasion of *xie qi*. The spicy flavour will be able to expel the *xie qi* upwards and outwards from the space between the skin and the muscle. Its dynamic will also open the pores, so *xie qi* can be driven out again. Excessive consumption of the spicy flavour can, however, damage Lung *yin*.

The Lung manifests with rotten odour

The odour that can be smelt when the Lung is out of balance can be translated into English as stale or rotten. The smell is rotten, as in rotten meat, fish or vegetables. It is the same smell that old rubbish bins or garbage trucks can have. This odour will be particularly noticeable when there is infected sputum in the Lung or a throat infection.

The Lung controls the voice

It is *zong qi* that gives the voice its strength. A person with Lung *qi xu* can have a weak voice that is lacking in strength, but they can also be taciturn and have little desire to talk. This is the body's subconscious attempt to conserve the Lung *qi*. The difference between these people and people with Heart imbalances is that people with Lung *qi xu* are not particularly uncommunicative, sullen or shy; they just appear to be quieter.

People who use their voice in their work – teachers, singers, actors, etc. – can have a tendency to have Lung *qi xu*, precisely because they are constantly using their voice.

The Lung manifests with a crying or weeping voice

The emotion of the Lung is sorrow. Grief can also be heard in a person's voice when there are Lung imbalances. There may be a slight choking of the words. The voice will sound as if the person is on the verge of tears. An extreme version of this voice is when a child is telling you something just after they have been crying. In Lung imbalances the voice may be lacking in strength and the sentences can have a tendency to ebb out before they are completely finished. This is because *zong qi* is often weak in many Lung imbalances and therefore there will not be enough strength to complete the sentence.

The Lung is affected by grief, sorrow, worry and melancholy

The emotion that is a manifestation of the Metal Phase is grief. In fact, white, which is the colour associated with the Metal Phase, is the colour associated with mourning in China. Grief also encompasses sorrow and melancholy and is called *bei* in Chinese. Sorrow affects the Lung negatively because it depletes Lung *qi* and it knots and inhibits *qi* in the upper *jiao*.

That grief, sorrow and melancholy affect the Lung is seen, for example, in the fact that crying has a resonance of the Metal Phase. It is through tears and crying that grief is manifested and released. There is a view that the Lung resonates with grief due to its association with *po*, the *shen* aspect that has its residence in the Lung. *Po*'s existence ends together with the physical body at death. This mortality is seen by some as being a reason that the Lung has a resonance with sorrow and the loss of something valuable.

The Lung has a relationship with drawing things in and letting things go. For example, the Lung inhales fresh air and exhales the old, spent air. The Lung also assists the Large Intestine in expelling the stools. We must defecate if there is to be space in the alimentary canal so that new nourishment can be ingested. It is not only impure air and stools, though, that the Lung helps us to let go of. It also helps us to release our emotional ties. It is when we are not able to let go of these attachments that grief arises. Letting go of these emotional attachments is an absolute necessity to be able to move forward. It is only when we let go of an emotional attachment that we are capable of making new emotional ties. Traditionally, when there was a death in the family in China, specific periods of time were set aside for grieving and certain rituals were adhered to in these periods. This created a space so a person could express their grief. It is important not to suppress or deny these emotions, but at the same time it is important to let go of these emotions again afterwards.

Another negative emotion that affects the Lung is the emotion that is called *you* in Chinese. This character is difficult to define clearly in English. This is further complicated by the fact that different authors translate *you* differently into English. For example, Giovanni Maciocia (2009) translates *you* as 'worry', which is the word that many other writers use to translate the character *si*. I have chosen to use Father Larre and Elisabeth Rochat de la Vallee's translation (1996). Here, *you* is translated as oppression, grief, restraint and anguish. They are of the opinion that in *you* there is a pronounced aspect of oppression. It is a more powerful emotion than normal grief or sadness. *You* can affect the free movement of *yang* in all *zang* organs, but it does this especially in the Lung, Spleen and Liver.

Worry and speculation (*si* in Chinese) is the emotion that is frequently associated with the Spleen. It is not only the Spleen, however, that is adversely affected by worry. Worry also 'knots' Lung *qi*. The knotting of Lung *qi* results in *qi* not descending or spreading, but accumulating in the upper *jiao* where it stagnates *zong qi*.

The Lung has reverence as its virtue

The virtue that is an aspect of the Lung is reverence and awe. It is the ability to experience each and every moment as being unique. This is linked to *po* and the ability to be in the moment. It is the ability to experience the beauty in each moment and every object. It is the reason we cry when we are confronted with extreme beauty.

The Lung is the residence of po

Po is the more *yin* material aspect of *shen*. It is the body's corporeal spirit. The Lung's *po* has a *yin/yang* relationship with Liver *hun*, which is the ethereal spirit in the body. The corporeal *po* helps to anchor the ethereal *hun* and keep it inside of the body.

Whereas there were originally believed to be three *hun*, there are seven *po*. These have responsibility for the daily, rhythmic functions in the body. *Po* controls all the aspects of the body that are not controlled by the conscious mind. It is the part of us that makes sure that the lungs inhale and exhale, that the stomach empties and that wounds heal; in short all the things that the body does without us having to think consciously about it. It is our instincts, our reflexes and our responses to physical stimuli. It is the *po* that reacts when the body is physically stimulated, such as when the skin is touched. It is said that *po* experiences pain but not suffering. This is because pain is an experience and suffering is our awareness of, and response to, it. On the whole, our sense of touch is related to *po*.[8] *Po*, like the Lung itself, is the point of contact between the body's interior and the physical world around it.

Po experiences things in the moment. Due to its *yin* nature, *po* is connected to space and time. This is part of the reason that it can anchor and balance the *yang hun*, whose visions for the future and whose ideas and dreams draw us out of the present moment. Whereas *hun* looks ahead and sees other opportunities and possibilities, *po* keeps us focussed in the present moment and helps us appreciate the now. This is one of the reasons many meditation techniques focus on the breath. This strengthens *po* and thereby helps to keep *hun* in check, so we can be present in the now.

Po has a close relationship with *jing*. Whereas *hun* and *shen*, being more *yang*, follow each other on a mental-emotional level, *jing* and *po* follow each other in the more physical, day-to-day maintenance and operation of the body.[9]

Po enters the body just after conception and is activated by the first breath. This reflects its close relationship to *jing*, helping to control the physical processes and growth of the foetus.

At death, *hun* rises upwards to the universe and survives the death of the physical body. *Po* is inextricably linked to the physical body. It ceases to exist together with the physical and sinks into the earth. *Hun* ascends and leaves the body through the most *yang* acupuncture point in the body, Du 20. *Po* descends and leaves the body through the *yin* rectum. The rectum was also known as *pomen* – *po* door or *po* gate – in the past.[10]

Po is connected to the place of birth. According to traditional Chinese philosophy, a person should preferably die in the vicinity of their place of birth. This is because *po* should return to the ground from which it came. Traditionally, it was thought that if you die a violent death before your time and if you die far from home, *po* can have difficulty returning to its birthplace and can therefore become a *gui* – a ghost.

The Lung's relationship to other organs

The Lung and the Liver

The Liver and the Lung have both a *qi/qi* relationship and a *qi/xue* relationship.

The Lung sends *qi* downwards and is dependent on the Liver's function of controlling *qi*. On the other hand, Liver *qi* is supported in its function of spreading *qi* by the Lung, which spreads and descends *qi*. Lung *qi* and *zong qi* are the driving force behind channel *qi*. Without *zong qi*, *qi* would stagnate in the channels.

Liver *qi* stagnation can interfere with the Lung *qi ji*. This is because Liver *qi* stagnation will cause Lung *qi* to stagnate, not just by preventing the overall free movement of *qi*, but also because the Liver is located directly below the Lung. A stagnation of *qi* here will in itself block the *qi* that is being sent down from the Lung. Energetically, the Liver is conceived of as being on the left side of the body and the Lung on the right. The Lung sends its *qi* downwards and the Liver its *qi* upwards. This creates a harmonic movement of *qi* up and down. If one of these organs' *qi* becomes out of balance, then it will interfere with the other organ's *qi ji*.

The Liver and the Lung *qi/xue* relationship is not as apparent as their *qi* relationship. The Liver regulates and stores *xue*. Lung *qi* and *zong qi* move *xue* through the channels and vessels.

In pathological situations, Liver Fire can flame up and invade the Lung.

The Lung and the Heart

In its simplest form, the Lung and Heart represent the fundamental relationship that there is between *qi* and *xue*. Qi moves *xue*, and *xue* nourishes *qi*. Lung *qi* and *zong qi* are used by the Heart to move *xue* through the channels and vessels. Heart *xue* nourishes the Lung. Without *qi*, *xue* would stagnate, and *qi* can only move through vessels and channels if there is *xue* to 'concentrate' and anchor it.

Because the Heart is dependent on Lung *qi* to drive *xue* through the vessels, it is said that 'the Lung controls the hundred vessels'. This means that the Lung has a significant influence on the movement of *xue* in the vessels. The Heart not only circulates *xue* through the vessels, but it also has an influence on the structure of the vessels. The structure of vessels can, to a certain degree, be seen as a natural extension of the Heart.

Whilst the Heart is the Emperor, the Lung is the Prime Minister with responsibility for regulation. Heart *shen* is mental consciousness. Lung *po* controls the somatic functions of the body that do not require conscious thought.

The Lung's control of rhythmic breathing can be used to calm the *shen* if it is unsettled. If a person is upset and completely beside themselves, one of the best things you can do is to get them to breathe calmly – breathing deeply down in the lower abdomen. By regulating Lung *qi*, the Heart *qi* is also regulated.

The Lung and the Kidneys

The Lung and the Kidneys cooperate closely with each other in relation to both respiration and with fluid physiology.

During respiration, the Lung sends *qi* downwards through the body where it is grasped by the Kidneys. For cooperation to work optimally, both organs' *qi* must be strong enough and Lung *qi* must not be blocked by exogenous *xie qi*, Phlegm or other forms of stagnation. If the Kidneys or the Lung are disrupted in their collaboration, breathing difficulties will arise.

The Kidneys' and the Lung's collaboration with regards to fluid physiology consists of the Lung sending impure fluids from the upper *jiao* down to the Urinary Bladder, where they are transformed by Kidney *yang*. Kidney *yang* in return sends pure *jinye* up again to the Lung to keep them moist, so that they do not dry out. Lung imbalances can therefore result in oedema and urinary problems. Likewise, Kidney imbalances can lead to the Lung drying out and thereby becoming *yin xu*.

Zong qi and *yuan qi*, which have a very close relationship to the Lung and the Kidneys respectively, also have a relationship to each other. *Yuan qi* ascends to the upper *jiao* to transform *zong qi* into *zhen qi*. *Zong qi* descends to the lower *jiao*, where it nourishes *yuan qi* and assists the Kidneys.

The Lung and the Spleen

The Spleen transforms the food that has been consumed into *gu qi*. *Gu qi* is sent up from the middle *jiao* to the upper *jiao*, where the Lung combines it with *da qi* from the air around us to create *zong qi*. This means that the Lung and the Spleen are the two sources of post-heaven *qi*, and that the Lung is dependent on the production of *gu qi* from the Spleen.

Spleen *qi xu* can have two main consequences for the Lung. First, a reduced production of *gu qi* will result in a reduced production of *zong qi*, which the Lung is dependent on in order to carry out its activities. On the other hand, Dampness and Phlegm are often a consequence of the Spleen's failure to transform optimally. This is the root of the statement that 'Phlegm is created in the Spleen, but is stored in the Lung' and 'to treat the Lung, you must treat the Spleen'. Many patterns of imbalance in the Lung are caused by Spleen *qi xu* or the consumption of Damp- and Phlegm-producing foods that the Spleen has difficulty transforming.

The Spleen is dependent on the Lung. This is both because of the Lung's role in *qi* production and because the Lung sends its *qi* downwards. By sending *qi* downwards, space is created for the *qi* that is sent up by the Spleen. Furthermore, the descending Lung *qi* supports the Spleen's partner organ, the Stomach, in its function of sending *qi* downwards through the Intestines.

It is not only *gu qi* that the Spleen sends up to the Lung. The two organs also have a collaboration with regards to the transformation of fluids. The Spleen separates the pure from the impure fluids and sends the pure aspect up to the Lung, which further transforms them. From here, the Lung distributes the transformed *jin* throughout the body as a fine mist and it sends the dirty residue down to the Urinary Bladder, where Kidney *yang* carries out the final transformation before the remaining useless residue is excreted.

The Spleen and the Lung also have a channel relationship; they are both aspects of the *taiyin* channel.

The Lung and the Large Intestine

The Large Intestine and the Lung are each other's *yin/yang* partner organ. In addition to having a direct channel relationship with each other, they also have a relationship to each other through their *qi*. The Large Intestine is dependent on the Lung sending its *qi* downwards to be able to expel the stools from the body. Constipation in the elderly can often be due to Lung *qi xu*. They simply do not have enough Lung *qi* to be able to press the stool out of the body. They will often feel exhausted and short of breath and will sweat spontaneously when they finally have passed the stool. Conversely, if a person is very constipated, it can block the descent of the Lung *qi*. This will result in a person being short of breath and having difficulty in breathing deeply.

THE LIVER

Chinese medicine assigns the Liver to the lower *jiao*. This is despite the fact that anatomically the Liver is located in the middle *jiao*. This is due to the fact that the Liver's functional activity relates to the lower *jiao*, and in Chinese medicine it is function rather than anatomy that is of greatest importance. The Liver has a very close relationship with the Kidneys. It is said that Liver *yin* and Kidney *yin* have a common root. Furthermore, there is a close relationship between *jing* and *xue*, which nourish each other, and each can transform into the other. All of this means that the Liver is defined as being an organ of the lower *jiao*. Its physical location is, however, not without significance. For example, the pulse positions and the areas of the tongue that relate to the Liver are to be found in the areas of the pulse and tongue that correspond to the middle *jiao*. In addition, acupuncture points such as Liv 14 and UB 18 have a powerful effect on the Liver. These acupuncture points are located close to the anatomical Liver.

Again in contrast to its anatomical location, it is said that 'the Liver arises on the left side of the body'. The positioning of the Liver on the left side of the body is a reflection of its Five Phase relationship. The Fire Phase, which is the most *yang* phase, is located at the summit of the *sheng* cycle. Fire is the ultimate *yang*. This is where the sun is to be found in the middle of the day. The Sun, and thereby young *yang*, rises in the East. East is on your left when you stand looking South towards the Fire Phase. Furthermore, the left middle pulse position (*guan* position) and left-hand side of the tongue relate to the Liver.

The Liver is partnered with the Gall Bladder. These two organs have a close relationship and functional cooperation. Their close relationship is also seen pathologically in that many Liver patterns of imbalance manifest in the Gall Bladder's channel or organ, whilst Liver *qi* stagnation is often a significant factor in many Gall Bladder imbalances.

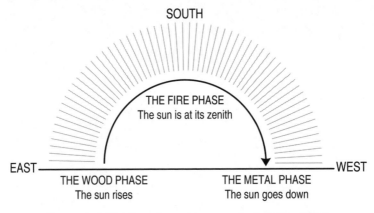

Figure 3.1 The Liver's position on the left-hand side

The functions of the Liver

Huang Di Nei Jing – Su Wen, chapter eight, describes the Liver as being a General who is responsible for plans and strategies. The Wood Phase is defined as being young *yang*. Being *yang* that is in growth gives the Liver a forward-looking, focussed dynamic. It is this dynamic that is needed in order to be able to make decisions and to have the strength and focus to carry out these decisions. This is why the Liver is known as the 'resolute organ'.

It is the Liver's *shen* aspect, known as *hun*, which has the greatest influence on our ability to plan and make decisions. One of the most important aspects of *hun* is that it enables us to have vision – to be able to visualise something in the future that is not manifest at the moment. This is what we do when we make plans and lay strategies. We have a vision of what the future will look like. People with a strong *hun* have clear ideas of what they want. They have goals in life and they pursue them, regardless of the cost. *Hun* is that which gives us a direction in life. People whose *hun* is weak can lack direction, vision and goals in life.

Boundaries are an aspect of the Liver. If the Liver is strong, a person will be assertive and can set their boundaries. If the Liver is weak, they will often get stepped upon and they will have difficulty being assertive and saying stop to other people. A weakness in one of the Liver aspects can mean that they do not have a strong enough vision of what they want or they lack the courage to pursue their goals. The moment someone with a more powerful Liver crosses their path they let themselves be brushed aside by the other person's momentum and determination, and they then compromise their own goals. On the other hand, if a person's Liver is overactive, they often overstep other people's boundaries. Their needs come first. Again, it is because they have a clear vision of what they want, and they don't care about other people's visions if they are in the way of their own aims. It is equally important that a General has the insight and the necessary flexibility it requires to be cautious when the situation requires it, and not just to blindly rush forward crushing everything in their path.[11]

Many politicians, captains of industry and CEOs have a strong *hun*. They have a clear vision of the future and they can be relentless in their pursuit of this vision. These people are willing to sacrifice other people to achieve their objectives.

A strong *hun* is also seen in many top-level athletes and sports persons. Again, they have a clear vision of what they want to achieve, which enables them to force themselves beyond their physical limits. This tendency can also be seen in some patients. These are people who push themselves harder than their physical body (i.e. *qi*, *xue* and *jing*) is capable of in the long term. They end up physically exhausting themselves.

Artists are another group who often have a strong *hun*. They look at a block of wood or a blank canvas and visualise a work of art that they then are able to manifest.

The Liver and *hun* not only create visions and dreams in a metaphorical sense – they also create our physical vision and allow us to see the world around us. It is also *hun* that creates the dreams we have when we sleep at night.

The Liver is not directly involved in the production of *qi* or *xue*. The Liver does, however, have a crucial influence on both substances. The Liver maintains the free movement of *qi* and *xue*, and the Liver is a reservoir for *xue*.

The functions and relationships of the Liver can be summarised as follows.

The Liver

- ensures the smooth flow of *qi*
- stores *xue*
- controls the sinews
- manifests in the nails
- opens to the eyes
- influences vision
- controls tears
- relates to Wind

- is affected by, and manifests with, anger
- manifests with a rancid odour
- is affected by the sour flavour
- manifests with a shouting voice
- is affected by, and manifests with, the green colour
- has benevolence as its virtue
- is the residence of *hun*

The Liver ensures the smooth flow of qi

The Liver sends its own *qi* outwards and slightly upwards, but the Liver's most important relationship to *qi* is that it ensures the free flow of *qi* throughout the body. Many patterns of imbalance result from Liver *qi* stagnation disrupting other organs' *qi*. It is important to remember, though, that this is a pathological situation. When the Liver is in balance, it supports the *qi ji* of the other organs. Also, and very importantly, not all stagnations of *qi* are due to Liver *qi* stagnation. An organ's *qi* can stagnate, because the organ is *qi xu* or the organ's *qi* is blocked by *xie qi*. In fact, situations can arise where Liver *qi* stagnates precisely because *qi* is stagnant elsewhere in the body. These stagnations prevent the Liver from being able to ensure the free flow of *qi* without hindrance.

When Liver *qi* flows freely, *qi* transformations take place as they should and *qi* moves in the right direction and at an appropriate speed. When Liver *qi* stagnates, *qi* transformations and movements can become choppy, delayed or disrupted.

Stagnations of Liver *qi* will on the physical level often disrupt the *qi ji* or *qi* dynamic of the Stomach, Spleen, Intestines and Lung. This can manifest as abdominal distension, nausea, constipation, diarrhoea, tightness of the chest, shortness of breath, etc.

The Liver has a close relationship to its partner organ, the Gall Bladder. The Gall Bladder is dependent on the free movement of Liver *qi* in order to be able to excrete bile in the right quantity and at the right times. Liver *qi* stagnation can interfere with this function and result in problems of digesting fats, loose stools, jaundice, nausea or pain in the hypochondriac region.

It is not only on the physical level that Liver *qi* ensures the free flow of *qi*. On the mental-emotional level, the free movement of *qi* is also of crucial importance.

When Liver *qi* is stagnant, people can be very inflexible in their mental attitude. Liver *qi* stagnation often manifests with irritability, impatience, mood swings or depression. The Liver has, in general, a close relationship to the emotions. Emotions are nothing other than movements of *qi*. Each emotion has its own *qi* dynamic. For example, anger makes *qi* ascend and fear makes *qi* descend. The emotions are in balance when they are free flowing and harmonious, are neither too strong nor too weak and are appropriate to the situation. The Liver can easily be affected adversely, if the emotions are not allowed to flow freely, as this will interfere with the Liver freely moving *qi* in all directions.

Liver *qi* is a very dynamic energy. It is young *yang*. This means that when you have a vision of what you want, Liver *qi* is the dynamic and driving force that enables you to reach your goal. It is this focussed determination that can be seen when a dandelion forces its way through the asphalt and up into the light.

All of this is difficult, however, when you live in a society with other people. These people also have ideas and visions of how their lives and the world should be. Just as when two trees grow up next to each other one will usually be forced to compromise and accommodate the will of the other. When the dynamic *qi* of the Liver is prevented from expanding outwards, it creates a stagnation of Liver *qi*. A person who feels inhibited or is in some way dominated by others, and whose emotions and opinions remain unexpressed, will find that their Liver *qi* stagnates. The degree of stagnation depends on how powerful their own Liver *qi* and *hun* are and how much the person is able to accommodate and accept these limitations. That is why we need another quality of the Wood Phase – flexibility. Having a clear goal and vision is important, but we must also have flexibility – flexibility to bend and adapt when needed, without giving up and losing sight of our objectives.

A person with a powerful Liver *qi* will be a person who is used to getting their way and realising their ideas. They are fine as long as they decide and as long as things conform to their vision. If things go against them, or if they no longer are able to decide or get their own way, the accumulated Liver *qi* can explode. They will be furious. People with Liver *qi* stagnation are often quick tempered and easily angered.

The Liver stores xue

The Liver is not directly involved in the production of either *qi* or *xue*, but it does have a very close relationship to both: *qi*, because the Liver continuously ensures that there is a free movement of *qi* in the body, and *xue*, because it is in the Liver that *xue* is stored.

It is said that the Liver is a reservoir for *xue*. This is where *xue* returns to and is stored when it is not in circulation in the body. The Liver ensures that there is always the appropriate quantity of *xue* needed by the body in circulation. The quantity of *xue* circulating through the muscles, channels and vessels should be appropriate in relation to the level of activity. When we are physically active, *xue* is sent out into the body to nourish the muscles. When we sleep and when we are resting, *xue* returns to the Liver, as it is no longer needed out in the body. The Liver's function as a reservoir for *xue* is also of great importance to the menstrual cycle. *Xue* is stored in the Liver before it is sent down to the Uterus or *bao* via *chong mai* to create a menstrual bleeding.

This constant regulation of *xue* is yet another aspect of the Liver's role of being a 'General with responsibility for planning and strategies'. It is a general's responsibility that there is always the appropriate amount of troops and that they are in the right place at the right time.

Xue nourishes and moisturises the Liver. This means that when a person is *xue xu*, it can result in their Liver being rigid and inflexible. This lack of flexibility can lead to Liver *qi* stagnation. This is a very typical cause of Liver *qi* stagnation in women. Women tend to be *xue xu* due to menstrual bleeding and births.

The Liver can, though, have a negative effect on *xue*. The Liver ensures that *qi* is constantly moving freely and without hindrance throughout the body. Liver *qi* thereby also ensures that *xue* moves freely and without hindrance, because it is *qi* that moves *xue*. This means that Liver *qi* stagnation, in the course of time, can lead to *xue* stagnation. Also, because *xue* is stored in the Liver, Heat conditions of the Liver, such as Liver Fire or Liver *qi* stagnation Heat, can lead to *xue* Heat. This can often be the cause of many menstrual problems and some skin conditions.

The Liver controls the sinews

Each *zang* organ is ascribed a relationship to a particular body tissue in Five Phase theory. These relationships are not arbitrary – they exist because there is an energetic resonance between the two, and particularly because the *zang* organ usually has a physiological relationship to this type of tissue.

The Liver has a Five Phase relationship with sinews. It is Liver *xue* that nourishes the sinews and tendons in the body. Furthermore, Liver *qi* ensures the free movement of *qi* and *xue* in the sinews and tendons. If there is Liver *xue xu* or Liver *qi* stagnation, tendons and sinews can become stiff and inflexible, resulting in problems in the joints.

Some sources, particularly Danish books, say that the tissue that is ascribed to the Liver is muscles and tendons. They state that the Liver relates to muscles in the torso and the Spleen to the muscles in the limbs. This is not entirely correct. The Spleen relates more to the muscles' form and structure and the Liver relates more to their function. Spleen *qi xu* can, for example, manifest with underdevelopment and weakness in the muscles. This will mainly be seen in the arms and legs. Liver imbalances have more of a tendency to manifest themselves as stiffness, cramping and tightness of the muscles and tendons.

The Liver manifests in the nails

Nails are considered to be an extension of the sinews in Chinese medicine. Liver imbalances can manifest in the nails, especially the fingernails. Liver *xue* nourishes the nails, and Liver *xue xu* can therefore result in undernourished nails. This will typically manifest with fingernails that are soft, break easily or are dry and ridged. Liver *xue* stagnation can manifest with fingernails that are bluish or purple.

The Liver opens to the eyes

The Liver has a significant influence on the eyes. Liver *xue* nourishes the eyes. *Hun*, which is the Liver's *shen* aspect, travels up to the eyes during the day and returns to the Liver at night. This is why the Liver has such an influence on the vision. Liver *xue xu* can result in difficulty focussing and blurred vision. The eyes can also feel dry. Liver *xue xu* can also manifest with sensitivity to bright light and night-blindness. Liver *shi* conditions such as Liver Fire and Liver *yang* rising will often manifest with symptoms and signs that relate to the eyes. This could be a headache, where the pain is located behind the eyes, pressure in the eyes, red eyes or a stinging, burning sensation in the eyes. It is important to remember that other organs also have an influence on the eyes, especially the Kidneys.

The Liver influences vision

The Liver ensures that the eyes are supplied with *xue*. This is why Liver *xue xu* can manifest with poor vision and other forms of visual disturbance. Most people have at some time experienced standing up too quickly and seeing stars or small dots in their vision. This is due to *xue* not rising up to eyes quickly enough, resulting in the eyes lacking *xue*. The Liver's *shen* aspect, *hun*, is present in the eye during the day, helping to create vision. This is why the sense of vision is attributed to the Wood Phase.

The Liver controls tears

The Liver controls tears in the sense that the Liver controls the aspect of tears that keeps the eyes moist and the tears that rinse foreign matter out of the eyes.

When there is Liver *xue xu* and Liver *yin xu*, there can often be a sensation of dry eyes or a gritty sensation in the eyes. Wind, which is the climate that has a negative effect on the Wood Phase, can make the eyes start to water. Most people experience this if it is very windy, but some people with Liver imbalances experience it even when they just step outside or ride on a bicycle.

The Liver relates to Wind

People with Liver imbalances may be negatively affected by climatic wind. As written above, wind can make the eyes water when there is Liver *xue xu*. Some people also become aggressive (which is an aspect of anger – the Liver's emotion) when it is windy. This can, for example, be seen when the sirocco wind blows across Spain from North Africa.

Liver imbalances can in themselves generate internal Wind in the body. Internal Wind is similar in many ways to climatic wind. Internal Wind is also a form of *xie qi*, but it has a different aetiology and other manifestations than exogenous climatic wind. See Part 6 on causes of disorder (page 691) for a further discussion of this.

The Liver is affected by, and manifests with, anger

The Liver is adversely affected by anger. Anger should be interpreted broadly and includes more than just anger. It also includes emotions such as frustration, irritation and aggression. Anger itself causes *qi* to rise upwards. This is something that Liver *qi* has a tendency to do already, due to its young *yang* dynamic.

Anger can affect the Liver in two main ways. Anger can cause Liver *qi* to rise up, resulting in patterns of imbalance such as Liver *yang* rising and Liver Fire. If the anger is not expressed, this dynamic energy, which is expansive and ascending in its dynamic, will be held back. This will stagnate Liver *qi*. Repressed emotions will in general have a stagnating effect on Liver *qi*, because every emotion is a movement of *qi*. When this movement of *qi* is hindered or blocked, it will stagnate Liver *qi*. This also means that every time a person has the experience that someone oversteps their boundaries or when they don't say stop to others, it will have a negative effect on their Liver *qi*.

Conversely, when our anger and aggression is fully expressed, we tend to overstep other people's boundaries.

If Liver *qi* does not flow freely and harmoniously, it can result in irritability, frustration, tetchiness or impatience. Conversely, if the Liver is in balance, a person will be emotionally balanced and be able to express their opinions when it is appropriate to do so. They will be in a position to set boundaries to other people and at the same time be able to respect other people's boundaries.

As is the case with all emotions, it is important to regard them as being neither negative nor positive in themselves. An emotion is only negative if it is too powerful or too weak, if it is persistent or if it is inappropriate to the situation. Anger and aggression are negative when they are too extreme and when they are inappropriate. On the other hand, anger is justified and correct in other situations. An imbalance in the Liver can be observed when a person is irascible, irritable and impatient, but also when a person lacks anger, represses their anger or does not even feel it at all. In addition, aggression can be the necessary dynamic that brings about change. It is young *yang*. Young *yang* and spring break the standstill that is characteristic of old *yin* and the winter. A gust of wind can clear foetid and stagnant air.

The Liver manifests with a rancid smell

The rancid smell is the smell that animals or urine can have. It is rancid, as in rancid butter or other rancid oils. The smell is also described by Hicks *et al.* (2004) as smelling like newly mown grass, but without this being a pleasant smell.

The Liver is affected by the sour flavour

The sour flavour resonates with the Wood Phase in general and with the Liver in particular. This is seen in Chinese herbal medicine, where herbs with a sour taste have an effect on the Liver. It is also seen in people who suffer from migraines that have their root in a Liver imbalance. Red wine can often be a triggering factor in their migraines. This is because red wine has a sour flavour and is energetically hot, causing Liver *yang* to ascend.

The most typical taste in the mouth in Liver imbalances is, however, the bitter taste, which can be experienced when there is Liver Fire.

The Liver manifests with a shouting voice

When the Liver is in balance, the voice is neither too hard nor too soft. The voice is resonant without it being shouting.

When the Liver is in imbalance, it can give a person's voice a very hard tone. It will have a shouting quality. The voice sounds sharp and it has force and direction. It is a voice that has no problem being heard and is not hesitant. It is the tone that is heard when someone is angry.

Liver *xu* imbalances, on the other hand, can manifest with a voice that lacks these resonant and hard qualities that the Liver *qi* gives to the voice. The voice will be too soft and will lack clout.

If a person's Liver *qi* is stagnant, this can be heard in their voice. The words will be clipped and voice will be staccato. It will sound a bit like a machine gun firing when they are talking. It is not necessarily because they speak quickly, but their voice is hard and the words sound sharp or clipped. Liver *qi* ensures that Heart *qi* and *zong qi* flow freely and without hindrance. When Liver *qi* is stagnant, it will cause the speech to lose its free-flowing quality and, because it is a Liver imbalance, the voice will also assume a harsher quality.

A voice that sounds aggressive is also a hard voice, and again this can occur when there is a Liver imbalance. It may be a general tone that their voice has, or it may be heard when they are talking about certain subjects or of certain people.

The Liver is affected by, and manifests with, the green colour

The colour that is associated with the Wood Phase is green. This is seen clearly in the spring, when all of nature explodes in green. The resonance of the green colour with the Wood Phase can also be seen in some Liver imbalances that manifest with areas of the face having a slightly greenish tint. This is easiest to see in the area around the mouth and the temple.

Green-leafed vegetables have a resonance with the Liver. In general, these vegetables are both cooling and *xue* nourishing. This means that they are recommended both when there is *shi* Heat and when there is *xue xu* or *yin xu* Liver imbalances.

The Liver has benevolence as its virtue

The Liver's potential is kindness, benevolence, humanity and righteousness. It requires a higher vision to be able to see both sides of a case and see what is best for the common good. This requires that a person is capable of seeing beyond their own needs and what benefits them. It is *hun* that can give us the vision – the vision of being something other and greater than our own individual needs. Selfishness can, on the other hand, be a sign of a *hun* imbalance.

The Liver is the residence of hun

Hun, which is often translated as the ethereal spirit, is one of the five *shen*, together with Heart *shen*, Spleen *yi*, Kidney *zhi* and Lung *po*.

It is said that *hun* resides in the Liver. *Hun*, which is *yang*, needs to be anchored and nourished by Liver *xue*. During the day *hun* travels to the Liver's sensory organ, the eyes, and at night *hun* returns to the Liver.[12]

There is a mutual *yin/yang* relationship between *hun* and *po*. *Hun* is *yang* in relation to *po*, and they are conceived of as being *shen's yin* and *yang* aspects. *Hun* and *po* balance and harmonise each other, thereby creating a harmonious *shen*. *Po* assists in anchoring and holding *hun* down in the body. *Hun* helps to activate *po*. *Hun* is referred to as the ethereal spirit. *Po* is the corporeal spirit that is related to reflexes, physical activity and all the things that the body does without the need to think about it. *Hun* has, as we will see in a moment, more of a relationship to visions, dreams and ideas.

The ethereal *hun* survives the physical body on death and rises up to the universe through the acupuncture point Du 20 on the top of the head. *Po* dies together with the physical body and leaves the body through the rectum and sinks into the earth. There are different opinions of when *hun* enters into the body. Some think that it enters the body in the eighth month of pregnancy, others that it enters the body at birth and others again that it comes first into the body after three days. Some sources also say that *hun* enters and leaves the body through the acupuncture point *Hunmen* (UB 47).

Hun's functions are closely linked to the functions of the Liver. As previously written, the Liver is the 'General with responsibility for planning and strategy'. Here, *hun's* ability to see and to have visions and dreams is of crucial importance.

It is also said that the Liver is the resolute organ. Liver *hun's* ability to plan and create strategies also requires a general's determination to carry out these plans. People with Liver *xue xu* can be indecisive. They have difficulty visualising what they want to do or be. To make a decision requires that you have an idea of where you want to go. *Hun* gives us direction in life.

However, it is not enough to have a plan and to take decisions. You must also have the courage to implement these plans. This courage comes from the Liver's partner organ, the Gall Bladder. It is not uncommon to hear people say that they have had enough, that they will not put up with something any more, but they then carry on without doing anything about it, because they do not have the courage to bring about the confrontation that is required to make a change. It is not the Liver's planning and strategies that are lacking – it is the courage to stick with their plans. Kidney *zhi* – willpower – is also an important factor. We must be able to hold fast in our projects, even when the going gets tough and we are exhausted.

Hun's vision is also behind the attributes of imagination and creativity. It is the ability to see something that is not there yet. *Hun*'s ability to create visions is what makes some people creative, artistic and imaginative.

Just as *hun* has to do with our dreams in life – our objectives – it is also *hun* that creates the dreams we have at night.

In the same way that Heart *shen* is anchored by Heart *xue* and Heart *yin*, *hun* is anchored by Liver *xue* and Liver *yin*. Both *shen* and *hun* return to their respective organs at night, where they rest quietly. During sleep, *hun* should be at rest in the Liver, but if the *yin* aspects of the Liver (which include Liver *xue*) are weak or if there is Heat in the Liver, *hun* can become agitated, disturbing the sleep pattern and resulting in excessive dreaming. During REM sleep the eyelids flutter rapidly, because *hun* has travelled up to the eyes, creating activity in the eyes and in the world of dreams. If *hun* is very agitated and is not anchored, it can even leave the body and the person may have an 'out of body experience' or the person can end up sleepwalking. During sleepwalking, *hun* has also activated *po*, so the body starts to walk. *Shen*, on the other hand, is not active whilst sleepwalking. This is witnessed by the fact that the person is not conscious whilst walking and you cannot talk to them.

Hun is also our subconscious – that which is not our conscious mind. It is often through dreams and whilst sleeping that we get ideas and solve problems.

Hun's ability to have a vision and see a possible future is what enables the Liver to be able to make 'plans and strategies'. This is because *hun* has a clear idea – a dream. Whereas *po* is *yin* and is rooted in space and time, *hun* does not have this limitation. This is why *hun* can look ahead and see other possibilities. If *hun* is not anchored or is agitated, a person can have too many ideas and dreams, seldom achieving any of them.

It is said that *hun* and *shen* follow each other in their 'entering and exiting'.[13] This reflects their relative *yang* nature, whereas *po* and *jing*, which are relatively *yin*, follow each other in their 'entering and exiting'. By following each other in their 'entering and exiting' we can see that they have a very close relationship to each other and complement each other in their functions. Also, *hun* 'sees' for *shen*. Our vision is the only sense that we can focus on specific objects.

There are three *hun*. One or more of these can leave the body temporarily, either because they are not anchored, because they are agitated by Heat or because they have been scattered by shock.

Hun is a part of the family or clan *hun*. It is linked to the family name, and it is the spirit that was worshipped when Chinese people made sacrifices to their ancestors.

Hun's functions can be summarised as follows.

Dreams	*Hun* must be rooted in Liver *xue* at night to ensure a deep and quiet sleep. *Hun* creates the dreams that are dreamt at night whilst sleeping. During the day *hun* creates aspirations.
Planning and strategies	*Hun* enables a person to be able to make plans and have the necessary strategic vision to be able to plan their lives so that they can achieve their dreams. *Hun* gives a person a direction in life.
Vision	*Hun* makes vision possible, both on the physical level through its relationship with its eyes and on the psychological level. By having psychological vision, it is possible to have imagination and creativity. It is possible to see that which is not yet manifest.

The Liver's relationship to other organs

The Liver has a functional relationship to all the other organs. This is because the Liver ensures the unimpeded and free flow of *qi*. Liver *qi* stagnation will, therefore, interfere with all organs' *qi ji*. The Liver does, though, have a specific functional relationship to certain organs.

The Liver and the Lung

The Liver and the Lung have both a *qi/qi* relationship and a *qi/xue* relationship.

The Lung sends its *qi* downwards and is dependent on the Liver's overall function of ensuring the free flow of *qi*. On the other hand, Liver *qi* is supported in its function of spreading *qi* by the Lung. *Zong qi* is the driving force behind channel *qi*. Without *zong qi*, *qi* will stagnate in the channel system.

Liver *qi* stagnation can interfere with the Lung's *qi ji*. This will happen when Liver *qi* stagnation causes Lung *qi* to stagnate by not ensuring the free flow of *qi*. Furthermore, because the Liver is located just below the Lung, a stagnation of *qi* here will block the descent of *qi* from above.

The Liver is energetically located in the left side of the body and the Lung on the right-hand side. The Lung sends its *qi* downwards and the Liver its *qi* upwards. This creates a harmonic movement of *qi* up and down. If one of these organs' *qi* becomes imbalanced, it will begin to interfere with the other organ's *qi ji*.

The Liver and the Lung's *qi/xue* relationship is not as apparent. The Liver regulates and stores *xue*. By creating *zong qi*, the Lung drives *xue* through the channels and vessels.

The Liver and the Heart

Both the Liver and the Heart have a close relationship with *xue*. The Heart governs *xue* and the Liver regulates and stores *xue*. It is very common to see Heart *xue xu* and Liver *xue xu* concurrently. This is, in fact, more the rule than the exception. For this reason, symptoms and signs that relate to both the Heart and the Liver will frequently be seen when there is *xue xu*.

As well as both organs having a close relationship to *xue* in that they govern, store and regulate *xue*, *xue* itself has a huge influence on both of these organs' *shen* aspects. *Hun* and *shen* are nourished, anchored and travel together with Liver and Heart *xue* respectively. This is why both organs' *shen* aspects are easily affected by *xue* imbalances.

The close relationship of *shen* and *hun* to each other is something other and more than just their common relationship to *xue*. Their relationship is summarised in the following statement: 'Shen and hun follow each other in their entering and exiting.' In practice, this means that if *shen* is not anchored or is agitated, then *hun* can start to 'wander'. If *hun* is blocked by stagnation, then *shen* can also become blocked.

Hun is *shen's* eyes. The eyes are the only sensory organ that can be focussed and that can be directionally determined. You think first and then the eyes follow where the mind wants to look. The other senses cannot be controlled and focussed so precisely. The eyes can focus on specific objects. When we consciously want to observe something, we move our eyes and the vision is focussed on the object. This is not something we are able to do with our hearing or smell, for example. Neither can we close our other sensory organs in the same way that we can close our eyes.

Shen imbalances can be seen clearly in the eyes. In depressive conditions where *shen* is blocked or lacks nourishment, the eyes are often glazed, without expression and with a blank stare, because there is no movement of *hun*. In Heat imbalances where *shen* is agitated, there can be a lot of eye movement, with the eyes constantly darting left and right, as *hun* comes and goes too quickly.

On the emotional level, there is a close relationship between the Liver and the Heart. Both organs are easily disturbed by emotional influences. The Liver is sensitive to stress, frustration and anger and when there are emotions that do not get expressed. These will create stagnations of *qi* or generate Heat in the Liver. Both of these conditions will eventually affect the Heart. All emotional imbalances that are chronic or extreme will affect the Heart. Liver *qi* stagnation and Liver Fire will, however, have a specifically negative effect on the Heart. Liver *qi* should support the movement of the Heart *qi*. Stagnations of Liver *qi* will lead to Heart *qi* stagnations. Heat from the Liver will quickly create imbalances in the Heart. This is because the Liver is physically located very near to the Heart. The Heat from the Liver will rise up to the Heart and create Heat here. In addition, when there is Heat in the Liver, *xue* can become Hot. *Shen*, which has its residence in Heart *xue*, will easily become agitated when there is *xue* Heat because of its *yang* nature.

The Liver, the Spleen and the Stomach

The Liver plays a central role in supporting the Spleen and Stomach in sending their *qi* up and down from the middle *jiao*. When Liver *qi* stagnates, it often disturbs this *qi ji*. This is the reason why there are often symptoms and signs such as nausea, bloating and problems with defecation when there is Liver *qi* stagnation.

The Spleen and Stomach produce *gu qi*, which is an antecedent to *xue*. The Liver, which is a reservoir for *xue*, is dependent on sufficient amounts of *xue* being produced. This means that Spleen and Stomach *qi xu* can lead to Liver *xue xu*.

The Liver and the Intestines

In the same way that the free flow of Liver *qi* supports the Stomach in sending its *qi* downwards, Liver *qi* supports the Large Intestine and Small Intestine in sending the remaining dregs from the digestion process down through the Intestines. If Liver *qi* stagnation disturbs the Intestines in this function, there will be symptoms and signs such as abdominal distension, abdominal pain and problems with the stools.

The Liver and the Kidneys

The relationship between the Kidneys and the Liver is reflected in the relationship between *jing* and *xue*, which mutually nourish each other. It is said that Liver and Kidney *yin* have a common root. This can be seen in practice by the fact that when there is *yin xu* in one of these organs there will usually also be a *yin xu* condition in the other. Furthermore, Liver *xue xu* can lead to Kidney *yin xu*, because Liver *xue* is an aspect of Liver *yin* and because Liver *xue* nourishes Kidney *jing*.

The Liver and the Gall Bladder

Liver *qi* ensures the free and unimpeded excretion of bile. This is important to aid digestion. Furthermore, a stagnation of Liver *qi* can contribute to the formation of gallstones.

On the mental-emotional level, there is a close cooperation and relationship between the Liver and the Gall Bladder. The Liver provides us with the ability to plan and to take the decisions, but it is the Gall Bladder that gives us the courage to carry out these decisions.

The Liver and Gall Bladder's close relationship to each other can be seen at the channel level, where many of the Liver imbalances manifest themselves with symptoms in the Gall Bladder channel. An example of this is a unilateral migraine due to ascending Liver *yang*.

The Liver and the Uterus

The Liver has, by virtue of its function of being a reservoir for *xue*, an important relationship to the *bao* (the Uterus).

Xue is stored in the Liver before it is sent down via *chong mai* to the Uterus to create a menstrual bleeding. Liver *qi* stagnation, Liver *xue* stagnation, Liver Fire and Liver *xue xu* can all have a disruptive effect on the menstrual cycle and menstrual bleeding. There can be disturbances of the cycle's rhythm and length and the quality and quantity of the menstrual blood, as well as menstrual pain.

THE HEART

The Heart is an aspect of the Fire Phase and thereby an expression of the most extreme *yang qi* in the body. This is reflected, amongst other things, in the fact that the Heart is located in the upper part of the upper *jiao*. The brain, which includes some of the Heart's functions in the Western sense of the word, is also located in the highest part of the body. The Heart's *yang* nature and its relationship to the Fire Phase is also seen in that the Heart is very easily affected by Heat. This is because Heat is itself an aspect of the Fire Phase, and Heat, because of its *yang* nature, will naturally ascend. This means that Heat, no matter where it is located, will also affect the upper aspects of the body. This means that Heat in other organs will nearly always affect the Heart and *shen* in some way.

Yang's nature is to govern and dominate, whereas *yin* is passive and nourishing. In the hierarchy of the internal organs, the ultimate *yang* organ is therefore assigned the role of the Emperor of the body's realm. The Heart is a true emperor – it does not do that much, but it is still vital for the well-being of the entire realm. If you look at which functions the Heart performs, the Heart does very little compared with the Spleen or the Liver, for example. Nevertheless, the Heart is the most important organ in the entire body.

The Emperor is responsible for the entire realm, so therefore he must be aware of everything. His omniscience is continuously utilised so that the necessary and appropriate action is taken in any situation. It is the Emperor's responsibility that the whole of the dominion functions. Without his guiding hand, there would be chaos and rebellion in the realm. It would all go into dissolution. If the Emperor is weak or demented, he will not be able to control his kingdom. This is exactly the same with the Heart. If the Heart is unstable, chaos starts to arise in the body and the mind. This is why there are many protective agencies around the Heart. It is important that an invasion does not penetrate into the Emperor's residence.

The functions of the Heart

As stated above, the Heart is viewed as being the body's most important organ. This is despite the fact that the tasks it performs are relatively limited, compared with other *zang* organs. The Heart is the most important organ in the body, because it is here that *shen* has its residence. *Shen* has the same role in the body that the Emperor had in ancient China. Just like the Emperor, *shen* is aware of everything that is going on in the body. The other organs' duty is to obey and serve the Emperor. They perform the Emperor's orders and constantly report information back to him. The Heart has a constant awareness and knowledge of all the events, influences and activities in the body, even though these take place in other organs. In reality, this is no different from the Western medicine physiological model. When, for example, we burn our fingers, the damage occurs in the fingers, but it is our brain that perceives and interprets the signals from the nerve endings in the fingers. The brain makes us aware of what has happened and then orders the body to take appropriate action. When we hear a sound, it is the ears that hear the sound wave, but it is our *shen* that makes us conscious that we have heard a sound, as well as what significance this sound has.

It is not only in relation to the body physiology that the Heart and *shen* have this function – it is also on the emotional level. The consequence of this is that all emotional influences will have an impact, not only on the organ that these emotions affect, but also on the Heart itself.

Shen, which is the most *yang* aspect of the Heart, has a very close relationship to Heart *xue*, which is a part of the Heart's *yin* aspect. There is a classic *yin/yang* relationship between these two aspects, where Heart *xue*, which is *yin*, both nourishes and controls *shen*, which is *yang*.

The Heart's relationship to *shen* is central to our understanding of the Heart itself in Chinese medicine. This becomes even more apparent in pathology and diagnosis, where Heart imbalances usually manifest with signs relating to the mind, mood, behaviour, sleep, memory, etc.

Heart *shen* is a refraction of the universal *shen* or *dao*. When our *shen* is in contact with the universal *shen*, we feel secure and peaceful and have a feeling of belonging. When our *shen* loses this connection, either because it is undernourished, agitated or blocked, we will experience loneliness, desolation, anxiety and a nagging sense of foreboding or of something not being right.

The Heart enables us to open ourselves to other people. It is through the Heart that we communicate with others, and it is the Heart that makes a connection with other people. This connecting to, and communicating with, other people is therefore a central aspect of the Heart. It is also the reason that speech is the 'sense' that relates to the Heart and the reason that the tongue is the sensory organ of the Heart. Equally as important as the ability to open the Heart and communicate and connect to others is the ability to close the Heart when this is relevant and not to over-communicate. People with Heat agitating the Heart have a tendency to talk too much and to express too much inappropriate or irrelevant information when talking to other people.

On the physical level, the Heart also has a close relationship to *xue*. The Heart is not directly involved in the production of *xue*, but the transformation of *gu qi* to *xue* takes place in the Heart under the influence of *yuan qi* from the Kidneys. The fire aspect of the Heart imparts the red colour to *xue*. In addition, the Heart governs the blood vessels. Together with *zong qi* from the Lung, the Heart rhythmically circulates *xue* through vessels and channels.

The functions and relationships of the Heart can be summarised as follows.

The Heart

- governs *xue*
- controls the blood vessels
- controls sweat
- manifests in the complexion
- opens to the tongue
- controls speech
- is affected by the bitter flavour
- is affected by Heat

- manifests with a burnt or scorched odour
- is affected by, and manifests with, the red colour
- is affected by joy
- manifests with a joyful or laughing voice
- has *li* as its virtue, which is propriety or appropriate behaviour
- is the residence of *shen*

The Heart governs xue

In the same way that the heart controls blood in Western medicine physiology, the Heart governs *xue* in Chinese medicine physiology. The Heart's governing of *xue* is carried out in cooperation with the Lung. The Lung creates *zong qi*, and it is *zong qi* that is the driving force behind the Heart's circulation of *xue* through blood vessels and the channel system.[14] At the same time, *zong qi* contributes to the Heart beating rhythmically and with the appropriate strength. Here we again see the close relationship that there is between *xue* and *qi*. From a diagnostic perspective, palpitations and irregularities of the heartbeat will therefore always be a sign of a Heart imbalance.

The Heart also has a relationship to *xue*, in that it is in the Heart that *yuan qi* transforms *gu qi* into *xue* and the Heart imparts the red colour to *xue*.

The Heart controls the blood vessels

It is not only *xue* flowing through the blood vessels that is governed by the Heart – the blood vessels themselves are also under the overall control of the Heart. In fact, they can be seen as being a natural extension of the Heart, because all blood vessels are directly connected to, and have their beginning and end in the chambers of, the Heart. This means that the vessels are a part of the Heart itself and will therefore naturally be governed by the Heart. The Heart's function of governing *xue* and the blood vessels is specifically reflected in the pulse. The most important qualities that a pulse should have are that it has vitality, that it is soft but at the same time has force, and that it is regular. This will reflect that the Heart is in balance and governs *xue* and the blood vessels as it should. This quality in pulse diagnosis is known as the pulse having *shen*.

Other organs do of course have an influence on the vessels, not least the Spleen, which ensures that *xue* is kept inside the vessels. Also Heat and *xue* stagnation can cause the walls of the blood vessels to rupture. This means that disorders relating to the structure of the vessels will usually be caused by other factors than imbalances in the Heart itself, even though the vessels are an aspect of the Heart.

The Heart controls sweat

Sweat is the body fluid that relates to the Fire Phase and to the Heart. Other organs, though, play key roles in the production, distribution and controlling of sweat. *Wei qi*, for example, controls the opening and closing of the pores, in relation to the body temperature and in relation to the presence of *xie qi*. The Kidneys, *san jiao*, the Lung, the Urinary Bladder, the Stomach and the Spleen are all involved in fluid physiology, but it is the Heart that has the overall responsibility of controlling sweat. This is seen clearly in nervousness and insecurity. When *shen* and the Heart are unsettled, a person will sweat spontaneously. The areas where a person sweats the most when nervous are the armpits and the palms of their hands. These are at the start and end of the Heart channel. Heart *yin xu* often manifests with night sweats.

Both sweat and *xue* are under the overall control of the Heart. There is a *yin/yin* relationship between *xue* and *jinye*, which sweat is an aspect of. *Jinye* and *xue* have a common root and complement each other in their functions. In addition, *jinye* can be transformed into *xue* and *jinye* thins *xue*, so *xue* does not become too thick and sticky. On the other hand, *xue* is weakened by excessive or persistent sweating.

According to the theory of the Six Stages, a direct invasion of exogenous *xie* Cold can occur at the *shaoyin* stage (Heart/Kidney) if a person is cooled by a breeze or the wind whilst sweating.

The Heart manifests in the complexion

The condition of the Heart is reflected in the complexion. Red cheekbones, for example, are a characteristic sign of Heart *yin xu*. Heart *xue xu* on the other hand will often result in a very pale and wan complexion. Heart *yang xu* can result in the face being pale and dull, while Heart *xue* stagnation can make the face look matt, dark and even purplish. This will also be apparent in the lips. When the Heart is in balance, the face will be neither too pale nor red, with the exception of the cheeks, which should be slightly rosy. The face as a whole should be lustrous and radiate vitality.

There are several reasons that the Heart influences the colours in the face. First, all organs and all vital substances have in some way or another an influence on the colours in the face and their distribution. Because the Heart governs *xue* and the blood vessels, the Heart will have a particularly significant influence on the complexion. The skin on the face is very fine and the blood vessels are very superficial. This means that changes in *xue*, which is governed by the Heart, will be more easily observed here than in many other places on the surface of the body. The quality of *shen*, which has a close relationship to Heart *xue*, can also be observed in a person's face. The colours and the complexion should have vitality and radiance.

The Heart opens to the tongue

The sensory organ that relates to the Heart is the tongue. There is a direct connection from the Heart to the tongue via the Heart's *luo* channel, which connects to the root of the tongue. It is through the Heart *luo* channel that the tongue is supplied with *xue*. This means that Heart *xue* and Heart *qi* will have an influence on the tongue's shape, colour and structure. This is clearly seen when there is Heat in the Heart, in particular the imbalance pattern known as Heart Fire. Heart Fire can, for example, manifest with blisters and ulcers on the tongue. As we will see below, the Heart controls speech. The tongue physically enables a person to speak.

The Heart controls speech

Each organ has a direct relationship to both a sensory organ and one of the body senses. The Liver's sensory organ, for example, is the eyes and the Liver controls vision. The Heart differs in several ways from the other organs. The other organs are considered to be more physical[15] and their sensory organs are hollow. This means that their sensory organs can be filled with sensory impressions. The Heart is fundamentally different. This is related to the Heart's relationship to *shen*. For the Heart to be filled with the universal *shen* or *dao*, it must be empty. This is why the Heart's sensory organ is solid in its structure. The Heart should not be filled up with sensory impressions. Instead, the tongue is used to talk with and thereby to 'empty the heart'.

The Heart's relationship to speech is also related to one of the Heart's most important functions, which is the ability to open up to and communicate with other people. This is something that we use speech to do. Many Heart imbalances manifest with changes in the speech. When a person is anxious and *shen* is unsettled, they often start to stammer. If there is Heat in the Heart, the person talks both a lot and quickly. They tend to over-communicate. Heart *qi xu* and Heart *qi* stagnation, however, often manifest with a person being taciturn and reserved. Phlegm blocking the orifices of the Heart can make the speech confused and muddled, with the person sometimes thinking one thing but saying something else.

The Heart is affected by the bitter flavour

The bitter flavour is used in herbal medicine particularly to drain Damp-Heat downwards and out of the body, but the bitter flavour also has a special resonance with the Fire Phase and the Heart. The bitter flavour can therefore guide a particular influence to the Heart. This can be seen with coffee, which has a bitter taste. The strong, stimulating effect of coffee affects the functions of the Heart and *shen*. The bitter taste relates not only to the Heart, but also to the Fire Phase in general. This explains why many people experience a bitter taste in the mouth when there is Liver Fire and Stomach Fire, because they are Fire imbalances.

The Heart is affected by Heat

Heat by virtue of its *yang* nature has an ascending dynamic. This means that when there is Heat, whether it is *shi* or *xu* Heat, it will always rise upwards. The Heart is located in the upper *jiao* and therefore the Heart is always in some way affected when there is Heat. The Heart is an aspect of the Fire Phase and thereby is very *yang* in nature. This means that the Heart is easily affected by Heat. Heat has a tendency to agitate and over-activate the Heart and *shen*.

Heat can have a further negative effect on the Heart, in that Heat can cause sweating, which can weaken Heart *qi*.

The Heart manifests with a burnt or scorched odour

The burnt or scorched odour is a manifestation of the Fire Phase and will manifest both when there are Fire imbalances and when there are Heart imbalances. The burnt or scorched odour is called *zhuo* in Chinese. Hicks *et al.* (2004) describe this odour as being like toast that has burnt, clothes that have just come out of a tumble dryer, a shirt that has been burnt with an iron or vegetables that have boiled dry in a saucepan. In the same way that the smell varies depending on what it is that has burnt, the burnt odour can vary from person to person and from imbalance to imbalance. The odour can often be smelt when a person has a high fever.

The Heart is affected by, and manifests with, the red colour

The red colour is an obvious aspect of the Fire Phase. Fire and flames are red in colour. A room that is painted red subjectively feels warmer than a blue room. Patterns of Heat and Fire usually manifest with redness of the face and head, whereas lack of physiological heat, such as when there is Heart *yang xu*, will manifest with a face that is pale. The red colour in the face – or lack of it – is often seen when *shen* is affected. We blush due to embarrassment and become totally pale when scared or nervous.

The Heart is the organ that relates to joy and pleasure. Both the red colour and the Heart represent passion, enthusiasm, desire and lust in many cultures. Red hearts represent being in love. In China, red and not white has traditionally been the colour that is used at weddings. It is not coincidental that the classic colour for sports cars is red, because red represents speed, lust, passion and enthusiasm, all of which are extreme *yang* qualities.

The Heart is affected by joy

When the Heart and *shen* are in balance, there is a natural, calm happiness and satisfaction in a person. When the Heart is in imbalance, however, there can either be a lack of pleasure, as in depression, or there may be an excessive elation and ecstasy, as in mania. The Heart, therefore, can be affected both negatively and positively by joy. Both laughter and cheerfulness have a proven, beneficial effect on the heart in Western medicine, and a lack of joy can have a similar negative effect. Too much happiness having a negative effect on the Heart sounds slightly counter-intuitive. It is important to remember that all emotions are in themselves just movements of *qi*. Emotions are neither negative nor positive, but are just something that affects the organism. It is our mind that assigns the various emotions positive or negative associations. An emotion is only negative when it is inappropriate to the situation, when it is excessive or lacking or when it is persistent, i.e. stuck. Joy is seen as being an aetiological factor in Heart imbalances. Here there will be an uncontrolled or excessive joyfulness. This could have arisen in connection with an abuse of stimulants, too much partying, too much sex or in a general over-stimulation of the senses. Excessive pleasure and elation weakens Heart *qi*, and thereby dulls the movement of Heart *qi*.

As is the case with sensory impressions, all emotions affect the Heart and *shen*, and not only the organs that the individual emotion resonates with or is an expression of. Again, this is because it is *shen* that makes us conscious of the emotion that we are currently experiencing. Anger causes Liver *yang* to rise upwards, but it is *shen* that makes us aware of the fact that we are angry. Without *shen* consciousness, anger would be a purely physiological condition in the body. This means that any long-term emotional imbalance will over time damage the Heart.

The Heart manifests with a joyful or laughing voice

The voice should preferably have a natural, happy quality when a person speaks. The joy in the voice should not be false or overexcited, but there should be a happiness in the voice that indicates that the Heart and *shen* are in harmony. This quality is usually heard when a person talks of a happy event. The voice will have vitality. When there are Heart *xu* imbalances or Heart stagnations, the voice will usually lack this quality. There will be a flatness and sadness in the voice. Conversely, when there is Heat in the Heart, the voice can sound artificially happy. There may be a constant, nervous giggling while talking. It can also be a 'life and soul of the party' voice – the person who constantly laughs loudly and makes jokes. The voice should also be appropriate to what is being talked about. If a person's voice is happy and lively, or they laugh, while they are talking about something sad, infers that there is a Heart imbalance. Similarly, it is an indication of a Heart imbalance when a person talks about something joyful in a sad and flat voice.

The Heart has li as its virtue, which is propriety or appropriate behaviour

Originally, *li* denoted the court rites performed to sustain social and cosmic order. In traditional Chinese society, it was the Emperor's main responsibility to follow dutifully and perform the appropriate rituals and ceremonies at the correct moment in time. He constantly had to behave correctly with regards to the universe so that the Empire, and thereby the population, were favoured by Heaven.

Li is reflected in the body by *shen* adapting our responses and behaviour to our surroundings and to the society around us. *Shen* makes us aware of what is normal and what is not normal, what is right and wrong and what is appropriate and inappropriate. When *shen* is in imbalance, a person can lose this ability to adapt to correct or normal standards of behaviour.

The Heart is the residence of shen

Shen is a difficult concept to translate. Even in Chinese medicine, *shen* has multiple interpretations and the word *shen* is translated differently by different authors. This reflects that there are varying definitions or rather aspects of *shen*, but also the emphasis that various authors place on these aspects.

Shen can be defined as the sum of all the mental, emotional and spiritual activities in the body, whilst our *shen* is simultaneously an individual refraction of the universal *shen*.

Each *zang* organ has its own individual *shen* aspect, and together these five aspects form a person's *shen*. This means that the concept of *shen* is used both as the sum of the five organs' *shen* aspects whilst at the same time denoting the specific aspect of *shen* that is unique for the Heart. This specific aspect of the Heart can be translated into English as something similar to the concept of the mind or consciousness. It is our cognitive powers. *Shen* is what enables us to comprehend what is happening to us and to understand this and integrate it. *Shen* is our mental activities and our emotions. Although certain feelings are connected to the specific organs, all emotions affect the Heart. It is through the Heart that we experience emotions and become aware of them.

The Heart *shen* makes us aware of sensory impressions. For example, the ears and thus the Kidneys are responsible for hearing, but it is *shen* that makes us aware of what we have heard. This is not dissimilar to Western medicine physiology, where the nerve receptors in the various sensory organs are stimulated by sound, smell, taste, etc., but it is the brain that makes us aware of what it is we are hearing, smelling, tasting and so on.

The Heart governs *xue*, and *shen* is both nourished and anchored by Heart *xue*. It is also said that *shen* resides in Heart *xue* and that *shen* flows with *xue* throughout the body. This close relationship between *xue* and *shen* is seen in that many *xue* imbalances manifest with emotional or psychological signs and symptoms, such as insomnia when there is *xue xu* or manic behaviour when there is *xue* Heat. Heart *xue* has, via its relationship to *shen*, a great influence on memory and the ability to concentrate.

Shen is one of the Three Treasures – *jing*, *qi* and *shen*. *Jing* and *qi* are relatively *yin* in comparison to *shen* and they are the root of *shen*. It is from these that *shen* is created. These three each have a close relationship to a specific organ in each of the three *jiao* – the Kidney, Spleen and Heart – and they also reflect the continuum of Earth, Man and Heaven. *Jing* and *shen* are the most extreme forms of *yin qi* and *yang qi* in the body respectively. In the same way that Water/Fire and *yin/yang* have a reciprocal relationship, so do *jing* and *shen*. *Shen* activates *jing*, and *jing* is the material base from which *shen* is created.

As previously stated, *shen* is the most *yang* form of *qi* in the body. *Shen* is anchored in the body by the body's *yin* aspects, especially *xue*, but due to its *yang* nature, *shen* is also to a certain extent outside the body. This can be experienced, for example, when you can feel that a person is staring at you, without you having seen them do it, or if you instinctively know that a person sitting in the carriage of a train is mentally disturbed without them having said a word. There is something about that person's *shen* that makes our own *shen* unsettled, even if there has been no form of contact with the other person.

A healthy and balanced *shen* is reflected in a person being happy and content and calmly resting in themselves. They are happy without being manic. They will talk calmly without being effusive or uncommunicative. They will be naturally outgoing without being either too brash and uninhibited or excessively shy. Their memory and their sleep will be good and they will be mentally alert and clear in the head. Emotionally, they will be harmonious and they will be able to both experience and manifest the various emotions without any of these getting out of hand.

When *shen* is in balance, we are able to enter into healthy relationships with other people.

In pathological conditions, *shen* can be weakened, blocked or agitated.

Even though each of the five *shen* are discussed in the relevant chapters about the various *zang* organs, I would like to sum up and provide an overview of the five *shen* here.

Heart shen

Shen has its residence in the Heart and vessels. *Shen* is anchored and nourished by Heart *xue* and Heart *yin*.

Shen encompasses the Western concept of the mind and is the sum of our mental abilities and emotional feelings. It is *shen* that makes us aware of what we are experiencing. It is, for example, *po* that feels that the skin is being touched or that we are touching something. It is the Liver that is affected by anger and it is our ears that hear the various sounds, but it is Heart *shen* that makes us aware of all these experiences.

Whereas *po* dies together with the body and *hun* rises up to the universe, *shen* is constant. It has never been separated from the Universe or the Earth. It just is. It is timeless and formless. It is the ultimate *yang*. Whereas *hun* is three in number and *po* is seven, *shen* is infinite and cannot be measured.

Shen also has the function of adapting our behaviour and responses to the environment and the society around us. It is what makes us aware of what is normal and abnormal – what is appropriate and inappropriate.

Liver hun

Hun has its residence in the Liver. *Hun* is nourished and anchored by Liver *yin* and Liver *xue*. During the day *hun* is in the eyes and 'sees' for *shen*. At night *hun* returns to the Liver. *Hun* is termed the ethereal spirit. At death *hun* rises up and out of the body through the acupuncture point Du 20. *Hun* survives the physical body. *Hun* remains in the world for three generations before it returns to the universe.

Hun creates our visions and dreams, both whilst we are awake and whilst we sleep. *Hun* enables us to see future possibilities. The ability of *hun* to create visions is the source of creativity and imagination in people who are artistic. *Hun* is also the subconscious – that which is not the conscious mind.

When sleeping, *hun* rests in the Liver, but if the Liver's *yin* aspects (which include Liver *xue*) are weak or if there is Heat in the Liver, *hun* will be activated, resulting in disturbed sleep and excessive dreaming. In REM sleep the eyelids flutter because *hun* has come up to the eyes. If *hun* is very agitated and is not anchored, it can even leave the body and the person may have an 'out of body experience'. On the other hand, it is often through dreams and whilst sleeping that people get ideas and solve problems.

Hun has the ability to create a vision and see a possible future; it enables the Liver to make 'plans and strategies'. This is because *hun* has a clear idea – a 'dream'. Whereas *po* is *yin* and is fixed in time and space, *hun* does not have this attachment. This is why *hun* can look forwards and see other possibilities. If *hun* is not anchored or if it is agitated, a person can have too many ideas and dreams without achieving any of them.

Lung po

Po has its residence in the Lung and *po* is the animal or corporeal spirit. *Po* ensures the physical functions and reflexes in the body. It is *po* that reacts when the body is exposed to physical impulses such as contact to the skin, which is an aspect of Metal. *Po* is that which ensures that the Lung draws in each breath, that the Stomach empties and that the body heals when it is wounded. It is all the things that the body does without us having to think consciously about it. It is our instincts, reflexes and responses to physical stimuli. *Po* is the contact point between the body and the world around it.

Po experiences things in the present moment. *Po*, by virtue of its *yin* nature, is anchored in space and time. It is for this reason that *po* experiences pain but not suffering. This is because pain is the experience and suffering is our response to it.

Po is the *yin* aspect of *shen* and *po* is *yin* in relation to *hun*, which is thereby *yang*. *Po* helps to anchor and hold the *yang hun* inside the body. *Hun* naturally seeks to rise upwards and back to the universe. Whereas *hun* has a close relationship to *qi* and *xue*, *po* has a close relationship to *jing*. This is similar to the relationship between *hun* and *shen*, which follow each other in their movements.[16] Whereas *shen* and *hun* follow each other in our inner relationship to the outside world and on a more mental-emotional plane, *jing* and *po* follow each other in the more physical aspects of existence and in the day-to-day maintenance and growth of the body.

By virtue of the fact that *po* is *yin* and is anchored in space and time, it anchors and balances *hun*, which does not have the same connection. Whereas *hun* sees into the future and visualises other possibilities, *po* enables us to be present in the moment and appreciate what is now.

Po enters into the body just after conception and is activated by the first breath. *Po* exits the body through the rectum (some say that it enters and leaves the body through the acupuncture point *Pohu* – UB 42). When *hun* rises up to Heaven and the Universe, *po* sinks into the ground.

Spleen yi

The Spleen's *shen* aspect is called *yi*. *Yi* can be defined as our mental faculties, our intellectual focus. *Yi* enables us to digest information so that we can reflect on our experiences and impressions. *Yi* also enables us to focus on one task and channel our *qi* in a certain direction, for example when we carry out certain acupuncture techniques.

Yi is used in, but can also be burdened by, studying, thinking and meditating.

Kidney zhi

Zhi, which has its residence in the Kidneys, can be translated as willpower. As well as being associated with willpower, *zhi* is also associated with concepts such as perseverance, motivation and memory. If the Kidneys are strong, we have the willpower and perseverance to carry out the projects we have started, i.e. the projects that the Liver and *hun* have visualised and decided upon. Without *zhi*, *hun* would just be empty ideas that would amount to nothing. *Zhi* is also that which gives us stability. It keeps us on track so that we do not keep wandering off and following every new idea.

There is also a close relationship between the Spleen's *yi* and the Kidneys' *zhi*. *Yi* is the intention that is used to focus *qi* when we need to start with a project. *Zhi* gives us the perseverance needed to complete the project.

Zhi is seen in the desire to live. It is the desire to grow that is seen in a sprout. The sprout determinedly grows up into the light. It is also the will to continue life that manifests as sexual desire and lust.

The Chinese character *zhi* also has a definition of memory. This makes sense when we take into account the fact that the brain is nurtured by and created from *jing*. Problems with the memory, especially the short-term memory, can arise when *jing* is weakened.

The Heart's relationship to other organs

The Heart and the Kidneys

The Heart and the Kidneys' relationship is a reflection of the fundamental relationship that there is between Fire and Water, up and down, *shen* and *jing* and *yang* and *yin*. Together they form the central, vertical axis in the body.

Shen is created and nourished by *jing*, but at the same time *shen* activates *jing*. Kidney *yin* both nourishes and anchors Heart fire. If Kidney *yin* is weak, Heart *yin* is not nourished and Heart fire will not be controlled.

The *yang* fire of the Heart flows down to the Kidneys, where it warms and activates the Kidneys' *yin* aspects.

The menstrual cycle is dependent on the communication and interaction between the Heart fire and Kidney water. This cooperation is a part of the foundation for the transformations from *yang* to *yin* and *yin* to *yang* that take place all through the cycle. The Heart is connected to *bao* (the Uterus) via a channel that is called *bao mai*. Another channel, called *bao luo*, connects the Kidneys and *bao*. *Tian gui* or 'Heavenly Water', which is the foundation of fertility and fecundity, is created when Heart *yang* fire flows down through *bao mai* to the *bao*. Here it transforms the *yin jing*, which the Kidneys have sent up via *bao luo*.

The Heart also ensures that the *bao* opens at the right times during the cycle, and the Kidneys ensure that the *bao* closes when it is appropriate.

The Heart is also dependent on Kidney *yang* performing its duties in relation to the transformation and transportation of fluids in the body. The Heart can be burdened and flooded by fluids when there is a condition of kidney *yang xu*.

The Heart and the Kidneys also have a relationship to each other in that they are both aspects of the *shaoyin* channel.

The Heart and the Lung

The relationship between the Heart and the Lung reflects the relationship between *qi* and *xue*. *Qi* moves *xue*, and *xue* nourishes *qi*. Lung *qi* and *zong qi* are used by the Heart to drive *xue* through the vessels, and Heart *xue* nourishes the Lung. Without *qi*, *xue* would stagnate, and *qi* can only flow through the channels and vessels if there is *xue* present to 'concentrate' and anchor it.

Even though it is said that the Heart governs the blood vessels, it is dependent on the *zong qi* that the Lung has created to be able to carry out its task of circulating *xue* rhythmically through the vessels and channels. It is therefore said that 'the Lung controls the hundred vessels'. This means that the Lung has a determining influence on the movement of *xue* in the vessels. It is therefore also common to see respiratory problems in cardiac disorders, disturbances of the breathing by cardiac disease and an increase in the speed of the pulse when there is Heat in the Lung.

The Heart is the Emperor; the Lung is the Prime Minister with responsibility for regulation. While Heart *shen* controls the mental consciousness, the Lung *po* controls the somatic and rhythmic functions in the body that do not require conscious thought.

The Lung's rhythmic control of breathing can also be used to calm *shen* if it is unsettled. One of the best ways to calm a person who is upset and agitated is to get them to breathe calmly and deeply into the lower abdomen. By regulating Lung *qi*, the Heart *qi* is regulated.

The Heart and the Liver

Whereas the relationship between the Lung and the Heart is characterised by a *qi/xue* relationship, the relationship between the Heart and the Liver is characterised by them both having a close relationship to *xue*. The Heart governs *xue*, and the Liver regulates and stores *xue*. It is very common to see Heart *xue xu* and Liver *xue xu* concurrently. This is actually more the rule than the exception. This is also the reason that there are symptoms and signs relating to both the Heart and the Liver when there is *xue xu*. Both organs will also often be affected when there is *xue* Heat.

As well as both organs having an influence on *xue* by governing it and storing it, *xue* also has a significant influence on these organs' *shen* aspects. *Hun* and *shen* are nourished and anchored by, as well as travelling together with, Liver and Heart *xue*. This is why both organs' *shen* aspects are easily affected by *xue* imbalances.

Shen and *hun* have a close relationship to each other. This relationship is greater than their common relationship to *xue*. Their relationship is summarised in the following statement: 'Shen and hun follow each other in their entering and exiting.' One of the consequences of this is that if *shen* is not firmly anchored or if *shen* is agitated, *hun* begins to wander, and if *hun* is blocked, *shen* will also become blocked.

Hun is the eyes for *shen*. The eyes are the only sense organ that can be focussed and that can be directionally orientated. You think first and then the eyes follow. We cannot control the other senses in the same way. The eyes can focus on specific objects. When you consciously want to observe something, you move your eyes and the vision focuses on the object. This is not something that can be achieved with the sense of smell or hearing, for example. Neither can we close our ears or nose in the same way that we can close our eyes.

Shen imbalances can be seen clearly in the eyes. In depressive conditions where *shen* is either blocked or lacks nourishment, the eyes will often be glazed, without expression or blankly staring, because there is no movement of *hun*. When Heat agitates *shen*, the eyes become restless, darting to the left and right, and the person cannot maintain eye contact for more than short periods of time, because *hun* is coming and going too quickly.

On the emotional level, there is a close relationship between the Liver and the Heart. Both organs are easily disturbed by emotional influences. The Liver is sensitive to stress, frustration, anger and emotions that are not expressed. These will create stagnations of *qi* or generate Heat in the Liver. Both of these conditions will over time affect the Heart. Even though all long-term or powerful emotional imbalances affect the Heart, Liver *qi* stagnation and Liver Fire can have a particularly negative effect on the Heart. Liver *qi* should support the flow of Heart *qi*. Stagnations of Liver *qi* will lead to Heart *qi* stagnation. Heat from the Liver will also quickly create imbalances in the Heart. This is because the Liver is located close to the Heart. Heat from the Liver will rise up to the Heart and create Heat here. In addition, Heat in the Liver can result in *xue* Heat, because the Liver stores *xue*. *Shen*, which has its residence in Heart *xue* and because of its *yang* nature, is easily agitated by *xue* Heat.

The Heart and the Spleen

The Spleen and the Heart both have a relationship to *xue*. The Heart governs *xue*, and *shen* is anchored and nourished by *xue*. The Spleen creates *gu qi* and is therefore the root of *xue*. This means that Spleen *qi xu* can lead to Heart *xue xu* with a subsequent impact on the person's *shen*. This is something that is commonly seen in the clinic.

THE PERICARDIUM

This *zang* organ has been translated into English in a number of ways – Pericardium, Heart Protector, Heart Governor, Heart Master and even circulation/sex. This is because this organ has been given more than one name in the various classical texts – *xin bao*, *xin bao luo* and *xin zhu*, but also because each of these names has been translated differently into English, German and French.

To get an idea and an understanding of what the Pericardium is, and what the difference between it and the Heart is, it is a good idea to look at the Chinese characters and what these mean. *Xin* means heart, and it is the same character that is used for the *zang* organ – the Heart. *Bao* means an envelope or wrapping – something that is placed around something precious, something that protects or covers. *Luo* here is the same *luo* as before, as in a *luo* vessel. *Luo* therefore tells us something about communication. The Pericardium is considered to be an ambassador for the Heart – someone who is responsible for the communication between the Emperor and the outside world. The Pericardium ensures that information, messages and orders are passed back and forth. At the same time, the Pericardium is a kind of bodyguard for the Emperor and protects the Emperor from being attacked.

The Pericardium is called *xin zhu* or Heart Master, and the Heart is called *xin jun*. *Jun* means sovereign, such as when a king or an Emperor is sovereign and decides everything. Thereby the Heart is *xin jun* or Heart Emperor. A *zhu* or master would have been the person who has the authority to perform the Emperor's wishes and orders. That is why the Pericardium is *xin zhu* or Heart Master.[17]

An emperor should be omniscient and omnipotent. This makes the Emperor the single most important person in the entire realm. The Emperor cannot be in direct contact with his subjects and his servants. All communication and contact takes place through an ambassador. In the body it is the Pericardium that performs this function. This is why the Pericardium was given the title of Ambassador in the organ hierarchy. The Ambassador acts on the Emperor's command. The difference between an Ambassador and a Prime Minister (which is the Lung) is that the Prime Minister has been assigned certain powers by the Emperor. The Prime Minister can therefore work independently, within a certain framework. The Ambassador on the other hand is completely dependent on the Emperor's instructions. The Ambassador has no independent functions. The Pericardium has, as its sole purpose, to be an ambassador and protect the Heart. This means that it is difficult to separate clearly their functions and characteristics from each other.

One significant difference between the Heart and the Pericardium can however be seen in their Chinese characters. In the character for the Heart, there is no flesh radical in the character. All the other *zang* organs, including the Pericardium, have this radical. This indicates that there is a crucial difference between the Heart and the other five *zang* organs; the Heart is not physical in the same way that the other organs are. The Pericardium is the more physical aspect of the Heart, i.e. its muscle and tissue. The Heart is the void that these muscles and tissues embrace. In Daoist thinking, the void that is the Heart should be filled by *shen* – the emptiness that encompasses everything and is the potential for everything. The Pericardium is the physical expression and manifestation of this emptiness.

In the oldest classical medical texts, such as the *Huang Di Nei Jing*, there is only mention of five *zang* organs. This is because the Pericardium was not considered to be an independent organ but was something that protected the Heart from being attacked by exogenous *xie qi*. On the other hand, it is the Pericardium channel, in the *Huang Di Nei Jing*, that is used when treating the Heart. This is again based on an understanding of the Pericardium as being something that protects the Heart and that it is through the Pericardium that the Heart communicates with the outside world. Therefore the Pericardium channel and not the Heart's own channel was used when trying to affect the Heart.

The functions of the Pericardium

Although the Heart and the Pericardium are nowadays conceived of as being two independent organs in Chinese medicine, they are still considered as having a very close and almost symbiotic relationship. This is seen in particular by the fact that their physiological functions are almost identical and many of their acupuncture points have almost the same actions and indications.

As described above, the Pericardium is the Heart's ambassador. It is its duty to carry out a large part of the Emperor's work and be a protective agency between the Emperor and the outside world. It is a type of bodyguard, because if the Emperor is attacked and dies, the whole kingdom will collapse. The Pericardium protects the Heart against invasions of exogenous *xie qi*, shock and emotional trauma.

As well as providing protection, the Pericardium also supports the Heart. It does this by governing *xue* and housing *shen*.

It is extremely important that there is free communication in and out of the Heart. In pathological situations, the Pericardium can be blocked by Phlegm or *xue* stagnation. This blockage will mean that the Heart *shen* will be blocked.

The functions and relationships of the Pericardium can be summarised as follows.

The Pericardium

- has a very close relationship to the Heart
- protects the Heart against attacks of exogenous *xie qi*
- governs *xue*
- has a major influence on the chest and *zong qi*
- is the residence of *shen*

The Pericardium has a very close relationship to the Heart

As written above, the Heart and the Pericardium have a very close relationship, where the Heart is dependent upon the Pericardium for protection, as well as being assisted in its communication with the outside world.

Their close relationship is also seen in that the Pericardium has almost no independent patterns of imbalance. The Pericardium's patterns of imbalance can in general be seen as being the same as those of the Heart. Heart imbalances are, though, often treated by using acupuncture points on the Pericardium channel. The only patterns of imbalance that specifically relate to the Pericardium are found in the two diagnostic models for 'Diagnosis according to the four levels' and 'Diagnosis according to the three *jiao*'. In both of these analyses, exogenous *xie qi* has invaded the body and either disrupted or blocked the Pericardium. These diagnostic models and treatment methods are described in detail in *The Art of Diagnosis* (Ching 2009).

The Pericardium protects the Heart against attacks of exogenous xie qi

If the Emperor is weakened, wounded or even dies, it will have consequences for the entire realm. That is why the Pericardium has the role of a kind of bodyguard. When exogenous *xie qi* invades the body, overcomes the body's *zheng qi* and penetrates deeper inwards, the Pericardium will be the deepest level *xie qi* can reach. The Pericardium prevents *xie qi* from reaching the Heart. As written above, this is also the reason that the only specific Pericardium patterns of imbalance relate to the treatment of invasions of exogenous *xie qi*.

The Pericardium governs xue

The Pericardium, which is the muscle of the Heart, helps to pump *xue* around the body.[18] Here we see again the close relationship and cooperation between the Heart and the Pericardium. The Pericardium channel is used primarily for the treatment of stagnation of *xue* in the Heart and the upper *jiao*, as well as to cool Heart *xue*.

The Pericardium has a major influence on the chest and zong qi

The Pericardium channel is used in the treatment of stagnations in the chest. There are several reasons for this. First, the Pericardium's primary and *luo* channels connect to the centre of the chest. This means that acupuncture points on the Pericardium channel will have a direct influence on this area of the body. Furthermore, as we saw with the Heart, there is a close relationship between *zong qi* and the functions of the Heart in circulating *xue* throughout the body. This means that the Pericardium channel can be used to treat *xue* stagnations, due to its relationship to Heart *xue*, as well as the treatment of *qi* stagnations in the chest, due to the relationship that there is between Heart *xue* and *zong qi*.

The Pericardium is the residence of shen

Because the Pericardium is an aspect of the Heart, it is also the place where *shen* has its residence. This also manifests when *xie* Heat that has invaded the Pericardium agitates *shen*. The Heat will agitate *shen*, as well as creating Phlegm, which blocks the movement of *shen* in and out of the Heart. Furthermore, the relationship between the Pericardium and *shen* can be seen in that there are many important points for the treatment of *shen* imbalances along the Pericardium channel.

The Pericardium's relationship to other organs

The Pericardium and the Heart have a mutual and internal relationship to each other by virtue of the Pericardium being an aspect of the Heart. This also means that the Pericardium's relationship to the other *zang* organs is very similar to the Heart.

FU ORGANS

THE STOMACH

Of all the *fu* organs, the Stomach is seen as being the most important. This is because the Stomach plays a key role in the production of post-heaven *qi*. The Stomach has a very close functional cooperation with its *yin* partner organ, the Spleen. The two are virtually indistinguishable in their collaboration in the production of the post-heaven *qi*. The Stomach and Spleen's *qi ji* or *qi* dynamic is like a crankshaft in the middle of the body, where the Stomach sends *qi* downwards and the Spleen sends *qi* upwards through the body. This *qi ji* is of great importance, not only for their own *qi* communication to and from the middle *jiao*, but also for *qi* communication throughout the whole of the body. All communication upwards and downwards in the body has to pass through the middle *jiao*.

The functions of the Stomach

The majority of the Stomach's functions are carried out in cooperation with the Spleen. Also, many of the Spleen's functions are dependent on this cooperation with the Stomach. The Stomach is the first organ that receives the ingested food and liquids. The Stomach has the task of 'ripening and rotting' the food so that the pure essences can be extracted and sent upwards in the body to where they will be used. The remaining impure residues are sent down from the Stomach to the Small Intestine for further transformation and separation. This means that the production of *qi*, *xue* and *jinye* is dependent on the Stomach and its *qi*, and that the Stomach is capable of being filled and emptied as it should. If the Stomach cannot send the impure residues down to the Small Intestine, there will come a point when it will no longer be possible to eat anything and the production of *gu qi* will come to a halt. The Stomach is also one of the only *fu* organs that can be *qi xu*, i.e. have a deficiency condition.

The functions and relationships of the Stomach can be summarised as follows.

> **The Stomach**
>
> - controls the receiving of food
> - ripens and rots the food
> - transports essences from the food out into the body
> - sends *qi* downwards
> - is the root of *jinye*
> - prefers moisture and dislikes dryness
> - has a tendency to Heat

The Stomach controls the receiving of food

The Stomach is directly connected to the exterior through the mouth and throat. The Stomach is the place where the ingested food and drink is retained until the process of transformation begins. By virtue of its function of storing food and drink, the Stomach is called 'the great breadbasket' and 'the sea of food'.

The Stomach must, like other *fu* organs, 'fill and empty'. This is why the Stomach functions optimally when there is regularity, i.e. when a person eats regularly and when they do not eat too much at a time. If too much food is eaten or if the Stomach does not get enough time to empty, food will stagnate in the Stomach. If there is too long between meals, or if there is insufficient food, then *qi xu* can arise. Furthermore, as it is the Stomach that receives the food, the Stomach will also be sensitive to what it is that is eaten. Food that is very spicy, or food and liquids that are very hot in their energy, can easily engender Heat in the Stomach or injure Stomach *yin*.

The Stomach ripens and rots the food

It is said that the Stomach 'rots and ripens' the food. To rot and ripen means that the ingested food and liquids start to get broken down in preparation for the transformation process. As in a compost heap or a fermentation chamber, the ingested food and liquids are broken down in the Stomach. This prepares the food so the Spleen can extract the pure essences from it. It is for this reason that the Stomach and the Spleen are known as the 'post-heaven root of *qi*'. It is here that the production of *qi* from the food that we eat begins.

Fermentation and composting require the right conditions. It should be neither too cold nor too dry. Both conditions will cause the fermentation process to stop. This is not dissimilar to the transformation process. Spleen *yang qi* is damaged by cold, and Stomach *yin* is damaged by dryness.

The Stomach transports essences from the food out into the body

The Stomach and the Spleen work very closely together to send the pure, transformed essence of food and liquids that have been consumed out into the body to where it is needed. Here again we see the inseparability of the Stomach and Spleen in their functionality.

The Stomach sends qi downwards

The impure and untransformed residues from the food and liquids that the Stomach and Spleen have processed are sent down by the Stomach to the Small Intestine. A further separation of the pure and the impure is carried out in the Small Intestine. This *qi ji* in the middle *jiao*, where the Spleen sends *qi* upwards and the Stomach sends *qi* downwards, means that the middle *jiao* is like an axle or a pivot in the middle of the body. This *qi ji* is of great importance, not only in aiding digestion, but also for the flow of *qi* in the whole body. This is why it is important that the Stomach and Spleen are functioning optimally. It is of great importance for the communication between the lower and the upper *jiao* and between the Kidneys and the Heart that this passage is open and that *qi* can flow freely.

The Stomach is the root of jinye

In the same way that the Stomach is the first stage in the production of post-heavenly *qi*, the Stomach is also the first stage in the production of *jinye*. The Stomach receives the liquids that have been consumed. The Stomach retains the liquids until they are transformed by the Spleen. The Spleen sends the pure aspect of these fluids up to the Lung. The impure remainder that has not been transformed is sent down to the Small Intestine together with the remaining untransformed food. In the Small Intestine there will be a further transformation separating the pure and the impure aspects from each other. It is because of its role in the initial stage of the fluid transformation that the Stomach is called the root of *jinye*.

The Stomach prefers moisture and dislikes dryness

In addition to being the root of *jinye*, the Stomach has in general a close relationship to *jinye*. The Stomach and the Large Intestine constitute the *yangming* aspect of the body. *Yangming* organs have the task of integrating climatic dryness in the body. This, though, also means that both the Stomach and the Large Intestine can be easily damaged by dryness. Dryness has a damaging effect on the Stomach *yin* aspect. The Stomach is also dependent on there being a sufficiently moist environment so that it can carry out its function of ripening and rotting the food. It is not only a lack of body fluids and liquids that can damage the Stomach; spicy food will often have a drying effect on Stomach *yin*. Food and drink that have a hot energy will also generate Heat in the Stomach and thereby create dryness in the Stomach.

The Stomach has a tendency to Heat

The Stomach and the Spleen are mutually dependent on each other, but they are also each other's opposites in many respects. As we saw above, the Stomach prefers a moist environment and is damaged by Dryness. The Spleen is the opposite. It is burdened by Dampness and too much moisture and thrives in a dry environment. The Spleen is also damaged by Cold and requires physiological heat from *mingmen* to be able to carry out its functions of transformation. The Stomach for its part is damaged by pathological Heat and by substances that have a hot energy, such as alcohol, strong spices, painkillers, etc. The Stomach can also be disrupted in its functions by Cold, but this disruption will be due to Cold preventing the Spleen from transforming the food in the Stomach.

Apart from Stomach *yin* being easily damaged by pathological Heat, the Stomach itself has a tendency to Heat. *Xu* and *shi* Heat in the Stomach often arise when there is a long-term consumption of food and substances that have a hot energy. This will typically be alcohol, strong spices, fried food, lamb and some medications such as painkillers. These all have a hot energy. Heat can also arise in the Stomach when there are invasions of exogenous *xie qi*. The Heat can either directly invade the Stomach, such as in food poisoning, or it may be *xie qi* that has penetrated deeper into the body after it has overcome the body's *wei qi*. Finally, Heat in the Stomach can arise when the Stomach is invaded by Heat from the Liver.

The Stomach's relationship to other organs

The Stomach has a relationship to all the other organs in that it sends pure essences from the ingested food and liquids to the rest of the body. Furthermore, the Stomach is the root of all the fluids in the body. This means that all organs are dependent on the Stomach operating optimally. The Stomach has specific relationships with the Spleen, the Liver, the Small Intestine, the Large Intestine and the Kidneys.

The Stomach and the Spleen

The Stomach and the Spleen are each other's *yin/yang* partner organs. Whereas some *zangfu* organs' *yin/yang* relationships can appear tenuous, other organs' *yin/yang* relationships are very logical and straightforward. The Stomach and the Spleen are so integrated and inseparable in their cooperation around the production of *qi* and *jinye* that each is totally dependent on the other to be able to perform its functions. This symbiosis means that it is less common that there is a *qi xu* condition in one of these organs without there also being *qi xu* in the other.

The Stomach receives, rots and ripens the food. The Stomach breaks down the food and prepares the food for transformation so that the Spleen can extract the pure essences. This is the same process that occurs with the fluids. If the Stomach does not carry out its functions, then the Spleen will not be able to carry out its functions and vice versa.

The two organs also send their *qi* in separate directions. The Stomach sends *qi* downwards, whilst the Spleen sends *qi* upwards. This *qi ji* is like a wheel, where the one side goes up while the other side goes down. If one of the organs is not able to send its *qi* up or down, it will result in the other organ having difficulty sending its *qi* in the opposite direction. The wheel will eventually grind to a halt. This dynamic is important, not only for the Stomach and the Spleen's internal relationship, but for the flow of *qi* in the body as a whole. The Stomach and the Spleen's *qi ji* is the central axle. If this *qi ji* breaks down or becomes blocked, the communication between the upper and lower *jiao* and between the Kidneys, the Lung and the Heart will be disturbed.

Furthermore, the Stomach and the Spleen's *yin/yang* relationship is not only seen in their dependence on, and support of, each other, but also in that they are, in some respects, each other's opposites. The Spleen is dependent on physiological heat and is damaged by the *yin* pathogens of Dampness and Cold. The Spleen also tends to become *yang xu* when it is chronically weakened. The Stomach, on the other hand, tends to Heat and is damaged by substances that are hot or dry in their energy. These will either generate Fire or damage the Stomach's *yin* aspect.

The Stomach	The Spleen
Damaged by Heat and consuming substances that have a hot energy.	Damaged by Cold and consuming substances that have a cold energy or temperature.
Damaged by Dryness.	Damaged by Dampness.
Tends to Heat and Fire (*yang shi*) and *yin xu*.	Tends to Dampness (*yin shi*) and *yang xu*.
Sends its *qi* downwards.	Sends its *qi* upwards.

The Stomach and the Kidneys

The Stomach and the Kidneys have a relationship to each other centred on *yin* and *jinye*.

Stomach *yin* and Kidney *yin* are mutually dependent on each other. Stomach *yin* is dependent on Kidney *yin*, as this is the root of all *yin* in the body. The Kidneys, on the other hand, are dependent on the production of *jinye*, whose production cycle starts in the Stomach.

Kidney *yang* supports Spleen *yang* in its transformation and transport of the fluids, which are received by the Stomach. This means that a condition of Kidney *yang xu* can contribute to fluids in the Stomach not being transformed by the Spleen.

The Stomach and the Liver

The Stomach's function of sending *qi* downwards is supported by the Liver, which ensures that *qi* flows freely and without hindrance in the body and that *qi* flows in the right direction. Liver *qi* stagnation can lead to Liver *qi* becoming rebellious and 'invading' the Stomach, i.e. instead of supporting the Stomach's *qi ji*, the Liver *qi* disrupts and blocks Stomach *qi*. This is why it is common to see signs that the Stomach is imbalanced when there is Liver *qi* stagnation. This could be symptoms and signs such as nausea, vomiting, abdominal distension, abdominal pain and constipation.

The Stomach and the Small Intestine

After the Spleen has transformed food and liquids in the Stomach and sent the pure aspects upwards, the Stomach sends the untransformed residues down to the Small Intestine for further processing. The Small Intestine is thus dependent on the Stomach sending its *qi* downwards to be able to carry out its functions.

The Stomach and the Large Intestine

The Large Intestine and the Stomach constitute the *yangming* aspect of the body. One of the important tasks that *yangming* carries out is to integrate dryness in the body. It is important that there is the right balance with neither too much nor too little dryness. The Stomach and the Large Intestine have a regulatory effect on the body's moisture and dryness. The Large Intestine absorbs fluid from the stool, and the Stomach is the root of *jinye*. When the Stomach is in imbalance, especially when there is Heat, there will often be signs of dryness, such as thirst, constipation and a dry tongue coating. Also Stomach *yin* is damaged by food and substances that are dry in their energy.

THE SMALL INTESTINE

The Small Intestine has a *yin/yang* relationship to the Heart. Some organ partnerships are very logical due to their functional cooperation; other pairs can seem slightly more incomprehensible. The closest link between the Heart and Small Intestine is probably on the mental level. Just as it does on the physical plane, the Small Intestine enables us to separate the pure from the impure. This means that it helps us to understand and to see things more clearly. By separating the relevant from the irrelevant, we can make decisions. It is of great importance to our mental clarity that we can filter information from the outside world so that we can integrate it in our minds.

In having a *yin/yang* relationship, the Heart and the Small Intestine have what is called a *biaoli* or external/internal relationship. This means that their respective channels have an internal branch that connects to both of the organs. Their channels' external branches are also connected to each other. The Heart channel connects to the start of the Small Intestine channel on the little finger. The two channels are also connected through their *luo*-connecting channels. Pathological Fire in the Heart can drain down to the Small Intestine via the channel's internal connections.

The functions of the Small Intestine

Many of the functions attributed to the small intestine in Western medicine physiology are attributed to the Spleen and the Stomach in Chinese medicine. This is why disorders such as diarrhoea, constipation, bloating, etc. are, as a general rule, treated by the use of the Stomach and Spleen channels.

The Small Intestine's main function in Chinese medicine physiology is to receive the untransformed residues from the Stomach. The Small Intestine separates the pure from the impure, the clear from the murky. The pure fluids and *qi* are sent up through *san jiao*, and the impure fluids and dross are sent downwards to the Urinary Bladder and the Large Intestine respectively.

Although these processes take place in the Small Intestine, they are carried out under the influence of Kidney *yang* and the Spleen.

The functions and relationships of the Small Intestine can be summarised as follows.

The Small Intestine

- controls receiving and transforming
- separates the pure and impure

The Small Intestine controls receiving and transforming

The Small Intestine receives the residues of the food and liquids that remain after the Spleen has performed its functions of transformation in the Stomach. These residues contain still usable *qi* and *jinye*. The Small Intestine's task is to separate the pure and usable aspects. The pure aspects that the Small Intestine separates are transported around the body via *san jiao* to where they are needed. The impure residue that remains will be sent to the Large Intestine and the Urinary Bladder to be further processed and expelled from the body.

The Small Intestine separates the pure and impure

As written above, there will still be usable residues of *qi* and *jinye* in the impure residue that is sent down to the Small Intestine from the Stomach. The Small Intestine carries out a further separation of the pure and impure aspects of these residues. In cooperation with the Spleen, the pure essences of the food are sent out into the body. The pure fluids that are separated out are sent up through *san jiao*, where they spread through the body. The impure dregs that remain after this further separation of pure and impure are sent down to the Urinary Bladder and the Large Intestine. In the Urinary Bladder there will be a further transformation of the impure fluids, after which the impure dregs are driven out of the body as urine. The Large Intestine receives the impure residue from the Small Intestine. In the Large Intestine the last traces of fluid are absorbed from the stools, before the stools are expelled from the body. In this way there is an optimal exploitation of the food and liquids that were consumed through the mouth.

The Small Intestine also separates the pure from the impure on the mental level. In order to make a decision and to be able to act upon it, it is necessary to have an overview. The Small Intestine helps to create this mental clarity by enabling us to separate the relevant and useful information from the irrelevant.

The Small Intestine's relationship to other organs

The Small Intestine has a direct relationship to the Stomach, the Large Intestine, the Urinary Bladder and the Heart. The Liver and the Kidneys also have an influence on the Small Intestine's activities.

The Small Intestine and the Heart

Although they are *yin/yang* partner organs, there is a relatively limited functional relationship between the Small Intestine and the Heart. As written above, there is cooperation on the mental level, where the Small Intestine assists the Heart by separating the relevant and useful information from the irrelevant. The Heart and the Small Intestine can affect each other when there is pathological Heat. Fire and Heat can be transmitted from one organ to the other via their internal channel connections.

The Small Intestine and the Stomach

The Stomach sends impure residues from the production of *qi* and *jinye* down to the Small Intestine for further processing. In addition, the Small Intestine is dependent on the Stomach sending its *qi* downwards to be able to send the remaining dregs down to the Large Intestine.

The Small Intestine and the Large Intestine

The Small Intestine sends the untransformed dross that is left after the production of *qi* and *jinye* downwards. These are received by the Large Intestine.

The Small Intestine and the Urinary Bladder

The impure fluids that were separated by the Small Intestine during the production of *jinye* are sent to the Urinary Bladder. In the Urinary Bladder there will be a further separation of pure and impure. The Small Intestine and the Urinary Bladder together constitute the *taiyang* aspect of the body and have a relationship to cold. The *taiyang* channel is the outer aspect of the body and protects the body against exogenous cold. It is in the *taiyang* channel that the first signs of an invasion of Wind-Cold manifest themselves.

The Small Intestine and the Kidneys

The Kidneys and the Small Intestine have a relationship with regards to fluid physiology. The Small Intestine is dependent on *yuan qi* from the Kidneys to carry out its functions of separating the pure and impure fluids from each other, as well as sending the pure fluids upwards and the impure fluids to the Urinary Bladder.

The Small Intestine and the Liver

In common with other organs, the Small Intestine is dependent on the Liver ensuring that *qi* is flowing freely and without hindrance in the body. Stagnant Liver *qi* can invade the Small Intestine with resultant symptoms such as abdominal distension, constipation and pain.

THE LARGE INTESTINE

The Large Intestine is the final section of the digestive tract and it is from here that the dross that is of no value and that was not transformed during the production of *qi* and *jinye* is separated from the body.

The functions of the Large Intestine

Just as was the case with the Small Intestine, many of the functions that Western medicine attributes to the large intestine are performed by the Spleen and the Stomach in Chinese medicine.

The main action that the Large Intestine performs is to receive the residue from the Small Intestine and absorb the last traces of pure fluids from the stool before expelling the stool from the body.

The functions and relationships of the Large Intestine can be summarised as follows.

The Large Intestine

- controls reception from the Small Intestine and sends the stool downwards
- absorbs fluid from the stool
- helps us to let go

The Large Intestine controls reception from the Small Intestine and sends the stool downwards

The Large Intestine receives the remaining residue that the Small Intestine has itself received from the Stomach. The Spleen and the Small Intestine have extracted all the useful *qi* from the food and most of the pure fluids from the liquids. If these organs have performed their functions optimally, there will only be a little residue of pure fluid remaining in the dross that the Large Intestine has received. The Large Intestine ensures that the last remaining pure fluids are absorbed by the body before the Large Intestine sends the remaining dross out of the body as faeces.

The Large Intestine absorbs fluid from the stool

The Large Intestine absorbs the pure fluids from the remnants that are left over after the production of *qi* and *jinye*. After the Large Intestine has performed this task, it expels the remaining dross from the body.

The Large Intestine helps us to let go

The mental-emotional aspect of the Large Intestine is similar to its function on the physical level. The Large Intestine helps us to let go of old emotions. It is important that we are able to let go of, and not hold on to, old relationships and emotions. By letting go, we are then able to let something new come into our lives. This allows us to be present in the moment and not to get stuck in the past.

This is connected to the mental-emotional aspect of the Large Intestine's partner organ, the Lung. The Lung has a resonance with grief and melancholy. It is normal and correct to be sad and grieve when something ends or when we lose someone or something, but in order to move on we must also be able to let go of it again.

The Large Intestine's relationship to other organs

The Large Intestine and the Lung

The Large Intestine has a *yin/yang* relationship to the Lung. Apart from them both being Metal Phase *zangfu* organs, there is also a functional relationship between the two. The Large Intestine is dependent on the Lung sending *qi* downwards through the body to be able to expel the stool from the body. This is clearly seen by the fact that we breathe in and press down from the diaphragm when we defecate. Elderly people, whose Lung *qi* is *xu*, often have difficulty passing stools and experience spontaneous sweating and exhaustion when trying to defecate. On the other hand, people who suffer from constipation can experience shortness of breath and difficulty breathing deeply when they are constipated.

On the mental-emotional level, both organs are involved in letting go so that we take something new in. This reflects the function that the Lung and the Large Intestine have on the physical level of expelling waste products from the body to create the space for the absorption of new nourishment. This is the same process that we see on the emotional level. The emotion that is attributed to the Lung is sorrow and melancholy. We experience sorrow when we are not able to let go of emotions and relationships. In order to create the space for something new, you have to be able to let go of that which has died or is no longer beneficial.

The Large Intestine and the Small Intestine

The Large Intestine receives the untransformed residues from the production of *qi* and *jinye* that have been sent down from the Small Intestine.

The Large Intestine and the Liver

In common with other organs, the Large Intestine is dependent on the Liver ensuring that *qi* flows freely and without hindrance in the body. Stagnant Liver *qi* can disrupt the functioning of the Large Intestine and lead to symptoms such as bloating, constipation and intestinal pain.

The Large Intestine and the Stomach

The Large Intestine and the Stomach constitute the *yangming* aspect of the body. One of the most important functions of *yangming* is to integrate dryness in the body. It is important that there is the right balance, with neither too much nor too little. This function is reflected in the Large Intestine's function of absorbing the last traces of pure fluid from the stool before it is expelled from the body. Imbalances of the Large Intestine will often manifest with too much or too little fluid in the stool.

The Stomach is at the root of *jinye*. When there is imbalance in the Stomach, especially if there is Heat, there are often signs of dryness, such as thirst, constipation and a dry tongue coating.

The Large Intestine and Stomach also have a channel relationship. They are, as stated above, both aspects of *yangming* and thereby their channels are also the arm and leg aspect of the *yangming* channel. The circulation of *qi* in the twelve-channel *qi* cycle continues from the Large Intestine channel to the Stomach channel in the face.

SAN JIAO

San jiao is in many ways a difficult concept. This is because *san jiao* is an organ that does not exist in the Western sense. This though is also an advantage, because it then becomes obvious how an organ should be understood in Chinese medicine – that function is more important than physical form.

Some classical texts say that '*san jiao* is an organ that has function, but does not have form', i.e. *san jiao* is an organ that cannot be seen but is understood through its functioning. In reality this is no different than is the case for all the other *zangfu* organs. The only real difference between *san jiao* and the other organs is that the other organs have a Western medicine counterpart that has a concrete, anatomical structure. Nevertheless, these organs will often have completely different properties and functions than they have in Chinese medicine, and it is their functions that define them as an organ in Chinese medicine.

As there is no Western counterpart to *san jiao*, this has resulted in this organ having many different names in Western acupuncture books. *San jiao* may be termed Triple Heater, Triple Burner, Triple Endocrine, Endocrine, the Three Burning Spaces, etc. In addition to describing the functions it carries out, some Western writers have not just interpreted, but also extrapolated, the characteristics that *san jiao* is attributed. Some write that *san jiao* is equivalent to the endocrine system, the lymphatic system or the thermal regulation of the body. Others write that *san jiao* is the connective tissue or the cavities that surround the internal organs, or *san jiao* is the organs that are located in the various areas of the chest and abdomen. To get a real understanding of what *san jiao* is, it is necessary to look at what the classic texts have written about *san jiao*.

The discussion on what *san jiao* is is in no way new. For nearly two thousand years Chinese doctors have discussed whether *san jiao* has a form or whether it is only the functions of *san jiao* that define it as an organ.

If *san jiao* is defined as having a form, then one of its definitions is that it is a threefold division of the body – the area above the diaphragm is the upper *jiao*, the area between the diaphragm and the navel is the middle *jiao*, and the area from the navel downwards is the lower *jiao*. It is important to remember when trying to understand the concept of *san jiao* that it is not the organs in each *jiao* that are this *jiao* but the space around them. For example, the Lung and the Heart are not the upper *jiao*, but the upper *jiao* is the cavity that surrounds the Lung and the Heart.

With regard to the locations of the organs, it is important to be aware of the fact that the Liver is considered to belong to both the middle *jiao* and the lower *jiao*. This is because the Liver is physically located in the middle part of the body, but its functional activities relate to the lower *jiao*. The Liver has a very close relationship to both the Kidneys and the Uterus (*bao*).

Some authors have gone a step further. They believe that *san jiao* is not only the cavities around the internal organs, but also that *san jiao* is all spaces in the body, as well as the space between our muscles and the gap between the skin and the connective tissue. These spaces in the tissues and between the skin and muscles are called the *cou li* in Chinese.[19] This definition of the *san jiao* makes a lot of sense when you look at the functions and activities that *san jiao* performs in relation to the transport and distribution of *yuan qi*, *ying qi*, *wei qi*, *jinye* and the impure liquids.

The functions of *san jiao*

San jiao transports and distributes fluids and it regulates the temperature of the body through perspiration and urination. *San jiao* is an avenue of *yuan qi*, *wei qi* and *zhen qi*, thereby having a very important relationship to all the other organs. *San jiao* ensures that *qi*, especially *yuan qi* and fluids, are distributed to where they should be. At the same time, *san jiao* ensures that *qi* from the various organs flows in the direction it should.

San jiao in general, and each of the three *jiao*, are defined by the functions they perform.

Huang Di Nei Jing – Ling Shu, chapter eighteen, describes the upper *jiao* as a mist: 'The upper *jiao* opens outwards, spreading the five flavours from the food, filling the body and permeating and moisturising the skin. It is like a mist.' This refers mainly to the functions that the Lung and the Heart have with regards to the production and distribution of *qi*, *xue* and *jinye*.

The same chapter in *Huang Di Nei Jing – Ling Shu* states that the middle *jiao* 'receives *qi*, expels waste products, evaporates body fluids, transforms the refined essences of the food and connects up to the Lung'. This is the Stomach and the Spleen's functions, which the middle *jiao* has the overall responsibility for.

The chapter goes on to describe the lower *jiao* like a drain or a ditch: 'Food and drink are first received in the Stomach and the waste products are sent down to the Large Intestine in the lower *jiao*. From here they seep downwards and the Large Intestine separates fluids and sends them to the Urinary Bladder.'

San jiao's role is similar to that of a municipal clerk who organises the work of the council workers on the street – the people who empty the bins, bring food out to the elderly, paint lines on the roads, etc. All these people are council workers, but it is important that it is the right person who comes to the right place at the right time. It is a problem if the home-helper empties the food into the garbage truck or the dustman empties the dustbin onto Mrs Jensen's plate. It is the individual employee who carries out the job, but there is an official in City Hall who has the overall responsibility for their daily itinerary. This official ensures that the right employee is in the right place at the right time. *San jiao* has the same function in relation to the internal organs. It is the individual organs that perform the tasks, but it is *san jiao* that coordinates and provides the communication between the various organs. In general, *san jiao* should be conceived of as being the invisible coordinator behind all the complex physiological processes in the body. *San jiao* is a genuine public servant – invisible and essential. He is not visible, but without him the whole system would collapse into chaos.

The functions and relationships of the *san jiao* can be summarised as follows.

San jiao

- is an avenue for *yuan qi*
- controls the movement of *qi*
- controls the water passages

San jiao is an avenue of yuan qi

Yuan qi has its origin in the space between the Kidneys. From here *yuan qi* travels upwards through *san jiao* to where it is needed by the body. *San jiao* is therefore an avenue or a passage for *yuan qi*. *San jiao* leads *yuan qi* both to the internal organs and to the twelve channels, where it enters the channels via their *yuan*-source points. Through its role as an avenue of *yuan qi*, *san jiao* ensures that *yuan qi* separates and assumes different forms. This means that *yuan qi* arrives in the place and in the form that is needed by the various places in the body. This enables *yuan qi* to perform the functions it should.

San jiao controls the movement of qi

San jiao ensures that *qi* moves up and down and in and out. *San jiao* controls the transport and distribution of *qi*. This means that *qi* arrives where it should so that the tasks *qi* should perform are carried out. The result is seen in the production of *zong qi*, *xue*, *jinye*, *ying qi* and *wei qi*.

San jiao not only controls the organs' *qi*, it also controls the movement of *qi* in all the spaces in the body, i.e. in *cou li*.

San jiao controls the water passages

San jiao ensures that fluids are transformed, transported and expelled correctly.

San jiao's title in organ hierarchy is the 'official responsible for drains and irrigation'; this refers to its role in fluid physiology. As mentioned above, *san jiao* is responsible for *yuan qi* arriving at the place and in the form that is needed. The whole production process of *jinye* is dependent on *yuan qi*. The Spleen, the Small Intestine, the Lung, the Kidneys and the Urinary Bladder all use *yuan qi* to transform and transport the fluids. Furthermore, *san jiao* ensures the passage of and directs the fluids up and down and in and out of the body. *San jiao* ensures that fluids arrive where they should.

San jiao has different responsibilities depending on which area of the body is being discussed. The upper *jiao* is described as a mist. *Jin* is dispersed from the upper *jiao* as a fine mist through the body in the cavity between the skin and muscles. The middle *jiao* is like a fermentation chamber or a bubbling pot. It is here that the fluids are first 'rotted and ripened' before being transformed and sent up to the upper *jiao*. The lower *jiao* is described as a drain or a ditch. It is here that the impure fluids are drained down to, and it is from here that the impure fluids are expelled from the body.

San jiao is, as stated, all the spaces in the body, including the spaces in the tissues and the spaces in the joints. *San jiao* controls the movement of fluid in these spaces and, for example, ensures that the joints are kept lubricated.

San jiao's relationship to other organs

San jiao is directly related to all the organs, because *san jiao* is the space around them and ensures that the organs' *qi* is transported to where it should be. *San jiao* and the Kidneys have a specific and close cooperation in relation to *yuan qi*. *Yuan qi* is generated and stored in the Kidneys, and *san jiao* distributes *yuan qi* throughout the body and makes sure that *yuan qi* arrives in the form that needs to be used.

San jiao and the Gall Bladder

The most important relationship that there is between the Gall Bladder and *san jiao* is that they constitute the body's *shaoyang* aspect. This means that their channels are an extension of each other and that they energetically comprise the pivot between the body's interior and its external aspects. It is in the *shaoyang* aspect that exogenous *xie qi* can become trapped.

THE GALL BLADDER

The Gall Bladder is unique amongst the internal organs. This is because the Gall Bladder is classified as being one of the regular *fu* organs whilst at the same time being classified as one of the six so-called extraordinary *fu* organs. Extraordinary *fu* organs have the structure of a *fu* organ but have the characteristics of a *zang* organ. Like a *zang* organ, the Gall Bladder is not in direct contact with the exterior. The Gall Bladder also stores a pure substance – bile – which is again a characteristic of a *zang* organ. The Gall Bladder is also not involved in receiving food or transporting waste products, which are normal *fu* organ functions.

The functions of the Gall Bladder

The Gall Bladder's main function is to store bile that is to be used to aid digestion. The Gall Bladder also has an important role on the mental-emotional level in that it gives a person the courage to carry out decisions. Both of these functions are dependent on a close cooperation with the Gall Bladder's partner organ, the Liver. The Gall Bladder also has a cooperation with the Liver in relation to the sinews.

The functions and relationships of the Gall Bladder can be summarised as follows.

> **The Gall Bladder**
>
> - stores bile
> - controls the sinews
> - controls courage and resoluteness

The Gall Bladder stores bile

The Gall Bladder stores bile, which is a pure substance or essence in Chinese medicine. This is one of the reasons that the Gall Bladder is classified as an extraordinary *fu* organ – it is normally only *zang* organs that store pure essences.

Bile is produced in the Gall Bladder's partner organ, the Liver. Liver *qi* ensures the free flow of bile from the Gall Bladder to the Intestines, where it assists with the digestion.

The Gall Bladder controls the sinews

The Gall Bladder ensures the free flow of *qi* in the sinews. This is the reason that the Gall Bladder's *he*-sea point, GB 34, is also the *hui*-gathering point for the sinews.

Both the Liver and the Gall Bladder have an influence on the tendons and help to make the joints flexible and strong. The Liver's primary relationship to the tendons is to nourish them with Liver *xue*. The Gall Bladder mainly ensures the free flow of *qi* in the tendons.

The Gall Bladder controls courage and resoluteness

Whereas the Liver is known as the 'General with responsibility for planning and strategies', the Gall Bladder is an 'upright official with responsibility for decisions'. It is also written in *Huang Di Nei Jing – Su Wen*, chapter nine, that 'the eleven organs depend on the Gall Bladder for decision making. This is due to its integrity and its *yang* Wood energy, that can break through obstacles.' In China, a person is said to have a 'small Gall Bladder' if they are shy or lack courage, whereas a person with a 'large Gall Bladder' is a person who is brave.

The Gall Bladder provides the courage to implement the decisions and plans that the Liver has made. Many will be able to recognise the image of a person who repeatedly makes a decision, to challenge their boss for example, only to put off the action because they lack the courage and resolution to carry out the decision. This is an example of a weak Gall Bladder.

It might be relevant to look at how a decision is taken and carried out, as seen from a Chinese medicine perspective. A decision requires the cooperation and coordination of several organs. If there is a tendency for a process to repeatedly break down in the same place, this could indicate an imbalance in that particular organ.

First of all, to be able to think clearly requires that *shen* is nourished by *jing* and *xue* and that *shen* is not blocked by Phlegm or stagnant *xue*. A blocked or malnourished *shen* will diminish the ability to think or perceive things clearly. If *shen* is agitated by Heat, there can be problems concentrating due to mental restlessness. Both the Spleen and the Small Intestine are involved in sorting the information that comes into the head. They differentiate the pure from the impure, the relevant from the irrelevant. If a person is Spleen *qi xu* or has Dampness, their thoughts will tend to go round in circles and they will constantly speculate without being able to come to a decision. It is as if everything has to be analysed again and again. They are not able to separate the pure from the impure. Their *yi* is not clear. This separation of pure and impure information is carried out in cooperation with the Small Intestine. As stated above, *shen* must be lucid if a person is to have an overview and understanding of a situation. The Liver must be capable of making a plan and having a strategy. This is *hun*'s function of being able to see a vision of the situation. When you have a vision of the future, you can focus on the development of a strategy and plan for how to get there. In order to carry out this plan, however, you need the courage to act on your decisions and manifest them in reality. This is the role of the Gall Bladder, which gives the person this courage. Finally, it requires *zhi* or willpower from the Kidneys to be able to carry through the project and not to give up when there are obstacles in the way or when the energy starts to run low.

The Gall Bladder's relationship to other organs

The Gall Bladder's main relationship is to its partner organ, the Liver. The two organs have a very close and integrated cooperation where their functions are almost overlapping.

The Gall Bladder and the Liver

Bile is created in the Liver and is sent from here to the Gall Bladder. Liver *qi* ensures the free and unimpeded excretion of bile to the Intestines, where it supports the digestive process. This also means that a stagnation of Liver *qi* can lead to the creation of gallstones.

On the mental-emotional level, there is a close cooperation and relationship between the Liver and the Gall Bladder. The Liver provides us with the ability to plan and to make decisions, but it is the Gall Bladder that gives us courage and resolution to carry out these decisions.

Both organs are involved in controlling the sinews. This is with regard to the free movement of *qi* in the sinews and because Liver *xue* nourishes the sinews.

The Liver and Gall Bladder's close relationship to each other can also be seen at the channel level. Many Liver imbalances manifest with symptoms along the Gall Bladder channel. An example of this is a unilateral headache, due to ascending Liver *yang*.

The Gall Bladder and san jiao

The most important relationship that there is between the Gall Bladder and *san jiao* is that they constitute the body's *shaoyang* aspect. This means that their channels are an extension of each other and that they energetically comprise the pivot between the body's interior and its external aspects. It is in the *shaoyang* aspect that exogenous *xie qi* can become trapped.

THE URINARY BLADDER

The Urinary Bladder is the *fu* organ of the Water Phase. The Urinary Bladder therefore has a *yin/yang* relationship to the Kidneys, with which it also has a very close functional cooperation.

The functions of the Urinary Bladder

The Urinary Bladder's functions in Chinese medicine are broader than those that it is attributed in Western medicine physiology. Just as in Western medicine, the Urinary Bladder stores urine until it is expelled from the body. In contrast to Western medicine, the Urinary Bladder is more than just a receptacle for the storage and excretion of urine. In Chinese medicine, the Urinary Bladder is also involved in the production and transformation of fluids.

As we will see in the following, the Urinary Bladder has a determining influence on the fluid level in the body. This influence on fluids is a result of the role that the Urinary Bladder plays both in fluid physiology and through its control of urination and its relationship to sweat.

It is not only fluid physiology that the Urinary Bladder has an influence on. The body also regulates the temperature through sweating. In this temperature regulation, we see an aspect of *taiyang*'s relationship to cold and how cold is controlled in the body.

The functions and relationships of the Urinary Bladder can be summarised as follows.

> **The Urinary Bladder**
>
> - receives impure fluids and sends pure fluids upwards
> - stores and expels urine from the body

The Urinary Bladder receives impure fluids and sends pure fluids upwards

Fluid physiology in the body is characterised by a constant refining of the fluids that have been consumed, where the pure and the impure parts are separated from each other. Each time the impure aspect is separated out, this aspect is further refined in order to extract the precious, pure aspects that remain in it. The Urinary Bladder carries out the final refining of the impure fluids. The pure part that is separated out in this final transformation is sent up through *san jiao* to the upper *jiao*, where it becomes sweat. These transformation processes in the Urinary Bladder are carried out by Kidney *yang*, and it is *yuan qi* from the Kidneys that sends the pure *jin* up through *san jiao*.

The Urinary Bladder stores and expels urine from the body

The murky, impure dregs that remain after the final transformation is the urine. Urine is retained inside the Urinary Bladder by Kidney *yang qi*, until the body is ready to expel it. Again, it is Kidney *yang qi* that drives the urine out of the body.

The Urinary Bladder's relationship to other organs

The Urinary Bladder's main relationship is to the Kidneys, with which it has a *yin/yang* organ and channel relationship. However, it also has a relationship to other organs, in particular the Lung, Small Intestine and *san jiao*.

The Urinary Bladder and the Kidneys

The Urinary Bladder and the Kidneys have a close functional relationship centred on fluid physiology. The Urinary Bladder 'stores and expels the urine from the body' and it 'receives the impure fluids and sends the pure liquids upwards'. These processes take place in the Urinary Bladder but are carried out by the Kidneys' *yang* aspect.

It is said that the Kidneys control the lower orifices. This means, amongst other things, that the Kidneys store the urine inside the Urinary Bladder. Kidney *yang* does this by keeping the urethra closed so that there is not involuntary or uncontrolled urination. Upon urination, it is again Kidney *yang* that drives the urine out of the Urinary Bladder. Both holding the urine inside the Urinary Bladder and expelling the urine are active *yang* processes that are controlled by Kidney *yang*. It is also Kidney *yang* that carries out the final transformation of fluids in the Urinary Bladder. In this final transformation, the last pure fluids are extracted and sent up through *san jiao* to form sweat, whilst the impure aspects form the urine.

The Urinary Bladder and the Small Intestine

The impure fluids that the Small Intestine separates out during the production of *jinye* are sent to the Urinary Bladder. In the Urinary Bladder there will be a further separation of the pure and impure fluids from each other. The Urinary Bladder and the Small Intestine also have a relationship to each other in that they are both *taiyang* organs. This means both that their channels are a direct extension of each other, but also that they are both involved in the *taiyang* aspect's integration of and protection from cold. It is usually the *taiyang* aspect that is affected when the body is invaded by exogenous Cold.

The Urinary Bladder and the Lung

The Lung sends impure fluids down to the Urinary Bladder when transforming the pure liquids that the Spleen has sent up from the Stomach. Kidney *yang* transforms these fluids in the Urinary Bladder and sends them back up through the body in the form of sweat.

The Urinary Bladder and the Liver

The Liver ensures that there is a free and unhindered flow of *qi* in the body. This is also important for the Urinary Bladder's processes. Furthermore, the Liver channel passes over the Urinary Bladder. This means that a stagnation of Liver *qi* can result in urinary difficulties and pain around the bladder upon urination.

THE SIX EXTRAORDINARY
FU ORGANS

In addition to the twelve regular *zangfu* organs, there are six 'extraordinary' *fu* organs. The extraordinary *fu* organs are characterised by having the form of a *fu* organ, i.e. they are hollow but have the function of a *zang* organ. *Zang* organs and extraordinary *fu* organs store pure substances or essences. Extraordinary *fu* organs are not involved in receiving food or expelling waste products. The six extraordinary organs are the Uterus (*bao*), the Bones, the Bone Marrow, the Brain, the Blood Vessels and the Gall Bladder.

The six extraordinary organs also differ from the regular *zangfu* organs in several ways. The extraordinary *fu* organs:

- do not have a *yin/yang* relationship to each other

- do not have a partner organ

- do not have an associated channel that traverses the surface of the body

- have no Five Phase relationship

- have a close relationship to the eight extraordinary vessels.

The Uterus

The Uterus is called *bao* in Chinese. *Bao*, however, encompasses more than just the Uterus. *Bao* is also the ovaries and the fallopian tubes. There is also a place called *bao* in men. This is the place where semen is produced and stored.

The Uterus has the structure of a *fu* organ. It is hollow. Furthermore, the Uterus empties like a *fu* organ. It does this by expelling the menstrual blood each month and it expels the baby at birth. At the same time the Uterus also has the functions of a *zang* organ. The Uterus stores pure, valuable substances. The Uterus stores the eggs, *tian gui* or Heavenly Water (menstrual blood) and the baby during pregnancy.

Bao in Chinese means something that envelops or wraps around something precious.

There is a connection to the Uterus from the Heart via a channel that is called *bao mai*. The Kidneys have a corresponding channel connection. This is called *bao luo*.

Menstrual blood is called *tian gui* (Heavenly Water). Some sources believe that *tian gui* is not the same as *xue*. They say that *tian gui* is created when Kidney *jing* rises up through *bao luo* to the Uterus, where it is transformed by Heart Fire that has travelled down through *bao mai*. Other historical sources say that *tian gui* is not only created by Kidney *jing*, but also is created from a surplus of *xue* after *xue* has circulated through the body and after *xue* has nourished and moistened the whole body. This is consistent with the fact that there is a reciprocal relationship between *jing* and *xue*, where *xue* nourishes *jing* and *jing* is an important part of *xue* production. This means that a *xue xu* condition will result in scanty menstrual bleeding. Furthermore, heavy menstrual bleeding can easily result in a condition of *xue xu*. My own personal interpretation is that *tian gui* is a prerequisite for fertility and thereby *tian gui* is different from the ordinary *xue*. An interpretation could be that *jing* is the pre-heavenly root of *tian gui* and that *xue* is the post-heavenly root of *tian gui*.

Tian gui in men is semen.

Tian gui has a major influence on a woman's physiology. When a girl reaches puberty and begins to menstruate, it is because there has been a sufficient surplus of *xue*, which has filled *chong mai* so much that it overflows and fills the Uterus with *tian gui*. Menstruation ceases when a woman is forty-nine years old, according to Chinese theories. This is because *mingmen* and the digestive fire started to decrease when she reached the age of thirty-five. This resulted in a poorer production of *xue*. Her Kidney *jing* has decreased so much when she is forty-nine that both the pre- and post-heavenly foundation of *tian gui* is no longer strong enough to create a menstrual bleeding.

The Uterus's relationship to other organs and channels

The Uterus has a close and complex relationship with many organs and channels. These connections are particularly relevant in the treatment of gynaecological disorders and infertility.

The Uterus and the Kidneys

The Uterus and the Kidneys are directly connected via the *bao luo* channel. The Kidneys store *jing*, which is the foundation of *tian gui*. This means that Kidney *jing* is fundamental for fertility and for menstrual blood.

Kidney *qi* holds the Uterus closed. This is an example of the Kidneys' function of keeping the lower orifices closed. This is important not only during pregnancy, but also through the whole menstrual cycle. If the Kidneys fail in this function there can be excessive bleeding or spotting during the cycle. The various transformation processes that take place during the cycle and in fertilisation are dependent on the heat of Kidney *yang*. Kidney *yang* is also used to release the egg at ovulation and to transport the egg through the fallopian tubes.

Kidney *xu* conditions can lead to infertility, miscarriages and irregular menstrual bleeding and spotting.

The Uterus and the Heart

Whilst the Kidneys have the task of keeping the Uterus closed, the Heart is responsible for opening the Uterus when this is appropriate. The Heart does this by sending *qi* and *xue* down through *bao mai*. It is important that the Uterus is able to open so fertilisation can take place and so menstrual bleeding can take place. If the Uterus does not open, it will not be possible for the man's *jing* to enter the Uterus. Stagnation conditions in the Heart can result in the Uterus not being able to open, with infertility being a consequence. Heart Fire, on the other hand, can cause the Uterus to open too much. This can result in spontaneous bleeding and miscarriages.

Another aspect of the Kidneys and the Heart's cooperation is seen in the production of *tian gui*, where Heart *yang* is sent down *bao mai* to transform Kidney *jing* in the Uterus.

All the physiological processes involved in menstruation, fertilisation and pregnancy depend on the balance between Water and Fire, the Kidneys and the Heart.

The Uterus and the Liver

The Liver is a reservoir for *xue*. *Xue* is stored in the Liver before it is sent down *chong mai* to the Uterus. The Uterus is thus dependent on the condition of the Liver *xue* and Liver *qi*. If there is Liver *xue xu*, there will not be enough *xue* to nourish the Uterus and to supplement *tian gui*. This will manifest with scanty menstrual bleeding and infertility. A fertilised egg is dependent on nourishment from *xue* in order to grow and develop. Women with Liver *xue xu* can have a thin endometrial lining, which means that it is difficult for a fertilised egg to attach itself and be nourished. Stagnations of Liver *qi* and Liver *xue* can lead to a stagnation of *xue* in the Uterus. This can manifest with fibroids, menstrual pain and infertility. Finally, Liver Heat and Liver Fire can lead to *xue* Heat. The Heat in the Liver can agitate *xue*, resulting in spontaneous bleeding, heavy bleeding or miscarriages.

The Uterus and the Spleen

The Spleen is the post-heavenly root of *xue*. The Uterus is, as we have seen above, dependent on there being sufficient *xue* to nourish the Uterus, and thus nourish a fertilised egg, and to supplement *tian gui*.

The Uterus and the Stomach

The Stomach and the Uterus have a direct channel connection to each other through *chong mai*. It is because of this connection that some women experience nausea and vomiting during pregnancy. There is a change in the flow of *qi* and *xue* in *chong mai* during pregnancy. This altered flow can result in rebellious *chong mai qi* upsetting the Stomach and causing the Stomach *qi* to ascend instead of descending.

The Uterus and *ren mai*

Ren mai has its origin in *bao*, i.e. in the Uterus in women and in the lower *jiao* in men. *Ren mai* has a very close and important relationship to the Uterus. *Ren mai* supplies the Uterus with *jing* and *qi*. This is of great importance for conception, pregnancy and the menstrual cycle. The first half of the menstrual cycle is particularly dependent on the condition of *ren mai*.

On the whole, women's physiology is heavily influenced by *ren mai*. Menstruation begins in puberty, when *ren mai* and *chong mai* are sufficiently full of *yin* and *xue* that they start to overflow. When *xue* and *yin* dry out in *ren mai* and *chong mai*, the menstrual bleeding stops and the woman is no longer fertile.

The Uterus and *chong mai*

Chong mai has its origin in *bao*, and it is *chong mai* that supplies the Uterus with *xue*. As we saw above, a girl first starts to menstruate when there is sufficient *xue* in *chong mai*. The menstruation stops and the woman enters menopause when *chong mai* dries up and she no longer has enough *xue* to enable *chong mai* to overflow. Because *chong mai* supplies the Uterus with *xue*, it will often be the cause of gynaecological disorders, especially when there is *xue* stagnation in *chong mai*. *Chong mai* channel points are therefore often used in the treatment of gynaecological problems when there is *xue* stagnation in the Uterus.

The Uterus and *du mai*

Just like *ren mai* and *chong mai*, *du mai* also has its origin in *bao*. Whilst *ren mai* and *chong mai* supply the Uterus with *yin*, *jing* and *xue*, *du mai* provides the Uterus with *yang* and heat. *Yang* and heat are required in all transformation processes in the Uterus and it keeps exogenous Cold out of the Uterus.

The Bones

Like several of the other extraordinary *fu* organs, the Bones have a close relationship to the Kidneys. The Bones are created from Kidney *jing*. This means that a person with a weak *jing* may have a weak bone structure. Furthermore, the bones become fragile and more porous in old age as *jing* decreases. The teeth, which are seen as being a surplus of the Bones, also tend to become loose and fall out in old age when *jing* is weak. Problems with bones in general will therefore be treated by nourishing Kidney *jing* or by treating UB 11, which is the *hui*-gathering point for Bones. Local skeletal problems will, however, be treated with local and distal acupuncture points along the channel that passes through the area.

The Bones are a part of the body's structural scaffolding, and at the same time the bones are a *fu* organ. Even though the Bones, like a *fu* organ, have a hollow structure, they do not have the functions that a *fu* organ has. The Bones do not transport impure substances, but they store pure essence in the form of the Bone

Marrow, which is conceived of as a substance that flows through the Bones. Giovanni Maciocia writes, '*Qi* moves in and out of the bones, on the way to and from the body's deeper energetic layer' (2005, p.83). Once again, we can see that the extraordinary organs are a deep-lying energetic aspect of the body. This also reflects the close relationship some authors think there is between the extraordinary vessels and the extraordinary *fu* organs.

The Bone Marrow

Like the Bones, the Bone Marrow is created from Kidney *jing*. There are three aspects of the Bone Marrow in Chinese medicine: the Marrow, which is found in the Bones; the spinal cord; and the Brain. The Bone Marrow is understood as being something that is fluid and moving, while the Brain is more dense and compact.

The Bone Marrow circulates in the Bones, which it nourishes and moistens. This is done in cooperation with *ye*, which is the *yin* aspect of the fluids.

Some sources believe that the Bone Marrow plays a role in the production of *xue* in the same way that the Bone Marrow produces blood in the Western physiological model.

The Bone Marrow is supplemented by nourishing Kidney *jing* and by treating GB 39, which is the *hui*-gathering point for the Bone Marrow.

The Brain

The Brain is considered both to be an independent organ and as an aspect of the Bone Marrow. The Brain is like a flower blossoming on top of the spinal cord. It is the densest form of Bone Marrow in the body. The Brain is also known as the 'Sea of Marrow' in some texts. The Brain is the great sea that is filled with the more mobile and fluid Bone Marrow, which flows into the Brain from the spinal cord. Just like the Bone Marrow, the Brain is also directly created from *jing*. This means that a person can experience problems with memory, concentration, intelligence and sensory impressions (sight, hearing, smell, etc.) when *jing* is weakened, either by old age or when there is *jing xu*.

Many of the Brain's functions overlap the functions that are attributed to *shen*. Both *shen* and the Brain are manifestations of *jing*, from which they both have been created. They are also both nourished by Heart *xue*.

Du mai has a close relationship to the Brain. *Du mai* passes through the spine and it is in the spine that the spinal cord, which is the root of the Brain, is found. At the same time, there is a branch of *du mai* that separates from the primary channel at the point Du 16 and enters the Brain. *Yin qiao mai* and *yang qiao mai* meet at the point UB 1 and continue their inner path into the Brain. This means that imbalances that can be related to the Brain are most often treated with points along the Kidney channel, Heart channel, *yin qiao mai*, *yang qiao mai* and *du mai*.

The Blood Vessels

The Blood Vessels are hollow in their structure, and it is through the Blood Vessels that *xue* flows. The Blood Vessels are involved in the distribution of *xue* and *ying qi* around the body. The Blood Vessels are mainly governed by the Heart. The Heart is the centre of the Blood Vessel network, and it is the Heart that drives *xue* through the vessels.

The Lung and the Spleen also have an influence on the Blood Vessels. The Lung ensures that there is a regular rhythm to the heartbeats. The Lung creates *zong qi*, which is used by the Heart to push *xue* through the Blood Vessels. This is one of the reasons why Lu 9 is the *hui*-gathering point of the Blood Vessels. The Spleen has an influence on the Blood Vessels in that it is Spleen *qi* that holds *xue* inside the Blood Vessels. The extraordinary vessel *chong mai* also has a relationship to the Blood Vessels. *Chong mai*, which is also known as the 'Sea of Blood', has a major influence on the movement of *xue* down to the Uterus and on the movement of *xue* in the Uterus.

The Gall Bladder

The Gall Bladder is both an ordinary *fu* organ and an extraordinary *fu* organ. This is because the Gall Bladder is different from the other *fu* organs in that it is the only *fu* organ that is not in direct contact with the exterior. Furthermore, the other *fu* organs are involved in the reception and transportation of impure substances. Once again, the Gall Bladder stands out because it does not receive untransformed substances. Instead the Gall Bladder stores a pure substance, bile, which is more characteristic of a *zang* organ. Bile is used to support transformation of the food in the intestines. The Gall Bladder also has more psycho-emotional characteristics than other *fu* organs. It is the Gall Bladder that gives us the courage and resolution to carry out our vision and decisions.

Part 4

THE CHANNEL SYSTEM

THE CHANNELS

Introduction

As well as the internal organs and the vital substances, the body also consists of a network of channels that have a direct relationship to the internal organs. This concept is unique to East Asian medicine. This system of energetic channels that *qi* and *xue* flow through is called *jingluo* in Chinese. The concept of *jingluo* is the foundation not only of acupuncture, but also of all the so-called 'channel'-based therapies, such as *shiatsu*, *tuina*, etc. *Jing* can be translated as a thread in a piece of cloth or something that passes through something else. It can also mean a channel that allows water to flow through the landscape. *Luo*, which means 'to attach' or 'a net', is often translated into English as 'collateral'. *Luo* are the network vessels that connect the *yin/yang* channel pairs with each other and connect the primary channel with another part of the body and are the fine network of minute vessels in the connective tissue and cutaneous regions. Together *jing* and *luo* form a fine-meshed network of channels that criss-cross the whole body.

Jingluo was originally translated as 'meridian' in the early French acupuncture books of the 1930s. When acupuncture textbooks were later published in English, the word meridian was therefore also used as a translation of *jingluo*. Most contemporary English textbooks choose to translate *jingluo* as 'channels'. This is because meridian is not a satisfactory translation of *jingluo*. Meridians are an imaginary grid system that arbitrarily divides the planet surface into lines of longitude and latitude. A channel is a naturally occurring structure in which water can flow from one place to another. *Qi* and *xue* flow in the channels from one part of the body to another. The word channel therefore gives a better description of what a *jing* is in a Chinese medicine context.

Western science has always had difficulty with the concept of both the channel system and the *qi* that flows through them. This is because *qi* and channels are not something that can be measured or weighed. Nevertheless, from a Chinese medicine perspective, a channel is something whose existence can be determined. The effects of their existence can be seen and they can be influenced with predictable results and consequences.

Chinese medicine often utilises images where many of the body's structures and substances are described using the image of water and watercourses. At the time that many of the theories relating to the body's physiology and structure were formulated, Chinese society was very dependent on the channelling and storage of water. This was because irrigation and the control of water levels in rivers was extremely important in the production of rice. Furthermore, how water behaves and the way that water affects and is affected by the landscape around it is a central theme in Daoism. Daoism was the prevailing philosophy during this period. The principles observed in nature and in the macrocosm were understood as being reflected in the microcosm of the human body. A twenty-first-century European analogy to describe the channel system would be the road network. One can understand *jing* as being the motorways and main roads that run through the countryside and connect the major cities. These roads also connect the external borders with the central areas of the country. *Luo* channels are the network of minor roads that connect the main roads with each other whilst also leading the traffic from the main roads to all the small villages and houses in the landscape. Whereas the road system transports people, goods, fuel supplies, ambulances, military troops, etc. through the country, the channel system transports the various forms of *qi*, *xue* and *jinye* through the body.

There are twelve so-called regular channels, which run bilaterally, i.e. twenty-four channels in total. These channels run vertically up or down. Each of these channels has an external/internal or *biaoli* relationship with a specific organ. A channel can in this way be understood as being an aspect or manifestation of the organ. In the Western literature, each of the regular channels is named after the organ that it has an internal/external relationship with. In China, the twelve regular channels are named after the twelve *zangfu* organs that they have a *biaoli* relationship with, but also as being the hand or foot aspect of one of the six 'great' channel pairs.

In China the channels are named:

- Small Intestine hand *taiyang* channel

- Urinary Bladder foot *taiyang* channel

- *san jiao* hand *shaoyang* channel

- Gall Bladder foot *shaoyang* channel

- Large Intestine hand *yangming* channel

- Stomach foot *yangming* channel

- Lung hand *taiyin* channel

- Spleen foot *taiyin* channel

- Heart hand *shaoyin* channel

- Kidney foot *shaoyin* channel

- Pericardium hand *jueyin* channel

- Liver foot *jueyin* channel.

This is a very important concept. It indicates that each channel has not only a *biaoli* relationship with a particular organ, but also is an aspect of a larger channel at the same time. For each channel that is located on the arm there is a corresponding channel on the leg. The channel on the leg will have a similar anatomical position as the one on the arm. It will also have similar characteristics and qualities as the channel on the arm that bears the same name. Their *qi* dynamic and resonance will

225

be the same. In this way, the same-name arm and leg channels can be understood as being an extension of each other. That is also why some people call them the extended channels. In Chinese they are simply called *liu jing* (the six channels) or – as it is often translated – the six great channels.

Of the twelve regular channels, six are *yang* in polarity and six of them are *yin*. Each *yang* channel has a specific *yin* partner channel and vice versa. The *yin/yang* channel relationships are the same as the *zang/fu* organ relationships, which again are the same pairings as in the Five Phases. The partnership between *yin* and *yang* channels is in no way coincidental. In addition to being connected to its own internal organ, each channel also connects to its partner's primary channel either at the beginning or end of its course and it connects to its partner's internal organ. Furthermore, there is also a vessel that flows between the two channels along their course on each side of the body. This means that the two *yin* and two *yang* channels are connected to each other and *qi* can flow between the two. This vessel is called a *luo*-connecting vessel.

Channel	English translation	Hand channel	Foot channel
Taiyang	Greater *Yang*	Small Intestine	Urinary Bladder
Shaoyang	Lesser *Yang*	*San jiao*	Gall Bladder
Yangming	*Yang* Brightness or Bright *Yang*	Large Intestine	Stomach
Taiyin	Greater *Yin*	Lung	Spleen
Shaoyin	Lesser *Yin*	Heart	Kidney
Jueyin	Terminal *Yin*	Pericardium	Liver

The channel system is a large circuit where each channel travels in certain directions in relation to the others. Where the one channel ends, the next begins. The sequence in the circulation is determined by the channel's Five Phase relationship and its 'great channel' relationship. For example, the *yin* Lung channel has its source in the chest and terminates in the thumb. Its *yang* Metal partner channel, the Large Intestine, continues the circuit from the tip of the index finger up to the face. As well as being the *yin/yang* partner of the Lung, the Large Intestine is also the hand *yangming* channel. The foot *yangming* channel, which is also known as the Stomach channel, continues the cycle by travelling down from the face to the toes. The *yin* Spleen channel travels from the toes back to the chest. The Spleen channel is not just the *yin* partner of the Stomach channel, it also has a relationship to the Lung channel that started this cycle. They are both *taiyin* channels.

The twelve regular channels in reality form three small circuits, which together unite into one large circuit. Each of these three small circuits starts in the chest area. *Qi* from the chest flows out to the fingertips along a *yin* channel. *Qi* then returns and flows up to the head along the *yang* channel that is partner to the channel that flowed out to the fingertips. *Qi* then flows from the head down to the feet along the *yang* channel that is the other *yang* half of the great channel that preceded it in this circuit.

Qi finally returns to the chest from the feet by travelling up the channel that is both the *yin* partner of the channel that flowed down the leg to the feet and at the same time is the other *yin* half of the great channel that initiated the circuit by flowing away from the chest and down the arm. From the chest, a new circuit begins, where *qi* flows out to the fingertip along a new *yin* channel.[1]

	From the chest along the arm to the fingertips	From the fingertips along the arm to the head	From the head down to the toes	From the toes to the chest
First circuit	Lung (hand *taiyin*)	Large Intestine (hand *yangming*)	Stomach (foot *yangming*)	Spleen (foot *taiyin*)
Second circuit	Heart (hand *shaoyin*)	Small Intestine (hand *taiyang*)	Urinary Bladder (foot *taiyang*)	Kidney (foot *shaoyin*)
Third circuit	Pericardium (hand *jueyin*)	*San jiao* (hand *shaoyang*)	Gall Bladder (foot *shaoyang*)	Liver (foot *jueyin*)

The sequence of this circuit, where each channel connects to the next channel, is also the basis of the so-called horary clock. Each channel has a two-hour period in the course of a day where *qi* is most powerful. Conversely, *qi* will be weakest in this channel twelve hours later. This is the same as the tidal flow of water, where there are periods of the day where the water in the sea is rising and periods where it is at its lowest. For example, the Stomach channel's *qi* is strongest from 7am–9am and is correspondingly weakest from 7pm–9pm.

Time period	Channel where *qi* is most powerful	Channel where *qi* is weakest
3am–5am	Lung	Urinary Bladder
5am–7am	Large Intestine	Kidney
7am–9am	Stomach	Pericardium
9am–11am	Spleen	*San jiao*
11am–1pm	Heart	Gall Bladder
1pm–3pm	Small Intestine	Liver
3pm–5pm	Urinary Bladder	Lung
5pm–7pm	Kidney	Large Intestine
7pm–9pm	Pericardium	Stomach
9pm–11pm	*San jiao*	Spleen
11pm–1am	Gall Bladder	Heart
1am–3am	Liver	Small Intestine

The channels connect the organs with the surface of the body. Each channel has a connection to at least one *zang* and one *fu* organ. Once again, a pattern emerges in the movement of *qi* in the channels, this time in the movement of channel *qi* between the exterior and the interior.

Hand *yin* channel	Hand *yang* channel	Foot *yang* channel	Foot *yin* channel
Starts in the interior of the body and connects to the fingertips.	Starts in the fingertips, a branch separates and connects to the interior of the body. The primary channel ends in the head.	Starts in the head, a branch separates and connects to the interior of the body. The primary channel ends in the feet.	Starts in the toes, a branch separates and connects to the interior of the body. The primary channel ends in the chest.

Already, we can see that the channel system is more complex and extensive than the general outlines represented on posters of the channels and on meridian models. These only chart the channels' exterior path. Each channel has several other aspects apart from the external pathway. As we will see below, there are several aspects to the channel system. As well as the primary channel that travels below the surface of the skin, there are also internal pathways, *luo*-connecting channels, *luo* vessels, sinew channels, divergent channels and cutaneous areas. All of these taken together comprise an individual channel.

In addition to the twelve regular channels, there are eight extraordinary vessels, as outlined in the table below. In Chinese these are called *qi jing ba mai* (eight extraordinary vessels). These are another and deeper aspect of the channel system. Even though they form a separate network, the eight extraordinary vessels are integrated with the twelve regular channels. In particular, they have a regulatory effect on the channel network in that they absorb, balance and distribute excesses and deficiencies of *qi* in the regular channels. The extraordinary vessels also connect pre-heaven and post-heaven *qi*. I will discuss and explain the functions of the eight extraordinary vessels in a separate chapter (page 331).

Chinese name	English translation
Du mai	Governing vessel
Ren mai	Directing vessel or Conception vessel
Chong mai	Penetrating vessel or Thoroughfare vessel
Dai mai	Belt vessel or Girdle vessel
Yin qiao mai	*Yin* heel vessel, *Yin* stepping vessel or *Yin* motility vessel
Yang qiao mai	*Yang* heel vessel, Yang stepping vessel or *Yang* motility vessel
Yin wei mai	*Yin* linking vessel
Yang wei mai	*Yang* linking vessel

The functions of the channels

The channels' main functions are:

- to connect different parts of the body with each other

- to transport the vital substances and distribute them around the body

- to harmonise *qi* in the body

- to protect the body against exogenous *xie qi*.

Connecting different aspects of the body to each other

The channels connect and integrate the various areas in the body with each other. It is the channels that ensure that the vital substances are distributed from their place of production or storage to every corner of the body.

It is through the channels that the various parts of the body communicate with each other. In addition, the channels ensure that there is a balance of *qi* between the various areas of the body. They channel excess *qi* away from areas with too much *qi* and to areas that have too little *qi*. In this way the channels harmonise *qi* in the body.

Connect the interior with the surface

Each *zangfu* organ is in contact with other *zangfu* organs and also with the exterior aspects of the body. At least two channels have a connection to each *zangfu* organ. Branches of the organ's own channel and that of its partner will pass through the organ. In addition, other channels' internal branches and divergent channels can connect to an organ.

This relationship between *zangfu* organs in the interior and the channel in the exterior is called a *biaoli* or an exterior/interior relationship. It is this relationship that results in imbalances in the organs, manifesting with changes in their channel on the surface of the body. This also explains how treatment of a channel can have a healing effect on the organ.

This relationship also explains how the vital substances, which are either produced or stored in one of the internal organs, can be circulated around the body.

It is, of course, not just a one-way communication between the interior and the surface. The communication and relationship is mutual. This, however, is not only positive. Exogenous *xie qi* can invade the body via the channel system.

Connect the interior to the interior

Some of the internal organs are in direct anatomical connection with each other. For example, the Small Intestine is in direct, anatomical connection with both the Stomach and the Large Intestine. Other organs are not directly connected with each other. The Stomach, for example, is not in direct contact with the Spleen, the

Heart, the Lung and the Liver. There are channel connections between the Stomach and these organs. The Stomach is connected to the Spleen through its own and the Spleen channel's course and the divergent channels. The Stomach is connected to the Heart through its divergent channel. In addition, there are direct channel connections between the Stomach and the Lung, the Small Intestine and the Liver.

Connect the surface to the surface

The channels connect the various aspects of the body surface with each other. This means that the right and left hand, the upper and lower parts of the body and the body's front and back are all connected to and communicate with each other. These various parts of the body are connected via the primary channels, the sinew channels and the *luo*-connecting vessels.

Connect up and down

The primary channels flow vertically up and down the body. The *yin* channels flow to and from the chest and connect to the extremities. The *yang* channels flow to and from the head, through the chest and the upper part of the back, and connect to the extremities. Although *yin* channels' main pathways do not flow to the head, there will still be a channel connection up to the head. For some *yin* channels, this will be via an internal branch of the channel flowing to the head. For other *yin* channels the connection may be through their *luo*-connecting channel. Finally, all *yin* divergent channels connect to their *yang* partner's divergent channel, which flows up to the head. The fact that all channels connect up and down is of great importance for the balance of the *yin* and *yang* in the body and in particular the balance of *qi* in the head, which is an extremely *yang* part of the body.

Transport

The channels are connected to the internal organs, where the vital substances are created and stored. The channels circulate and distribute the vital substances throughout the body, both in the body's interior aspects where the internal organs are located and through the exterior, i.e. the skin and muscles. There is no part of the body that is not supplied by the channel system. The channels' circulation of the vital substances, *qi*, *xue* and *jinye*, can nourish and moisten all tissue in the body. This is similar to the blood vessel system in Western medicine physiology. In Chinese medicine there is no clear separation between the channels and the blood vessels. Nevertheless, the channels and blood vessels are conceived as being separate anatomical structures.

Protection

As well as nourishing and harmonising the body, the channels have a very important protective function. *Wei qi*, which protects the body against exogenous *xie qi*, circulates in the area below the skin. This area consists of *cou li* (the space between the skin and the muscles), the sinew channels and the *luo* vessel network. As well as the circulating in the sinew channels and the *luo* vessel network, *wei qi* also has a very close relationship to *ying qi*, which circulates in the primary channels.

Channel pathology

As stated earlier, it is not entirely positive that the channels connect the internal aspects of the body with the exterior. Exogenous *xie qi* can invade the surface of the body, i.e. the skin and muscles. *Xie qi* can penetrate deeper into the body via the channel system. As we will see below, there are various levels in the channel system and different forms of *qi* circulate in these aspects. The most superficial channels are the small *luo* vessels, the sinew channels and the cutaneous regions. It is mainly here that *wei qi* circulates, protecting the body against invasions of exogenous *xie qi*. If exogenous *xie qi* succeeds in overcoming *wei qi* in these exterior aspects, then it can enter the primary channel and penetrate deeper into the interior aspects of the body. This can be seen, for example, when someone walks around in bare feet or with inappropriate footwear when it is cold and damp. Exogenous Damp-Cold can invade the channels in the feet and legs and from here proceed to the lower *jiao*, where Damp-Cold can penetrate the Urinary Bladder or the Intestines, resulting in diarrhoea or cystitis.

The various levels of the channel system

When you see an image of a channel network in various books or when you see an acupuncture model, it is generally only the twelve regular channels, together with *du mai* and *ren mai*, that have been illustrated. Only the primary channels that flow just below the skin are delineated. This is equivalent to a road map of England that only illustrates the main roads that connect the major cities and the motorways. In the classical texts, the channels' internal pathways and the branches that split away from the primary channel are also described. These are now also reproduced in many modern acupuncture books. In addition, the finely meshed *luo* vessel network is also described and this explains how *qi*, *xue* and *jinye* can diffuse through every nook and cranny in the body.

It is important to develop an understanding of the entire channel network and not only the primary channels. Understanding the channel's internal flow and the pathway of its secondary branches, as well as the divergent and sinew channel pathways, is diagnostically very important and also helps to explain many of the body's physiological mechanisms and relationships. It also provides a logic when trying to understand why certain acupuncture points have the effects that they have.

Jing zheng – the primary channel

The primary channel is the aspect of the channel that flows just below the surface of the skin. As stated, this is the aspect of the channel that is most often illustrated on a channel chart or acupuncture model. It is along the primary channel that acupuncture points are located. The primary channel flows from the first acupuncture point on the channel and terminates at the final acupuncture point on the channel. If a person stands with their arms raised above their head, all the *yang* channels flow downwards towards the ground. At the same time, all the *yin* channels will flow from the chest or toes up towards the sky.

The first acupuncture point on nine of the channels is located on the fingertips, the toes or adjacent to the eyes. From here, the channel flows towards the torso. Somewhere along the primary channel, a branch will split away. This branch will penetrate deeper into the body, where it will connect to two or more of the internal organs. These will include its own and its partner *zangfu* organ. There can also be several other branches along the path of the primary channel where the secondary channel either connects to the interior or the other channels.

The three hand *yin* channels, i.e. the Lung, Heart and Pericardium channels, start their pathway in the interior and flow through two or more organs before they surface at the first acupuncture point on the channel and become the primary pathway of the channel. The channel then proceeds to flow from the chest to the fingertips.

Each primary channel:

- is connected to its *yin/yang* partner channel via its own and its partner's *luo-connecting* channel

- is connected to its *yin/yang* partner channel at the beginning or end of the channel

- has at least one branch that splits away from the primary channel and connects to its own and its partner *zangfu* organ

- connects directly to the other half of its great channel in the toes, fingers or inside the chest

- connects to the previous and following channel in the horary or meridian clock.

Jing bie – the divergent channel

In addition to the branches that are mentioned above, each of the regular channels also has a so-called divergent channel. This is also a pathway that branches away from the primary channel and connects to the interior and the *zangfu* organs.

With the exception of the *san jiao* divergent channel, all the divergent channels branch away from their primary channel in the arms and legs. All divergent channels flow towards the body, even if their primary channel's flow is in the opposite direction.

Yang divergent channels separate from the main pathway of the primary channel and connect to their own and, as a rule, their partner organ, before reconnecting with their own primary channel in the head or neck area. *Yin* divergent channels branch away from the primary channel and connect at some point with their own organ, before merging with their *yang* partner's primary channel.

Divergent channels are yet another way that partner channels connect to each other and to their respective *zangfu* organs. The divergent channels are also one of the ways in which *yin* channels connect to the head and neck. The divergent channels can thus explain how points on *yin* channels can affect the head and neck.

Because the divergent channels flow deep inside the body, they have no acupuncture points. On the other hand, there are certain acupuncture points on some of the primary channels where the divergent channel branches away from the primary channel or where they meet each other again. These acupuncture points can be used to influence the divergent channel.

Luo mai – connecting vessels

Luo mai are the most superficial and microscopic branches of the channel network. *Luo* vessels help to make the channel network three-dimensional. The *luo* vessel network spreads through the area above and between the primary channels. This means that they play a very significant role in the distribution of *qi* and *xue* throughout the body, particularly in the body's more superficial aspects, i.e. the muscles and skin. This is of importance in the nourishment and moistening of the tissue. At the same time, *wei qi* also circulates in the microscopic *luo* vessels. This means that the *luo* vessels play a role in protecting the body against exogenous *xie qi*.

Luo vessels have three main aspects.

- They are the horizontal relationship between the *yin/yang* partner channel.

- They are the superficial branches that split away from the primary channel and connect to a different area of the body.

- They are the very fine branches of channel network that flow through the superficial aspects of the body.

The fifteen luo-connecting vessels

Each of the twelve regular channels has a horizontal connection to its partner channel. This vessel flows from a so-called *luo*-connecting point on the channel. *Luo* vessels are one of the ways in which the body can regulate and harmonise *qi* via the channel network. If there is too much or too little *qi* in a channel, it can be balanced by *qi* flowing to or from its partner channel. *Luo* vessels are yet another way that *yin* and *yang* partner channels and organs communicate with each other.

In addition to there being a horizontal vessel that connects the two regular channels, there is also a longitudinal vessel that branches away from the primary channel at the *luo*-connecting point. This vessel connects to a separate part of the body. Some connect to the internal organs, others to the head, while others yet again only have a short pathway to an adjacent area.

In addition to the twelve *luo*-connecting vessels that have their source in a *luo*-connecting point in the vicinity of the wrists, ankles or lower leg, there are an additional four *luo*-connecting vessels. These differ in that they have their origin in the torso. Three of them have traditionally been discussed together with the twelve regular *luo*-connecting vessels because they start their course from a specific *luo*-connecting point. That is why there is talk of fifteen *luo*-connecting vessels. Both *du mai* and *ren mai* have a *luo*-connecting vessel. The Spleen also has an extra *luo*-connecting vessel, which is also known as the great *luo*-connecting vessel. The great *luo*-connecting vessel originates in the acupuncture point Sp 21, which is therefore also known as the great *luo*-connecting point. Some sources believe that Sp 21 influences all *luo*-connecting vessels in the body. In addition to these three torso *luo*-connecting vessels that have a *luo*-connecting point, the Stomach also has an extra *luo*-connecting vessel. This vessel differs from the others in that its origin is in the interior in the Stomach itself and it does not have a *luo*-connecting point.

Superficial luo vessels – network vessels

The superficial *luo* vessels can be compared to the capillary network in Western medicine physiology. They are a sophisticated network of microscopic channels that flow through all the tissue in the body. They fill the space that is above and between the primary channels. They give a third dimension to the two-dimensional longitudinal channels.

The superficial *luo* vessels have the function of distributing and circulating *qi*, *xue* and *jinye* through all the tissues in the body, not just in the muscles and skin, but also in the internal organs.

There are three types of superficial *luo* vessels. *Sun luo* are the minute branches that flow vertically upwards. These split into the even smaller *fu luo*. *Fu luo* split again into even more microscopic lateral branches, which are called *xue luo*. This creates a very extensive and finely meshed network of microscopic vessels.

These small vessels can easily get blocked by exogenous *xie qi*. Stagnations of *qi* and *xue* will also have a tendency to manifest with a blockage of these vessels. This is because these vessels are extremely narrow and have the structure of a net. It is possible to observe changes visibly in these vessels when there are stagnations or invasions of exogenous *xie qi*.

Techniques such as *gua sha*, cupping, plum-blossom needling and trigger point treatments can be used to stimulate the superficial *luo* vessels directly when they are blocked. Stimulation of the primary channel's *luo*-connecting point will also affect the superficial *luo* vessels, as well as influencing the horizontal *luo*-connecting vessel. By creating a flow of *qi* in the horizontal *luo*-connecting vessel, *qi* can be balanced between two partner channels. Finally, stimulation of *luo*-connecting points is used to affect the area of the body that is under the influence of the longitudinal *luo* channel.

Jing jin – the sinew channel

The sinew channel is sometimes also called the muscle channel. It is important to remember that these sinew or muscle channels are not the same as the muscle and organ relationships that are described in kinesiology and reflexology. Kinesiology and reflexology relate specific muscles to specific organs. This is a different system, which is not based on the channel system.

The sinew channels are a very superficial aspect of the channel system. They are a network of small channels surrounding the muscles and tendons. The sinew channels all start in the hands and feet and generally follow the primary channel's superficial pathway. As we saw with the divergent channel, the sinew channels flow from the extremities inwards towards the torso. They differ from the primary channel in that they do not connect to their internal *zangfu* body or to other organs. They are much broader than the primary channel. Sinew channels will often follow the contours of groups of muscle, tendons and sinews along the course of the channel. The sinew channels do not have any acupuncture points along their course apart from the acupuncture points that are located on the primary channel. On the other hand, there will often be so-called 'a-shi' points and trigger points along their course when there is a disruption of the *qi* and *xue* flow in the sinew channel. The sinew channels are mainly activated by the use of techniques such as *gua sha*, cupping, plum-blossom needling and trigger point treatments.

The function of the sinew channel is to distribute *qi* and *xue* in the muscles and tendons. They also have a protective function and circulate *wei qi* in the muscles and tendons.

Pi bu – cutaneous regions

The skin, which is the most superficial aspect of the body, is divided into six broad longitudinal areas. These cutaneous regions are called *pi bu* in Chinese. These regions are not a part of the channel network, but they are the cutaneous areas that are situated above the primary channels and *luo* vessels. They are broad areas of the skin that follow the course of the primary channel. They are named after the six great channels, which are as follows – *taiyang, shaoyang, yangming, taiyin, shaoyin* and *jueyin*. It is these channels' small *luo* vessels that supply them with *qi* and *xue*.

The cutaneous regions' main function is to control the pores and to protect the body. *Wei qi* circulates in and below the cutaneous regions and protects the body against exogenous *xie qi*, whilst controlling the pores.

Imbalances in the internal organs can sometimes manifest with visible changes in the colour, moisture and structure of the cutaneous regions. The cutaneous regions can also be treated with superficial techniques to expel exogenous *xie qi*, as well as to spread stagnations of *qi* and *xue* in the skin and muscles.

In this way the body can be understood as being energetically like an onion, where the internal organs are in the centre and the skin is on the outside.

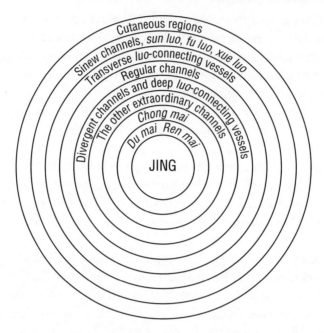

Figure 4.1 Energetic depths of the various aspects of the channel system

Depth or level	*Jingluo* aspect
Superficial	*Pi bu* (cutaneous regions)
	Sun luo *Fu luo* } *luo* vessels *Xue luo*
	Jing jin (sinew channel)
Middle depth	The fifteen *luo*-connecting channels
	Jing zheng (primary channel) superficial pathway
	Jing bie (divergent channel) superficial pathway
Internal	*Qi jing ba mai* (extraordinary vessel)
	Jing zheng (primary channel) internal pathway
	Jing bie (divergent channel) internal pathway

THE SIX GREAT CHANNELS

Before I start to describe the twelve regular channels individually, I would like to explain a little bit about the six great channels' fundamental qualities and their relationship to each other. As was seen in the introduction, each of the twelve regular channels has various relationships. They connect to their same-name *zangfu* organ and to their partner organ. They also connect to their *yin/yang* partner channel and to their hand/foot great channel extension.

Unlike *zangfu* organs, where *zang* organs are considered to be more important than *fu* organs, there is no difference in the *yin* and *yang* channels' relative importance. There is only a difference in their relative depths and dynamics. The six great channels can be understood as being six different energetic levels or stages. These aspects reflect both the *qi* that flows in the channel and the functions that channel's internal organ has. The three *yang* channels are more superficial and the three *yin* channels are thereby deeper. Furthermore, there is also a difference in depth between the individual *yin* channels and *yang* channels.

The six great channels can be understood as being stages that reflect changes in the *qi* that flows through the body, both in terms of the depth of *qi* and with regards to its quality and functionality. This is because the six channels are not static structures, but six levels that have an active relationship to each other and communicate upwards and downwards with each other. They are the stages in a process in which *qi* changes quality and functionality, depending on how deep or superficial it is.

The six great channels' relative depths

Taiyang is the most superficial and *yang* channel. Its *qi* circulates in the exterior aspects of the body. It is said that *taiyang* opens to the exterior, i.e. to the world that is outside of the body. *Taiyang* has, as will be explained later, a relationship with *wei qi* and thus protects the body against exogenous *xie qi*. *Wei qi* controls the pores and thereby the skin's 'openings' to the exterior.

Two levels down from *taiyang* is *yangming*. *Yangming* closes the outer *yang* aspect of the channel system and opens inwards towards the body's *yin* channels. This means that *yangming* has a close relationship with the internal *yin* aspects of the body. This is reflected by the fact that the Stomach channel flows down the *yin* side of the torso and the Stomach organ is closely involved in the production of the vital substances. In between these two *yang* levels is the *shaoyang* channel. *Shaoyang* is a hinge or a pivot point between the two *yang* levels. This means that *shaoyang* can regulate the movement of *qi* up and down between the *yang* levels.

Taiyin is similar to *taiyang* in that it opens outwards and upwards. The difference is, however, that where *taiyang* opens to the exterior, i.e. the world outside the body, *taiyin* opens to the more exterior or *yang* aspects of the channel system. This reflects the Spleen's and the Lung's functions of producing and distributing *qi*. *Taiyin* is thus also relatively more dynamic and *yang* than the other two *yin* channels. *Taiyin* sends nourishing *qi* upwards and outwards.

Shaoyin is similar to *shaoyang* in that it is a hinge or a pivot. This time the pivot or hinge is between two *yin* levels. This is also reflected by the *shaoyin* organs having a close cooperation with both the *taiyin* and *jueyin* organs.

The deepest and most *yin* level is *jueyin*. *Jue* means 'terminal' or 'returning'. It is here that *yin* has reached its extreme and is to 'terminate' or 'return' and become *yang*. This makes *jueyin* the deepest, most *yin* aspect of the interior.

Not all books place *jueyin* as the deepest level when they categorise the channels. For example, Giovanni Maciocia, in *The Channels of Acupuncture* (2006), categorises *shaoyin* as the deepest level and *jueyin* as being the hinge between the other two *yin* channels. It can be argued that *shaoyin* should be categorised as the deepest level. From a *zangfu* understanding of the organs, it is tempting to place *shaoyin* deepest, as this is where the Kidneys are. After all, it is in the Kidneys that *jing* is stored. The Kidneys are also known as the root of *yin* in the body. However, it is important to remember that the stages, as described above, reflect a dynamic process in the channels. The dynamic is to some extent a reflection of the *qi* and the functions of the *zangfu* organs, but the organs are not the same as the channels. The organs and channels connect to each other and are, in the end, manifestations of the same *qi*, but they are also two different aspects of this *qi*.

Professor Wang Ju Yi explains the discrepancy between the Kidneys' channel level and the fact that *jing*, which is stored in the Kidneys, is the deepest and most *yin* form of *qi* in the body as follows. Wang Ju Yi believes that *jueyin* is classified as the deepest and most *yin* level because the Liver is a reservoir that holds large quantities of *xue*. Both *xue* and *jing* are *yin* in nature, and even though *jing* is the most *yin* form of *qi* in the body, it is the volume of *xue*, which is stored in the Liver, that makes *jueyin* the most *yin*. Furthermore, he feels that the explanation of *jueyin*'s position is to be found in the relationship that there is between *jueyin* and its partner channel and organs. *Jueyin*'s partner channels constitute *shaoyang*, which is characterised by its *yang* movement. This is the *yang* movement that is the catalyst that transforms *yin* back to *yang* (Wang and Robertson 2008).

Personally, I think that there is also a logic when you look at the channel cycle in the body. The *yin* channels flow in the following sequence: Lung, Spleen, Heart, Kidney, Pericardium and Liver. In this sequence, the *jueyin* channels are the channels that are the final part of the *yin* channels' circuit before *qi* returns to the start of a new circuit.

Finally, it is also important to distinguish between relative depth, quantity and importance. *Jueyin* is the deepest *yin* level, which contains the largest quantity of *yin*, while the Kidneys and thus *shaoyin* are the most fundamental aspect of the *yin*, which is the foundation of all *yin* in the body.

Another difference in the sequence of the stages is seen in the sequence of the stages in the diagnostic model 'Diagnosis according to the six stages', which was presented in the book *Shang Han Lun*. In this model *yangming* and *shaoyang* are in opposite positions.[2]

Channel	Function	Level
Taiyang	Opens	Opens to the exterior
Shaoyang	Pivots	The hinge between *taiyang* and *yangming*
Yangming	Closes	Closes inwards to the external aspects of the interior
Taiyin	Opens	Opens to the internal aspects of the exterior
Shaoyin	Pivots	The hinge between *taiyin* and *jueyin*
Jueyin	Closes	Closes inwards to the interior

The relationship between the six great channels and the six forms of climatic *qi*

There are six forms of climatic *qi*: cold, summer-heat, dryness, dampness, heat and wind. All six climatic *qi* are needed to create a harmonious environment. Each season has a specific climatic *qi* that is dominant. These climatic *qi* come and go in a natural rhythm. It is only a problem if they become too dominant or if they are absent. Prolonged periods of rain can be detrimental to some plants, but so can a lack of rain. It also creates imbalances when there are sudden changes in the climatic *qi*. This is especially the case when there is a sudden climatic change that is not harmonious with a particular season. A sudden period of cold in summer, for example, can result in people catching colds. When climatic *qi* is the source of disease or imbalance it is called exogenous *xie qi*.

Nothing is ever random in the classical Chinese understanding of the universe. This is particularly true of numerical classification. There are six types of climatic *qi* and there are six great channels. Each of the six channels' *qi* resonates in a specific way, as do the six forms of climatic *qi*. The six channels integrate, transform and protect the body against these forms of *qi*. If a particular channel's *qi* is out of balance, it can have difficulty in transforming or protecting the body against precisely the type of climatic *qi* that it resonates with. Also, a predominance of this type of climatic *qi*, or a sudden change of the weather to this type of climatic *qi*, can create imbalances in the channel that has the task of protecting against or integrating this *qi*.

The six channels' relationships to the six types of climatic *qi* are as follows.

Channel	Climatic *qi*
Taiyang	Cold
Shaoyang	Summer-Heat
Yangming	Dryness
Taiyin	Dampness
Shaoyin	Fire
Jueyin	Wind

The six great channels' relative quantities of *qi* and *xue*

In addition to having varying energetic depths, the six channels are considered to have variable quantities of *qi* and *xue* circulating in them. Some have more *qi* than *xue*; others have the opposite, and *yangming* is characterised by being rich in both *qi* and *xue*. This is one of the reasons so many Stomach points are used in the treatment of *xu* conditions.

Channel	Relative relationship of *qi* to *xue*
Taiyang	Rich in *xue*, less *qi*
Shaoyang	Rich in *qi*, less *xue*
Yangming	Rich in *qi* and *xue*
Taiyin	Rich in *qi*, less *xue*
Shaoyin	Rich in *qi*, less *xue*
Jueyin	Rich in *xue*, less *qi*

Taiyang

Taiyang means greater *yang*. *Taiyang* is the most exterior and thereby the most *yang* channel. *Qi* cannot become more *yang*, so therefore it is '*tai*' *yang*. There are several reasons why *taiyang* is considered to be the 'greatest' *yang*. *Taiyang* is the regular channel that flows closest to the backbone and *du mai*. This is absolutely the most *yang* area of the body. The Urinary Bladder channel is also the greatest channel in length, with sixty-seven acupuncture points. Furthermore, the *taiyang* channel is also the 'greatest' *yang* because the *qi* that flows in the channel is more *yang* than the *qi* in the other *yang* channels. This *yang* polarity, combined with the *taiyang* channel being the most exterior channel in the body, is of great importance for its functionality. *Taiyang* opens to the exterior. *Taiyang* circulates warming and protective *wei qi* and is thereby involved in protecting the body against external climatic influences, especially cold. This is reflected in the acupuncture point combination UB 62, UB 10 and SI 3 being effective in treating invasions of external Wind-Cold.

Taiyang:

- opens to the exterior
- has a relationship to cold
- is rich in *xue*, but has less *qi*
- channels and organs have a relationship to *shaoyin* channels and organs.

Shaoyang

Shaoyang means lesser *yang*. *Shaoyang* is not as great a *yang* as *taiyang* or greater *yang*. *Shaoyang* is hinged between the two *yang* channel systems. It is the space between *taiyang*, which opens outwards to the world around the body, and *yangming*, which closes inwards towards the body's *yin* aspects. *Shaoyang* regulates and allows the passage of the heat that rises up through *yangming* from the interior to rise up to the surface, where it is distributed by *taiyang*. *Shaoyang* ensures that the vital substances that are created in the deeper *yin* levels circulate through the tissue as they should. *Shaoyang* governs and moves *qi* in the spaces of the body. When this regulation is blocked, there will often arise Heat and Dampness. Damp-Heat will at the same time block this regulation and movement of *qi*.

The climatic *qi* that *shaoyang* has a relationship to is Summer-Heat, whose characteristic is precisely the combination of Dampness and Heat.

Shaoyang organs and channels are partnered with *jueyin* organs and channels. The heat and motion that there is in *shaoyang* is used to activate the deep *yin* stillness that there is in *jueyin*.

Shaoyang:

- is hinged between *taiyang* and *yangming*

- has a relationship to Summer-Heat and thereby also Damp-Heat

- is rich in *qi*, but has less *xue*

- channels and organs have a relationship to *jueyin* channels and organs.

Yangming

The *yangming* channel is the deepest *yang* level in the six divisions. It is here that *yang* closes inwards towards the internal *yin* aspects of the body. *Yangming* means shining or bright *yang*.

Yangming's close relationship to the internal *yin* aspects of the body is also seen in the Stomach channel being the only *yang* channel that flows on the *yin* aspect of the body. On the front of the torso, the Stomach channel flows side by side with the Spleen channel. Here, it is a 'bright' *yang* channel among the *yin* channels. *Yangming*, which is the deepest *yang* channel, sends heat and *qi* that has been created in the interior *yin* areas upwards and outwards to the more active *yang* aspects of the body. It is also for this reason that *yangming* is described as being rich in *qi* and *xue*. It is from *taiyin's* transformation of *qi* that the wealth of *qi* and *xue* is drawn.

The close relationship between the inner *yin* aspects and outer *yang* aspects is reflected in the relationship between the organs and channels that are located on these levels. *Yangming* and *taiyin* have a close cooperation on several levels. Stomach, Spleen and Lung are all central organs in the production of *qi* and *xue*. Furthermore, all four *yangming* and *taiyin* organs also have a close cooperation in relation to the harmonious integration of dampness and dryness in the body. *Yangming* assimilates external dryness, but often develops dryness when it is imbalanced. The Stomach hates dryness, and constipation in the Large Intestine is often a consequence when there is dryness in the body. Conversely, when *yangming* is in balance it ensures that there is the necessary dryness so Dampness does not begin to dominate. This helps the Spleen, which is burdened by Dampness. *Taiyin* transforms and distributes *jinye*. This ensures that the body does not dry out. It is repeatedly seen in the six channels' *yin/yang* relationships how the pairs balance and support each other.

Yangming:

- closes inwards towards the interior *yin* channels

- has a relationship to dryness

- is rich in *qi* and *xue*

- channels and organs have a relationship to *taiyin* channels and organs.

Taiyin

Tai again means great or greater. This is the great *yin* channel. However, it must not be understood as 'great' meaning the most *yin* channel. On the contrary, great *yin* indicates that it is the most exterior *yin* channel. To be on the exterior is in reality a *yang* quality. *Taiyin* opens upwards and outwards in the same way that *taiyang* opens upwards and outwards, the difference being that *taiyin* opens up to the body's deepest *yang* aspects, whereas *taiyang* opens up to the exterior outside the body. *Taiyin* is also relatively *yang* in relation to the other *yin* channels. This is because it has a closer relationship with *qi* than it does with *xue*.

As we saw previously, there is a close relationship, cooperation and communication between *taiyin* and *yangming*, both in relation to the various transformation processes and the balance between dampness and dryness in the body. *Taiyin*'s relationship to dampness and moisture is seen by the fact that the Lung and the Spleen play key roles in the production and distribution of *jinye*, which is the physiological dampness in the body. Pathological Dampness easily arises when *taiyin*'s organs are in imbalance. In these situations, there is often a production and accumulation of Dampness and Phlegm. Furthermore, both these organs' physiological activity is constrained and burdened by the presence of Dampness.

Taiyin:

- opens to the *yang* channels

- has a relationship to Dampness

- is rich in *qi* and has less *xue*

- channels and organs have a relationship to *yangming* channels and organs.

Shaoyin

Shaoyin is the lesser *yin*. Like *shaoyang*, *shaoyin* is a hinge or a pivot between the other two *yin* channels. As written in the introduction to this section, it can be discussed which of the two deeper *yin* channels is the pivot and which of them closes inwards. I have chosen to follow the traditional, classical model. *Shaoyin* is placed in the classical model between *jueyin* and *taiyin*. *Shaoyin* has a very close relationship to both of these channels. *Shaoyin* has a more *yang* relationship to *taiyin*. This matches the more *yang* nature that *taiyin* has in relation to the other *yin* channels. *Mingmen* is the fire that supports the Spleen in its transformation of *qi* and *jinye*. The Heart and Lung have a close relationship with regards to the circulation of *qi* and *xue* in the body. *Shaoyin*'s relationship to *jueyin* is much more *yin* in nature. This is especially seen in that Kidney *yin* and Liver *yin* are considered to have a common root. Additionally, there is also a close relationship between Kidney *jing* and Liver *xue*.

Shaoyin has a close relationship to fire – both the pathological and physiological fire. The Heart is a Fire Phase organ, and it is in the Heart that the 'imperial fire' has its residence. The Kidneys' relationship to fire is seen by the fact that it is between the two Kidneys that the 'ministerial fire' *mingmen* is situated. This means that the body's activating heat has its root in *shaoyin*. It is this movement of heat and activity that makes *shaoyin* a pivot. This activity and movement is also seen in the Heart's rhythmic circulation of *qi* through the blood vessels. *Yuan qi*, which arises from the heat of *mingmen*, is circulated through the body in the *san jiao*, which is an aspect of *shaoyang*. Both pivots, *shaoyang* and *shaoyin*, are thus involved in circulating *yuan qi*, which is the fundamental catalyst of the body and is involved in all physiological processes.

As previously written, *shaoyin* also has a close relationship to pathological fire. The Heart has a tendency to develop both *xu* and *shi* patterns of Heat by virtue of its resonance with fire. In addition, the Heart is easily affected by Heat rising up from other organs or areas of the body. This is due to the Heart being located at the top of the torso, which is where Heat rises up to.

The Kidneys have the function of controlling Heart fire. The Kidneys also have a tendency to develop *yin xu* Heat.

We saw earlier that *shaoyin*'s partner, *taiyang*, has a relationship to cold. Once again, there is a close relationship between *yin* and *yang* pairs. *Taiyang* is dependent on the heat generated in the Kidneys to protect the body from cold. The Heart, on the other hand, drains Heat downwards via the Small Intestine to the Urinary Bladder, where it is expelled from the body, together with the urine.

Shaoyin:

- is the pivot between the two *yin* channels

- has a relationship to fire

- is rich in *qi* and has less *xue*

- channels and organs have a relationship with *taiyang* channels and organs.

Jueyin

Jueyin means terminal, absolute or returning *yin*. It is the deepest and most *yin* level. It is here that the *yin* polarity has reached its extreme before returning towards *yang*. *Jueyin* is the most internal aspect of the interior. Whereas *yangming* closes inwards towards the *yin* levels, *jueyin* closes inwards towards the interior of the body. *Jueyin's* function is to store and cultivate *yin*, whilst at the same time nourishing and regulating the distribution of *xue*. It is in *jueyin* that large quantities of *xue*, which is *yin*, is stored. The Liver is a reservoir for *xue*, and the *xue*-filled Pericardium ensures that the Heart has peace and quiet. This state of tranquillity and peace in *jueyin* balances wind, which is the climatic *qi* that *jueyin* integrates and controls. When there is an ample quantity of *xue*, the body is nourished and is thereby able to withstand invasions of Wind from the outside. When *xue* is weakened or agitated, internal Wind can arise. In Liver *xue xu* conditions, Wind can start to stir in the empty channels and vessels. This is like the wind that stirs in underground railway tunnels. When there are *shi* imbalances in the Liver, especially when there is Fire, Wind can also arise. This is likened to a fierce fire where the heat from the fire drives large amounts of air upwards.

It is said that the Liver dredges and drains the *qi* passages. This makes it possible for *yin xue* to flow freely. *Qi* is dependent on the nourishment that *xue* gives it. The Pericardium constantly ensures that there is a *yin* condition of tranquillity in the Heart by absorbing and calming emotional stress and traumas, whilst the Pericardium communicates externally with the surroundings and thereby also calms the Heart.

Jueyin:

- closes inwards towards the interior of the body

- has a relationship to Wind

- is rich in *xue* and has less *qi*

- channels and organs have a relationship to *shaoyang* channels and organs.

THE TWELVE
REGULAR CHANNELS

There are several good books in English, German and French with precise descriptions of channels' flow and the location of the acupuncture points. Not all the books are in one hundred per cent agreement about where the channels meet with each other or on the details of the internal pathways of the channels, etc. Furthermore, there are also variations in the precise localisation of some of the acupuncture points amongst some of the teachers I have had through the years. In the following descriptions of channels' pathways, I have mainly followed the descriptions presented in Claudia Focks's *Atlas of Acupuncture* (2008), Peter Deadman and Mazin Al-Khafaji's *A Manual of Acupuncture* (1998), Giovanni Maciocia's *The Channels of Acupuncture* (2006) and Hamid Montakab's *Acupuncture Point and Channel Energetics* (2014) and used these as reference books. When there was disagreement between these books, I have usually, though not always, followed Claudia Focks's book.

THE LUNG CHANNEL SYSTEM – *SHOU TAIYIN JING LUO*

Lung primary channel – *shou taiyin jing mai*

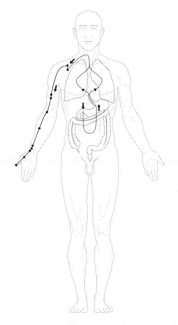

Figure 4.2 Lung primary vessel

The Lung channel is the first part of the great twelve-channel circuit. At the same time, it is the start of the first of three smaller circuits, where four channels flow sequentially from the chest to the fingertips, from the fingertips up to the head, from the head to the feet and from the toes back to the chest.

The Lung primary channel begins its pathway in the interior and flows through all three *jiao*, before it emerges on the surface at the acupuncture point Lu 1.

Pathway

- The Lung channel has its source in the Stomach in the middle *jiao.*

- From here it flows down and connects to its partner *fu* organ, the Large Intestine.

- From the Large Intestine the channel rises upwards through the Stomach.

- It passes through the diaphragm.

- It continues into its own *zang* organ, the Lung. The Lung channel meets with a branch of the Liver channel, which is the last channel in the twelve-channel cycle. This allows the cycle of *qi* through the twelve channels to continue uninterrupted.

- From the Lung the channel rises up to the throat area.

- The channel flows laterally to the area below the lateral end of the clavicle, level with the first intercostal space. The primary channel emerges on the surface at the acupuncture point Lu 1.

- It flows one *cun*[3] up to the acupuncture point Lu 2.

- It flows out to the front of the shoulder.

- From the shoulder the channel flows down along the lateral aspect of the arm.

- A branch of the channel separates away from the primary channel at the acupuncture point Lu 7, which is located on the styloid process of the radius one and a half *cun* from the wrist. This branch flows to the radial side of the index finger where it meets with the acupuncture point LI 1, which is the start of the Large Intestine channel.

- The primary channel continues its pathway from Lu 7 to the corner of the nail on the radial side of the thumb and the acupuncture point Lu 11, where the Lung channel terminates.

Lung *luo*-connecting vessel – *shou taiyin luo mai*

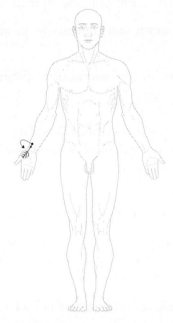

Figure 4.3 Lung *luo*-connecting vessel

The Lung *luo*-connecting vessel branches away from the primary channel at the channel's *luo*-connecting point, Lu 7, which is one and a half *cun* from the wrist on the styloid process of the radius. From here it connects in three directions.

Pathway

- It connects laterally to its partner channel, the Large Intestine channel.

- It connects vertically to the network of *sun luo, fu luo* and *xue luo*.

- It connects towards the palm of the hand, spreading across the thenar eminence.

Lung divergent channel – *shou taiyin jing bie*

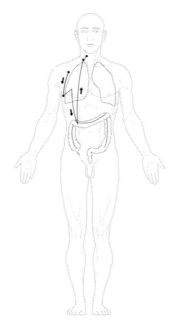

Figure 4.4 Lung divergent channel

The Lung divergent channel separates from the primary channel at the acupuncture point Lu 1.

Pathway

- From Lu 1 the divergent channel flows down to the acupuncture point GB 22 on the lateral aspect of the chest.

- It penetrates downwards into the thorax.

- It connects to its own *zang* organ, the Lung.

- It flows down to its partner *fu* organ, the Large Intestine.

- It flows upwards again up through the body to just below the clavicle at the acupuncture point St 12.

- It continues its course to the acupuncture point LI 18, where it merges with the Large Intestine channel.

Lung sinew channel – *shou taiyin jing jin*

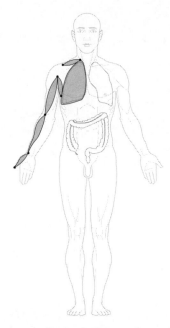

Figure 4.5 Lung sinew channel

The Lung sinew channel begins its flow in the thumb and travels in the opposite direction of the primary channel, inwards towards the torso.

Pathway

- From the thumb the sinew channel travels to the radial side of the wrist and the acupuncture point Lu 9.

- It follows the path of the primary channel up to the shoulder and past Lu 1.

- It travels down to the anterior aspect of the axilla where it meets the Pericardium and Heart sinew channels.

- It spreads around the pectoral muscles, before connecting to the acupuncture point St 12.

- It travels across the shoulder to the acupuncture point LI 15.

Lung channel connections

- *Yin/yang* partner channel: the Large Intestine channel.

- Hand/Foot channel: the Spleen channel.

- The twelve-channel *qi* cycle: the Liver and Large Intestine channels.

Yin/yang partner channel: the Large Intestine channel

- A branch separates from the primary channel at the *luo*-connecting point, Lu 7, which is one and a half *cun* from the wrist on the styloid process of the radius. This branch flows to the radial side of the index finger, where it meets with the acupuncture point LI 1, which is the start of the Large Intestine channel.

- The Lung *luo*-connecting vessel separates from the primary channel at the *luo*-connecting point, Lu 7, which is one and a half *cun* from the wrist on the styloid process of the radius. From here it flows laterally to the Large Intestine channel.

- The Large Intestine *luo*-connecting vessel branches away from the Large Intestine channel at its *luo*-connecting point LI 6, which is located three *cun* from the wrist on the radial side of the lower arm. From here it flows laterally and connects to the Lung channel.

Hand/Foot channel: the Spleen channel

- A branch separates from the Spleen channel at the acupuncture point Sp 20, which is located in the second intercostal space six *cun* lateral to the midline. From here it flows up to the acupuncture point Lu 1.

The twelve-channel qi cycle

- The previous channel in the cycle is the Liver channel. An internal branch of the Liver channel flows from the Liver and up to the acupuncture point Lu 1, which is the start of the Lung channel.

- The next channel in the circuit is the Large Intestine channel. A branch separates from the primary channel at the *luo*-connecting point, Lu 7, which is one and a half *cun* from the wrist on the styloid process of the radius. This branch flows to the radial side of the index finger, where it meets with the acupuncture point LI 1, which is the start of the Large Intestine channel.

Organ connections

The Lung channel connects to its own *zang* organ, the Lung, to its partner *fu organ*, the Large Intestine, and to the Stomach.

Meeting points with other channels

Lu 1	Spleen channel

THE LARGE INTESTINE CHANNEL SYSTEM – *SHOU YANGMING JING LUO*

Large Intestine primary channel –
shou yangming jing mai

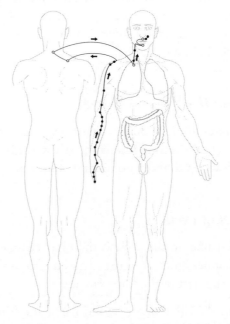

Figure 4.6 Large Intestine primary channel

The Large Intestine primary channel begins its course when a branch separates from the Lung channel at the *luo*-connecting point, Lu 7, which is one and a half *cun* from the wrist on the styloid process of the radius. This branch flows to the radial side of the index finger, where it meets with the acupuncture point LI 1, which is the start of the Large Intestine channel.

Pathway

- The channel flows from LI 1 along the radial side of the index finger.

- It continues over the radial side of the back of the hand to the upper radial side of the wrist.

- It travels up the radial side of the lower arm past the elbow's lateral side and continues up the lateral aspect of the upper arm to the anterior aspect of the shoulder joint.

- It crosses over the shoulder, meeting with the Small Intestine channel point SI 12 in the centre of the suprascapular fossa.

- It continues to acupuncture point Du 14, which is below the seventh cervical vertebra. The Large Intestine channel meets with the five other regular *yang* channels and *du mai* here.

- It flows back to the front of the shoulder and the clavicle, meeting with four other *yang* channels at the acupuncture point St 12.

- A branch separates from the primary channel at the acupuncture point St 12, penetrating down into the body where it connects with the Large Intestine's partner *zang* organ, the Lung. From here it continues down to its own *fu* organ, the Large Intestine. The internal branch of the channel continues its course from here down to the tibia, where it terminates in the Large Intestine's lower *he*-sea point St 37, located six *cun* below the patella on the lateral side of the tibia.

- The main branch of the primary channel continues its pathway from St 12 up the throat and across the jawbone.

- It meets with the Stomach channel and *ren mai* at the acupuncture point St 4, which is lateral to the corner of the mouth.

- It continues up above the upper lip.

- It crosses the midline of the face at the acupuncture point Du 26, where it meets with the Stomach channel and *du mai*.

- The external pathway of the channel ends on the lateral side of the naso-labial groove on the opposite side of the body to its source point.

- The channel continues up over the face, until it becomes the Stomach channel.

Large Intestine *luo*-connecting vessel – *shou yangming luo mai*

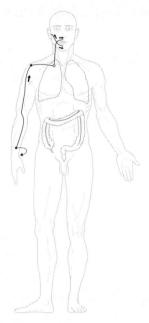

Figure 4.7 Large Intestine *luo*-connecting vessel

The Large Intestine *luo*-connecting vessel separates from the primary channel at the channel's *luo*-connecting point LI 6, which is located three *cun* from the wrist on the radial side of the lower arm. From here it connects in three directions.

Pathway

- It connects laterally to its partner channel, the Lung channel.

- It connects vertically to the network of *sun luo*, *fu luo* and *xue luo*.

- It connects to LI 15 on the shoulder joint. The vessel continues its course over the clavicle to St 12, travelling up the lateral aspect of the throat and past the jaw, where it divides into two branches. One branch connects with the teeth and the other enters the ear and connects with the Stomach, *san jiao*, Gall Bladder and Small Intestine channels that gather here.

Large Intestine divergent channel – *shou yangming jing bie*

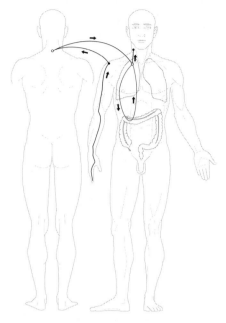

Figure 4.8 Large Intestine divergent channel

The Large Intestine divergent channel separates from the primary channel at the fingertips.

Pathway

- The divergent channel flows upwards from the hand to the acupuncture point LI 15 on the shoulder joint.

- The channel splits into two branches at LI 15. One branch travels down to the breast. The other branch passes over the shoulder to Du 14, which is located below the seventh cervical vertebra.

- It courses back to the front of the body to the acupuncture point St 12 above the clavicle.

- It penetrates down into the body where it connects to the Large Intestine's partner *zang* organ, the Lung, and to its own *fu* organ, the Large Intestine.

- It travels upwards again to St 12, from where it continues its path to the acupuncture point LI 18, which merges with the Large Intestine primary channel.

Large Intestine sinew channel – *shou yangming jing jin*

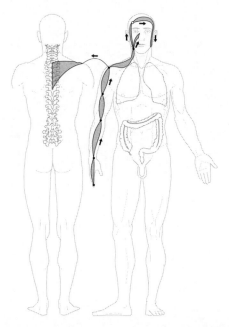

Figure 4.9 Large Intestine sinew channel

The Large Intestine sinew channel begins its pathway on the index finger and flows in a broad band alongside the primary channel up the arm to the head.

Pathway

- From the index finger the sinew channel passes over the back of the hand, along the lateral aspect of the wrist, to the acupuncture point LI 5.

- It follows the primary channel's pathway up along the arm's lateral, posterior aspect to the shoulder joint and the acupuncture point LI 15.

- At LI 15 a branch separates and courses over the shoulder and the scapula and connects to the spine from below the seventh cervical vertebra and down to the fifth thoracic vertebra.

- The other branch continues its path from LI 15 up the side of the neck to the jaw.

- The channel splits into two branches on the jaw.

- One branch travels to the lateral aspect of the nose.

- The other branch continues up the face in front of the Small Intestine channel to the acupuncture point GB 13, where it meets with the other *yang* sinew channels.

- It crosses the midline and flows down to the mandible on the opposite side.

Large Intestine channel connections

- *Yin/yang* partner channel: the Lung channel.

- Hand/Foot channel: the Stomach channel.

- The twelve-channel *qi* cycle: the Lung and Stomach channels.

Yin/yang partner channel: the Lung channel

- A branch separates from the Lung channel at the *luo*-connecting point, Lu 7, which is one and a half *cun* from the wrist on the styloid process of the radius. This branch flows to the radial side of the index finger, where it meets with the acupuncture point LI 1, which is the start of the Large Intestine channel.

- The Lung *luo*-connecting vessel separates from the primary channel at the *luo*-connecting point, Lu 7, which is one and a half *cun* from the wrist on the styloid process of the radius. From here it flows laterally to the Large Intestine channel.

- The Large Intestine *luo*-connecting vessel branches away from the Large Intestine channel at its *luo*-connecting point LI 6, which is located three *cun* from the wrist on the radial side of the lower arm. From here it flows laterally and connects to the Lung channel.

Hand/Foot channel: the Stomach channel

- The Large Intestine channel continues its course up to the medial corner of the orbit at the acupuncture point UB 1. From here the channel flows down to St 1, where the Stomach channel has its source.

The twelve-channel qi cycle

- The previous channel in the cycle is the Lung channel. A branch separates from the Lung channel at the *luo*-connecting point, Lu 7, which is one and a half *cun* from the wrist on the styloid process of the radius. This branch flows to the radial side of the index finger, where it meets with the acupuncture point LI 1, which is the start of the Large Intestine channel.

- The next channel in the cycle is the Stomach channel. The Large Intestine channel continues its course up to the medial corner of the orbit at the acupuncture point UB 1. From here the channel flows down to St 1, where the Stomach channel has its source.

Organ connections

The Large Intestine channel connects to its own *fu* organ, the Large Intestine, and its partner *zang* organ, the Lung.

Meeting points with other channels

LI 14	Small Intestine and Urinary Bladder channels and *yang wei mai*
LI 15	*Yang qiao mai*
LI 16	*Yang qiao mai*
LI 20	Stomach channel
Du 14	All the *yang* channels
St 4	Stomach channel, *yang qiao mai* and *ren mai*
St 12	*San jiao*, Small Intestine, Gall Bladder and Stomach channels and *yin qiao mai*
SI 12	Small Intestine, *san jiao* and Gall Bladder channels
Du 26	Stomach channel and *du mai*
Ren 24	Stomach channel, *du mai* and *ren mai*
Some sources state that the Large Intestine channel also connects to GB 5, GB 6 and GB 14.	

THE STOMACH CHANNEL SYSTEM
– *ZU YANGMING JING LUO*

Stomach primary channel – *zu yangming jing mai*

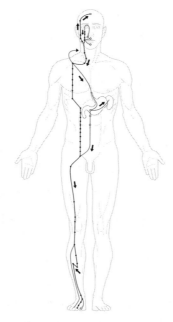

Figure 4.10 Stomach primary channel

The Stomach channel and the Large Intestine channel are the foot and hand sections of the *yangming* channel, respectively. The Stomach channel is a continuation of the Large Intestine primary channel, which terminates on the lateral side of the naso-labial groove. From here *qi* flows to the medial corner of the orbit at the acupuncture point UB 1. *Qi* then flows down to St 1, where the Stomach channel has its source.

Pathway

- The Stomach channel has its source on the lower edge of the orbit at the acupuncture point St 1.

- The channel descends down to the acupuncture point St 3, which is lateral to the naso-labial groove.

- It crosses over to the acupuncture point Du 26, on the midline of the face, between the nose and the upper lip. Here the Stomach channel meets with *du mai* and the Large Intestine channel and connects inwards to the gums.

- It crosses back to acupuncture point St 4, level with the corner of the mouth.

- It crosses back to the midline, this time between the lower lip and the chin and the acupuncture point Ren 24, where the Stomach channel meets with *ren mai* and the Large Intestine channel.

- It flows back over the mandible to the acupuncture point St 5, which is located on the anterior border of the masseter muscle, where the primary channel splits into two branches.

- One branch continues up over the cheek connecting to the Gall Bladder and Small Intestine channels at the acupuncture point GB 3 on the upper border of the zygomatic arch.

- It follows the Gall Bladder channel passing through GB 4, GB 5 and GB 6, meeting with the *san jiao*, Large Intestine and Gall Bladder channels.

- It continues up to St 8 on the corner of the forehead inside the hairline.

- It crosses from here to the midline to meet with *du mai* and the Urinary Bladder channel at the acupuncture point Du 24, which is located just behind the hairline. This branch of the primary channel terminates here.

- The other branch flows down from the mandible, across the lateral side of the neck and along the clavicle to the acupuncture point St 12, where it meets with four other *yang* channels and divides into three branches.

- The first branch passes over the shoulder to the seventh cervical vertebra, where it meets with all the *yang* channels at Du 14.

- The second branch penetrates into the body, where it first connects to its own *fu* organ, the Stomach, and then to its partner *zang* organ, the Spleen. Offshoots from the internal branch of the channel connect to the acupuncture points Ren 10, Ren 11 and Ren 12. The internal branch continues downwards through the abdominal cavity until it resurfaces just above the pubic bone at the acupuncture point St 30, where it rejoins the primary channel.

- A third branch continues down from St 12 over the nipple and down to the pubic bone through the inguinal area and down the lateral aspect of the leg.

- A branch of the channel separates from the primary channel at the acupuncture point St 36, three *cun* below the patella on the lateral aspect of the tibia, and travels down the lateral aspect of the leg to the middle toe.

- The primary channel continues its course down the lateral aspect of the tibia, through the ankle, passing through the acupuncture point St 42 (on the dorsum of the foot in the depression between the junction of the second and third metatarsal bones and the cuneiform bones) where a branch separates away and courses over to Sp 1, which is located on the medial corner of the large toenail, where the channel becomes the Spleen channel.

- The primary channel continues its pathway from St 42 down to the lateral corner of the nail on the second toe. The Stomach channel terminates its pathway here.

Stomach *luo*-connecting vessel – *zu yangming luo mai*

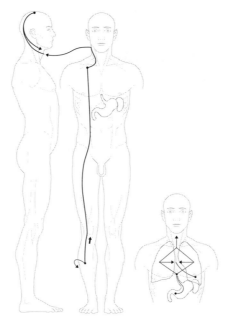

Figure 4.11 Stomach *luo*-connecting vessel

The Stomach *luo*-connecting vessel separates from the primary channel at the channel's *luo*-connecting point St 40, which is located midway along the lateral edge of the tibia. From there it connects in three directions.

Pathway

- It connects laterally to its partner channel, the Spleen channel.

- It connects vertically to the network of *sun luo*, *fu luo* and *xue luo*.

- It flows up along the lateral aspect of the leg, over the anterior aspect of the torso and up to the throat, where it splits into two branches. One branch continues up to the head, where it meets with *qi* from the other *yang* channels and terminates at the top of the head at Du 20. The other branch spreads across the throat.

Stomach great *luo*-connecting vessel – *zu yangming da luo mai*

Both the Stomach and the Spleen have an extra *luo*-connecting vessel. The Stomach great *luo*-connecting vessel starts in the interior and has no *luo*-connecting point.

Pathway

- It originates inside the chest and moves through the diaphragm.

- It connects to the Lung.

- It emerges at the surface by the left breast.

Stomach divergent channel – *zu yangming jing bie*

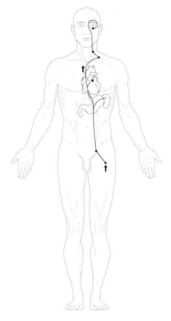

Figure 4.12 Stomach divergent channel

The Stomach divergent channel separates from the primary channel in the inguinal area at the acupuncture point St 31 and flows upwards in the opposite direction of the primary channel.

- It penetrates into the body above the pubic bone at the acupuncture point St 30.

- It passes through the abdominal cavity and connects to its own *fu* organ, the Stomach, and its partner *zang* organ, the Spleen.

- It continues upwards and connects to the Heart.

- It flows from the Heart up to the clavicle and through the throat.

- It merges with the primary channel at the acupuncture point St 9 on the lateral aspect of the throat.

- It travels up to the mouth and along the side of the nose to the eye, where it terminates at the acupuncture point St 1 on the lower edge of the orbit.

Stomach sinew channel – *zu yangming jing jin*

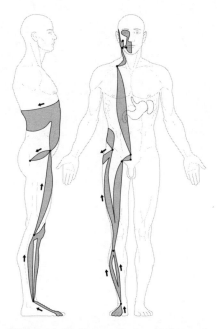

Figure 4.13 Stomach sinew channel

The Stomach sinew channel begins its course on the three middle toes. From here it flows in a broad band alongside the primary channel, but in the opposite direction to the flow of the primary channel, i.e. towards the head.

- The Stomach sinew channel flows from the three middle toes over the top of the foot to the ankle, where it divides into two main branches.

- One branch travels up alongside the tibia and thigh to the inguinal area, where it flows inwards to the pubic bone and up past the navel, across the breast to the clavicle and the acupuncture point St 12. From here it continues over the neck and jaw, where it divides into three branches, which flow to the ear, around the mouth and under the eye, spreading over the lower eyelid.

- The second branch travels up the leg, lateral to the first branch. A branch separates at the waist and flows round to the buttock and the acupuncture point GB 30. The rest of the channel continues up the abdomen and spreads across the lower edge of the ribs and towards the spine.

Stomach channel connections

- *Yin/yang* partner channel: the Spleen channel.

- Hand/Foot channel: the Large Intestine channel.

- The twelve-channel *qi* cycle: the Large Intestine and Spleen channels.

Yin/yang partner channel: the Spleen channel

- A branch separates from the primary channel at the acupuncture point St 42 (on the dorsum of the foot, in the depression between the junction of the second and third metatarsal bones and the cuneiform bones) and travels down to the acupuncture point Sp 1, which is located on the medial corner of the large toenail, where the channel becomes the Spleen channel.

- The Stomach *luo*-connecting vessel separates from the primary channel at the *luo*-connecting point St 40, which is located midway along the lateral side of the tibia. From here it flows medially, connecting to the Spleen channel.

- The Spleen *luo*-connecting vessel separates from the Spleen channel at its *luo*-connecting point Sp 4, which is located on the medial side of the foot inferior to the first metatarsal bone. From here it flows laterally and connects to the Stomach channel.

Hand/Foot channel: the Large Intestine channel

- The Large Intestine channel continues its course up to the medial corner of the orbit at the acupuncture point UB 1. From here the channel flows down to St 1, where the Stomach channel has its source.

The twelve-channel qi cycle

- The previous channel in the cycle is the Large Intestine channel. The Large Intestine channel continues its course up to the medial corner of the orbit at the acupuncture point UB 1. From here the channel flows down to St 1, where the Stomach channel has its source.

- The next channel in the cycle is the Spleen channel. A branch separates from the Stomach channel at the acupuncture point St 42 (on the dorsum of the foot, in the depression between the junction of the second and third metatarsal bones and the cuneiform bones) and travels down to the acupuncture point Sp 1, which is located on the medial corner of the large toenail, where the channel becomes the Spleen channel.

Organ connections

The Stomach primary channel connects to its own *fu* organ, the Stomach, and its partner *zang* organ, the Spleen. The Stomach divergent channel also connects to the Heart, and its great *luo*-connecting vessel connects to the Lung.

Meeting points with other channels

St 1	*Ren mai*, *yang qiao mai* and *du mai*
St 2	*Yang qiao mai*
St 3	*Yang qiao mai*
St 4	Large Intestine channel, *ren mai*, *yang qiao mai* and *du mai*
St 5	Gall Bladder channel
St 6	Gall Bladder channel
St 7	Gall Bladder channel
St 8	Gall Bladder channel and *yang wei mai*
St 9	Gall Bladder channel, *yang qiao mai* and *yin qiao mai*
St 12	Large Intestine, Small Intestine, *san jiao* and Gall Bladder channels and *yin qiao mai*
St 30	Gall Bladder channel and *chong mai*
LI 20	Large Intestine
UB 1	Urinary Bladder, *san jiao*, Small Intestine and Gall Bladder channels, *yin qiao mai*, *yang qiao mai* and *du mai*
GB 3	*San jiao* and Gall Bladder channels
GB 4	*San jiao* and Gall Bladder channels
GB 5	Large Intestine, *san jiao* and Gall Bladder channels
GB 6	Large Intestine, *san jiao* and Gall Bladder channels
Du 14	All the *yang* channels
Du 24	Urinary Bladder channel and *du mai*
Du 26	Large Intestine channel and *ren mai*
Ren 10	Spleen channel and *ren mai*
Ren 12	Small Intestine and *san jiao* channels and *ren mai*
Ren 13	Small Intestine channel and *ren mai*
Ren 24	Large Intestine channel, *du mai* and *ren mai*
Some sources state that the Stomach channel also connects to Du 28, GB 14 and GB 21.	

THE SPLEEN CHANNEL SYSTEM –
ZU TAIYIN JING LUO

Spleen primary channel – *zu taiyin jing mai*

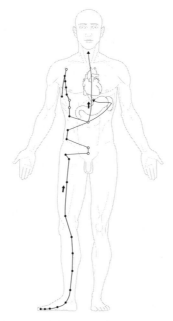

Figure 4.14 Spleen primary channel

The Spleen channel is the final section of the first channel circuit. So far three channels have flowed from the chest out to the fingertips, up to the head and then down to the toes. The Spleen channel flows from the toes back up to the chest to complete the first cycle. The Stomach and Spleen channels are *yin/yang* partner channels and they follow each other in the twelve-channel *qi* cycle. The Stomach channel has a branch that splits away from the main channel at the acupuncture point St 42 (on the dorsum of the foot, in the depression between the junction of the second and third metatarsal bones and the cuneiform bones). From here the channel flows down to the acupuncture point Sp 1, which is located on the medial corner of the large toenail, where the channel becomes the Spleen channel.

Pathway

- The Spleen channel has its source in the medial corner of the large toenail, where the acupuncture point Sp 1 is located.

- It flows along the medial aspect of the foot to the front edge of the medial malleolus.

- It continues up the medial aspect of the tibia, knee and thigh.

- It passes through the inguinal area crossing over to the midline, where it meets with the acupuncture points Ren 3 and Ren 4 located on the midline between the navel and the pubic bone.

- It passes back to a line four *cun* away from the midline of the abdomen and flows upwards to above the umbilicus, where it again courses into the midline and meets with Ren 10. At this point the channel sinks down into the body and connects to the Spleen's partner *fu* organ, the Stomach, its own *zang* organ, the Spleen, and up to the Heart. The Spleen channel connects to the Heart channel in the Heart. Some sources state that the internal channel flows up to the tongue from here.

- A branch separates from the primary channel internal pathway and resurfaces at the acupuncture point Sp 16 on the lower edge of the costal region.

- The channel continues upwards, passing through the acupuncture points GB 24 and Liv 14 along the way.

- A branch separates from the primary channel at the acupuncture point Sp 20, which is located in the second intercostal space, six *cun* lateral to the midline, connecting to Lu 1. Lu 1 is the first acupuncture point on the Spleen's *taiyin* channel partner, the Lung channel, and the first acupuncture point in the first *qi* circuit to and from the chest.

- It flows downwards and laterally to its final point Sp 21, which is located in the sixth intercostal space on the mid-axillary line.

Spleen *luo*-connecting vessel – *zu taiyin luo mai*

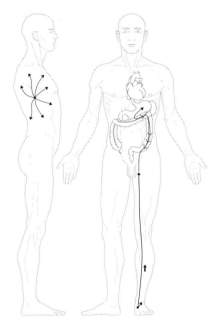

Figure 4.15 Spleen *luo*-connecting vessel

The Spleen *luo*-connecting vessel separates from the Spleen channel at its *luo*-connecting point Sp 4, which is located on the medial aspect of the foot, below the first metatarsal bone. From here it connects in three directions.

- It connects laterally to its partner channel, the Stomach channel.

- It connects vertically to the network of *sun luo*, *fu luo* and *xue luo*.

- It travels up the medial aspect of the tibia and through the inguinal area, where it penetrates into the body, connecting to the Large Intestine and the Spleen's partner *fu* organ, the Stomach.

Spleen great *luo*-connecting vessel – *zu taiyin da luo mai*

The Spleen has an extra *luo*-connecting vessel, which spreads out from the Spleen's large *luo*-connecting point Sp 21 over the sides of the costal region and the diaphragm.

Pathway

- It separates from the primary channel at the Spleen's great *luo*-connecting point, which is located in the sixth intercostal space on the mid-axillary line.

- It spreads over the ribs and the diaphragm.

Spleen divergent channel – *zu taiyin jing bie*

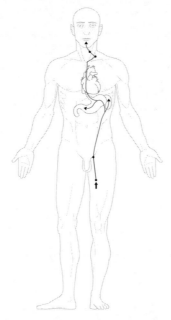

Figure 4.16 Spleen divergent channel

The Spleen divergent channel branches away from the primary channel on the front of the thigh at acupuncture point Sp 11.

Pathway

- It travels up from the thigh, through the inguinal area, to St 30 above the pubic bone, where it penetrates into the body.

- It connects to its partner *zang* organ, the Stomach, its own *zang* organ, the Spleen, and the Heart.

- It rises up to the clavicle and up to the front of the throat, where it merges with the Stomach primary channel at the acupuncture point St 9.

- It connects to the throat and the tongue.

Spleen sinew channel – *zu taiyin jing jin*

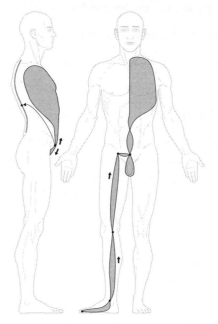

Figure 4.17 Spleen sinew channel

The Spleen sinew channel begins its pathway on the medial side of the big toe. From here it flows in a broad band alongside the primary channel, up to the chest.

Pathway

- It starts on the large toe and travels up the medial aspect of the foot to the front edge of the malleolus.

- It flows up the medial aspect of the tibia to the knee.

- It continues from the knee up along the medial side of the thigh to the inguinal area.

- It flows inwards to the midline.

- It splits in two branches at the acupuncture point Ren 3 located one *cun* above the pubic bone.

- One branch connects down to the external genitalia.

- The other branch continues up along the midline, past the umbilicus, and then spreads across the costal region and the chest.

Spleen channel connections

- *Yin/yang* partner channel: the Stomach channel.

- Hand/Foot channel: the Lung channel.

- The twelve-channel *qi* cycle: the Stomach and Heart channels.

Yin/yang partner channel: the Stomach channel

- A branch separates from the Stomach channel at the acupuncture point St 42 (on the dorsum of the foot, in the depression between the junction of the second and third metatarsal bones and the cuneiform bones) and travels down to the acupuncture point Sp 1, which is located on the medial corner of the large toenail, where the channel becomes the Spleen channel.

- The Stomach *luo*-connecting vessel separates from the primary channel at the *luo*-connecting point St 40, which is located midway along the lateral aspect of the tibia. From here it flows medially connecting to the Spleen channel.

- The Spleen *luo*-connecting vessel separates from the Spleen channel at its *luo*-connecting point Sp 4, which is located on the medial aspect of the foot inferior to the first metatarsal bone. From here it flows laterally and connects to the Stomach channel.

Hand/Foot channel: the Lung channel

- A branch separates from the Spleen channel at the acupuncture point Sp 20, which is located in the second intercostal space six *cun* lateral to the midline. From here it flows up to the acupuncture point Lu 1.

The twelve-channel qi cycle

- The previous channel in the cycle is the Stomach channel. A branch separates from the Stomach channel at the acupuncture point St 42 (on the dorsum of the foot, in the depression between the junction of the second and third metatarsal bones and the cuneiform bones) and travels down to the acupuncture point Sp 1, which is located on the medial corner of the large toenail, where the channel becomes the Spleen channel.

- The next channel in the cycle is the Heart channel. The internal branch of the Spleen primary channel flows to the Heart. In the Heart it connects to the source of the Heart primary channel.

Organ connections

The Spleen channel connects to its own *zang* organ, the Spleen, its partner *fu* organ, the Stomach, and to the Heart. The Spleen's *luo*-connecting vessels also connect to the Stomach and Large Intestine.

Meeting points with other channels

Sp 6	Liver and Kidney channels and *yin qiao mai*
Sp 12	Liver and *san jiao* channels and *yin wei mai*
Sp 13	Liver channel and *yin wei mai*
Sp 15	*Yin wei mai*
Sp 16	*Yin wei mai*
Lu 1	Lung channel
GB 24	Gall Bladder channel and *yang wei mai*
Liv 14	Liver channel and *yin wei mai*
Ren 3	Liver and Kidney channels and *ren mai*
Ren 10	Stomach channel and *ren mai*
According to some sources, Ren 17 also connects to the Kidney, Small Intestine and *san jiao* channels and *ren mai*.	

THE HEART CHANNEL SYSTEM – *SHOU SHAOYIN JING LUO*

Heart primary channel – *shou shaoyin jing mai*

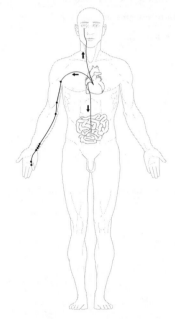

Figure 4.18 Heart primary channel

The Heart succeeds the Spleen channel in the twelve-channel *qi* cycle. At the same time, the Heart channel is the first channel in the second channel circuit to and from the chest. The Heart channel starts its flow inside the Heart, where it is a continuation of the internal branch of the Spleen channel.

Pathway

- It has its source in the Heart.
- It divides into three branches.
- The first branch flows downwards through the diaphragm and connects to the Heart's partner *fu* organ, the Small Intestine.

- A second branch flows up to the throat before dispersing in the area around the eyes. Some sources say that this branch continues from here into the brain.

- A third branch flows through the Lung and out to the centre of the axilla, where it surfaces at the acupuncture point He 1, which is the first point on the channel.

- It flows down the medial aspect of the inner arm, passing through the elbow, wrist and palm.

- The Heart channel terminates at He 9, which is located in the radial border of the base of the nail on the little finger.

- The pathway continues from He 9 to SI 1, which is on the base of the nail's opposite corner, thereby connecting the Heart channel to the Small Intestine channel's starting point.

Heart *luo*-connecting vessel – *shou shaoyin luo mai*

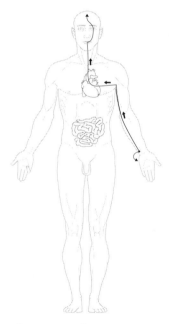

Figure 4.19 Heart *luo*-connecting vessel

The Heart *luo*-connecting vessel separates from the Heart channel at its *luo*-connecting point He 5, which is one *cun* above the wrist on the medial side of the forearm. From here it connects in three directions.

Pathway

- It connects around the forearm to its partner channel, the Small Intestine channel.

- It connects vertically to the network of *sun luo*, *fu luo* and *xue luo*.

- It flows up the anteromedial aspect of the arm to the axilla, penetrates into the body and connects into its own *zang* organ, the Heart, continues up to the root of the tongue and continues up to the eye. From the eye there is a branch that flows into the brain.

Heart divergent channel – *shou shaoyin jing bie*

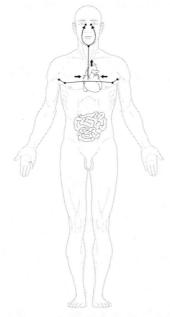

Figure 4.20 Heart divergent channel

The Heart divergent channel separates from the primary channel at He 1 in the centre of the axilla.

Pathway

- It flows downwards from the axilla three *cun* to the acupuncture point GB 22, where it penetrates into the chest.

- It connects to its own *zang* organ, the Heart.

- It rises up to the front of the throat and the acupuncture point Ren 23.

- It spreads over the cheeks and merges with its partner channel, the Small Intestine, at UB 1 in the inner edge of the orbit.

Heart sinew channel – *shou shaoyin jing jin*

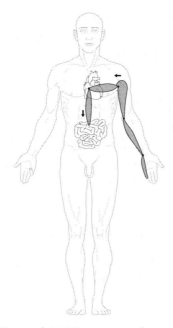

Figure 4.21 Heart sinew channel

The Heart sinew channel starts its flow on the radial side of the little finger. From here it flows in a broad band in the opposite direction of the primary channel, up to the chest and the abdomen.

Pathway

- From the little finger's radial side, the sinew channel flows to the radial aspect of the wrist.

- It flows up the anteromedial side of the arm to the axilla.

- It crosses from the axilla to the centre of the chest and the acupuncture point Ren 17.

- It flows from Ren 17 over the diaphragm and down to the umbilicus.

Heart channel connections

- *Yin/yang* partner channels: the Small Intestine channel.

- Hand/Foot channel: the Kidney channel.

- The twelve-channel *qi* cycle: the Spleen and Small Intestine channels.

Yin/yang partner channel: the Small Intestine channel

- The Heart channel continues from He 9 to SI 1, which are both located on opposite corners of the base of the little fingernail, thereby connecting the Heart channel to the Small Intestine's channel starting point.

- The Heart *luo*-connecting channel connects around the forearm to its partner channel, the Small Intestine channel.

- The Small Intestine *luo*-connecting vessel branches away from the Small Intestine channel at its *luo*-connecting point SI 7, which is located five *cun* above from the wrist on the ulnar aspect of the underarm. From here it flows laterally and connects to the Heart channel.

Hand/Foot channel: the Kidney channel

- An internal branch of the Kidney channel passes through the Liver and Lung before continuing up to the Heart, where it connects with the Heart primary channel.

The twelve-channel qi cycle

- The previous channel in the cycle is the Spleen channel. The internal branch of the Spleen primary channel flows to the Heart, where it continues its course into the Heart channel, thereby becoming the source of the Heart primary channel.

- The next channel in the cycle is the Small Intestine channel. The Heart channel continues from He 9 to SI 1, which are both located on opposite corners on the base of the little fingernail, thereby connecting the Heart channel to the Small Intestine channel's starting point.

Organ connections

The Heart channel connects to its own *zang* organ, the Heart, and its partner *fu* organ, the Small Intestine.

Meeting points with other channels

None.

THE SMALL INTESTINE CHANNEL SYSTEM – *SHOU TAIYANG JING LUO*

Small Intestine primary channel – *shou taiyang jing mai*

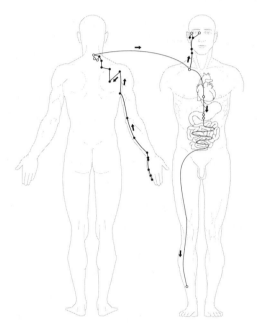

Figure 4.22 Small Intestine primary channel

The Small Intestine primary channel starts its course where the Heart channel continues from He 9 to SI 1, which are both located on opposite corners of the base of the little fingernail, thereby connecting the Heart channel to the Small Intestine primary channel's starting point.

Pathway

- The Small Intestine channel flows from SI 1 on the ulnar corner of the little fingernail's base, along the ulnar aspect of the little finger.

- The primary channel traverses the ulnar aspect of the wrist and flows up the ulnar aspect of the arm.

- It continues past the elbow and up to the posterior aspect of the shoulder joint.

- It flows in a zigzag fashion on the posterior aspect of the shoulder and scapula.

- It passes through the acupuncture points UB 11 and UB 41 and connects to the acupuncture point Du 14 (directly below the seventh vertical vertebra), where it meets with all the other *yang* channels.

- It crosses from Du 14 over the shoulder to the clavicle, where it meets with the Stomach, Large Intestine, *san jiao* and Gall Bladder channels at the acupuncture point St 12.

- From St 12 a branch separates from the main channel and penetrates inwards and downwards to the channel's partner *zang* organ, the Heart. The internal channel continues down through the Stomach to the Small Intestine. On its path downwards the internal branch connects to *ren mai* at Ren 17, Ren 13 and Ren 12. From the Small Intestine, the channel flows down to the tibia, where it connects to St 39 (one *cun* below the midpoint of the lateral edge of the tibia), which is the lower *he*-sea point of the Small Intestine.

- The primary channel's external branch continues its pathway from St 12 up the lateral aspect of the neck to SI 16.

- It continues up to SI 18 on the lower border of the zygomatic bone. The channel then splits into two branches.

- One branch flows up to the inner corner of the orbit, where it connects to its hand/foot channel, the Urinary Bladder.

- The other branch flows up to the outer corner of the orbit, where it connects with GB 1. From here it flows on to the ear. Some sources say that it connects to GB 11, SJ 20 and SJ 22, before the channel terminates in front of the ear at SI 19.

Small Intestine *luo*-connecting vessel – *shou taiyang luo mai*

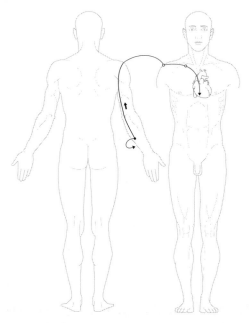

Figure 4.23 Small Intestine *luo*-connecting vessel

The Small Intestine *luo*-connecting vessel branches away from the primary channel at the channel's *luo*-connecting point, SI 7, which is located five *cun* above the wrist on the ulnar aspect of the lower arm. From here it connects in three directions.

Pathway

- It connects laterally to its partner channel, the Heart channel.

- It connects vertically to the network of *sun luo*, *fu luo* and *xue luo*.

- It flows up the medial aspect of the arm to the shoulder and acupuncture point LI 15, which is located anterior and inferior to the acromion. Some authors write that the *luo*-connecting vessel spreads outwards from here. Other authors write that the *luo*-connecting vessel continues its path from LI 15 along the clavicle to St 12, where it sinks into the body and connects to the channel's partner *zang* organ, the Heart.

Small Intestine divergent channel – *shou taiyang jing bie*

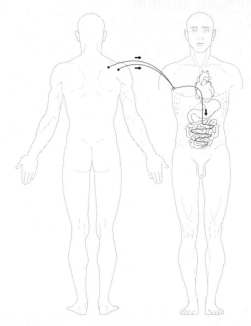

Figure 4.24 Small Intestine divergent channel

The Small Intestine divergent channel branches away from the primary channel at the shoulder.

Pathway

- There are differing opinions on where exactly the divergent channel branches away from the Small Intestine primary channel. Some sources state that it is in the region of SI 10; others that it is at SI 12.

- From the shoulder the divergent channel flows down to GB 22, which is located three *cun* below the axilla.

- It flows from GB 22 into the chest, where it connects with its partner *zang* organ, the Heart.

- The divergent channel flows from the Heart down through the diaphragm and into the Small Intestine.

Small Intestine sinew channel – *shou taiyang jing jin*

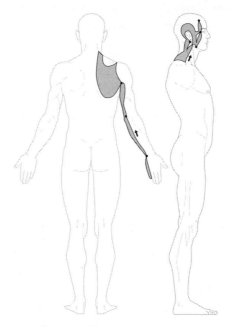

Figure 4.25 Small Intestine sinew channel

The Small Intestine sinew channel starts on the ulnar aspect of the little finger and flows in a broad band alongside the primary channel up the arm, over the scapula and up to the head.

Pathway

- It flows from the ulnar aspect of the arm from its source point on the little finger to the posterior aspect of the shoulder.

- It spreads across the scapula.

- It flows up the neck, over the ear and down to the jaw.

- It continues from the jaw up to the outer edge of the orbit and the side of the head.

Small Intestine channel connections

- *Yin/yang* partner channel: the Heart channel.

- Hand/Foot channel: the Urinary Bladder channel.

- The twelve-channel *qi* cycle: the Heart and Urinary Bladder channels.

Yin/yang partner channel: the Heart channel

- The Heart channel continues from He 9 to SI 1, which are both located on opposite corners of the base of the little fingernail, thereby connecting the Heart channel to the Small Intestine primary channel's starting point.

- The Heart *luo*-connecting channel connects around the forearm to its partner channel, the Small Intestine channel.

- The Small Intestine *luo*-connecting vessel branches away from the Small Intestine channel at its *luo*-connecting point SI 7, which is located five *cun* up from the wrist on the ulnar aspect of the underarm. From here it flows laterally and connects to the Heart channel.

Hand/Foot channel: the Urinary Bladder channel

- The Small Intestine's primary channel has a branch that flows from SI 18 on the zygomatic bone to UB 1 in the inner corner of the orbit, where the Small Intestine connects to the Urinary Bladder.

The twelve-channel qi cycle

- The previous channel in the cycle is the Heart channel. The Heart channel continues from He 9 to SI 1, which are both located on opposite corners of the base of the little fingernail, thereby connecting the Heart channel to the Small Intestine channel's starting point.

- The next channel in the cycle is the Urinary Bladder channel. The Small Intestine primary channel has a branch that flows from SI 18 on the zygomatic bone to UB 1 in the inner corner of the orbit, where the Small Intestine channel connects to the Urinary Bladder channel.

Organ connections

The Small Intestine channel connects to its own *fu* organ, the Small Intestine, and its partner *zang* organ, the Heart. There is also a connection to the Stomach.

Meeting points with other channels

SI 10	Urinary bladder channel, *yang wei mai* and *yang qiao mai*
SI 12	Large Intestine, *san jiao* and Gall Bladder channels
SI 18	*San jiao* channel
SI 19	Gall Bladder and *san jiao* channels
LI 14	Urinary Bladder channel and *yang wei mai*
Du 14	All the *yang* channels
UB 11	Urinary Bladder, *san jiao* and Gall Bladder channels and *du mai*
UB 41	Urinary Bladder channel
St 12	*San jiao*, Gall Bladder, Large Intestine and Stomach channels and *yin qiao mai*
Ren 12	*San jiao* and Stomach channels and *ren mai*
Ren 13	Stomach channel and *ren mai*
Ren 17	Spleen, Kidney and *san jiao* channels and *ren mai*
GB 1	*San jiao* and Gall Bladder channels
GB 11	Urinary Bladder, *san jiao* and Gall Bladder channels
SJ 20	Gall Bladder and *san jiao* channels
SJ 22	Gall Bladder and *san jiao* channels
UB 1	Stomach, Gall Bladder, *san jiao* and Urinary Bladder channels, *yang qiao mai, yin qiao mai* and *ren mai*

THE URINARY BLADDER CHANNEL SYSTEM – *ZU TAIYANG JING LUO*

Urinary Bladder primary channel – *zu taiyang jing mai*

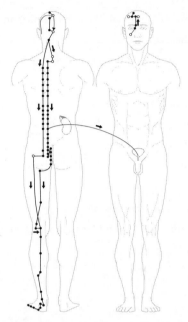

Figure 4.26 Urinary Bladder primary channel

The Urinary Bladder primary channel begins its course when a branch of the Small Intestine primary channel has a branch that flows from SI 18 on the zygomatic bone to UB 1 in the inner corner of the orbit, where the Small Intestine connects to the Urinary Bladder.

Pathway

- It flows from UB 1 in the inner corner of the orbit up over the inner edge of the eyebrow.

- It continues up and over the forehead to the hairline, where it connects with Du 24 and GB 15.

- It continues over the head one and a half *cun* lateral to the midline to UB 7 where the channel courses inwards and connects to Du 20.

- At Du 20 two branches split away from the primary channel.

- One branch flows outwards to the side of the head and connects to the Gall Bladder channel at the points GB 7, GB 8, GB 9, GB 10, GB 11 and GB 12.

- The second branch penetrates into the head, flowing through the brain before resurfacing at UB 8 or Du 17, depending on the source.

- The primary channel pathway continues from Du 20 to UB 8 and UB 9.

- From UB 9 the channel connects to Du 17.

- It continues from Du 17 to UB 10 one and a third *cun* lateral to the lower edge of the first cervical vertebra, where the channel splits into two branches.

- The inner branch connects down to Du 14 and Du 13 before continuing its pathway along the paraspinal muscle one and a half *cun* lateral to the spine. A branch separates from the channel level with the second lumbar vertebra and penetrates into the body. This internal branch connects to its channel's partner *zang* organ, the Kidneys, and its own *fu* organ, the Urinary Bladder. The main pathway continues down to the buttock. At the lower edge of the sacrum, the channel flows upwards and medially to the first posterior sacral foramen. From here the channel flows downwards again, along the posterior aspect of the thigh, down to UB 40 in the centre of the popliteal crease on the back of the knee, where the outer and inner branches of the primary channel meet each other again.

- The outer branch flows from UB 10 down to the upper part of the back, where it flows three *cun* to the spine, parallel with the inner branch. It continues its pathway from the back over the buttock to UB 54, which is three *cun* lateral to the sacral-coccygeal hiatus. It flows slightly downwards and laterally, connecting to GB 30. It continues down the posterior aspect of the thigh to UB 40 in the popliteal crease on the back of the knee, where the outer and inner branches of the primary channel meet each other again.

- The reunified channel travels down the posterior aspect of the gastrocnemius muscle to the lateral side of the ankle.

- It passes over the lateral aspect of the foot, terminating in the lateral corner of the little toenail border.

- From UB 67 a branch of the channel continues to the sole of the foot, between the second and third metatarsal bones, where Kid 1 is situated, which is the start of the Kidney channel.

Urinary Bladder *luo*-connecting vessel – *zu taiyang luo mai*

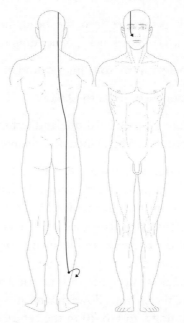

Figure 4.27 Urinary Bladder *luo*-connecting vessel

The Urinary Bladder *luo*-connecting vessel separates from the primary channel at its *luo*-connecting point UB 57, which is situated nine *cun* below the popliteal crease on the posterior aspect of the gastrocnemius muscle. From here it connects in three directions.

Pathway

- It connects laterally to its partner channel, the Kidney channel.

- It connects vertically to the network of *sun luo*, *fu luo* and *xue luo*.

- There are differences of opinion with regard to the longitudinal pathway of the Urinary Bladder *luo*-connecting vessel. Peter Deadman and Mazin Al-Khafaji (1998), for example, write that the Urinary Bladder *luo*-connecting vessel only connects to the Kidney channel. Claudia Focks (2008) on the other hand refers to Solinas *et al.*, who state that a branch of the *luo*-connecting vessel ascends to the back, continuing up to and over the head and connecting to the nose. This course is not directly referred to in the classical texts. There are, however, references to pathological conditions in this vessel that suggest that there is a pathway to the nose.

Urinary Bladder divergent channel – *zu taiyang jing bie*

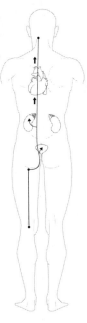

Figure 4.28 Urinary Bladder divergent channel

The Urinary Bladder divergent channel has its source in the centre of the popliteal crease on the back of the knee. From here it flows upwards, opposite the direction of the primary channel to the neck.

Pathway

- It separates from the primary channel at the acupuncture point UB 40, in the centre of the popliteal crease on the back of the knee.

- It flows up the posterior aspect of the thigh to UB 36 in the centre of the transverse gluteal crease.

- It sinks inwards and connects to the anus.

- It continues upwards and connects to its own *fu* organ, the Urinary Bladder.

- It ascends up the spine and connects to its partner *zang* organ, the Kidneys.

- It continues up the spine and connects to the Heart.

- From the Heart, the divergent channel continues its course up to the neck, where it meets with the Kidneys' divergent channel at UB 10, one and a third *cun* lateral to the lower edge of the first cervical vertebra.

Urinary Bladder sinew channel – *zu taiyang jing jin*

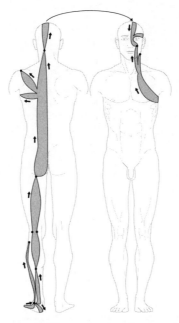

Figure 4.29 Urinary Bladder sinew channel

The Urinary Bladder sinew channel starts on the little toe and flows in a broad belt upwards, opposite the flow of the primary channel, traversing the posterior aspect of the body and terminating in the face.

Pathway

- It starts on the lateral aspect of the little toe.

- It flows to the lateral aspect of the ankle where two branches split away from the main branch of the sinew channel.

- One branch spreads across the heel.

- The other branch flows up the lateral aspect of the lower leg and connects with GB 34 situated one *cun* inferior and anterior to the head of the fibula.

- The main pathway of the sinew channel passes through the Achilles tendon, ascending up the back of the leg and across the buttock.

- It continues up along the spine to the area between the scapula, where two branches separate from the main channel.

- One branch passes over the scapula and ascends to the acromion and the acupuncture point LI 15.

- The other branch passes below the lower border of the scapula to the axilla and across the breast and nipple. It continues upwards and splits into two more branches at the clavicle. One branch ascends to GB 12 below the mastoid process. The other branch traverses the neck to the cheek and the jaw, where it meets with the other *yang* sinew channels at the acupuncture point SI 18 on the zygomatic bone.

- The main branch of the sinew channel continues upwards from the area between the scapula to the acupuncture point UB 10, one and a third *cun* lateral to the lower edge of the first cervical vertebra, where the channel splits into two branches.

- One branch descends into the head and connects to the root of the tongue.

- The second branch passes over the top of the head and down to the medial corner of the orbit, where it splits into two branches. One branch passes down alongside the nose and over the cheek to SI 18 on the zygomatic bone. The other branch spreads across the upper eyelid and connects with the Stomach sinew channel, which spreads over the lower eyelid.

Urinary Bladder channel connections

- *Yin/yang* partner channel: the Kidney channel.

- Hand/Foot channel: the Small Intestine channel.

- The twelve-channel *qi* cycle: the Small Intestine and Kidney channels.

Yin/yang partner channel: the Kidney channel

- From UB 67, which is located on the lateral corner of the border of the little toenail, the Urinary Bladder channel continues its flow to the sole of the foot, between the second and third metatarsal bones, where Kid 1 is situated, which is the start of the Kidney channel.

- The Urinary Bladder *luo*-connecting vessel separates from the primary channel at its *luo*-connecting point UB 57, which is situated nine *cun* below the popliteal crease on the posterior aspect of the gastrocnemius muscle. From here it flows medially towards the Kidney channel.

- The Kidneys' *luo*-connecting vessel separates from the Kidney channel at its *luo*-connecting point Kid 4, which is located on the medial aspect of the ankle on the anterior edge of the Achilles tendon half a *cun* below the top of the malleolus. From here it flows laterally and connects to the Urinary Bladder channel.

Hand/Foot channel: the Small Intestine channel

- The Small Intestine primary channel connects to the Urinary Bladder channel via a branch that ascends from the acupuncture point SI 18 on the zygomatic bone to the acupuncture point UB 1, in the medial corner of the orbit.

The twelve-channel qi cycle

- The previous channel in the cycle is the Small Intestine channel. The Small Intestine primary channel connects to the Urinary Bladder channel via a branch that ascends from the acupuncture point SI 18 on the zygomatic bone to the acupuncture point UB 1 in the medial corner of the orbit.

- The next channel in the cycle is the Kidney channel. From UB 67, which is located on the lateral corner of the border of the little toenail, the Urinary Bladder channel continues its flow to the sole of the foot, between the second and third metatarsal bones, where Kid 1 is situated, which is the start of the Kidney channel.

Organ connections

The Urinary Bladder channel connects to its own *fu* organ, the Urinary Bladder, and its partner *zang* organ, the Kidneys. In addition, there is a connection to the Heart via the Urinary Bladder divergent channel.

Meeting points with other channels

UB 1	Stomach, Gall Bladder, *san jiao* and Small Intestine channels, *yang qiao mai*, *yin qiao mai* and *ren mai*
UB 11	*San jiao* and Gall Bladder channels and *ren mai*
UB 12	*Ren mai*
UB 23	*Ren mai*
UB 31	Gall Bladder channel
UB 32	Gall Bladder channel
UB 33	Gall Bladder channel
UB 34	Gall Bladder channel
UB 41	Small Intestine channel
UB 59	*Yang qiao mai*
UB 61	*Yang qiao mai*
UB 62	*Yang qiao mai*
UB 63	*Yang wei mai*
Du 13	*Du mai*
Du 14	All the *yang* channels
Du 17	*Du mai*
Du 20	Gall Bladder, *san jiao* and Liver channels and *du mai*
Du 24	Stomach channel and *du mai*
GB 7	Gall Bladder channel
GB 8	Gall Bladder channel
GB 9	Gall Bladder channel
GB 10	Gall Bladder channel
GB 11	Gall Bladder, Small Intestine and *san jiao* channels
GB 12	Gall Bladder channel
GB 15	Gall Bladder channel and *yang wei mai*
GB 30	Gall Bladder channel
SI 10	Small Intestine channel, *yang wei mai* and *yang qiao mai*

THE KIDNEY CHANNEL SYSTEM – FOOT *SHAOYIN JING LUO*

Kidney primary channel – *zu shaoyin jing mai*

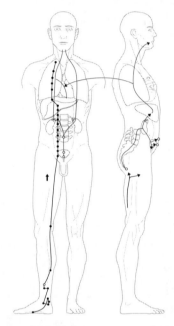

Figure 4.30 Kidney primary channel

The Kidney channel is the final section of the second circuit where two pairs of channels flow from the chest, out to the fingers, up to the head, down to the feet and back to the chest. The foot *shaoyin* channel thereby completes the circuit that the hand *shaoyin* channel initiated, and that the hand and foot *taiyang* channels continued. As well as completing the second cycle, the Kidney channel also initiates the third and final circuit. An internal pathway of the Kidney channel ascends from the Kidney organ and up through the Liver and Lung to the Heart, where it connects to the Pericardium channel and thereby starts the next circuit.

The Kidney channel is the *yin/yang* partner channel of the Urinary Bladder and follows this *taiyang* channel in the cycle.

The Urinary Bladder channel terminates at the acupuncture point UB 67, which is located in the lateral corner of the border of the little toenail. From here, a pathway flows to the sole of the foot between the second and third metatarsal bones, where Kid 1 is situated, which is the start of the Kidney channel.

Pathway

- The Kidney channel starts on the sole of the foot, between the second and third metatarsal bones, at the acupuncture point Kid 1.

- It flows up to the medial metatarsal bone.

- It continues diagonally to the acupuncture point Kid 3, which is located midway between the highest point of the medial malleolus and the Achilles tendon.

- It descends one *cun* to the acupuncture point Kid 5.

- It crosses horizontally to the acupuncture point Kid 6, 1 *cun* below the top of the medial malleolus.

- It ascends diagonally to the acupuncture point Kid 7 on the anterior edge of the Achilles tendon.

- It flows laterally one *cun* to the acupuncture point Kid 8.

- It ascends diagonally to the acupuncture point Sp 6, located three *cun* above the medial malleolus posterior to the edge of the tibia.

- It continues up the medial side of the leg to the inguinal area, where the channel divides into two branches.

- One branch penetrates into the body, crossing through to Du 1 between the tip of the coccyx and the anus. From Du 1, the channel ascends through the spine, before connecting to its partner *fu* organ, the Urinary Bladder, and to its own *zang* organ, the Kidneys. Small branches separate from the channel and connect to Ren 3, Ren 4 and Ren 7. A branch also ascends from the Kidneys and continues up to the Liver and the Lung. In the Lung the channel divides into two branches. One branch continues up to the throat and terminates its pathway in the root of the tongue. The other branch continues from the Lung to the Heart, where it connects to the Kidneys' hand/foot partner channel, the Heart channel. In the Heart the Kidney channel also connects to the Pericardium channel, which is the start of the next circuit of *qi* to and from the chest. Finally, the channel spreads from the Heart through the chest and connects to Ren 17, which is situated midway between the two nipples.

- The external branch continues upwards from the inguinal area to the pubic bone, from where it ascends up to the lower edge of the costal region, travelling in a pathway half a *cun* lateral to the midline.

- From the lower edge of the costal region the channel courses upwards in a pathway two *cun* lateral to the midline, terminating inferior to the clavicle.

Kidney *luo*-connecting vessel – *zu shaoyin luo mai*

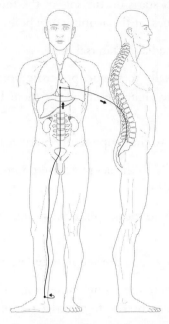

Figure 4.31 Kidney *luo*-connecting vessel

The Kidney *luo*-connecting vessel branches away from the Kidney channel at its *luo*-connecting point Kid 4, which is located half a *cun* inferior to the midpoint between the Achilles tendon and the tip of the medial malleolus, on the anterior border of the Achilles tendon. From here it connects in three directions.

Pathway

- It connects laterally to its partner channel, the Urinary Bladder.

- It connects vertically to the network of *sun luo*, *fu luo* and *xue luo*.

- It flows up the medial aspect of the leg, through the inguinal area, ascending up to the chest. At the acupuncture point Ren 17, situated midway between the nipples, the *luo*-connecting vessel penetrates into the body, passing through the thorax and travelling down through the spine to the lumbar vertebrae.

Kidney divergent channel – *zu shaoyin jing bie*

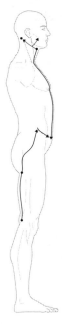

Figure 4.32 Kidney divergent channel

The Kidney divergent channel separates from the primary channel on the medial end of the popliteal crease at the acupuncture point Kid 10.

Pathway

- From its starting point at the acupuncture point Kid 10, the divergent channel connects to its partner channel at the acupuncture point UB 40 in the centre of the popliteal crease.

- It ascends along the posterior aspect of the thigh to the acupuncture point UB 36, located in the transverse gluteal crease.

- It travels inward to the anus and ascends upwards to its partner *fu* organ, the Urinary Bladder, and to the Kidneys themselves.

- It ascends to the acupuncture point UB 23 one and a half *cun* lateral to the inferior border of the second lumbar vertebra, where it meets with the extraordinary vessel *dai mai.*

- It follows *dai mai* around the waist to the anterior aspect of the abdomen.

- It ascends along the midline to the acupuncture point Ren 23 in the depression above the hyoid bone.

- From here it connects to the root of the tongue and the acupuncture point UB 10, situated one and a third *cun* lateral to the lower edge of the first cervical vertebra, where it merges with the Urinary Bladder channel.

Kidney sinew channel – *zu shaoyin jing jin*

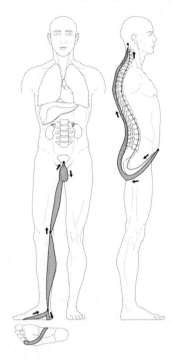

Figure 4.33 Kidney sinew channel

The Kidney sinew channel begins its flow on the inferior aspect of the little toe and travels in a broad band up the medial aspect of the leg to the external genitalia, before penetrating inwards, travelling up along the inner aspect of the spine and terminating below the occiput.

Pathway

- It has its source on the inferior aspect of the little toe and flows up the medial aspect of the foot to the medial malleolus.

- It divides into two branches at the malleolus.

- One of the branches connects down to the heel.

- The main branch ascends along the anterior, medial aspect of the leg to the genitalia.

- From the genitalia the sinew channel ascends to the area superior to the pubic bone and the acupuncture points Ren 2 and Ren 3.

- The sinew channel penetrates into the body at the acupuncture point Ren 3, which is located one *cun* superior to the pubic bone on the midline of the abdomen.

- It flows to the coccyx where it divides into two branches, which ascend posterior and anterior to the spine.

- The sinew channel terminates at the acupuncture point in the neck at the acupuncture point UB 10, located one and a third *cun* lateral to the lower edge of the first cervical vertebra.

Kidney channel connections

- *Yin/yang* partner channel: the Urinary Bladder channel.

- Hand/Foot channel: the Heart channel.

- The twelve-channel *qi* cycle: the Urinary Bladder and Pericardium channels.

Yin/yang partner channel: the Urinary Bladder channel

- From UB 67, which is located in the lateral corner of the border of the little toenail, the Urinary Bladder continues its flow to the sole of the foot, between the second and third metatarsal bones, where Kid 1 is situated, which is the start of the Kidney channel.

- The Urinary Bladder *luo*-connecting vessel separates from the primary channel at its *luo*-connecting point UB 57, which is situated nine *cun* below the popliteal crease on the posterior aspect of the gastrocnemius muscle. From here it flows medially towards the Kidney channel.

- The Kidneys' *luo*-connecting vessel separates from the Kidney channel at its *luo*-connecting point Kid 4, which is located on the medial aspect of the ankle on the anterior edge of the Achilles tendon half a *cun* below the top of the malleolus. From here it flows laterally and connects to the Urinary Bladder channel.

Hand/Foot channel: the Heart channel

- An internal branch of the Kidney channel ascends via the Liver and Lung to the Heart, where it connects to the Kidneys' hand/foot partner channel, the Heart channel. In the Heart the Kidney channel also connects to the

Pericardium channel, which is the start of the next circuit of *qi* to and from the chest.

The twelve-channel qi cycle

- The previous channel in the cycle is the Urinary Bladder channel. From the final acupuncture point on the Urinary Bladder channel, which is located on the lateral corner of the border of the little toenail, the Urinary Bladder channel continues its flow to the sole of the foot, between the second and third metatarsal bones, where Kid 1 is situated, which is the start of the Kidney channel.

- The next channel in the cycle is the Pericardium channel. There is an internal branch of the Kidney channel that ascends via the Liver and Lung to the Heart, where it connects to the source of the Pericardium channel.

Organ connections

The Kidney channel connects to its own *zang* organ, the Kidneys, its partner *fu* organ, the Urinary Bladder, and the Liver, Lung and Heart.

Meeting points with other channels

Kid 2	*Yin qiao mai*
Kid 6	*Yin qiao mai*
Kid 8	*Yin qiao mai*
Kid 9	*Yin qiao mai*
Kid 11–Kid 21	*Chong mai*
Sp 6	Liver and Kidney channels and *yin qiao mai*
Du 1	Gall Bladder channel, *ren mai* and *du mai*
Ren 3	Liver and Spleen channels and *ren mai*
Ren 4	Liver and Spleen channels and *ren mai*
Ren 7	*Chong mai* and *ren mai*
Ren 17	Spleen, Small Intestine and *san jiao* channels and *ren mai*

THE PERICARDIUM CHANNEL SYSTEM – *SHOU JUEYIN JING LUO*

Pericardium primary channel – *shou jueyin jing mai*

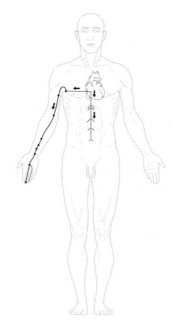

Figure 4.34 Pericardium primary channel

The Pericardium channel initiates the final circuit of the three circuits to and from the chest. The Pericardium channel follows the Kidney channel, which completed the second circuit. An internal branch of the Kidney channel passes through the Heart and meets with the start of the Pericardium channel in the centre of the chest. The Pericardium hand/foot *jueyin* partner channel is the Liver. An internal branch of the Liver channel connects to the Pericardium channel at the acupuncture point Pe 1.

Pathway

- It has its source in the centre of the thorax at the same level as the acupuncture point Ren 17.

- It divides into two branches.

- The first branch descends down through the abdomen and connects to all three *jiao*.

- The other branch flows laterally from the centre of the thorax and surfaces at the acupuncture point Pe 1, which is situated one *cun* lateral to the nipple. The Pericardium channel also connects to an internal branch of its hand/foot *jueyin* partner, the Liver channel, in the area below Pe 1.

- The channel ascends from Pe 1 to the front of the shoulder slightly superior to the axilla.

- It flows from the axilla along the middle of the anterior aspect of the arm, passing through the elbow, wrist and palm.

- A branch separates from the primary channel, at the acupuncture point Pe 8, which is situated between the second and third metacarpal bones. This branch connects to the ring fingernail border's ulnar corner. This is where the *san jiao* channel has its source.

- The Pericardium channel terminates at the acupuncture point Pe 9, which is located on the tip of the middle finger.

Pericardium *luo*-connecting vessel – *shou jueyin luo mai*

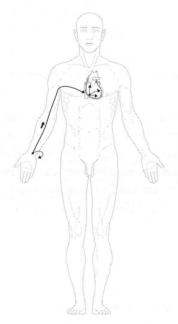

Figure 4.35 Pericardium *luo*-connecting vessel

The Pericardium *luo*-connecting vessel separates from the Pericardium channel at its *luo*-connecting point Pe 6, which is situated between the tendons of the palmaris longus and the flexor carpi radialis, two *cun* above the wrist. From here it connects in three directions.

Pathway

- It connects around the forearm to its partner channel, the *san jiao* channel.

- It connects vertically to the network of *sun luo*, *fu luo* and *xue luo*.

- It travels up the anterior medial aspect of the arm alongside the primary channel and flows to the chest. At the acupuncture point Ren 17 the channel penetrates into the chest and connects to the Heart and the Pericardium.

Pericardium divergent channel – *shou jueyin jing bie*

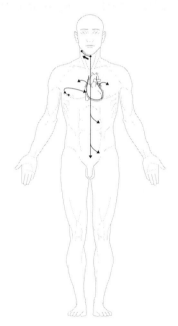

Figure 4.36 Pericardium divergent channel

The Pericardium divergent channel has its source one *cun* lateral to the nipple at the acupuncture point Pe 1.

Pathway

- From Pe 1 the channel flows laterally to GB 22, which is situated three *cun* below the axilla on the mid-axillary line.

- It penetrates into the thorax and connects it to the Heart, where it divides into two branches.

- One branch flows downwards through the abdomen, connecting to the upper, middle and lower *jiao*.

- The other branch ascends to the throat and connects to Ren 23 above the hyoid bone.

- It flows laterally from Ren 23 and merges with its partner channel, the *san jiao* channel, at SJ 16, on the posterior border of the sternocleidomastoid muscle.

Pericardium sinew channel – *shou jueyin jing jin*

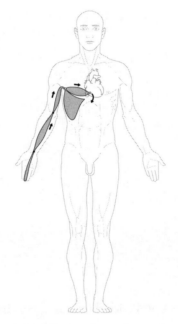

Figure 4.37 Pericardium sinew channel

The Pericardium sinew channel begins its pathway at the tip of the middle finger. From here it flows in a broad band opposite the flow of the primary channel to the chest and costal region.

Pathway

- From the tip of the middle finger the sinew channel flows along the anterior aspect to the centre of the wrist.

- It flows upwards along the anterior, medial aspect of the arm to the axilla.

- It connects to GB 22, three *cun* inferior to the axilla on the mid-axilla line, where it divides into two branches.

- One branch crosses over the chest to the midpoint between the nipples and the acupuncture point Ren 17.

- The other branch spreads across the lateral aspect of the ribs.

Pericardium channel connections

- *Yin/yang* partner channel: the *san jiao* channel.

- Hand/Foot channel: the Liver channel.

- The twelve-channel *qi* cycle: the Kidney and *san jiao* channels.

Yin/yang partner channel: the san jiao channel

- A branch separates from the Pericardium channel at the acupuncture point Pe 8, which is situated between the second and third metacarpal bones. This branch connects to the ring fingernail border's ulnar corner. This is where the *san jiao* channel has its source.

- The Pericardium *luo*-connecting vessel separates from the Pericardium channel at its *luo*-connecting point Pe 6, which is situated between the tendons of the palmaris longus and flexor carpi radialis, two *cun* from the wrist. From here it connects around the arm to the *san jiao* channel.

- The *san jiao luo*-connecting vessel separates from the *san jiao* channel at its *luo*-connecting point SJ 5, which is situated two *cun* from the wrist, between the radius and the ulna, on the radial side of the extensor digitorum communis tendons. From here it flows around the arm and connects to the Pericardium channel.

Hand/Foot channel: the Liver channel

- An internal branch of the Liver channel connects with the Pericardium channel, immediately below the acupuncture point Pe 1, which is located one *cun* lateral to the nipple in the fourth intercostal space.

The twelve-channel qi cycle

- The previous channel in the cycle is the Kidney channel. There is an internal branch of the Kidney channel that passes through the Liver, Lung and Heart. Here the channel connects with the source of the Pericardium channel, which flows up to the acupuncture point Ren 17, midway between the two nipples.

- The next channel in the cycle is the *san jiao* channel. A branch separates from the Pericardium channel, at the acupuncture point Pe 8, which is situated between the second and third metacarpal bones. This branch connects to the ring fingernail border's ulnar corner. This is where the *san jiao* channel has its source.

Organ connections

The Pericardium channel connects to its own *zang* organ, the Pericardium, to its partner *fu* organ, *san jiao*, and to the Heart.

Meeting points with other channels

Pe 1	Liver, *san jiao* and Gall Bladder channels

THE SAN JIAO CHANNEL SYSTEM – SHOU SHAOYANG JING LUO

San jiao primary channel – *shou shaoyang jing mai*

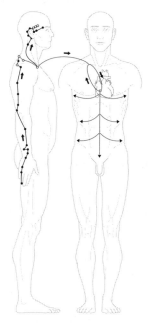

Figure 4.38 *San jiao* primary channel

The *san jiao* primary channel follows its *yin/yang* channel partner, the Pericardium channel, in the twelve-channel *qi* cycle. A branch separates from the Pericardium channel at the acupuncture point Pe 8, which is situated between the second and third metacarpal bones. This branch connects to the ring fingernail border's ulnar corner. This is where the *san jiao* channel has its source.

Pathway

- The channel has its source at SJ 1, which is located on the ring finger at the junction of the ulnar border and the base of the nail.

- It flows along the fourth and fifth metacarpal bones on the dorsum aspect of the hand.

- It passes over the wrist and travels up the posterior aspect of the arm between the radius and the ulnar bones to the elbow.

- It passes through the elbow at the olecranon and travels up the lateral, posterior aspect of the upper arm to the shoulder.

- It traverses the shoulder at the acupuncture point SJ 14, which is situated posterior and inferior to the lateral end of the acromion.

- It passes over the posterior aspect of the shoulder to the acupuncture point SJ 15 in the suprascapular fossa. From SJ 15, the channel connects inferiorly to SI 12 and medially to Du 14 on the lower edge of the seventh cervical vertebra, where it meets with all the other *yang* channels.

- The channel courses back from Du 14 to GB 21 on the apex of the shoulder and down to the clavicle, where it connects with the acupuncture point St 12, where the channel penetrates into the body and meets with its partner channel at Ren 17.

- The channel divides into two separate branches at Ren 17.

- One branch travels downwards and spreads out through the three *jiao*. A branch descends from the lower *jiao* to the popliteal fossa, where it connects to the acupuncture point UB 39, which is the lower *he*-sea point of *san jiao*.

- The other branch ascends upwards, returning to St 12, where the *san jiao* channel continues its course flowing up to SJ 16 on the posterior border of the sternocleidomastoid muscle on the lateral side of the neck.

- It continues its ascent to SJ 17 in the depression between the mastoid process and the mandible.

- It flows around the border of the temporal bone.

- A branch separates from the primary channel at the apex of the ear and connects to the acupuncture points GB 6, GB 5 and GB 4 before it descends down the cheek and jaw. The channel then ascends again to the acupuncture point SI 18 on the zygomatic bone, terminating in the infraorbital region.

- At SJ 17, a branch of the primary channel penetrates into the ear and then emerges anterior to the tragus, where it meets with SI 19.

- It traverses from the ear to the lateral border of the eyebrow, where the external pathway of the channel terminates at the acupuncture point SJ 23.

- A pathway continues from SJ 23 to the acupuncture point GB 1 on the lateral border of the orbital margin. GB 1 is the starting point of the following channel in the circuit. The Gall Bladder channel is also the leg aspect of the *shaoyang* channel.

San jiao luo-connecting vessel – *shou shaoyang luo mai*

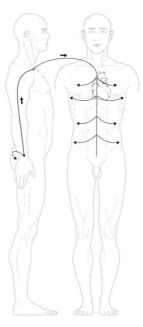

Figure 4.39 *San jiao luo*-connecting vessel

The *san jiao luo*-connecting vessel separates from the primary channel at the channel's *luo*-connecting point, SJ 5, which is located two *cun* proximal to the wrist, in the depression between the radius and the ulnar. From here the vessel connects in three directions.

Pathway

- It connects laterally to its partner channel, the Pericardium channel.

- It connects vertically to the network of *sun luo*, *fu luo* and *xue luo*.

- It flows up the posterior, lateral aspect of the arm to the acupuncture point St 12, superior to the clavicle. From St 12 the vessel penetrates into the body and spreads through the upper *jiao*, where it connects to its partner *zang* organ, the Pericardium. It continues its descent and spreads out through the middle and lower *jiao*.

San jiao divergent channel – *shou shaoyang jing bie*

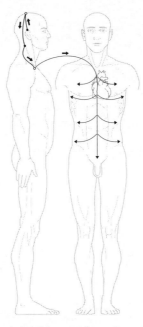

Figure 4.40 *San jiao* divergent channel

The *san jiao* divergent channel separates from the primary channel at SJ 20 superior to the apex of the ear.

Pathway

- It ascends from SJ 20 to Du 20 on the vertex of the head.

- It descends from Du 20 to SJ 16 on the posterior border of the sternocleidomastoid muscle, where it connects to the primary channel.

- It descends from SJ 16 to St 12 superior to the clavicle, where the divergent channel penetrates into the thorax.

- It spreads through the upper *jiao*, where it connects to its partner *zang* organ, the Pericardium. The divergent channel continues downwards and spreads out through the middle and lower *jiao*.

San jiao sinew channel – *shou shaoyang jing jin*

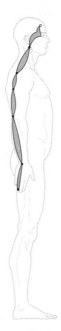

Figure 4.41 *San jiao* sinew channel

The *san jiao* sinew channel begins its flow on the ulnar aspect of the ring finger and flows in a broad band alongside the primary channel up the arm, over the posterior aspect of the shoulder and up to the head.

Pathway

- The sinew channel has its source at the acupuncture point SJ 1, on the ulnar aspect of the ring finger at the junction of the ulnar border and base of the fingernail.

- It courses up the posterior aspect of the arm, over the elbow and along the posterior aspect of the upper arm to the posterior aspect of the shoulder.

- It continues up the posterior, lateral aspect of the neck to the angle of the mandible, where it divides into two branches.

- One branch penetrates inwards and connects to the root of the tongue.

- The other branch ascends anterior to the ear and flows to the outer canthus of the eyes, before ascending to the temple and the frontoparietal region where it ends its pathway and connects to the other three 'hand' *yang* sinew channels.

San jiao channel connections

- *Yin/yang* partner channel: the Pericardium channel.

- Hand/Foot channel: the Gall Bladder channel.

- The twelve-channel *qi* cycle: the Pericardium and Gall Bladder channels.

Yin/yang partner channel: the Pericardium channel

- A branch separates from the Pericardium channel at the acupuncture point Pe 8, which is situated between the second and third metacarpal bones. This branch connects to the ring fingernail border's ulnar corner. This is where the *san jiao* channel has its source.

- The Pericardium *luo*-connecting vessel separates from the Pericardium channel at its *luo*-connecting point Pe 6, which is situated between the tendons of the palmaris longus and flexor carpi radialis, two *cun* from the wrist. From here it connects around the arm to the *san jiao* channel.

- The *san jiao luo*-connecting vessel separates from the *san jiao* channel at its *luo*-connecting point SJ 5, which is situated two *cun* from the wrist between the radius and the ulna, on the radial side of the extensor digitorum communis tendons. From here it flows around the arm and connects to the Pericardium channel.

Hand/Foot channel: the Gall Bladder channel

- The Gall Bladder channel is the hand/foot *shaoyang* partner of the *san jiao* channel, as well as succeeding the *san jiao* channel in the twelve-channel *qi* cycle. A branch continues, flowing from SJ 23, which is the last acupuncture point on the *san jiao* channel to the acupuncture point GB 1 on the lateral border of the orbital margin. GB 1 is the source point of the Gall Bladder channel.

The twelve-channel qi cycle

- The previous channel in the cycle is the Pericardium channel. A branch separates from the Pericardium channel at the acupuncture point Pe 8, which is situated between the second and third metacarpal bones. This branch connects to the ring fingernail border's ulnar corner. This is where the *san jiao* channel has its source.

- The next channel in the cycle is the Gall Bladder channel. A branch continues flowing from SJ 23, which is the last acupuncture point on the *san jiao* channel to the acupuncture point GB 1 on the lateral border of the orbital margin. GB 1 is the source point of the Gall Bladder channel.

Organ connections

The *san jiao* channel connects to its own *fu* organ, *san jiao*, and its partner *zang* organ, the Pericardium. Furthermore, by spreading through all three *jiao*, the *san jiao* channel connects to all the *zangfu* organs.

Meeting points with other channels

SJ 13	Gall Bladder channel and *yang wei mai*
SJ 15	Gall Bladder channel and *yang wei mai*
SJ 20	Gall Bladder and Small Intestine channels
SJ 22	Gall Bladder and Small Intestine channels
SI 12	Small Intestine, Large Intestine and Gall Bladder channels
SI 18	Small Intestine channel
SI 19	Gall Bladder and Small Intestine channels
UB 11	Urinary Bladder, Gall Bladder and Small Intestine channels and *du mai*
St 12	Gall Bladder, Small Intestine, Large Intestine and Stomach channels and *yin qiao mai*
GB 1	Gall Bladder and Small Intestine channels
GB 3	Stomach and Small Intestine channels
GB 4	Gall Bladder and Stomach channels
GB 5	Large Intestine, Stomach and Gall Bladder channels
GB 6	Large Intestine, Stomach and Gall Bladder channels
GB 11	Small Intestine, Urinary Bladder and Gall Bladder channels
GB 14	Large Intestine, Stomach and Gall Bladder channels
GB 20	Gall Bladder channel, *yang wei mai* and *yang qiao mai*
GB 21	Gall Bladder and Stomach channels and *yang wei mai*
Du 14	All the *yang* channels
Ren 12	Kidney and Stomach channels and *ren mai*
Ren 17	Spleen, Kidney and Small Intestine channels and *ren mai*

THE GALL BLADDER CHANNEL SYSTEM – *ZU SHAOYANG JING LUO*

Gall Bladder primary channel – *zu shaoyang jing mai*

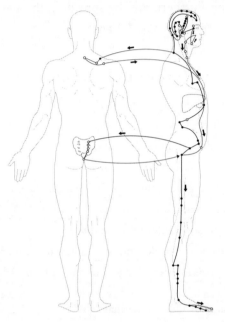

Figure 4.42 Gall Bladder primary channel

The Gall Bladder primary channel begins its pathway when a branch of the *san jiao* channel flows from SJ 23, which is the last acupuncture point on the *san jiao* channel to the acupuncture point GB 1 on the lateral border of the orbital margin.

Pathway

- It starts its pathway at GB 1, which is located on the lateral border of the orbital margin.

- It flows laterally to GB 2 anterior to the intertragic notch.

- It ascends to St 8 on the corner of the forehead.

- From St 8 the channel traverses downwards to the acupuncture point SJ 22 at the upper border of the root of the ear.

- From SJ 22 the channel flows to SJ 20 superior to the apex of the ear, before ascending 1 *cun* to the acupuncture point GB 8.

- From GB 8 the channel curves downwards to the acupuncture point GB 12, posterior and anterior to the mastoid process.

- From GB 12 the channel courses back to the forehead and the acupuncture points GB 13 (half a *cun* within the hairline, directly superior to the outer canthus of the eye) and GB 14 (one *cun* superior to the middle of the eyebrow).

- At GB 14 the channel changes direction again and traverses the lateral aspect of the head and then descends down to the acupuncture point GB 20, located on the lower border of the occiput in the depression between the origins of the sternocleidomastoid and trapezius muscles.

- An internal branch separates from the primary channel at GB 20 and traverses to the acupuncture point SJ 17 in the depression between the mastoid process and the mandible. At SJ 17 a branch of the primary channel penetrates the ear and then emerges anterior to the tragus, where it meets with SI 19 and continues medially through St 7 to GB 1 on the lateral border of the orbital margin. From GB 1 the channel flows down to St 5 in the depression on the anterior border of the masseter muscle. The channel ascends to the infraorbital region to meet with the *san jiao* channel, before descending again to St 6 on the prominence of the masseter muscle. The internal branch of the channel continues down the neck through the acupuncture point St 9 and down to the clavicle, where it reunites with the primary channel at the acupuncture point St 12.

- The main branch of the primary channel continues down from GB 20 to the acupuncture point GB 21 on the crest of the trapezius muscle, midway between the lower border of the seventh vertebra and the lateral extremity of the acromion.

- It descends one *cun* to the acupuncture point SJ 15 before travelling medially to the acupuncture point Du 14 on the lower border of the seventh vertebra, where it meets with all the *yang* channels.

- From Du 14 the channel courses outwards, passing through the acupuncture points UB 11 (one and a half *cun* lateral to the lower border of the first thoracic vertebra) and SI 12 (in the centre of the suprascapular fossa), before crossing the shoulder to the acupuncture point St 12, which is superior to the clavicle.

- The channel divides into two branches at St 12.

- An internal branch penetrates down into the thorax, connecting to the Pericardium channel at Pe 1 (one *cun* lateral to the nipple in the fourth intercostal space) and continues through the diaphragm, connecting to its partner *zang* organ, the Liver, and to its own *fu* organ, the Gall Bladder. From the Gall Bladder the internal channel continues down to the acupuncture point St 30 (two *cun* lateral to the midline, directly superior to the pubic bone). From St 30 the channel continues to the external genitalia, before passing through the body to the first sacral vertebra. It flows out to the buttock and the acupuncture point GB 30 (one third of the distance from the prominence of the great trochanter and the sacral hiatus), where it meets with the outer branch of the channel.

- The primary channel descends from St 12, passing over the side of the ribs through the acupuncture points GB 22 (three *cun* inferior to the apex of the axilla on the mid-axillary line), GB 23 (one *cun* medial to GB 22), GB 24 (located in the seventh intercostal space, on the mamillary line) and Liv 13 (anterior and inferior to the tip of the eleventh rib).

- It flows posteriorly to the acupuncture point GB 25 (anterior and inferior to the tip of the twelfth rib), before switching back to the front of the abdomen again and the acupuncture points GB 26 (directly inferior to Liv 13, level with the umbilicus), GB 27 (in the depression medial to the anterior superior iliac spine) and GB 28 (0.5 *cun* inferior and anterior to GB 27).

- It travels diagonally downwards to GB 30 (one third of the distance from the prominence of the great trochanter and the sacral hiatus), where it reunites with the internal branch of the channel.

- It descends along the lateral aspect of the leg to the anterior aspect of the lateral malleolus.

- It continues along the dorsum of the foot to the acupuncture point GB 41 in the junction between the fourth and fifth metatarsal bones. A branch travels from the Gall Bladder to the junction of the lateral border and the base of the large toenail, where it connects to the acupuncture point Liv 1 and the start of the Liver channel.

- The primary channel continues to the junction of the lateral border and the base of the fourth toenail, where the Gall Bladder channel terminates at the acupuncture point GB 44.

Gall Bladder *luo*-connecting vessel – *zu shaoyang luo mai*

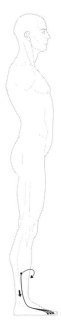

Figure 4.43 Gall Bladder *luo*-connecting vessel

The Gall Bladder *luo*-connecting vessel separates from the primary channel at its *luo*-connecting point GB 37, which is situated five *cun* above the lateral malleolus on the anterior border of the fibula. From here the vessel connects in three directions.

Pathway

- It connects medially to its partner channel, the Liver channel.

- It connects vertically to the network of *sun luo*, *fu luo* and *xue luo*.

- It flows downwards over the dorsum of the foot to the third, fourth and fifth toes.

Gall Bladder divergent channel – *zu shaoyang jing bie*

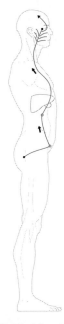

Figure 4.44 Gall Bladder divergent channel

The Gall Bladder's divergent channel has its source in the buttock and ascends to the head.

Pathway

- It separates from the primary channel at the acupuncture point GB 30, one third of the distance from the prominence of the great trochanter and the sacral hiatus.

- It penetrates into the body and crosses the Liver divergent channel at the acupuncture point Ren 2, which is located immediately superior to the pubic bone on the midline.

- It ascends to the acupuncture point Liv 13, anterior and inferior to the tip of the eleventh rib.

- It continues up to its own *fu* organ, the Gall Bladder, and its partner *zang* organ, the Liver, and on up to the Heart.

- It ascends to the neck and the jaw before dispersing over the face.

- It connects with the primary channel and the Liver divergent channel at the acupuncture point GB 1 on the lateral border of the orbital margin.

- It penetrates into the eye and continues into the brain.

Gall Bladder sinew channel – *zu shaoyang jing jin*

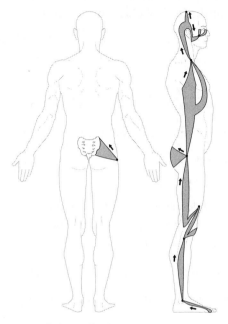

Figure 4.45 Gall Bladder sinew channel

The Gall Bladder sinew channel starts on the lateral aspect of the fourth toe, flowing in a broad band, opposite the flow of the primary channel up the lateral aspect of the leg and the lateral aspect of the torso and neck before terminating on the lateral aspect of the head.

Pathway

- It starts at the lateral aspect of the fourth toe.

- It flows to the anterior aspect of the lateral malleolus.

- It flows up the lateral aspect of the leg, binding at the lateral aspect of the knee.

- Just above the knee a branch binds to the acupuncture point St 32, six *cun* superior to the lateral border of the patella.

- The sinew channel continues upwards, dividing into two branches at the great trochanter, spreading over the buttock and binding at the sacrum.

- The other branch ascends up the lateral aspect of the body, dividing into two branches at the lower border of the costal region.

- One branch ascends over the lateral aspect of the costal region to the acupuncture point St 12, superior to the clavicle, where it meets with the second branch of the Gall Bladder sinew channel.

- The second branch ascends along the mid-axillary line connecting to St 12, superior to the clavicle, where it meets with the first branch of the sinew channel.

- It ascends up the lateral aspect of the neck and curves around the ear.

- Superior to the apex of the ear, the sinew channel divides into two branches.

- One branch ascends to the vertex of the head and the acupuncture point Du 20.

- The second branch descends in front of the ear and traverses to the zygomatic bone and the acupuncture point SI 18, where it meets the other two foot *yang* sinew channels and divides into two branches.

- One branch flows to and terminates on the edge of the nostril.

- The other branch flows to and terminates at the outer canthus of the eye.

Gall Bladder channel connections

- *Yin/yang* partner channel: the Liver channel.

- Hand/Foot channel: the *san jiao* channel.

- The twelve-channel *qi* cycle: the *san jiao* and Liver channels.

Yin/yang partner channel: the Liver channel

- A branch separates from the Gall Bladder channel at the acupuncture point GB 41 in the junction between the fourth and fifth metatarsal bones. This branch flows to the junction of the lateral border and the base of the large toenail, where it connects to the acupuncture point Liv 1 and the start of the Liver channel.

- The Gall Bladder *luo*-connecting vessel separates from the primary channel at its *luo*-connecting point GB 37, which is situated five *cun* above the lateral malleolus on the anterior border of the fibula and connects laterally to the Liver channel.

- The Liver *luo*-connecting vessel separates from the primary Liver channel at its *luo*-connecting point Liv 5, which is located five *cun* superior to the prominence of the medial malleolus, posterior to the border of the tibia. From here it flows laterally and connects to the Gall Bladder channel.

Hand/Foot channel: the san jiao channel

- The Gall Bladder channel is the hand/foot *shaoyang* partner of the *san jiao* channel. At the same time the Gall Bladder is also the next channel in the twelve-channel *qi* cycle. A branch continues the flow from the acupuncture point SJ 23 (located on the lateral border of the eyebrow), which is the last acupuncture point on the *san jiao* channel to the acupuncture point GB 1 on the lateral border of the orbital margin. GB 1 is the source point of the Gall Bladder channel.

The twelve-channel qi cycle

- The previous channel in the cycle is the *san jiao* channel. A branch continues the flow from the acupuncture point SJ 23 (located on the lateral border of the eyebrow), which is the last acupuncture point on the *san jiao* channel, to the acupuncture point GB 1 on the lateral border of the orbital margin. GB 1 is the source point of the Gall Bladder channel.

- The next channel in the cycle is the Liver channel. A branch separates from the Gall Bladder channel at the acupuncture point GB 41 in the junction between the fourth and fifth metatarsal bones. This branch flows to the junction of the lateral border and the base of the large toenail, where it connects to the acupuncture point Liv 1 and the start of the Liver channel.

Organ connections

The Gall Bladder channel connects to its own *fu* organ, the Gall Bladder, and its partner *zang* organ, the Liver. In addition, there are connections to the Heart via the divergent channel.

Meeting points with other channels

GB 1	Small Intestine and *san jiao* channels
GB 3	*San jiao* and Stomach channels
GB 4	*San jiao* and Stomach channels
GB 5	*San jiao*, Large Intestine and Stomach channels
GB 6	*San jiao*, Large Intestine and Stomach channels
GB 7	Urinary Bladder channel
GB 8	Urinary Bladder channel
GB 9	Urinary Bladder channel
GB 10	Urinary Bladder channel
GB 11	Small Intestine, *san jiao* and Urinary Bladder channels
GB 12	Urinary Bladder channel
GB 13	*Yang wei mai*
GB 14	Stomach, Large Intestine and *san jiao* channels and *yang wei mai*
GB 15	Urinary Bladder channel and *yang wei mai*
GB 16	*Yang wei mai*
GB 17	*Yang wei mai*
GB 18	*Yang wei mai*
GB 19	*Yang wei mai*
GB 20	*San jiao* channel, *yang qiao mai* and *yang wei mai*
GB 21	Stomach and *san jiao* channels and *yang wei mai*
GB 23	Urinary Bladder channel
GB 24	Spleen channel and *yang wei mai*
GB 26	*Dai mai*
GB 27	*Dai mai*
GB 28	*Dai mai*
GB 29	*Yang qiao mai*
GB 30	Urinary Bladder channel
GB 35	*Yang wei mai*
St 5	Stomach channel
St 6	Stomach channel
St 7	Stomach channel
St 8	Stomach channel and *yang wei mai*
St 9	Stomach channel, *yang qiao mai* and *yin qiao mai*
St 12	Small Intestine, Large Intestine, *san jiao* and Stomach channels and *yin qiao mai*
St 30	Stomach channel and *chong mai*
SI 12	*San jiao*, Large Intestine and Small Intestine channels

SI 19	*San jiao* and Small Intestine channels
UB 1	Stomach, Small Intestine, *san jiao* and Urinary Bladder channels, *yang qiao mai*, *yin qiao mai* and *du mai*
UB 11	*San jiao* and Urinary Bladder channels
UB 31	Urinary Bladder channel
UB 32	Urinary Bladder channel
UB 33	Urinary Bladder channel
UB 34	Urinary Bladder channel
Pe 1	Liver, *san jiao* and Pericardium channels
SJ 15	*San jiao* channel and *yang wei mai*
SJ 17	*San jiao* channel
SJ 20	Small Intestine and *san jiao* channels
SJ 22	Small Intestine and *san jiao* channels
Liv 13	Liver channel and *dai mai*
Du 1	Kidney channel, *du mai* and *ren mai*
Du 14	All the *yang* channels
Du 20	Urinary Bladder, *san jiao* and Liver channels and *du mai*

THE LIVER CHANNEL SYSTEM – ZU JUEYIN JING LUO

Liver primary channel – *zu jueyin jing mai*

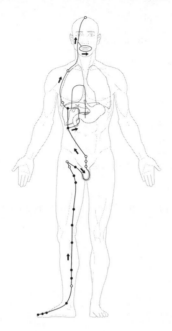

Figure 4.46 Liver primary channel

The Liver channel is the final section of the third cycle of channels flowing to and from the chest. It is also the final section of the twelve-channel *qi* cycle. The Liver channel follows its *yin/yang* partner channel, when a branch separates from the Gall Bladder at the acupuncture point GB 41 in the junction between the fourth and fifth metatarsal bones. This branch flows to the junction of the lateral border and the base of the large toenail, where it connects to the acupuncture point Liv 1 and the start of the Liver channel.

The flow of *qi* through the channels does not end when the Liver channel terminates its pathway. An internal branch of the Liver channel connects to the Lung channel in the interior of the thorax, thereby initiating a new circuit of *qi* through the twelve channels.

Pathway

- The Liver channel starts its pathway on the junction of the lateral border and the base of the large toenail, at the acupuncture point Liv 1.

- It travels up and over the dorsum of the foot to the anterior aspect of the medial malleolus at the acupuncture point Liv 4.

- It ascends the medial aspect of the leg and connects to the other leg *yin* channels at the acupuncture point Sp 6, which is located three *cun* above the prominence of the medial malleolus, posterior to the edge of the tibia.

- It continues flowing up the medial aspect of the leg to the inguinal area.

- It connects to the acupuncture points Sp 12 and Sp 13 in the inguinal area.

- The primary channel circles around the external genitalia.

- It ascends along the midline of the abdomen through the acupuncture points Ren 2, Ren 3 and Ren 4, which lie zero *cun*, one *cun* and two *cun*, respectively, above the pubic bone.

- It ascends diagonally lateral to the acupuncture point Liv 13, inferior and anterior to the tip of the eleventh rib.

- It flows diagonally medial to the acupuncture point Liv 14 on the mamillary line, four *cun* from the midline in the sixth intercostal space, where the exterior pathway of the primary channel terminates its flow.

- An internal branch of the channel separates from the primary channel at the acupuncture point Liv 13, inferior and anterior to the tip of the eleventh rib. The internal branch penetrates into the abdomen, passing through the Stomach, its own *zang* organ, the Liver, and its *fu* organ, the Gall Bladder. From the Gall Bladder, the channel continues up to the Lung, where it connects with the Lung channel, which is the next channel in the twelve-channel *qi* cycle. The internal branch of the channel continues its pathway from the Lung by flowing laterally to the acupuncture point Pe 1, situated 1 *cun* lateral to the nipple. At Pe 1, the Liver channel connects to the Pericardium channel, which is the hand *jueyin* partner of the Liver and the channel that initiated the third channel cycle to and from the chest. The internal branch then ascends through the neck, behind the trachea and up to the eye. A branch of the channel separates and flows down the face and encircles the mouth. The rest of the channel penetrates into the brain before flowing up the forehead and terminating in the vertex at the acupuncture point Du 20.

Liver *luo*-connecting vessel – *zu jueyin luo mai*

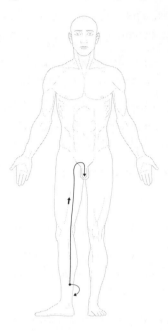

Figure 4.47 Liver *luo*-connecting vessel

The Liver *luo*-connecting vessel separates from the primary Liver channel at its *luo*-connecting point Liv 5, which is located five *cun* superior to the prominence of the medial malleolus, posterior to the border of the tibia. From here it connects in three directions.

Pathway

- It connects laterally to its partner channel, the Gall Bladder channel.

- It connects vertically to the network of *sun luo, fu luo* and *xue luo*.

- It ascends along the medial aspect of the leg, alongside the primary channel, to the inguinal area, where the *luo*-connecting vessel descends, spreading over the external genitalia.

Liver divergent channel – *zu jueyin jing bie*

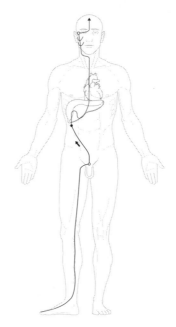

Figure 4.48 Liver divergent channel

The Liver divergent channel separates from the primary channel on the dorsum of the foot.

Pathway

- It ascends from the dorsum of the foot along the medial aspect of the leg to the inguinal area.

- It meets with the Gall Bladder divergent channel at the acupuncture point Ren 2 on the midline immediately superior to the pubic bone.

- It ascends diagonally to the acupuncture point Liv 13, which is located inferior and anterior to the tip of the eleventh rib, where it penetrates into the body and connects to its own *zang* organ, the Liver, and to its partner *fu* organ, the Gall Bladder.

- It continues up to the Heart.

- It ascends from the Heart to the neck and jaw, spreading over the face.

- A branch continues up to the acupuncture point GB 1 on the outer canthus of the eye, where the divergent channel unites with the Gall Bladder primary channel.

- It penetrates through the eye into the brain.

327

Liver sinew channel – *zu jueyin jing jin*

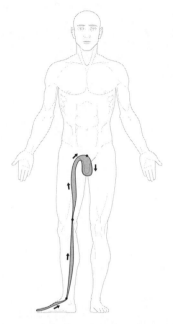

Figure 4.49 Liver sinew channel

The Liver sinew channel has its source on the dorsum of the big toe and flows in a broad belt alongside the primary channel to the inguinal area, before descending to the external genitalia.

Pathway

- It has its source at the dorsum of the big toe, then flows to the anterior aspect of the medial malleolus.

- It ascends the medial aspect of the leg to the inguinal area, before descending to the external genitalia.

Liver channel connections

- *Yin/yang* partner channel: the Gall Bladder channel.

- Hand/Foot channel: the Pericardium channel.

- The twelve-channel *qi* cycle: the Gall Bladder and Lung channels.

Yin/yang partner channel: the Gall Bladder channel

- A branch separates from the Gall Bladder channel at the acupuncture point GB 41 in the junction between the fourth and fifth metatarsal bones. This branch flows to the junction of the lateral border and the base of the large toenail, where it connects to the acupuncture point Liv 1 and the start of the Liver channel.

- The Gall Bladder *luo*-connecting vessel separates from the primary channel at its *luo*-connecting point GB 37, which is situated five *cun* above the lateral malleolus on the anterior border of the fibula and connects laterally to the Liver channel.

- The Liver *luo*-connecting vessel separates from the primary Liver channel at its *luo*-connecting point Liv 5, which is located five *cun* superior to the prominence of the medial malleolus, posterior to the border of the tibia. From here it flows laterally and connects to the Gall Bladder channel.

Hand/Foot channel: the Pericardium channel

- An internal branch of the Liver channel connects with the Pericardium channel, immediately below the acupuncture point Pe 1, which is located one *cun* lateral to the nipple in the fourth intercostal space.

The twelve-channel qi cycle

- The previous channel in the cycle is the Gall Bladder channel. A branch separates from the Gall Bladder channel at the acupuncture point GB 41 in the junction between the fourth and fifth metatarsal bones. This branch flows to the junction of the lateral border and the base of the large toenail, where it connects to the acupuncture point Liv 1 and the start of the Liver channel.

- The next channel in the cycle is the Lung channel. An internal branch of the Liver channel connects to the Lung channel in the interior of the thorax, thereby initiating a new circuit of *qi* through the twelve channels.

Organ connections

The Liver channel connects to its own *zang* organ, the Liver, and its partner *fu* organ, the Gall Bladder. In addition, the Liver channel connects to the Stomach and the Heart.

Meeting points with other channels

Liv 13	Gall Bladder channel and *dai mai*
Liv 14	Stomach channel and *yin wei mai*
Sp 6	Kidney and Spleen channels and *yin qiao mai*
Sp 12	*San jiao* and Spleen channels and *yin wei mai*
Sp 13	Spleen channel and *yin wei mai*
Pe 1	*San jiao* and Pericardium channels
Ren 2	*Ren mai*
Ren 3	Kidney and Spleen channels and *ren mai*
Ren 4	Kidney and Spleen channels and *ren mai*
Du 20	Urinary Bladder, Gall Bladder and *san jiao* channels and *du mai*

THE EIGHT EXTRAORDINARY VESSELS – *QI JING BA MAI*

Qi jing ba mai is sometimes referred to as the eight extra meridians. This can make them sound as if they are a supplement or an attachment to the regular channel system. These vessels are in fact a more primal and fundamental aspect of the body's physiological structure. They are more of an underpinning of the channel system than a superstructure. It is for this reason that I have followed the example of most contemporary authors and have utilised the more accurate translation of *qi jing ba mai* – the eight extraordinary vessels. *Qi* in this context is a completely different word than *qi* as in vital substance. *Qi* here means 'extraordinary', 'fantastic', 'surprising' and 'unique'. *Jing* is the same as in *jingluo* or channel, i.e. *jing* being 'a longitudinal thread in a piece of cloth' and 'a channel, or something that connects two things', *ba* is the number eight and *mai* means 'vessel', as in blood vessels. This infers that these vessels are something other and more than the regular channels. The regular channels are called *zheng*, which means 'correct' or 'normal'.

The eight extraordinary vessels are mentioned in the *Huang Di Nei Jing*, but it was not until the *Nanjing* that they were systematically presented as a complete and coherent system. It is also from these works and Li Shi Zhen's book *Qi Jing Ba Mai Kao* (*A Study of the Eight Extraordinary Vessels*, 1578 CE) that most of the knowledge that forms the basis for the interpretation of these channels comes. Compared with the regular channels, historically not much has been written about the eight extraordinary vessels. This means that the comprehension of them is much more open to interpretation, assumptions and, in certain instances, guesswork.

As stated above, the eight extraordinary vessels are more primal than the regular channels. Many people are of the opinion that the eight extraordinary vessels arise immediately after conception. In the Daoist understanding of how the universe emerged, there was originally 'nothingness', i.e. an all-embracing void that contained the potential for everything. Out of this void arose the first primary, fundamental forces – the two complementary opposites *yin* and *yang*, which everything in the universe consists of. Before the egg is fertilised there is 'nothing', but in this 'nothingness' there is also the potential for everything – the potential for life itself. Immediately after fertilisation the egg divides into two cells. It is in this division that the first channels, *du mai* and *ren mai*, arise. *Du mai* and *ren mai* divide the body vertically into two halves, creating left and right sides. *Du mai* and *ren mai* are the basic *yang* and *yin* governing vessels. *Du mai* and *ren mai* have the overall control of *yang* and *yin* and they influence all of the other channels.

The body's first *yang* channel, *du mai*, is the *yang* governing vessel. This is also reflected by the fact that the acupuncture points that have the greatest influence on *yang* are located on *du mai*. This is especially true of the acupuncture points Du 4, Du 14 and Du 20. *Ren mai*, which is the primary *yin* channel, also has a similar relationship to *yin qi* in the body. This relationship is valid in both the foetal stage and the rest of a person's life.

In general, it is not only in the period after conception that the eight extraordinary vessels are governing and active. The functions that the eight extraordinary vessels carry out in the period after conception form the basis for their functions throughout life. As we will see, this has relevance both structurally and in relation to physiology. It is through the eight extraordinary vessels that the pre-heaven *jing* integrates with the post-heavenly *qi*.

The third channel to arise is *chong mai*. In the same way that *qi* in the universe is created by the tension between the two fundamental forces of *yin* and *yang*, *chong mai* arises from the interaction of *yin* and *yang* in the fertilised egg. *Chong mai* is the foundation for the further development of the rest of the channel system. Therefore, it is said in Chinese medicine that *chong mai* is 'the Sea of the Twelve Channels'.

Du mai, *ren mai* and *chong mai* all have their origin in the area between the two Kidneys. In this way we can see that they have a deep, fundamental relationship to *jing*.

The fourth channel to arise is *dai mai*. *Dai mai* is the only horizontal or lateral channel in the body. *Dai mai* encircles and embraces the other channel and thereby integrates *yin* and *yang*.

There are still no limbs on the embryo after the initial divisions. When the limbs start to form, the last four extraordinary vessels are also formed. These are *yin qiao mai*, *yang qiao mai*, *yin wei mai* and *yang wei mai*. *Yin qiao mai* and *yang qiao mai* coordinate the movement of *yin* and *yang* upwards and downwards in the body, and they regulate the rhythm and the alternation that there is between *yin* and *yang* in the diurnal cycles. This is why they have such an impact on the body's ability to fall asleep and wake up in the morning. *Yang wei mai* and *yin wei mai* coordinate and balance *yin* and *yang*. They do this by controlling and coordinating the movement of *yin* and *yang* inwards and outwards in the body. This is also reflected in the names of the two acupuncture points that are used to activate *yin wei mai* and *yang wei mai* – *neiguan* or inner gate, and *waiguan* or outer gate.

Because they arise immediately after conception and because they are the first channels that form in the embryo, the eight extraordinary vessels create a structure or a framework around which the body is built. At the same time they are responsible for the circulation of *jing*, which is used to create the skeleton.

Furthermore, it is the extraordinary vessels that circulate *jing*, *qi* and *xue* until the organs and the regular channel network are operational and able to provide the body with *qi* and *xue*.

The extraordinary vessels are formed immediately after conception and are involved in the construction of the body from the very start. They constitute some of the deepest aspects of the body's energetic structure. In a way the channel system can be understood as being a series of concentric rings, i.e. that the different aspects

332

of the channel system can be seen as energetic layers. The core in the middle of the rings is Kidney *jing* and *mingmen*, the next ring is *du mai* and *ren mai*, and then comes *chong mai*. The next ring is the rest of the eight extraordinary vessels. Further out energetically come the divergent channels, the internal branches of the regular channels and the internal branches of the *luo* vessels. More superficial are the regular channels' primary pathways, and above these come the lateral *luo*-connecting vessels. The most exterior ring is the sinew channels, the *sun luo*, *fu luo* and *xue luo* vessels and the cutaneous regions.

Relationship to the regular channels

The extraordinary vessels are fundamentally different from the regular channels in several ways, even though they are completely integrated with each other. The regular channels are characterised by the fact that they have more fixed relationships. Regular channels have a Five Phase relationship, a *yin/yang* relationship to another channel and a foot/hand relationship to another channel. In addition, they have a *biaoli* or external/internal relationship to a specific same-name organ. Each of the regular channels has a relationship to a specific climatic factor and type of *xie qi*, as well as periods of the day and the year. In addition, the regular channels relate to each other as levels, i.e. they open outwards or inwards, or are a pivot between two other channel levels.

The eight extraordinary vessels have none of these relationships. Even though channels such as *yin qiao mai* and *yang qiao mai*, for example, have the same names and their functions reflect each other, they are not *yin/yang* pairs in the same way that the regular channels are. There are no internal and external relations between them and there are also no *luo* connections. As we will see in a moment, the extraordinary vessels have a relationship to the regular channel network, but their functions are very different. Also, even though the extraordinary vessels have a relationship with the internal organs, they do not have specific, individual relationships in the style of the *biaoli* relationships that the regular channels have to specific organs.

The extraordinary vessels operate on a different level. Generally, they are energetically deeper than the regular channels. With the exception of *ren mai* and *du mai*, they do not have their own independent channel pathways and they do not have their own acupuncture points, but they do connect across the regular channels. *Dai mai* is also the only lateral or horizontal channel in the body.

Something that is a characteristic of the extraordinary vessels is that they have a so-called 'opening point'. Some authors state that these acupuncture points must be used to activate the extraordinary vessel in treatment. Furthermore, some authors are of the opinion that the extraordinary vessels must be activated in pairs. The following pairs are typically activated together: *du mai/yang qiao mai*; *ren mai/yin qiao mai*; *chong mai/yin wei mai* and *dai mai/yang wei mai*. The opening point of the extraordinary vessel and its partner vessel's opening point will be used together and be inserted in a specific order. As we will see later, there can also be other approaches to activating the extraordinary vessels.

Functions of the eight extraordinary vessels

Jing

The extraordinary vessels have a very close relationship to the Kidneys and to the *jing* that is stored in them. One of the extraordinary vessels' important functions is to circulate *jing* in the body. *Jing* is utilised in the formation and development of the first structures in the embryo in the same way that *jing* in a seed is utilised in the growth and development of a seedling. This is extremely important in the development of the body. However, it is not only in its embryonic stages that this relationship is relevant. The extraordinary vessels' circulation of *jing* has a determining influence on a person's development throughout their life. This can be seen in the seven- and eight-year cycles of women and men respectively. For example, the *Huang Di Nei Jing – Su Wen*, chapter one, states that a girl starts to menstruate when she is fourteen years old, because *ren mai* begins to flow and *chong mai* is flourishing. Also, when she is forty-nine, *chong mai* is empty, *ren mai* is depleted and her menstruation stops.

The extraordinary vessels also integrate pre- and post-heaven *qi* in the body by connecting the various aspects of the regular channel system with each other. The extraordinary vessels' relationship to *jing* means that some people are of the opinion that the eight extraordinary vessels should be used with caution, especially when there is a deficiency, such as when there is *qi xu* and *jing xu*.

The extraordinary vessels' relationship to the Kidneys, and thereby to *jing*, is also seen in the fact that *ren mai*, *du mai* and *chong mai* all have their source in the space between the Kidneys. *Chong mai* flows through a large section of the Kidney channel and shares many acupuncture points with the Kidneys. *Yin qiao mai* and *yang qiao mai* also flow together with the Kidney and Urinary Bladder channels during the initial stages of their course. *Yin wei mai* and *yang wei mai* have Kidney and Urinary Bladder acupuncture points as their source points.

This means, in practice, that the extraordinary vessels can be used to regulate *jing* and *yuan qi* and to influence the deepest energetic aspects of the body.

Lifecycles

The extraordinary vessels, especially *du mai*, *ren mai* and *chong mai*, are closely involved in the seven- and eight-year *jing* cycles of women and men. This is very obvious in women, where the state of *chong mai* and *ren mai* has a determining influence on when menstruation begins and ends. These vessels are therefore often treated to regulate the transition between these stages in life, for example in the treatment of menopausal disorders. The extraordinary vessels may also be used if there is a delay in the development process from one stage to the next, for example when menstruation does not start in puberty.

Reservoir

The *Nanjing* describes the extraordinary vessels as a reservoir. This means that one of their functions is to absorb excesses of *qi* and be a reservoir that can be drawn upon when there is a deficiency of *qi*. They can also be drawn on in situations where there is a sudden need to mobilise large quantities of *qi*, for example when there is shock. The name extraordinary vessel is not coincidental. These vessels are used to regulate extraordinary situations.

The extraordinary vessels are particularly well suited to this function of being a reservoir, as they connect the regular channels in a criss-cross pattern and because they connect to the Kidneys and *jing*, where the body's fundamental reserves are stored.

Yin qiao mai and *yang qiao mai* are the primary channels involved in absorbing excesses of *yin qi* and *yang qi* from the channel system. *Yin qiao mai* and *yang qiao mai*, especially, regulate the balance of *yin qi* and *yang qi* between the upper and lower parts of the body. They have a close relationship to the head and they are therefore used to regulate *yin qi* and *yang qi* to and from the eyes, the brain and the head. *Yin wei mai* and *yang wei mai* connect all the *yin* and all the *yang* channels respectively. *Yin wei mai* and *yang wei mai* can therefore regulate surpluses and deficiencies between the channels and between the internal and external aspects of the body.

Connect the twelve regular channels

As stated above, the extraordinary vessels intercross the regular channels. In this way they can integrate the pre- and post-heaven *qi*, whilst at the same time creating a balance between the channels themselves.

We saw in the chapter describing the channels (page 224) how the *luo*-connecting vessels linked the *yin/yang* channel partners with each other and thereby could harmonise them when they were no longer in balance with each other. The extraordinary vessels, on the other hand, can create balance between several channels at one time. *Yin wei mai* links all the *yin* channels and can therefore harmonise them when they are out of balance with each other. *Yang wei mai* can have the same effect on the *yang* channels. This is why it is said that *yin wei mai* dominates the interior and *yang wei mai* dominates the exterior.

Also, all the *yang* channels meet at the *du mai* acupuncture point Du 14. All three of the *yin* leg channels meet at the *ren mai* acupuncture points Ren 3 and Ren 4. *Dai mai* encircles the body at the waist and thereby connects all of the channels that travel up and down the body.

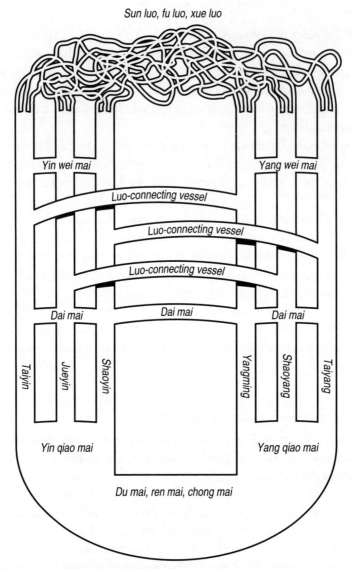

Figure 4.50 The relationship between the regular
channels and the extraordinary channels

Link the pre- and post-heaven qi

As we have seen in the previous section, the extraordinary vessels connect to the regular channels, which circulate *zhen qi*, *xue* and *jinye*. The extraordinary vessels also connect to the Kidneys and thus *jing* and *yuan qi*. This means that they are able to integrate the pre- and post-heaven *qi*. This also means that a treatment of the extraordinary vessels will have a deeper energetic effect than an ordinary acupuncture treatment.

Structure

As stated previously, the eight extraordinary vessels are an energetic framework for the body. They do not just control the development of our physical structure, but they also maintain it. This can be seen, for example, in skeletal disorders such as Scheuermann kyphosis, scoliosis, uneven hips and shoulders, etc., which can be a manifestation of imbalances in the extraordinary vessels. The extraordinary vessels can therefore be used in the treatment of structural imbalances in the body.

- *Ren mai* and *yin qiao mai* affect the anterior aspect of the body and the face.

- *Du mai* and *yang qiao mai* affect the posterior aspect of the body, the neck and the head.

- *Chong mai* and *yin wei mai* affect the medial aspect of the legs, the abdomen and the chest.

- *Dai mai* and *yang wei mai* affect the lateral aspects of the body.

Wei qi

The eight extraordinary vessels are ascribed a close relationship with *wei qi*. Among the functions that *ren mai*, *du mai* and *chong mai* are attributed is the spreading and circulating of *wei qi* in the chest, abdomen and back. Furthermore, Li Shi Zhen writes in the book *Qi Jing Ba Mai Kao* that the surplus of *qi* that flows in the extraordinary vessels 'flows in the space between the skin and muscles'. This space is the area that *wei qi* circulates in. Use of the extraordinary vessels can therefore circulate *wei qi*.

Both *wei qi* and the extraordinary vessels have a close relationship to *jing*. *Jing* is the pre-heavenly root of *wei qi*. *Jing* is the root of *yuan qi*, which transforms *zong qi* to *zhen qi* and thus *wei qi*. Use of the extraordinary vessels can therefore affect the pre-heavenly root of *wei qi*.

Wei qi is the most *yang* aspect of *zhen qi*. *Du mai* is the *yang* governing vessel and thereby has a close relationship to *wei qi*. This relationship is reflected in the acupuncture point Du 14 being one of the most important acupuncture points to stimulate *wei qi*.

Summary of the functions of the extraordinary vessels

- circulate *jing*
- control lifecycles
- reservoir for *qi*
- link the twelve regular channels
- connect the pre- and post-heaven *qi*
- govern the structure of the body
- partial control of *wei qi*

Activating the vessels

There is not only disagreement about when and what the extraordinary vessels should be used for – there are also varying opinions with regard to how the extraordinary vessels should be activated.

The most popular approach to activating the extraordinary vessels is to use combinations of so-called opening points. These acupuncture points, which are not usually located along the course of the extraordinary vessel, can be understood as being a key that activates the *qi* in the extraordinary vessel. In this approach, the opening point will either be used alone to activate the vessel or it will be used in combination with acupuncture points along the channel.

The opening points that most people agree upon when activating the extraordinary vessels are as follows:

- *du mai* – SI 3

- *ren mai* – Lu 7

- *chong mai* – Sp 4

- *dai mai* – GB 41

- *yang qiao mai* – UB 62

- *yin qiao mai* – Kid 6

- *yang wei mai* – SJ 5

- *yin wei mai* – Pe 6.

Not everyone agrees that it is these acupuncture points that should be used. Some people think[4] that Liv 3 is a more logical acupuncture point to use when activating *chong mai*. This is due to the Liver's relationship to *chong mai* and also because the name of the point is *taichong* – the great *chong*. Furthermore, a branch of *chong mai* terminates at Liv 3.

In addition to using the opening point of an extraordinary vessel, most people recommend coupling the opening point with a so-called partner point. These acupuncture points are also opening points, but for one of the other extraordinary vessels that is believed to have a relationship to the vessel that is to be activated.

The most common approach is to insert the first needle of the treatment in the opening point of the extraordinary vessel that is to be activated. The next acupuncture point that is needled will then be the opening point of the partner vessel. Only after these needles have been inserted, and in this order, will the remaining needles be inserted in the other acupuncture points that are to be utilised in the treatment. At the end of the treatment, the needles will be removed again in reverse order, i.e. the needle inserted in the partner channel's opening point will be taken out as the penultimate needle to be removed, and the channel's own opening point as the final point.

Giovanni Maciocia (2005) writes that the opening point should be used on the right-hand side of women and the partner opening point on the left-hand side. For men this will be the other way round, with the opening point being activated on the left-hand side and the partner opening point on the right-hand side. Personally, I generally use the opening and partner opening points bilaterally, but will still insert the first needle in the opening point of the extraordinary vessel on the left-hand side in men and right-hand side in women, because there is no reason not to do it in that order.

Below is the most common presentation of opening point/partner opening point relations among the extraordinary vessels:

- Lu 7 (*ren mai*)/Kid 6 (*yin qiao mai*)

- SI 3 (*du mai*)/UB 62 (*yang qiao mai*)

- Sp 4 (*chong mai*)/Pe 6 (*yin wei mai*)

- GB 41 (*dai mai*)/SJ 5 (*yang wei mai*).

This, however, is not the only possibility. Some people work with a more three-dimensional model,[5] with the channel relations being like the corners of a cube.

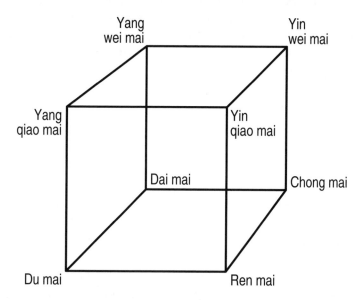

Figure 4.51 The three-dimensional model of the extraordinary channels' relationships

This means that each channel has a relationship to three sides. For example, if you want to activate *ren mai*, you would use Lu 7 as the opening point, but you could either use Kid 6 (*yin qiao mai*), SI 3 (*du mai*) or Sp 4 (*chong mai*) as the partner vessel opening point. The choice of partner will depend upon the symptoms and signs that the person manifests and what your treatment strategy is. This approach allows a greater flexibility in practice. Personally I often use this model, a typical example of this being the combination Kid 6, UB 62 and UB 1 in the treatment of insomnia. This treatment creates balance between *yin qiao mai* and *yang qiao mai* by using their opening points (Kid 6/UB 62) and their meeting point (UB 1).

Alternative presentation of the opening points and partner opening points

- *ren mai* (Lu 7) – *yin qiao mai* (Kid 6), *du mai* (SI 3), *chong mai* (Sp 4)
- *du mai* (SI 3) – *yang qiao mai* (UB 62), *ren mai* (Lu 7), *dai mai* (GB 41)
- *chong mai* (Sp 4) – *yin wei mai* (Pe 6), *ren mai* (Lu 7), *dai mai* (GB 41)
- *dai mai* (GB 41) – *yang wei mai* (SJ 5), *chong mai* (Sp 4), *du mai* (SI 3)
- *yin qiao mai* (Kid 6) – *ren mai* (Lu 7), *yang qiao mai* (UB 62), *yin wei mai* (Pe 6)
- *yang qiao mai* (UB 62) – *du mai* (SI 3), *yin qiao mai* (Kid 6), *yang wei mai* (SJ 5)
- *yin wei mai* (Pe 6) – *chong mai* (Sp 4), *yin qiao mai* (Kid 6), *yang wei mai* (SJ 5)
- *yang wei mai* (SJ 5) – *dai mai* (GB 41), *yang qiao mai* (UB 62), *yin wei mai* (Pe 6)

There is disagreement about which acupuncture points are to be used as opening points and partner points, as well as in which order these points should be inserted. There is also disagreement as to whether only extraordinary vessel points should be used during a treatment or whether regular channel points can also be used. It could be argued that it is most appropriate to only use extraordinary vessel opening points, partner points and acupuncture points on these vessels, when treating an extraordinary vessel. This is because the treatment of the extraordinary vessels operates on a deeper *qi* level. This would thereby exclude the use of acupuncture points on the regular channels in the same treatment. This approach is not as restrictive as it might sound. There are many acupuncture points that are both points on a regular channel and points on an extraordinary vessel. An acupuncture point such as GB 20 is, for example, a meeting point of the Gall Bladder and *san jiao* channels, as well as being a point on *yang qiao mai* and *yang wei mai*.

Personally, I often begin a treatment where I am going to activate one or more of the extraordinary vessels by only using the opening points, the partner opening points where appropriate and the acupuncture points along the extraordinary vessel at the beginning of the treatment. Ten to fifteen minutes later, I add the rest of the acupuncture points that are exclusively situated on the regular channels.

As is the case with the regular channels, you can, of course, use local and distal points along the pathway of the vessel to affect an area of the vessel. For example, it is possible to use Du 3 and Du 4 as *du mai* local points and Du 26 as a distal point in the treatment of lower back pain. This can be done both with or without the use of the vessel's opening and partner opening point.

DU MAI

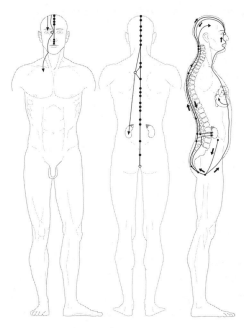

Figure 4.52 *Du mai*

Du mai is often translated into English as 'Governing vessel'. This is the reason that many books use the abbreviation GV for *du mai* acupuncture points. *Du mai* is the most *yang* channel in the body. It is also called the 'Sea of *yang*'. This is because of its governing function with regard to *yang qi* in the body. Furthermore, *du mai* passes through the spine and up to the top of the head. These are the body's most extreme *yang* areas.

Nevertheless, it is possible to see how *yin* and *yang* are integrated and inseparable. Although *du mai* is the most *yang* channel in the body, it has its source in *bao*, which is in the deepest aspect of the interior of the body, and the first point on the channel is the acupuncture point Ren 1, which is situated in the perineum, which is one of the most *yin* areas of the body.

Both *du mai* and *ren mai* are unique as extraordinary vessels in that they are the only extraordinary vessels that have their own independent channel pathways and channel points. For this reason they are often mentioned in conjunction with the regular channels as being two of the 'fourteen channels'.

Pathway

- *Du mai* has three separate branches.

- The primary branch of *du mai* has its origin in *bao* or the space between the Kidneys.

- *Du mai* flows down from *bao* to the perineum where it surfaces at the acupuncture point Ren 1.

- The primary channel travels posteriorly to Du 1, which is located between the anus and the tip of the coccyx.

- It ascends up the spine to the acupuncture point Du 16, inferior to the external occipital protuberance.

- A branch separates from the main channel and enters into the brain. This branch continues its course upwards, reuniting with the primary channel at Du 20 on the vertex.

- The primary channel continues its path from Du 16 along the midline of the cranium through the vertex and forehead and down along the nose to Du 26 located in the philtrum, where it penetrates the upper gum and the acupuncture point Du 28, meeting with *ren mai* and ending its pathway.

- *Du mai's* second branch also has its source in the *bao* or the space between the Kidneys.

- From here it flows down to Ren 1 in the perineum.

- This branch of *du mai* travels in front of and winds around the external genitalia.

- It flows up the midline of the body, through the umbilical region, and up to the Heart, which it passes through.

- It continues up the throat before winding around the mouth.

- It ascends from the mouth up to the middle of each eye.

- *Du mai's* third branch has its source in the eye and emerges at the acupuncture point UB 1 on the medial border of the orbit.

- It follows the Urinary Bladder channel over the forehead and to the acupuncture point Du 20 on the vertex, where it penetrates downwards and into the brain.

- It descends through the brain and resurfaces at the acupuncture point Du 16, inferior to the external occipital protuberance.

- It splits into two parallel branches at Du 16 and travels down to the acupuncture point UB 12, one and a half *cun* lateral to the lower border of the second thoracic vertebra.

- It descends down the back and enters the Kidneys.

Du mai and *ren mai* differ from the other extraordinary vessels by having a *luo*-connecting vessel.

- The *du mai luo*-connecting vessel separates from the primary channel at the acupuncture point Du 1, which is located between the anus and the tip of the coccyx.

- It ascends bilaterally alongside the spine. It connects to the Urinary Bladder between the scapula and spreads into the spine. It continues simultaneously up to the occiput and the neck where it spreads outwards.

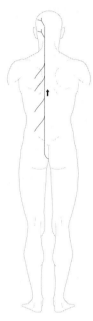

Figure 4.53 *Du mai luo*-connecting vessel

Organ connections

Du mai connects to *bao*, the Brain, the Kidneys and the Heart.

Point categories

Opening point	SI 3
Partner opening point	UB 62
Source point	Ren 1
Luo-connecting point	Du 1

Meeting points with other channels

Du 1	*Ren mai*, Kidney and Gall Bladder channels
Du 13	Urinary Bladder channel
Du 14	Large Intestine, Stomach, Small Intestine, Urinary Bladder, Gall Bladder and *san jiao* channels
Du 15	*Yang wei mai*
Du 16	*Yang qiao mai* and *yang wei mai*
Du 17	Urinary Bladder channel
Du 20	Urinary Bladder, *san jiao*, Gall Bladder and Liver channels
Du 24	Stomach and Urinary Bladder channels
Du 26	Large Intestine and Stomach channels
Du 28	Stomach channel and *ren mai*
Ren 1	*Ren mai* and *chong mai*
Ren 24	Large Intestine channel, *du mai* and *ren mai*
UB 1	Stomach, Small Intestine, Urinary Bladder, Gall Bladder and *san jiao* channels, *ren mai*, *yin qiao mai* and *yang qiao mai*
UB 11	Urinary Bladder, Small Intestine, *san jiao* and Gall Bladder channels
UB 12	Urinary Bladder channel
UB 23	Urinary Bladder channel
St 1	Stomach channel, *yang qiao mai* and *ren mai*

Areas of usage

Du mai can be used in the treatment of many and varied types of disorders and imbalances. Depending on the situation, the opening points can be used alone or in conjunction with channel points. Points along the channel can also be used alone without the use of the opening points.

Du mai influences yang qi

Du mai is the *yang* governing vessel and thereby has an effect on all the aspects of *yang qi* in the body and all the *yang* channels. This means that *du mai* and its acupuncture points are used both to strengthen and regulate *yang qi*.

This can be seen in practice in several ways.

- All *yang* channels meet at the acupuncture point Du 14, and this acupuncture point can be used to regulate all *yang* channels in the body. In addition, Du 14 can be used to regulate *wei qi*, which is one of the most *yang* forms of *qi* in the body. Du 14 is at the same time one of the body's most important acupuncture points to drain *shi* Heat, which is a *yang* pathogen.

- *Du mai* acupuncture points are often used both to tonify *yang qi* and to regulate various forms of *yang qi*.

- ○ The use of moxa on Du 4 is, for example, one of the best ways to warm *mingmen* and thereby tonify *yang qi*.

- ○ Du 20 sends *yang qi* down from the head and is used, amongst other things, to calm *shen* when it is agitated by *yang* Heat. It calms Wind that has risen to the head and it sends ascendant *yang qi* downwards again.

- ○ Du 16 is one of the primary acupuncture points used to extinguish internal Wind.

- ○ Du 14, as we have just seen, is one of the body's most important *yang qi*-regulating and Heat-draining acupuncture points.

- ○ Du 26 is used to resuscitate a person who has lost consciousness.

- • *Du mai* can be used to strengthen *yang* and thereby raise *yang* in the body. It can be used to treat organ prolapse, a sensation of heaviness or poor posture of the body.

Treatment of structural problems

The treatment of the *du mai* channel and points is often a determining factor in the treatment of problems relating to the body's physical structure, especially when they are located in the spine. These problems may be fundamental and congenital abnormalities, such as Scheuermann, scoliosis, etc., or they can be acquired problems such as spinal disc herniation, acute or chronic lumbago, neck pain, whiplash injuries, etc. *Du mai* acupuncture points can be used in the treatment of both *xu* and *shi* conditions. The determining factor for treatment is that the problem is located along the pathway of *du mai*.

Du mai expels exogenous Wind

Du mai and *wei qi* have a relationship to each other on several levels. *Du mai* is the *yang* governing vessel and it has a governing influence on all forms of *yang qi*, including *wei qi*. *Du mai* is also responsible for spreading *yang qi* through the back. Many *du mai* acupuncture points have the specific action of activating *wei qi* or expelling exogenous *xie qi*. Du 14, for example, is used to activate *wei qi*, and all *du mai* acupuncture points from Du 12 to Du 24 expel Wind.

Treatment of disorders along the path of the channel

In common with all channels, *du mai* and its channel points can be used to treat ailments that manifest along or in the vicinity of the channel's pathway. This is because an acupuncture point on a channel can be used to treat symptoms caused by imbalances in a channel's *qi*. At the same time, any acupuncture point on a channel will also have an effect on *qi* in the local area. This means, therefore, that acupuncture points can be used to treat symptoms manifesting in the surrounding area, even though these symptoms have no direct relationship to the channel itself. *Du mai* acupuncture points can be used for any symptom that is located in the vicinity of the primary channel. Normally, this will be problems manifesting in the lumbar region, along the spine or in the neck or head, but it can also be a problem with the uterus, the external genitalia and the urinary tract, due to the channel's anterior pathway. In addition, *du mai* points can be used to treat problems of the sensory organs and the rectum, for example haemorrhoids.

Treatment of zang organ disorders

Du mai acupuncture points located at the same level as back-*shu* points on the Urinary Bladder channel often have similar actions and indications to this back-*shu* point. This means these *du mai* points can be used to treat disorders of the *zang* organs, the organ's functionality and its sensory organ.

Du mai affects the Brain and the Marrow

The Brain and the Marrow are two of the extraordinary *fu* organs. Both of these organs have a very close relationship to *du mai*. *Du mai* flows up through the spinal cord and enters the brain. This means that *du mai* acupuncture points are often used both to nourish these organs and to treat imbalances that relate to them. This is seen in practice when acupuncture points such as Du 16, Du 20 and Du 24 are used for problems that relate to the brain. Even though modern acupuncture texts state that *shen* has its residence in the Heart, there are some traditions that attribute this role to the Brain. There is definitely an overlap between many of the processes that are attributed to the brain in Western medicine physiology and *shen* in Chinese medicine. *Du mai* in fact unites these two different approaches. Through its flow, *du mai* connects the Heart and the Brain. In practice, acupuncture points such as Du 11, Du 20 and Du 24 are used to calm the *shen*.

Treatment of gynaecological problems

Despite the fact that it is *chong mai* and *ren mai* that are most often referred to in the discussion of gynaecological problems, *du mai* also plays a crucial role in women's physiology. This is why the treatment of *du mai* acupuncture points is also relevant in gynaecological disorders.

Du mai affects gynaecological processes in several ways. First of all, all transformations in the body are dependent on *yang qi*, which is governed by *du mai*. *Du mai* also passes through the *bao* and thereby the uterus, ovaries and fallopian tubes. Many gynaecological problems are caused by either a lack of *yang* or invasions of exogenous Cold. In both cases, *du mai* can be utilised. Du 4 can, for example, be used to strengthen and warm *mingmen*, either to expel Cold or to increase the quantity and the strength of *yang*.

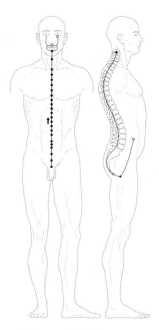

Figure 4.54 *Ren mai*

Ren mai is often translated into English as 'Directing vessel' or 'Conception vessel'. This is why many acupuncture books use the abbreviation CV for *ren mai* acupuncture points. *Ren mai* and *du mai* are the most *yin* and *yang* channels in the body, and this is reflected in their pathways being on opposite sides of the body. Whereas *du mai* travels up the midline of the back and thereby along the most *yang* aspect of the body, *ren mai* flows up the midline of the front of the body, the body's most *yin* aspect. Furthermore, *ren mai* originates in the deepest aspect of the interior, between the two Kidneys, and its source point is Ren 1, which is situated in the perineum, one of the most *yin* locations in the body.

Pathway

- *Ren mai* has two separate branches.

- The main channel has its source in the *bao* or the space between the Kidneys.

- From the *bao* the channel travels down to the perineum, where it surfaces at the acupuncture point Ren 1.

- *Ren mai* ascends along the midline on the front of the body to the throat and chin.

- It penetrates into the mouth at its final acupuncture point Ren 24, which is situated in the centre of the mentolabial groove. It connects with *du mai* at the acupuncture point Du 28 in the upper gum.

- It divides into two branches, which ascend up to the eyes and the acupuncture point St 1 in the centre of the infraorbital ridge. The vessel then flows medially to UB 1 on the medial edge of the orbit, where it terminates.

- The other branch of *ren mai* also starts its flow in the *bao* or in the space between the two Kidneys.

- It descends to the acupuncture point Ren 1 in the perineum.

- It flows posteriorly and ascends up through the spine.

Du mai and *ren mai* differ from the other extraordinary vessels in that they have a *luo*-connecting vessel.

- The *ren mai luo*-connecting vessel separates away from the primary channel at Ren 15, one *cun* inferior to the sternocostal angle.

- It spreads outwards and downwards from Ren 15.

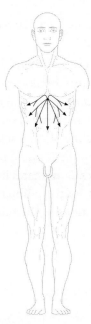

Figure 4.55 *Ren mai luo*-connecting vessel

Organ connections

Ren mai connects to the *bao* and the Kidneys.

Point categories

Opening point	Lu 7
Partner opening point	Kid 6
Source point	Ren 1
Luo-connecting point	Ren 15

Meeting points with other channels

Ren 1	*Du mai* and *chong mai*
Ren 2	Liver channel
Ren 3	Spleen, Kidney and Liver channels
Ren 4	Spleen, Kidney and Liver channels
Ren 7	Kidney channel and *chong mai*
Ren 10	Spleen channel
Ren 12	Stomach, Small Intestine and *san jiao* channels
Ren 13	Stomach and Small Intestine channels
Ren 17	Stomach, Small Intestine, Kidney and *san jiao* channels
Ren 22	*Yin wei mai*
Ren 23	*Yin wei mai*
Ren 24	Large Intestine and Stomach channels and *du mai*
St 1	Stomach channel, *yang qiao mai* and *du mai*
St 4	Large Intestine and Stomach channels and *yang qiao mai*
Du 1	Kidney and Gall Bladder channels and *du mai*
Du 28	Stomach and Liver channels and *du mai*

Areas of usage

Ren mai is the *yin* controlling vessel. It is said that *ren mai* is 'the Sea of *yin*', in the same way that *du mai* is 'the Sea of *yang*'. This means that *ren mai* has a similar influence on *yin qi* that *du mai* has on *yang qi*. Although there is not an acupuncture point on *ren mai* that is similar to Du 14 where all the *yang* channels meet, there are two *ren mai* points, Ren 3 and Ren 4, where all three of the leg's *yin* channels meet. These leg channels are in direct connection with the arm *yin* channels through the three 'great' or foot/hand *yin* channels. This means that *ren mai* is directly connected to all the *yin* channels through Ren 3 and Ren 4.

Ren mai has a determining influence on women's physiology, through its relationship to *yin* and due to the pathway of the vessel. This is of considerable importance, both in relation to fertility and especially during pregnancy. *Ren mai* and *chong mai* ensure that the foetus is nourished by *qi*, *xue* and *jing*, so that it develops as it should.

Ren mai can be used in the treatment of many and varied types of disorders and imbalances. Depending on the situation, the opening points can be used alone or in conjunction with channel points. Points along the channel can also be used alone, without the use of the opening points.

Ren mai influences yin qi

Ren mai is 'the Sea of *yin*'. It thereby has influence on all forms of *yin qi* in the body and on all the *yin* channels. *Yin qi* includes *yin*, *jinye*, *jing* and *xue*. This means that *ren mai* and its acupuncture points can be used to both nourish and regulate *yin qi*.

This can be seen in practice in several ways.

- *Ren mai* opening points can be utilised to activate and nourish *yin* in the body. This is especially relevant in conditions of generalised *yin xu*.

- Several acupuncture points along *ren mai* nourish *yin* in specific organs and can be utilised when there are conditions of *yin xu* in these organs: Ren 4 nourishes Kidney and Liver *yin* and *jing*; Ren 12 nourishes Stomach *yin*; Ren 14 and Ren 15 nourish Heart *yin*; and Ren 17 nourishes Heart and Lung *yin*.

- *Yin qi* includes *jing*. *Jing xu* is difficult to treat, because the pre-heavenly *jing* is something that is created at conception. It is also therefore difficult to replenish *jing*, which is lost through an inappropriate lifestyle. What can be done is to nourish and support the remaining *jing*. An acupuncture point such as Ren 4 can be used for this purpose. *Jing* is the root of *yuan qi*, and Ren 6 is often used to tonify *yuan qi*.

- *Ren mai* can be used to regulate *jing* and its seven- and eight-year cycles in women and men. *Ren mai* is often used in the treatment of women with problems relating to the menstrual cycle, amenorrhoea, fertility problems or menopausal syndrome.

- *Ren mai* is often used in the first half of the menstrual cycle, as it has a nourishing effect on *yin* and *xue*, thereby helping to replenish the *yin* and *xue* that has been lost during menstrual bleeding. It is also beneficial to strengthen *ren mai* after a birth.

Ren mai influences yang qi

Although *ren mai* is the *yin* controlling channel, it also has an influence on *yang*. This is because *yin* and *yang* are inextricably linked to each other and because *yin* is at the root of *yang*. This means that the use of acupuncture points such as Ren 4 and Ren 6 with moxa will specifically tonify Kidney *yang* whilst tonifying *yang* in the whole body. In addition, some *ren mai* acupuncture points activate *yang*. Ren 6 and Ren 8 can be stimulated with moxa to rescue *yang* when it has collapsed.

Ren mai influences the female genitalia

Ren mai has a significant influence on the female genitalia and their physiology. This influence is a result of the channel's pathway, which transverses the internal and external genitalia, and is also due to its relationship to *yin* substances in general and through this their influence on the female physiology.

This means that *ren mai* and its channel points are often used in the treatment of gynaecological disorders. As previously written, *ren mai* points and opening points are used in the treatment of infertility, menstrual disorders and menopausal syndrome. *Ren mai* points are used both when there are *xu* conditions and when there is stagnation.

Ren mai points can also be used for problems that manifest in the genitalia, such as vaginal discharge, itching and vaginal dryness.

Treatment of problems along the channel

Like regular channels, *ren mai* points can be used to treat disorders that manifest in the local area near the channel or along its path. *Ren mai* points have, in particular, a significant influence on the regulation of *qi* in all three *jiao*. Many *ren mai* points are used to regulate stagnant or rebellious *qi*.

- Ren 1 and Ren 2 regulate *qi* in and around the genitalia.

- Ren 3, Ren 5 and Ren 7 activate and circulate *qi* in the lower *jiao* and can therefore be used for stagnations of *qi* in this area.

- Ren 6, Ren 10, Ren 11, Ren 12 and Ren 13 regulate *qi* in the middle *jiao* and can be used for stagnations of *qi* in this area. Ren 13, Ren 14 and Ren 22 especially are used in the treatment of rebellious, ascending Stomach *qi*.

- Ren 17 and Ren 22 are often used for stagnations of *qi* in the upper *jiao* and to regulate Lung *qi*.

- Ren 22 and Ren 23 are used for stagnations of *qi* in the throat.

Ren mai is characterised by having relatively many *mu*-collecting points on its channel. This means that in addition to being able to regulate *qi* locally, many *ren mai* acupuncture points also have a strong effect on several of the internal organs.

The following *ren mai* acupuncture points are *mu*-collecting points:

- Ren 3 – Urinary Bladder

- Ren 4 – Small Intestine

- Ren 5 – *San jiao*

- Ren 12 – Stomach

- Ren 14 – Heart

- Ren 17 – Pericardium.

Regulation of the water passages

There are several *ren mai* acupuncture points that have both direct and indirect influence on fluid physiology and the regulation of the water passages. As we have just seen, many *ren mai* points have a significant influence on the flow of *qi* in all three *jiao*. This in itself is crucial for the transportation and transformation of fluids in the three *jiao*. At the same time, *ren mai* points can stimulate all the organs that are involved in fluid physiology and they can also be used to strengthen *yuan qi*, which is a vital component in all parts of the process.

The *ren mai* points that have a specific, direct influence on fluid physiology are as follows.

- Ren 3 is the *mu*-collecting point for the Urinary Bladder. Ren 3 is therefore often used to regulate the Urinary Bladder's functions, especially its ability to store and expel urine from the body.

- Ren 4 can be used with moxa to tonify Kidney *yang*, which is important in many of the processes involved in fluid physiology, but especially in keeping the urine inside the Urinary Bladder and in expelling the urine out of the Urinary Bladder when urinating.

- Ren 5 is the *mu*-collecting point of *san jiao*. Ren 5 can be used to influence *san jiao*, which has the overall responsibility for the transformation and distribution of fluids. *San jiao* is also responsible for the distribution of *yuan qi*, which is vital in fluid physiology. Ren 5 is also an acupuncture point that has a major influence on the lower *jiao* and it can therefore influence the transformation fluids and urination.

- Ren 6 tonifies *yuan qi*, which is vital in fluid physiology.

- Ren 9 opens the water passages. Ren 9 is an important acupuncture point in the treatment of oedema, especially if there is an accumulation of fluids in the abdominal cavity.

- Ren 12 can be used to tonify the Spleen and Stomach, both of which are involved in fluid physiology.

- Ren 17 and Ren 22 can affect the Lung, which both spreads fluids throughout the body and sends impure fluids down to the Kidneys and the Urinary Bladder.

CHONG MAI

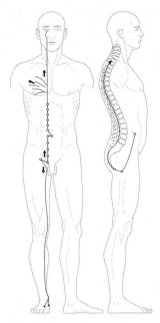

Figure 4.56 *Chong mai*

Chong mai is often translated into English as the 'Thoroughfare vessel' or 'Penetrating vessel'. *Chong mai*, like most extraordinary vessels, does not have its own independent pathway. Therefore, there are no independent *chong mai* points. There are, though, many acupuncture points along its course that can be utilised to activate and treat *chong mai*. Many of these points are Kidney channel points, as *chong mai* shares a common pathway with the Kidney channel on the abdomen.

Chong mai has its origin in the *bao*, as does *ren mai* and *du mai*. Whereas *du mai* and *ren mai* arose as the first manifestations of *yang* and *yin* in the body, *chong mai* arose from the interaction of the primal *yin* and the primal *yang*. This interaction of *yin* and *yang* gave rise to the physical body. For this reason, *chong mai* is called 'the Sea of the Twelve Channels' and 'the Sea of *Yin* and *Yang*'. Another name that is used to describe *chong mai* in the classic texts is 'the Sea of *Xue*'. This is a reference to *chong mai* having the overall responsibility for *xue* in the deep *luo* vessels. Furthermore, *chong mai* also influences the supply and movement of *xue* in the *bao*. This means that the condition of *chong mai* is of great importance for the menstrual cycle. *Chong mai* imbalances can affect the length and rhythm of the cycle and quantity and quality of the menstrual blood. The relationship between *chong mai* and *xue* can also be seen in the difference between women's and men's body hair. Women lose *xue* through menstrual bleeding, as well as there being a general downward movement of *xue* to the *bao* via *chong mai*. Men, on the other hand, do not lose *xue* through monthly bleeding. This means that their *chong mai* is richer in *xue*. At the same time there is not the same downward movement of *xue*. *Xue* nourishes the growth of hair. Men therefore often have a copious growth of hair on the chest and around the mouth, which are along the pathway of *chong mai*. Women do not have this growth of hair in these regions, due to the relative paucity of *xue* in their *chong mai*. On the other hand, when a woman's menstruations stop, she often starts to develop a slight growth of hair in these regions. This is due to the dynamic of *xue* in *chong mai* changing during the menopause, because *xue* is no longer sent downwards to create a menstrual bleeding. *Chong mai* is still relatively *xue xu* in post-menopausal women, compared with men, so the hair growth is also relatively sparse.

Chong mai integrates the pre- and post-heavenly *qi* by connecting the Kidney organ and channel with the Stomach channel. The relationship of *chong mai* to the post-heavenly *qi* is also seen in the fact that *chong mai* spreads *wei qi* in the chest and abdomen.

Pathway

- *Chong mai* has two separate branches.

- The main pathway has its source in the *bao* or the space between the Kidneys.

- It descends down to the perineum where the channel surfaces at the acupuncture point Ren 1.

- It ascends from Ren 1 to the acupuncture point St 30, two *cun* lateral to the midline, immediately superior to the pubic bone. The channel then divides into two branches.

- One branch flows down the medial aspect of the leg to the medial malleolus, where it splits in two. One branch travels to Liv 3 on the dorsum of the foot between the first and second metatarsal bones. The second branch flows down to Kid 1 on the sole of the foot between the second and third metatarsal bones.

- The second branch that separated away at St 30 flows medially to the acupuncture point Kid 11, half a *cun* lateral to the midline, immediately superior to the pubic bone.

- *Chong mai* shares the pathway of the Kidney channel up the lower abdomen to the acupuncture point Kid 15 (one *cun* inferior to the umbilicus, half a *cun* lateral to the midline), where it courses medially and connects to the acupuncture point Ren 7.

- It returns to the Kidney channel pathway and ascends to the acupuncture point Kid 21 (six *cun* superior to the umbilicus, half a *cun* lateral to the midline), where it spreads out across the chest.

- A branch of the main channel continues to ascend to the throat, encircles the mouth and continues up to the eyes.

- The second branch of *chong mai* also has its source in the *bao* or in the space between the two Kidneys.

- It descends to the perineum and the acupuncture point Ren 1.

- It flows posteriorly to Du 1 (midway between the anus and the coccyx), where it ascends up through the spine.

Organ connections

Chong mai connects to the *bao* and the Kidneys.

Point categories

Opening point	Sp 4
Partner opening point	Pe 6
Source point	Ren 1

Meeting points with other channels

Ren 1	*Du mai* and *ren mai*
Ren 7	Kidney channel and *ren mai*
St 30	Stomach channel
Kid 11–21	Kidney channel

Areas of usage

Chong mai has a regulatory effect on *qi* and *xue*. This is reflected in some of the titles *chong mai* has been assigned through the ages, for example 'the Sea of the Twelve Channels' and 'the Sea of *Xue*'.

Chong mai has a particularly close relationship to the *bao*. *Chong mai* is therefore often used in the treatment of gynaecological disorders, especially when the disorder is caused by *xue* imbalances.

Chong mai is utilised in treatment either through the use of its opening points alone or in combination with acupuncture points along the pathway of *chong mai*. The acupuncture points along the channel's pathway can also be used without the use of the opening points.

As mentioned earlier, some people argue that Liv 3 can be used at the opening point of *chong mai*, either instead of or in conjunction with Sp 4.

Chong mai calms and regulates rebellious qi

Chong mai is used to treat rebellious *qi*, especially rebellious *qi* in the abdomen and chest. One of the more quaint disease names in Chinese medicine is 'running piglet *qi* syndrome' (*ben tun qi bing*). Even though there are very few European patients who seek treatment for 'running piglet *qi*', it is a symptom that many experience, especially female patients. Running piglet *qi* is a bubbling feeling of unease, similar to the sensation we in English also give a zoological name – butterflies. This sensation will often start in the lower abdomen and ascend up to the chest and throat. It is often accompanied by a tightness or choking sensation in the throat, emotional unease and/or palpitations. Panic attacks can sometimes be an aspect of this syndrome and vice versa. The pathway of the symptoms is reflective of *chong mai's* course. Treatment of running piglet *qi* will usually focus on regulating rebellious *qi* in *chong mai*.

Chong mai normally sends *qi* and *xue* down to the *bao*, but this downward movement of *qi* can be disturbed at the start of a pregnancy. This can result in *qi* in *chong mai* becoming rebellious, rising upwards and interfering with the Stomach's function of sending *qi* downwards. This can result in nausea and/or vomiting.

Chong mai controls and moves xue

Chong mai regulates *xue* in all channels, but particularly in the deep *luo* vessels. It also has a major influence on the supply of *xue* to the *bao* in women. *Chong mai* is involved in the transformation of *jing* to *tian gui* or menstrual blood. This means that the treatment of *chong mai* is often central in the treatment of gynaecological disorders, where the underlying cause is *xue xu*, *xue* Heat or *xue* stagnation. We will see in a moment that there is also a close relationship between *chong mai* and the Heart. This means that it is also possible to use *chong mai* points when treating problems that relate to Heart *xue*.

Treatment of gynaecological disorders

As written above, *chong mai* is frequently used in the treatment of gynaecological disorders, due to its relationship with *xue* and *tian gui* and because it flows through the *bao*. For example, it is not uncommon for some women to experience menstrual pain that radiates out from the uterus to the lumbar region and down the medial aspect of the thigh. This pain is caused by stagnation of *qi* and *xue* in *chong mai*.

Treatment of Heart problems

Chong mai and the Heart have a close relationship, especially as they both have a close relationship to *xue* and its movement. *Chong mai* is 'the Sea of *Xue*', and the Heart governs *xue*. Furthermore, *chong mai* encircles the Heart when it spreads out across and through the chest. *Chong mai* can therefore be used for the treatment of Heart disorders, especially when these are due to *xue* imbalances.

Treatment of weak or underdeveloped muscles in the legs

Chong mai has a branch that descends down the medial aspect of the leg. *Chong mai* therefore helps to nourish the muscles along its course. *Chong mai* can be used to activate and strengthen the muscles on the inside of the leg when there is weakness or atrophy.

DAI MAI

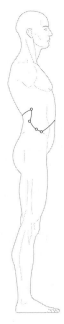

Figure 4.57 *Dai mai*

Dai mai can be translated into English as 'Girdle vessel' or 'Belt vessel'. *Dai mai* is unique in that it is the only horizontal or laterally flowing channel in the body. *Dai mai* is the fourth extraordinary vessel to develop after fertilisation. Whilst *chong mai* arises from the interaction of primal *yin* and primal *yang* in *ren mai* and *du mai*, *dai mai* arises out of the need to integrate *yin* and *yang*. This is reflected in its horizontal pathway around the body, where it connects all six regular foot/leg channels, as well as *du mai* and *ren mai*.

Whereas *ren mai*, *du mai* and *chong mai* have a close relationship to the Kidneys and *bao*, *dai mai* has a close relationship to the Liver and Gall Bladder. This relationship is reflected both in its opening point and in the acupuncture points on its pathway, which are exclusively Liver and Gall Bladder channel points.

Dai mai is called the belt vessel, not only because it traverses the waist like a belt, but also because some of its functions are similar to the functions of a belt. *Dai mai* can become like a belt that is too tight in *shi* conditions. This will block the movement of *qi* up and down through the vertical channels. This will often result in a significant difference in temperature between the upper and lower parts of the body. At the same time, there will often be a tight or distended sensation in the area of the waist.

A belt can also be too loose. When there are *xu* conditions in the *dai mai*, there can be organ prolapse, hernias, muscle atrophy and spontaneous abortions.

Dai mai is also described as a gutter for Dampness. *Dai mai* imbalances can result in Dampness or Damp-Heat draining downwards and causing symptoms such as vaginal discharge and urinary dysfunctions.

Pathway

- *Dai mai* has its source at Liv 13, inferior and anterior to the tip of the eleventh rib.

- It flows diagonally downwards and medially to the acupuncture points GB 26 (directly inferior to Liv 13, level with the umbilicus), GB 27 (in the depression medial to the anterior superior iliac spine) and GB 28 (0.5 *cun* inferior and anterior to GB 27).

- It crosses the midline of the body and connects to the acupuncture point GB 28.

- It continues through GB 27, GB 26 and Liv 13.

- It continues around the side of the body, travelling laterally across the back and crossing through the spine, returning to its source point, Liv 13.

Point categories

Opening point	GB 41
Partner opening point	SJ 5
Source point	Liv 13

Meeting points with other channels

Liv 13	Gall Bladder and Liver channels
GB 26	Gall Bladder channel
GB 27	Gall Bladder channel
GB 28	Gall Bladder channel

Areas of usage

As written in the introduction, *dai mai* is a belt that encircles and links the longitudinal, vertical channels in the body. This is also reflected in its applications. When *dai mai* is in imbalance, the 'belt' can often be either too tight or too slack. This will affect communication between the upper and lower parts of the body. *Dai mai* is also a 'gutter' that drains Dampness. This means that *dai mai* can be used to treat Dampness and Damp-Heat.

Dai mai regulates the circulation of qi in the legs

Dai mai encircles and flows through all the channels that connect to and from the legs. This means that *dai mai* influences the circulation of *qi* in the legs. *Dai mai* can therefore be used in the treatment of muscle dysfunction or atrophy in the legs.

Dai mai can also be used when there is a significant difference in the perception of temperature in the legs compared with the upper body. The classic description of this feeling is that the person has the sensation that they are sitting in a bath full of cold water, i.e. that they have a cold and possibly clammy sensation in the legs and the lower part of the body.

Dai mai can also be used to treat tight and tense muscles in the legs.

Treatment of imbalances in the hip and waist area

Disturbance of the circulation of *qi* in *dai mai* will not only affect communication upwards and downwards in the body – it will also affect the areas that *dai mai* traverses. This means that *dai mai* can also be used for disorders such as pain, discomfort, distension, etc. in the hip and waist area, especially when symptoms manifest along the pathway of the channel.

Treatment of Dampness and Damp-Heat in the lower jiao

The *yin* nature of Dampness will mean that Dampness and Damp-Heat can have a tendency to seep downwards to the lower *jiao* when *dai mai* fails to carry out its function of being a 'gutter' that drains Dampness.

The treatment of *dai mai* is of particular relevance in the treatment of gynaecological disorders that are caused by Dampness and Damp-Heat. *Dai mai* is primarily used in the treatment of all forms of vaginal discharge. It can also be used for other disorders resulting from Dampness and Damp-Heat in the lower *jiao*, for example Damp-Heat in the Urinary Bladder.

Dai mai harmonises the Liver and Gall Bladder

Dai mai has a very close relationship to the Gall Bladder and the Liver. This is reflected in the opening point of *dai mai* being GB 41 and in all of the *dai mai* acupuncture points also being Liver and Gall Bladder channel points. *Dai mai* is especially used in *shi* imbalances, such as Liver *qi* stagnation and Damp-Heat in the Liver and Gall Bladder.

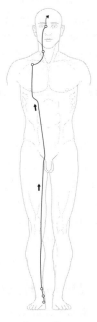

Figure 4.58 *Yin qiao mai*

Yin qiao mai and *yang qiao mai* are the two extraordinary vessels whose names are translated into English differently by different authors. To add to the confusion, Giovanni Maciocia (2005) has changed the translation of their names in his later books from the translation he used in his earlier books. The Chinese character *qiao* has an aspect of a foot that is lifting upwards from the ground. This is seen in the three most common translations into English of *qiao mai*: Heel vessel, Stepping vessel and Motility vessel.

Yin qiao mai and *yang qiao mai* do not just share the same name. Their functions are also very closely integrated. They have a *yin/yang* relationship to each other and they control and integrate the same *qi* in the body. It is crucial for the balance of *yin* and *yang*, especially in the head and the eyes, that they are in harmony. The closeness of their relationship is seen by the fact that they both have the task of absorbing excesses of *yin* and *yang qi* in the body, especially from the head. They also supply the body and head with *yin* and *yang qi*. They both have a close relationship to the eyes and to sleep. The two channels meet with each other at the acupuncture point UB 1. This means that the *qi* in the two respective channels is in direct contact. *Yin qiao mai* and *yang qiao mai* have the essential function of regulating the cycles of *yin* and *yang* through the course of the day. They help to ensure that *yang qi* starts to dominate in the morning when *wei qi* rises up through *yang qiao mai* to

UB 1 and flows twenty-five times in the exterior. In the evening they ensure that *yin qi* waxes and that *yang qi* wanes when *wei qi* returns via UB 1 and *yin qiao mai* enters the interior, where it will circulate twenty-five times during the night. This can be utilised in practice when the two channels are used in the treatment of both insomnia and somnolence.

The *yin/yang* relationship between *yin qiao mai* and *yang qiao mai* can be seen in their respective pathways and their influence on the muscles on the medial and lateral aspects of the legs.

Yin qiao mai has a close relationship to the Kidneys. *Yin qiao mai* has its origin in the Kidney channel and flows through the Kidney channel during the initial stages of its course. The Kidneys are also the root of *yin* in the body, and *yin qiao mai* has the function of absorbing and releasing *yin qi*.

Pathway

- *Yin qiao mai* has its source at the acupuncture point Kid 2, located on the medial side of the foot, distal and inferior to the navicular tuberosity.

- It ascends to the acupuncture point Kid 6, one *cun* below the prominence of the medial malleolus.

- It continues its ascent to the acupuncture point Kid 8, two *cun* superior to the medial malleolus, posterior to the medial border of the tibia.

- It ascends along the medial aspect of the leg, through the inguinal area, abdomen and chest, to the clavicle, where the vessel passes through the acupuncture point St 12.

- It ascends to the acupuncture point St 9, one and a half *cun* lateral to the prominence of the larynx.

- It traverses the face from St 9, travelling to the acupuncture point UB 1 on the edge of the medial aspect of the orbit.

- It penetrates into the brain.

Point categories

Opening point	Kid 6
Partner opening point	Lu 7
Source point	Kid 2
Xi-cleft point	Kid 8

Meeting points with other channels

Kid 2	Kidney channel
Kid 6	Kidney channel
Kid 8	Kidney channel
Sp 6	Kidney, Spleen and Liver channels
St 9	Stomach and Gall Bladder channels and *yang qiao mai*
St 12	Stomach, Large Intestine, Small Intestine, *san jiao* and Gall Bladder channels
UB 1	Urinary Bladder, *san jiao*, Small Intestine, Stomach and Gall Bladder channels, *yang qiao mai* and *du mai*

Areas of usage

Yin qiao mai is a reservoir for *yin qi*. It absorbs excesses of *yin qi* from the body and sends *yin qi* up to the throat, the eyes and the brain. This is done in close cooperation with *yang qiao mai*. These two extraordinary vessels ensure that *yin* and *yang qi* dominate and manifest correctly at the right moments during the day and night. *Yin qiao mai* also has a relationship to the leg muscles and the *bao*, which is also seen in its applications.

Treatment of insomnia and somnolence

Yin qiao mai points are often used in the treatment of insomnia. These points will often be combined with points that affect *yang qiao mai*, the aim being to create harmony between *yin* and *yang* in the brain and the eyes. In the morning *yang wei qi* rises up through *yang qiao mai* to UB 1 and causes the eyes to open before flowing out to circulate twenty-five times in the exterior aspects of the body. In the evening *wei qi* returns to UB 1 and flows back down into the interior through *yin qiao mai* and the eyes close. *Wei qi* then circulates twenty-five times in the interior. Problems with falling asleep or waking are therefore often related to excesses and deficiencies of *yin qi* and *yang qi* or to *yin qiao mai* and *yang qiao mai* being blocked or disrupted. When there is insomnia, *yin qiao mai* should be tonified, and when there is somnolence, it should be drained.

Treatment of mental restlessness

Yin qiao mai nourishes *yin qi* in the head and in the brain. At the same time, it can control *yang qi*. Tonifying *yin qiao mai* can help to create calmness of the mind and can be used both when there are *xu* and *shi* forms of mental restlessness.

Treatment of the eyes

As well as influencing the opening and closing of the eyes, *yin qiao mai* also has an influence on the supply of the *yin qi* to the eyes in general. This means that *yin qiao mai* can also be used for red and, in particular, dry eyes.

Treatment of the throat

Yin qiao mai can be used when there is too little Kidney and Lung *yin* to nourish *yin* in the throat or when *yin* in the throat has been damaged by *shi* Heat. These conditions will often manifest with a dry or itchy throat. *Yin qiao mai*'s opening point Kid 6 is typically used in these situations and is often combined with its partner opening point Lu 7, which is the opening point for *ren mai*.

Treatment of constipation

Kid 6, the opening point of *yin qiao mai*, is often used in combination with Sp 6 in the treatment of constipation where the underlying cause is *yin xu*. The combination of these two acupuncture points generates *yin* and leads this *yin qi* to the lower *jiao* and the Intestines.

Used to increase the strength and tone of the muscles on the inside of the leg

When *yin qiao mai* is *xu*, there can be weakness, poor tone or atrophy of the muscles on the inside of the leg. Conversely, when there is a *shi* condition in the channel, the muscle could be tight and tense. Once again, there is a close relationship between *yin qiao mai* and *yang qiao mai*. It is therefore usually appropriate to treat both of them at the same time if muscles on the inside and outside of the leg are weak or tight.

Treatment of structural imbalances between the left and right sides of the body

As stated in the introduction to the chapter, the extraordinary vessels have a huge influence on the physical structure of the body. They have been a framework during the development of the foetus. When the hips or shoulders are uneven, treating *yin qiao mai* and *yang qiao mai* will often be a relevant treatment strategy.

However, it is not only congenital anomalies that can be treated by utilising the extraordinary vessels. Structural imbalances that have arisen later in life can also be influenced through the use of these channels.

Furthermore, it is not only structural imbalances between the right and the left sides of the body that can be treated through the use of *yin qiao mai* points. They can also be used if there is a difference in temperature between the right and left legs or feet or if a person only sweats unilaterally.

Used to stop bleeding from the uterus

The primary action of Kid 8, which is the *xi*-cleft point of *yin qiao mai*, is to stop the bleeding from the uterus. That is why it can be used for irregular menstrual bleeding, such as spotting, heavy bleeding and prolonged bleeding.

Treatment of stagnations of xue, qi, Dampness and Damp-Heat in the lower jiao

Yin qiao mai can be used to treat stagnations of Dampness, *xue* and *qi* in the lower *jiao*. These conditions will manifest with symptoms such as urinary disorders, oedema in the abdominal cavity, genital itching, vaginal discharge, fibroids in the uterus, etc.

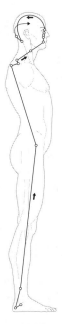

Figure 4.59 *Yang qiao mai*

Yin qiao mai and *yang qiao mai* have, as written in the introduction to *yin qiao mai*, a close relationship with each other. An imbalance in the one will often result in an imbalance in the other, due to their *yin/yang* relationship. This is fully in keeping with the fundamental principles of *yin* and *yang*. In practice, this means that they are often used for the treatment of the same disorders and will often be used together in the same treatment.

Whereas *yin qiao mai* has its origins in the Kidney channel, *yang qiao mai* has its origins in the Kidneys' *yang* partner channel, the Urinary Bladder channel.

Yang qiao mai has both an influence on the body's structure and the important function of regulating the amount of *yang qi* in the head and absorbing excesses.

Pathway

- *Yang qiao mai* has its origin at the acupuncture point UB 62, one *cun* inferior to the lateral malleolus.

- It follows the pathway of the Urinary Bladder channel through the acupuncture points UB 61 (on the calcaneum on the lateral aspect of the heel) and UB 59 (three *cun* superior to the lateral malleolus, on the anterior edge of the Achilles tendon).

- It ascends along the lateral aspect of the leg to the hip and the acupuncture point GB 29 (midway between the anterior superior iliac spine and the prominence of the greater trochanter).

- It ascends to the acupuncture point SI 10 on the posterior aspect of the shoulder, superior to the posterior axillary crease.

- It courses anteriorly to the acupuncture points LI 15 (anterior and inferior to the acromion) and LI 16 (medial to the acromion).

- It continues up the acupuncture point St 9, one and a half *cun* lateral to the larynx.

- It ascends to the face, flowing through the acupuncture points St 4 (four tenths of a *cun* lateral to the corner of the mouth), St 3 (lateral to the nasio-labial groove), St 2 (in the infraorbital foramen) and St 1 (above the infraorbital foramen, on the edge of the infraorbital ridge).

- It ascends to the acupuncture point UB 1 on the medial edge of the orbit, where *yang qiao mai* meets with *yin qiao mai*.

- It ascends up over the head and then down to the acupuncture point GB 20, below the occiput, between the sternomastoid and trapezius muscles.

- It flows medially to the acupuncture point Du 16 immediately below the occipital protuberance and continues into the Brain.

Point categories

Opening point	UB 62
Partner opening point	SI 3
Source point	UB 62
Xi-cleft point	UB 59

Meeting points with other channels

UB 1	Urinary Bladder, *san jiao*, Small Intestine, Stomach and Gall Bladder channels, *yin qiao mai* and *du mai*
UB 59	Urinary Bladder channel
UB 61	Urinary Bladder channel
UB 62	Urinary Bladder channel
GB 29	Gall Bladder channel
SI 10	Small Intestine and Urinary Bladder channels and *yang wei mai*
LI 15	Large Intestine channel
LI 16	Large Intestine channel

St 9	Stomach and Gall Bladder channels and *yin qiao mai*
St 1	Stomach channel, *ren mai* and *du mai*
St 2	Stomach channel
St 3	Stomach channel
St 4	Stomach and Large Intestine channels, *ren mai* and *du mai*
St 12	Stomach, Large Intestine, Small Intestine, *san jiao* and Gall Bladder channels
UB 1	Urinary Bladder, *san jiao*, Small Intestine, Stomach and Gall Bladder channels, *yin qiao mai* and *du mai*
GB 20	Gall Bladder and *san jiao* channels and *yang wei mai*
Du 16	*Du mai* and *yang wei mai*

Areas of usage

Yang qiao mai is a reservoir for *yang qi*. It absorbs excesses of *yang qi* and can be used to drain *yang qi* down from the head. Like *yin qiao mai*, *yang qiao mai* influences the physical structure of the body.

Treatment of insomnia and somnolence

Yang qiao mai is often used together with *yin qiao mai* in the treatment of sleeping disorders. Whereas the opening points of *yin qiao mai* are tonified when there is insomnia and drained when there is somnolence, the opposite is the case with *yang qiao mai*. In insomnia, the opening points of *yang qiao mai* are drained so that *yang qi* is drained away from the eyes. This enables the eyes to close. At the same time, *yang qi* will be drained down from the brain so that it is easier to relax and the brain can 'shut down'.

When there is increased and uncontrollable drowsiness, *yang qiao mai* should be tonified so that there will be more *yang qi* rising up to the eyes and the brain.

Treatment of yang shi conditions in the head

Yang qiao mai absorbs excesses of *yang qi* from the head. Using a draining technique on needles that have been inserted into the opening point of *yang qiao mai* – UB 62 – or on *yang qiao mai* points in the head will drain *yang qi* downwards. The ascending nature of *yang qi* causes it to have a tendency to accumulate in the head. This can be seen when there is internally generated Wind, rebellious *yang qi*, such as ascendant Liver *yang*, and Fire. This means that *yang qiao mai* points can be used in the treatment of disorders such as headache, epilepsy, strokes, facial paralysis, mental restlessness, mania, etc.

Used to expel invasions of exogenous Wind

It is not only internally generated Wind that *yang qiao mai* can control. *Yang qiao mai* can also be used to expel invasions of exogenous Wind, especially when these affect the head.

Treatment of mental restlessness

The opening points of *yang qiao mai* can be used alone or, as is often the case, together with the opening points of *yin qiao mai* to calm the mind.

Treatment of the eyes

Yang qiao mai meets up with *yin qiao mai* in the corner of the eye at the acupuncture point UB 1. This means that, as well as being able to be used for insomnia, *yang qiao mai* can also be used to drain *yang qi* down from the eyes. This could be relevant when, for example, there are red, stinging, itchy eyes or there is a feeling of pressure behind or in the eyes.

It gives strength and tone to the muscles on the outside of the leg

If *yang qiao mai* is *xu*, it can result in weakness, poor muscle tone or atrophy of the muscles on the outside of the leg. Conversely, the muscles can be tight and tense in *shi* conditions. Again, there is often a close relationship between *yin qiao mai* and *yang qiao mai*. This means that it is often appropriate to treat both of them when the muscles on the outside of the leg are either weak or tight.

Treatment of structural imbalances between the left and right sides of the body

Like *yin qiao mai*, *yang qiao mai* can influence the physical structure of the body, both during the development in the uterus and later in life. Because *yin qiao mai* and *yang qiao mai* mirror each other in their pathway up the body, they are often together used to treat the same imbalances in the body's physical structure, i.e. uneven hips and shoulders, as well as unilateral sweating and differences in temperature between the right and left sides of the body.

Treatment of hip pain and sciatica

Yang qiao mai shares a common pathway with both the Urinary Bladder and the Gall Bladder channels. This means that *yang qiao mai* points can be used to optimise the treatment of sciatica when the pain radiates down the posterior and lateral aspects of the leg. Also, because of its pathway through the hip, *yang qiao mai* points can be used to treat hip pain.

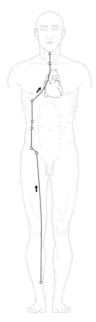

Figure 4.60 *Yin wei mai*

Yin wei mai is called the '*yin* linking vessel' in English.

Wei is a type of rope that connects and binds things together, as in the mesh of a net. *Wei* provides stability. *Yin wei mai* has this binding and stabilising effect on all *yin* in the body, both *yin* substances and the *yin* channels. Whereas *ren mai* arises as the original *yin* in the body, *yin wei mai* has the task of coordinating and regulating *yin*. On the level of the channels, *yin wei mai* links the three great *yin* channels – *shaoyin*, *taiyin* and *jueyin* – as well as *ren mai*. This enables *yin wei mai* to have a regulatory effect and balance *qi* in all the *yin* channels in the body.

It is said that *yin wei mai* 'controls the interior of the body'. This is also reflected in the name of its opening point Pe 6, which is called *neiguan*, 'the inner gate' or 'the gate to the interior'. By connecting and regulating all the *yin* channels, it will have an influence on all the *yin* aspects of the body. It is also felt that *yin wei mai* has an influence on the *yin* substances in the body, especially *xue* and *yin*.

Pathway

- *Yin wei mai* has its origin in Kid 9, five *cun* superior to the medial malleolus, one *cun* posterior to the medial border of the tibia.

- It ascends along the medial aspect of the leg to the inguinal area and the acupuncture points Sp 12 (three and a half *cun* lateral to the midline, level with the upper border of the pubic bone) and Sp 13 (four *cun* lateral to the midline and seven tenths *cun* superior to the upper border of the pubic bone).

- It ascends along the abdomen to the acupuncture points Sp 15 (four *cun* lateral to the umbilicus), Sp 16 (four *cun* lateral to the midline, three *cun* superior to the umbilicus) and Liv 14 (four *cun* lateral to the midline in the sixth intercostal space).

- It ascends diagonally across the chest to meet with *ren mai* at the acupuncture point Ren 22, in the suprasternal fossa.

- It terminates above the hyoid bone at the acupuncture point Ren 23.

Point categories

Opening point	Pe 6
Partner opening point	Sp 4
Source point	Kid 9
Xi-cleft point	Kid 9

Meeting points with other channels

Kid 9	Kidney channel
Sp 12	Liver, *san jiao* and Spleen channels
Sp 13	Liver and Spleen channels
Sp 15	Spleen channel
Sp 16	Spleen channel
Liv 14	Stomach and Liver channels

Areas of usage

Yin wei mai is used mainly in the treatment of cardiac problems and problems manifesting in the thorax, especially when these are due to *yin xu* or *xue xu* conditions. *Xue xu* and *yin xu* are in general the underlying cause of disorders, where the use of *yin wei mai* is recommended. This reflects *yin wei mai*'s function of coordinating and regulating *yin*.

Treatment of pain in the heart, chest and ribs

Yin wei mai passes through the costal region and thorax and across the cardiac region. *Yin wei mai* can therefore be used in the treatment of pain and discomfort arising from stagnations of *qi* and *xue* in these areas. Treating *yin wei mai* is particularly relevant when there is an underlying *yin xu* or *xue xu* imbalance.

Treatment of mental-emotional imbalances

As well as being relevant in the treatment of physical discomfort in the Heart, *yin wei mai* can be used to treat the Heart's mental-emotional aspects. This could be nervousness, anxiety, fear, depression, melancholy and constant worrying. The use of *yin wei mai* is again indicated when there is an underlying condition of *yin xu* or *xue xu* and when there are physical symptoms that manifest along the path of the channel.

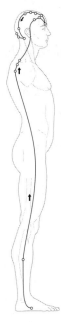

Figure 4.61 *Yang wei mai*

Yang wei mai is called the '*yang* linking vessel' in English.

Yang wei mai has a similar relationship to the *yang* channels and *yang qi* that *yin wei mai* has with the *yin* channels and the *yin* substances. Whereas *yin wei mai* 'controls the interior of the body', *yang wei mai* controls the exterior aspects. The relationship between the two *wei mai* and the body's internal and external aspects is also reflected in the names of their opening points. Pe 6, which is the opening point of *yin wei mai*, is called *neiguan* – 'the gate to the interior', while *yang wei mai*'s opening point SJ 5 is called *waiguan* – 'the gate to the exterior'. Pe 6 has a strong regulatory effect on *qi* and *xue* in the middle and upper *jiao* and calms *shen*, whilst SJ 5 is one of the major points to 'open to the exterior' and activate *wei qi*. It is also said that *yang wei mai* has a close relationship to *wei qi*, while *yin wei mai* has a similar relationship to *ying qi*.

In the classic texts, there is no definitive description of the pathways of *yang wei mai* and *yin wei mai*. *Nanjing*, Difficulty Twenty-Eight, for example, does not describe their pathway, as it does with the other six extraordinary vessels. *Yin wei mai* and *yang wei mai* are in fact described together and not separately, as is the case with the other extraordinary vessels. The focus in the text is on their function of coordinating and harmonising the channels and *yin* and *yang qi* in the body, their function seemingly being of greater relevance than their physical location. Therefore, they should possibly be interpreted as being more of an organising principle than as specific channels.

Li Shi Zhen has in his book an extra branch of *yang wei mai* in the upper arm. He also describes the primary channel as flowing in the opposite direction on the head than it is described as doing in most other texts. The pathway described below is the one most frequently described in modern textbooks.

Pathway

- *Yang wei mai* has its origin on the lateral aspect of the foot, proximal to the tuberosity of the fifth metatarsal bone, at the acupuncture point UB 63.

- It ascends along the lateral aspect of the leg to the acupuncture point GB 35, on the posterior border of the fibula, seven *cun* superior to the lateral malleolus.

- It continues upwards along the lateral aspect of the leg, hip and torso to the acupuncture point SI 10 on the posterior aspect of the shoulder, one *cun* superior to the posterior axilla groove.

- It ascends to the apex of the shoulder and the acupuncture points SJ 15 (in the suprascapular fossa, midway between the seventh cervical vertebra and the tip of the acromion) and GB 21 (on the apex of the shoulder, midway between the seventh cervical vertebra and the tip of the acromion).

- It continues up the neck, passing in front of the ear and ascending to the acupuncture point St 8, half a *cun* superior to the anterior hairline, four and a half *cun* lateral to the midline.

- It traverses one and a half *cun* laterally to the acupuncture point GB 13 and then down to the acupuncture point GB 14, one *cun* superior to the midpoint of the eyebrow.

- It follows the Gall Bladder channel over the head to the acupuncture point GB 20, inferior to the occipital bone, between the trapezius and sternocleidomastoid muscles.

- It flows inwards to the acupuncture point Du 16 immediately inferior to the occipital protuberance, before terminating at the acupuncture point Du 15, below the first cervical vertebra.

Point categories

Opening point	SJ 5
Partner opening point	GB 41
Source point	UB 63
Xi-cleft point	GB 35

Meeting points with other channels

UB 63	Urinary Bladder channels
GB 13	Gall Bladder channel
GB 14	Stomach, Large Intestine and *san jiao* channels
GB 15	Gall Bladder and Urinary Bladder channels and *yang wei mai*
GB 16	Gall Bladder channel
GB 17	Gall Bladder channel
GB 18	Gall Bladder channel
GB 19	Gall Bladder channel
GB 20	*San jiao* and Gall Bladder channels and *yang qiao mai*
GB 21	Gall Bladder, Stomach and *san jiao* channels
GB 24	Gall Bladder and Spleen channels
GB 35	Gall Bladder channel
St 8	Stomach and Gall Bladder channels
SI 10	Small Intestine and Urinary Bladder channels and *yang qiao mai*
SJ 13	*San jiao* and Gall Bladder channels
SJ 15	*San jiao* and Gall Bladder channels
Du 15	*Du mai*
Du 16	*Du mai* and *yang qiao mai*

Areas of usage

Yang wei mai has a close relationship to the *shaoyang* channel with which it shares several acupuncture points and has SJ 5 as its opening point. This is also reflected in the situations that *yang wei mai* is used to treat. *Yang wei mai* can also be used to expel invasions of exogenous *xie qi*, due to its relationship with *wei qi*.

Treatment of invasions of exogenous xie qi

It is said that *yang wei mai* controls the exterior and *yang qi*. *Yang wei mai* also has a close relationship with *wei qi*, and the opening point SJ 5 is termed 'the gate to the exterior'. All of this means that *yang wei mai*, and in particular its opening point, can be used to expel invasions of exogenous *xie qi* that disturb the circulation and functions of *wei qi*. This will typically manifest as chills and an aversion to cold. It is important to remember that aversions to cold and chills are seen in all invasions of exogenous *xie qi* and not just invasions of Wind-Cold. The chills and aversion to cold are due to *wei qi* being blocked and no longer warming the skin. GB 20, which is one of the most important acupuncture points to expel invasions of Wind, is also an acupuncture point on *yang wei mai*. I personally choose to use *yang wei mai* in the treatment of invasions of exogenous *xie qi* when there are other symptoms and signs that relate to *yang wei mai*, such as acute earache or a unilateral headache.

Yang wei mai can also be used in the treatment of exogenous *xie qi* that is locked in the *shaoyang* level in the diagnostic model 'diagnosis according to the six stages'.[6] This reflects both the relationship that *yang wei mai* has to *wei qi* and the close relationship it has with the Gall Bladder and *san jiao* channels.

It affects the ears

Yang wei mai can be used for problems with the ears, particularly earache. This is due to the close relationship that *yang wei mai* has to the Gall Bladder and *san jiao* channels, both of which connect to the ear.

Treatment of pain along the side of the body

Yang wei mai influences the lateral aspect of the body. This means that it can be used for the treatment of pain and discomfort that manifests itself in this aspect. This could be sciatica, hip pain, neck and shoulder problems, unilateral headache, etc.

A person who is Gall Bladder *qi xu* will often be shy and afraid of confrontations.

Part 5

THE ACUPUNCTURE POINTS

ACUPUNCTURE POINTS

Acupuncture points are a central concept in acupuncture and Chinese medicine. These are places that are usually, but not always, situated along the course of a channel. 'Acupuncture point' is not a satisfactory name for these places. First, these sites can be used therapeutically for many other purposes apart from acupuncture. Second, and more importantly, the word 'point' gives a false perception of what these places actually are. In many ways, it is the same problem that was previously discussed in the introduction to the chapter on the channels (page 224). The English word 'point' that is used to translate the Chinese term *xue shu* is not adequate. It is in fact misleading – a point is something that is two-dimensional. The word point does not create an image of movement, activity or of a place where something is happening. Despite these reservations I have chosen to use the term acupuncture point, as this is the most commonly used term in English for these sites.

The Chinese word for these places along the channel is *xue shu*.[1] *Xue*[2] has two definitions in Chinese. The first meaning of the word *xue* is the common definition of an acupuncture point.[3] The second and older sense of the word is: a hole, a hollow, a cave, a nest, a dragon's lair or a cavern. This reflects the fact that acupuncture points are often situated between bones, tendons and muscles. *Shu* is the same word as in back-*shu* points and the five *shu*-transport points. *Shu* means: to transport, conveyance or fluid movement.

This gives a more three-dimensional impression. Acupuncture points are places that can be palpated and places where there is activity and movement.[4] This is important, as it gives an understanding of the *qi* dynamic that is found in these places. It also makes it easier to find acupuncture points with the fingers. This is because, energetically, acupuncture points are dynamic places where you will be able to sense that there is something different with the fingertips. In fact, there is a lower electrical resistance in these places, which means that acupuncture points can also be located by using an electrical point detector.

Professor Wang Ju Yi defines acupuncture points as being 'places on the body surface from which there is transformation and transportation of information, regulation of channel and organ function, irrigation of surrounding tissues, and connectivity to the channel system as a whole' (Wang and Robertson 2008, p.422). This means that when you insert a needle into an acupuncture point it affects not only the local area, but also the channel as a whole, including the channel's internal pathways, and thereby the point will also affect the *zangfu* organ system.

In older acupuncture books, the channels and acupuncture points were not drawn very precisely – they were sketches. This is in stark contrast to the fantastically detailed illustrations in modern acupuncture books, where a point is unambiguously located in relation to the muscles, bones, tendons, nerves and blood vessels. These images are anatomically very precise. However, there is a pitfall in these modern depictions, and it was perhaps for exactly this reason that the old texts were more sketchy in their images of acupuncture points. It should be remembered that acupuncture points are places where *qi* collects and are not anatomical structures. *Qi* is dynamic and will flow where there is a natural channel, in the same way that water flows through the landscape. This is often seen with the regular channels. They often course between two muscles in the same way that a river flows between two hills or ridges. Acupuncture points often feel like small depressions in the tissue. Acupuncture points are also often situated between two muscles or tendons, adjacent to the end of a bone, in depressions in the skull bone or similar places. In reality we should think of the depictions that we see of the channels and their associated acupuncture points as being a map of a landscape. When you want to find a specific spot in the landscape, you follow the map until you come to the area that is in the vicinity of the spot. When, according to the map, you are near to the site, you use your eyes to find the exact spot instead of slavishly measuring the ground in relation to the map. The same is the case with acupuncture points – instead of using our eyes, we use our fingertips. That does not mean you should not follow the measurements and descriptions given in acupuncture manuals and charts when finding acupuncture points. These instructions should be used to find the area where the point is located, but you should then use your fingertips to sense *qi* sensations in the area where you expect that the acupuncture point should be. Exactly how the acupuncture point feels is different from acupuncture point to acupuncture point, and perhaps also from person to person. It is something that is best learnt through practical instruction from an experienced teacher. Typical sensations that I look for when I am looking for acupuncture points are changes in the physical and energetic resistance whilst I very gently draw my fingers across the surface of the skin. In the beginning, the fingers should only just touch the skin, without there being any physical pressure downwards. What I am trying to sense here are changes in the skin's temperature and moistness. Afterwards I palpate slightly deeper, but still very superficially and with a very light touch, to sense whether there is a difference in tissue quality and whether there is a hollowness, a tightness, a slight elevation or any other physical differences in the structure or resistance of the tissue whilst I draw my finger lightly through the surface of the tissue. It is important that you only use an extremely light touch before palpating a little deeper. By palpating with more than a minimum of pressure, you will change the dynamics of the *qi* and therefore you will not be able to sense a difference or, more accurately, the act of palpation will itself create a difference in *qi*, but the difference will be the result of the finger's pressure. The image that I usually give to my students is that it is like looking out onto a garden after it has snowed and you want to find a certain object. Your eyes can survey the surface of the snow looking for hollows and bumps that will tell you something about what is on the ground below the surface of the snow. You could also walk around on the lawn, using your feet to prod the snow, and in this way try to find the object beneath the snow. The problem is that once you have started walking around in the snow, you can no longer step back and use your eyes to survey the surface of the snow. The same is true of the tissue below the skin. Once you physically palpate the area with the fingers, you have disrupted and altered the flow of *qi* in the tissue so that it temporarily collects and stagnates in some places and is dissipated away from other areas. All this can make acupuncture point localisation sound esoteric and complicated, but it is in fact something that is relatively easy to learn. It just requires practice and an open mind.

In the following chapters, I will discuss some of the classical acupuncture point categories. I will also describe acupuncture points' individual actions and indications, but I will not describe their locations. To find acupuncture points requires the use of a good acupuncture manual. Claudia Focks's *Atlas of Acupuncture* (2008) or Peter Deadman and Mazin Al-Khafaji's *Manual of Acupuncture* (1998) are excellent examples of such books.

YUAN-SOURCE POINTS

Yuan-source points are acupuncture points that are found on all the regular channels. There is, however, a difference between the actions and indications that *yuan*-source points have on *yin* and *yang* channels. Before we look at the *yuan*-source points and their qualities, it would be appropriate to focus briefly on *yuan qi*. *Yuan qi* is created when *jing* is transformed by *mingmen* in the lower *jiao*. *Yuan qi* is a fundamental form of *yang qi*, which is used as a catalyst in transformations of *qi* and *xue*. It is also the motivating force that is the basis for the organs' functional activity.

Yuan qi is distributed throughout the body from its place of origin between the Kidneys via *san jiao*. *San jiao* differentiates and separates *yuan qi*, so that it can take on different forms and perform different functions around the body as required. *Yuan qi* is sent, for example, to all the organs, where it is the motivating force that enables them to carry out their functions. *Yuan qi* is also distributed by *san jiao* to the individual channels via their *yuan*-source points.

Huang Di Nei Jing – Ling Shu lists only five *yin yuan*-source points, the Heart being treated via the Pericardium channel at the time. *Nanjing*, Difficulty Sixty-Six, also describes two additional *yuan*-source points – one for *gao* (fatty tissue) and one for *huang* (membranes).

Yuan-source points

- Lung: Lu 9
- Large Intestine: LI 4
- Stomach: St 42
- Spleen: Sp 3
- Heart: He 7
- Small Intestine: SI 4
- Urinary Bladder: UB 64
- Kidney: Kid 3
- Pericardium: Pe 7
- *San jiao*: SJ 4
- Gall Bladder: GB 40
- Liver: Liv 3
- *Gao*: Ren 15
- *Huang*: Ren 6

Yuan-source points are therefore points where *yuan qi* enters the channel and places where *yuan qi* can be accessed. *Yuan*-source points on the *yin* channels have a very powerful tonifying effect on the channel's same-name organ. *Yuan*-source points are therefore also some of the most commonly used acupuncture points in Chinese medicine.

The *yin* channels' *yuan*-source points are identical to the channel's *shu*-stream and Earth point. *Yuan*-source points on the *yang* channels are not considered to have the same tonifying effect on their corresponding organ. *Yuan*-source points on *yang* channels are, on the other hand, a place where exogenous *xie qi* can have a tendency to invade the channel. This, though, also means that *yang* channel *yuan*-source points are points that are often used to expel exogenous *xie qi*.

Some modern Western authors believe that *yuan*-source points connect to their partner channel's *luo*-connecting point. This is not something that I have seen in texts that have their root in Chinese texts. Nevertheless, there are many situations where it is common to use a combination of the primary channel's *yuan*-source point with its partner channel's *luo*-connecting point. For instance, it is very typical to use Lu 7 and LI 4 in combination; likewise Sp 3 and St 40 is also a much used combination.

Yin yuan-source points

As written above, *yin yuan*-source points are some of the body's most important tonifying acupuncture points. Therefore they are often used in the treatment of chronic *xu* conditions, both in their channel's *zang* organ and in the body as a whole.

Yin yuan-source points' actions can be summarised as follows.

- They are the channel's primary point to tonify the corresponding *zang* organ. *Yin yuan*-source points are particularly used to tonify all *xu* conditions in their channel's *zang* organ, i.e. *yin xu*, *yang xu*, *xue xu* and *qi xu* conditions.

- They balance *yin* and *yang*. *Yuan*-source points are reasonably neutral and therefore they can be used to tonify both *yin* and *yang*. This can be seen clearly in Kid 3, which is used just as often to nourish Kidney *yin* as it is used to strengthen Kidney *yang*.

- They stabilise the emotions. Many *yuan*-source points are used in the treatment of emotional imbalances, especially the *yuan*-source points on the arm *yin* channels. Lu 9, He 7 and Pe 7 are all used in the treatment of *shen* imbalances. Liv 3, Kid 3 and Sp 3 are often used to treat the underlying causes of *shen* imbalances.

- They can be used diagnostically. If there are changes in the skin colour or texture or palpable changes in the tissue around the *yuan*-source point, this can be a sign of an imbalance in the channel's corresponding organ.

- They are often used in combination with other tonifying points, such as the organ's back-*shu* point.

Yuan-source points are often combined with other channels' *yuan*-source points and with *hui*-gathering points, as well as their own organ's back-*shu, mu*-collecting or *luo*-connecting points.

Yang *yuan*-source points

Yang channel *yuan*-source points do not have the same tonifying properties that *yuan*-source points on *yin* channels have. *Yang* channel *yuan*-source points are not identical to the channel's *shu*-stream and Earth points. *Yang yuan*-source points are situated between the channel's *shu*-stream and *jing*-river points. With the exception of GB 40, *yang* channel *yuan*-source points are the fourth or the fourth from last point on the channel, depending on the channel's direction of flow.

Yang channel *yuan*-source points' actions can be summarised as follows.

- They are most commonly used in the treatment of *shi* conditions. Whilst *yin* channel *yuan*-source points are commonly used in the treatment of *xu* conditions, *yang* channel *yuan*-source points are mainly used in the treatment of *shi* conditions. For example, LI 4 is used to expel Wind-Cold, St 42 drains Stomach Fire, GB 40 drains Gall Bladder Damp-Heat, SJ 4 expels Wind-Heat from the eyes and UB 64 spreads and disperses stagnant *qi* in the Urinary Bladder channel.

- They are often used to regulate the channel. *Yang* channel *yuan*-source points are often used as distal points when treating painful blockages of *qi* and *xue* further up the channel. These blockages typically manifest as disorders in the joints such as tennis elbow, frozen shoulder, knee pain, etc.

- They expel exogenous *xie qi* from the channel. Exogenous *xie qi* can invade *yang* channels through their *yuan*-source points. Exogenous *xie qi* can then subsequently block the joints further up the channel. This also means that these acupuncture points can be used to expel exogenous *xie qi* in *bi* syndromes (painful blockage syndromes).

- They can be used to tonify their own *fu* organ. This is not the primary usage area; nevertheless, it is possible to use LI 4 to tonify and activate *qi*, SJ 4 to tonify *yuan qi*, St 42 to tonify Stomach and Spleen *qi* or GB 40 to tonify Gall Bladder *qi*. It is, though, more typical to use *fu* organs' lower *he*-sea points to tonify the organ.

Other *yuan*-source points

Ren 15 is the *yuan*-source point for *gao* or fatty tissue and for the area under the Heart. Ren 15 is also regarded as being the *yuan*-source point for all *zang* organs. In particular, it is used to treat mental-emotional imbalances caused by *yin xu* conditions in *zang* organs.

Ren 6 is the *yuan*-source point for the area below the navel and *huang* or membranes. Ren 6 is also regarded as the *yuan*-source point for all *fu* organs. Ren 6 can therefore be used to treat *xu* conditions in *fu* organs and to tonify *yuan qi*.

LUO-CONNECTING POINTS

Luo means 'network' and is the same word as in *luo* channel or *luo* vessel. These points are called *luo*-connecting points because of their relationship to the *luo* vessels. *Luo*-connecting points are the place on a channel where the *luo*-connecting vessels separate from the main channel. The body has fifteen *luo*-connecting points all together. Each of the twelve regular channels, as well as *ren mai* and *du mai*, has a *luo*-connecting point. In addition to these fourteen points, there is a 'great' *luo*-connecting point on the Spleen channel, which is Sp 21.

> ### *Luo*-connecting points
>
> - Lung: Lu 7
> - Large Intestine: LI 6
> - Stomach: St 40
> - Spleen: Sp 4
> - Heart: He 5
> - Small Intestine: SI 7
> - Urinary Bladder: UB 58
> - Kidney: Kid 4
> - Pericardium: Pe 6
> - *San jiao*: SJ 5
> - Gall Bladder: GB 37
> - Liver: Liv 5
> - *Ren mai*: Ren 15
> - *Du mai*: Du 1
> - the Spleen great *luo*-connecting vessel: Sp 21

Luo-connecting points are the place where two vessels separate from the primary channel. The one vessel connects with its *yin/yang* partner channel, and the second vessel connects to a separate area of the body and sometimes to one or more of the internal organs. In addition to having an influence on these two vessels that separate from the primary channel, the *luo*-connecting point also influences the intricate and minute network of *luo* vessels that flow through the tissue below the surface of the body.

Treatment with *luo*-connecting points

Luo-connecting points are frequently used in the treatment of a wide range of disorders in the body. They have an influence on both their own and their partner's internal organ. They affect *qi* and *xue* in their own and their partner's channel. They affect their own longitudinal *luo* vessels and the areas that this *luo* vessel passes through, and they activate *qi* in the small intricate network of microscopic *luo* vessels that flow through all the tissue between the channel and the skin.

Treatment of imbalances in their own channel and organ and that of their partner

Each of the twelve regular channels has a horizontal connection to its partner channel. This vessel runs from the *luo*-connecting point on the channel. *Luo* vessels are one of the ways in which the body can regulate and harmonise *qi* in the channel network. When there is too much or too little *qi* in a channel, it can be balanced by *qi* flowing to or from its partner channel. In addition, *luo* vessels are yet another example of how *yin* and *yang* partner organs and channels communicate with each other. This means that *luo*-connecting points can be used in the treatment of imbalances in their own or their partner channel or organ. The *luo*-connecting point can be used to lead *qi* to or from the partner channel, both in *xu* and *shi* conditions.

It is common to use both the *luo*-connecting points and the *yuan*-source points when there is a *xu* condition. By using the channel's own *yuan*-source point, the channel or organ can be strongly tonified. This effect can be optimised by combining the *yuan*-source point with the partner channel's *luo*-connecting point, so that it can draw on the *qi* in the partner channel. This method is known as the 'guest-host' method.

Luo-connecting points can also be used unilaterally when treating stagnations of *qi* and/or *xue* in the partner channel on the other side of the body. For example, if a lot of Large Intestine channel points in the right arm have been used because the person has a repetitive strain injury in their right elbow or has pain in their right shoulder, Lu 7 can be used in the left arm to balance the treatment.

Treatment of imbalances related to the areas controlled by the channel's luo vessel

Each of the *luo*-connecting points is a source point for a longitudinal vessel that separates from the primary channel and connects to another area of the body. Some of these vessels connect to internal organs and others to the head, while others again have a short pathway in the local area. Treatment of *luo*-connecting points can thus be used to affect *qi* and *xue* in these areas. This explains some of the unique indications some *luo*-connecting points have – for example, the use of He 5 in the treatment of tongue problems and speech disorders or Liv 5 for problems with the external genitalia.

For a more comprehensive description of these longitudinal *luo* connections, the reader is referred to the appropriate section in the chapter describing the channels (page 224).

The areas that the longitudinal *luo* vessel connects to are as follows.

- Lung *luo* vessel: Thenar eminence and palm.

- Large Intestine *luo* vessel: Shoulder, jaw, teeth and ear.

- Stomach *luo* vessel: Front of the body, neck and head.

- Spleen *luo* vessel: Stomach and Intestines.

- Heart *luo* vessel: Heart, tongue, eyes and brain.

- Small Intestine *luo* vessel: Shoulder and clavicle.

- Urinary Bladder *luo* vessel: Around the leg.[5]

- Kidney *luo* vessel: Inguinal area, chest and lumbar region.

- Pericardium *luo* vessel: Thorax and Heart.

- *San jiao luo* vessel: The three *jiao*.

- Gall Bladder *luo* vessel: Lateral aspect of the dorsum of the foot to the third, fourth and fifth toes.

- Liver *luo* vessel: External genitalia.

- *Ren mai luo* vessel: Abdomen.

- *Du mai luo* vessel: Scapula and neck.

- Spleen great *luo* vessel: Thorax and ribs.

Expel xie qi and spread stagnations of qi and xue

One of the aspects of *luo* vessels that the *luo*-connecting points have an influence on is the intricate network of microscopic vessels that flow through all tissue in the body. There are three types of superficial *luo* vessels – *sun luo*, *fu luo* and *xue luo*. *Sun luo* are the small branches that ascend vertically from the main channel. These branches divide again into even finer *fu luo*. *Fu luo* will further divide into the even smaller lateral branches, which are called *xue luo*. This results in an extremely comprehensive network of fine-meshed microscopic vessels.

These small vessels fill the space above and between the primary channels. The superficial *luo* vessels have the task of spreading and circulating *qi*, *xue* and *jinye* in all the tissues in the body, in both the muscles and skin, but also in the internal organs.

These small pathways can easily be blocked by exogenous *xie qi*. Stagnations of *qi* and *xue* also have a tendency to disrupt these vessels. This is because the vessels themselves are extremely narrow and they have the structure of a net. Furthermore, *qi*, *xue* and *jinye* in these vessels can have difficulty passing through major joints. Stagnations of *qi* and *xue* in these vessels can sometimes manifest with the vessels becoming visible or with changes in the skin in the local area. *Luo*-connecting points can be used to spread stagnations and expel *xie qi* from these vessels. Bleeding of *luo*-connecting points is recommended when there are stagnations of *qi* and especially stagnations of *xue* in the *sun luo*, *fu luo* and *xue luo*.

Treatment of mental-emotional imbalances

This is particularly relevant for *yin* channels' *luo*-connecting points, as several of these have an influence on *shen*.

Examples of these *luo*-connecting points are:

- Lu 7: poor memory, uncontrolled or inappropriate laughter

- St 40: manic behaviour, uncontrolled laughter, singing, shouting or inappropriate behaviour, bipolar disorder

- Sp 4: bipolar disorder, mania, mental restlessness, insomnia, unrest in the body

- He 5: fear, sadness, depression, anxiety, mental unrest

- SI 7: bipolar disorder, anxiety, fear, fright, nervousness

- Kid 4: mental retardation, nervousness, somnolence, fear, wanting to stay indoors, depression

- Pe 6: insomnia, poor memory, anxiety, mania, depression

- Liv 5: 'plumstone' *qi* sensation in the throat, depression, anxiety, impotence, worry

- Ren 15: mania, bipolar disorder, anxiety, insomnia.

XI-CLEFT POINTS

Xi means cleft or hole in Chinese. It is the place where *qi* and *xue*, which until now have been flowing relatively superficially since the *jing*-well point, start to gather and plunge deeper. Each of the regular channels has a *xi*-cleft point, as do four of the extraordinary channels. All the *xi*-cleft points, with the exception of St 34, are located between the wrist and the elbow or between the knee and the ankle.

Xi-cleft points are mainly used:

- to treat acute and painful disorders along the path of the channel and in the corresponding organ

- in the case of *yin xi*-cleft points, to treat *xue* imbalances and bleeding that is related to their *zang* organ.

The use of these points to treat acute and painful disorders may be related to these points being clefts or deep holes. This is a place where the dynamic of a stream or a river would be very powerful. Changing the flow and the dynamic of movement here can subsequently create significant changes in the flow further along the course of a channel. Because they treat acute conditions and pain, they are usually used to treat *shi* conditions. This means that *xi*-cleft points are usually treated using a draining needle technique.

Examples of usage of these points are:

- Lu 6 in the treatment of acute asthma and bloody sputum

- St 34 to treat acute epigastric pain and vomiting

- Sp 8 to treat menstrual pain and bleeding from the uterus

- Pe 4 and He 6 for the treatment of cardiac pain and acute pain in the thorax

- Kid 8 to stop bleeding from the uterus.

Xi-cleft points can also be used diagnostically.

- They are often painful when palpated in *shi* conditions of the channel or the associated organ. They can also be red and/or swollen in these situations.

- They can be sunken or depressed, with a mild tenderness on palpation, when there are *xu* conditions in the channel or associated organ.

Xi-cleft points

- Lung: Lu 6
- Large Intestine: LI 7
- Stomach: St 34
- Spleen: Sp 8
- Heart: He 6
- Small Intestine: SI 6
- Urinary Bladder: UB 63
- Kidney: Kid 5
- Pericardium: Pe 4
- *San jiao*: SJ 7
- Gall Bladder: GB 36
- Liver: Liv 6
- *Yang qiao mai*: UB 59
- *Yin qiao mai*: Kid 8
- *Yang wei mai*: GB 35
- *Yin wei mai*: Kid 9

BACK-*SHU* POINTS

Back-*shu* points are a category of acupuncture points that are located along the Urinary Bladder channel's medial pathway on the back. This acupuncture point category is unique in that all the points are located on the same channel. *Shu* is the same word or character that is used in the title of the category of acupuncture points known as the five *shu*-transport points, i.e. the series of points that are located on the limbs, as well as the title of the third point in this series, the *shu*-stream point. *Shu* also means transport or conveyance in this context. Back-*shu* acupuncture points can transport *qi* directly to their organ. The individual back-*shu* points' names are composed of the name of an organ and the word *shu*. The Lung's back-*shu* point is, for example, called *feishu*, the Kidney back-*shu* point *shenshu*, etc. Each of the twelve *zangfu* organs has a back-*shu* point. In addition to these, there are another six back-*shu* points located on the Urinary Bladder channel that have a relationship to either specific areas of the body or a specific aspect of the body. The back-*shu* points are anatomically located at the same level as the organ is in the body or the area of the body that they are related to. The back-*shu* points are also situated almost opposite their organ's *mu*-collecting point. These two categories of points also have some common features.

Mu-collecting points and back-*shu* points both:

- can be used diagnostically and therapeutically

- are roughly in line with the corresponding organ

- have a direct impact on their corresponding organ.

Zangfu organs' back-*shu* points

- UB 13: Lung
- UB 14: Pericardium
- UB 15: Heart
- UB 18: Liver
- UB 19: Gall Bladder
- UB 20: Spleen
- UB 21: Stomach
- UB 22: *San jiao*
- UB 23: Kidney
- UB 25: Large Intestine
- UB 27: Small Intestine
- UB 28: Urinary Bladder

> **Other back-*shu* points**
>
> - UB 16: *Du mai*
> - UB 17: Diaphragm
> - UB 24: Sea of *qi*
> - UB 26: Lumbar region
> - UB 29: Sacrum
> - UB 30: Anus
> - UB 43: *Huang* or membranes

Treatment with back-*shu* points

Back-*shu* points communicate directly with their corresponding organ. This means that the use of these points in treatment will have a strong and direct effect on the organ and its functions, as well as the associated body tissue, sensory organs, *shen* aspects, etc. that this organ has an influence on. For example, treating the back-*shu* point UB 18 (*Ganshu*) has an effect not only on the Liver itself, Liver *qi*, Liver *xue*, Liver *yin* and Liver *yang*, but also on the eyes, *hun*, tendons, emotions such as anger and frustration, internal Wind, etc. This means that back-*shu* points have a very broad and comprehensive range of actions.

Back-*shu* points do not have a direct effect on the channel of the organ.

There are differing opinions amongst some practitioners as to how and when to use these acupuncture points. Some refer to *Nanjing,* chapter sixty-seven, where it states that *mu*-collecting points are used to treat *yang* disorders and back-*shu* points to treat *yin* disorders. This statement appears to infer that back-*shu* points should be used to treat chronic disorders, disorders in *zang* organs, *xu* disorders and Cold and Damp disorders. Even though all of these situations are conditions that back-*shu* points are able to treat, most practitioners also utilise these points to treat acute conditions, *shi* disorders, Heat and Wind conditions and disorders of *fu* organs. Furthermore, *mu*-collecting points are also used to treat both *yin* and *yang* types of imbalances. My own experience confirms this. For example, I will often use UB 13 to treat invasions of exogenous *xie qi* or Phlegm conditions in the Lung. I will also use UB 25 in the treatment of constipation, because it is the Large Intestine back-*shu* point. This means that I use back-*shu* points to treat both *shi* and *xu* disorders, as well as *zang* and *fu* organs. I therefore interpret the statement that back-*shu* points are used to treat *xu* disorders in *zang* organs as meaning that these points should be used at some stage in the treatment of these disorders.

Some authors, including Giovanni Maciocia (2005), recommend that the needles should only remain in place in the back-*shu* points for a maximum of ten minutes in both *xu* and *shi* conditions. A second approach is to insert a needle in a back-*shu* point, utilise a stimulating technique, remove the needle again and then continue the rest of the treatment by inserting needles in the regular channel points for fifteen to twenty minutes. When treating on a weekly basis, treatments can alternate between points on the front of the body and back-*shu* points.

As well as treating disorders of the *zangfu* organs, back-*shu* points can of course also be used to treat disorders in the local area and disorders along the pathway of the Urinary Bladder channel. This means that these points are commonly used in the treatment of back pain.

Diagnosis with back-*shu* points

Back-*shu* points can be used as a diagnostic tool. When an organ is in imbalance, its back-*shu* point can feel tense, sore or painful to touch. There can also be visible changes in the tissue or skin around the point.

MU-COLLECTING POINTS

Mu points are also termed as the 'alarm' points in some books. This is because they are often sore and tender when their corresponding organ is imbalanced, and because they can be used to treat acute conditions in their respective organ. *Mu* in Chinese means to gather, collect or recruit. *Mu* points have received their name because it is here that the organ's *qi* collects on the front side of the body.

In the same way that each *zangfu* organ has a back-*shu* point, they also have a *mu*-collecting point. *Mu*-collecting points are all located on the front of the body, with the exception of GB 25, and they will often be in the vicinity of their corresponding organ. They can be used diagnostically and therapeutically when there are imbalances in their organ. As was the case with back-*shu* points, it is only the organ, and not the channel, that is directly affected by these points.

Mu-collecting points are located on more than one channel, but half of them are to be found on *ren mai*.

The twelve *mu*-collecting points

- Lung: Lu 1
- Large Intestine: St 25
- Stomach: Ren 12
- Spleen: Liv 13
- Heart: Ren 14
- Small Intestine: Ren 4
- Urinary Bladder: Ren 3
- Kidney: GB 25
- Pericardium: Ren 17
- *San jiao*: Ren 5
- Gall Bladder: GB 24
- Liver: Liv 14

Mu-collecting points can be used both diagnostically and therapeutically. When there is an imbalance in their corresponding organ, the *mu*-collecting point will often be sore or painful upon palpation.

Despite the fact that the *Nanjing* states that these *yin* acupuncture points are used to treat *yang* diseases, they can also be used in the treatment of all types of imbalances in their corresponding organ, both *xu* and *shi*, chronic and acute. Many therapists in fact consciously combine the use of a body's *mu*-collecting point together with its back-*shu* point in the same treatment.

HUI-GATHERING POINTS

Hui can be translated as 'meeting', 'collect' or 'gather'. It is a place where certain types of *qi* collect or meet. Giovanni Maciocia (2005) chooses to translate the term into English as 'gathering', whereas Claudia Focks (2008) and Peter Deadman (Deadman and Al-Khafaji 1998) translate it as 'meeting'. I have chosen to follow Giovanni Maciocia's translation, because 'meeting' point is also used as a term for acupuncture points where two or more channels meet in the same point. There are eight *hui*-gathering points distributed over the body. They are acupuncture points that have a special influence on certain organs, substances or tissues, and can be used in the treatment of these.

The eight *hui*-gathering points are as follows.

Hui-gathering point	Area of influence	Is frequently used to treat
UB 11	Bones	Chronic *bi* syndrome, bone disorders, stiffness in the neck and spine
UB 17	*Xue*	*Xue xu*, *xue* stagnation, *xue* Heat
Liv 13	*Zang* organs	Tonifies the Spleen and thereby the production of post-heavenly *qi*. By strengthening the production of post-heavenly *qi*, Liv 13 tonifies all *zang* organs
Ren 12	*Fu* organs	Tonifies the Stomach and thereby *qi* in the Stomach and the Intestines
Ren 17	*Qi*	Tonifies and spreads *zong qi* and thereby also the production and movement of *qi*
Lu 9	Blood vessels	Harmonises *zong qi* and *xue*, which flow through the blood vessels. If *zong qi* is *xu*, *xue* stagnates, because it is not moved through the vessels
GB 34	Tendons	Influences the tendons
GB 39	Bone marrow	Tonifies the Marrow and thereby also the Brain

THE FIVE *SHU*-TRANSPORT POINTS

Each channel has five so-called *shu* points. *Shu* means transport or to convey. It is the same name that is used in the term back-*shu* points, and in both contexts the word has the same meaning. Elisabeth Rochat de la Vallee (2009, p.128) defines *shu* as 'a place where certain influences are gathering and from where influences may be transferred'. When we look at the individual *shu* points we can see that they have a relationship to communication from the exterior to the interior.

The five *shu*-transport points are described from a concept of the channel being like a water course that starts on a mountainside and flows down to the coast and into the ocean. The first *shu*-transport point is the *jing*-well point, where water bubbles up to the surface from its source deep within the ground. This is where *yin* and *yang* transform into each other in the channel. This is why there is almost no movement here, but at the same time there is a powerful dynamic. The next *shu*-transport point is called *ying*-spring, because it is like a mountain spring that flows down the mountainside. There is still a strong bubbling dynamic, as well as movement, but there is not much volume yet. The third *shu*-transport point is the *shu*-stream point. The bubbling dynamic is decreasing and the volume is increasing. There is now enough water in the riverbed, so things can float and be transported. This is why this *shu*-transport point is also called *shu*. The next *shu*-transport point on the channel is the *jing*-river point. The water course has now become a river. There is a lot more water in the channel, but the speed and the dynamic energy that the spring had is gone. The river is wider and deeper. The last *shu*-transport point is the *he*-sea point, where the river flows into the sea. The channel is wide and deep, but it is moving slowly. Compared with the water in the spring, the water is much richer and more nutritive. It is full of sediment, minerals and nutrients. It can give life to many things. The water that started up on the hill was very clean and clear, but it was not as nourishing. There is a difference in both the breadth and depth of the spring running down the mountainside and the river when it flows out into the sea.

Something that is difficult for many people to comprehend in the beginning is that the *shu*-transport points represent a different and at times contradictory *qi* dynamic to the general channel system. In this model, *qi* flows in the opposite direction in half of the channels in relation to the direction of the twelve-channel *qi* cycle. Unlike in Western science, Chinese medicine does not have a problem encompassing multiple and ostensibly contradictory explanations of the body's physiology. Chinese medicine is a science that has developed continuously over a period of three thousand years. This means that there have been various theories and ideas that have been prevalent at various times. Chinese thought is more pragmatic and its founding philosophies are more inclusive. If a theory matched the clinical reality, it was not rejected when a new theory was formulated. It was not seen as a problem to have two theories existing side by side. It is also often the case that it is only on the surface that the theories are contradictory. If approached with an open mind, it is usually possible to see that they are just describing different aspects of the same reality.

The flow of *qi* and the dynamics of the channel system are a case in hand. Most of the theories we use today with regard to the movement of *qi* through the channel system are based on a cyclic model. In this model *qi* starts its flow inside the chest and moves outwards from the chest via a *yin* channel to the fingertips. At the fingertips the polarity of *qi* changes and *qi* flows back up the arm to the head via a *yang* channel. From the head *qi* flows down a *yang* channel to the feet, where the polarity again changes and *qi* returns up the leg via a *yin* channel to the chest, where the next cycle starts with *qi* flowing out to the fingers via a new *yin* channel. In an older understanding of the channel system, the conception was that *qi* flowed into the body from Heaven and Earth through the tips of the fingers and the toes. *Qi* then flowed inwards along the arms and legs to the body. Whilst the contemporary system is a cyclic system, this earlier system is centripetal, i.e. *qi* flows inwards from the fingers and toes towards the centre. When a person stands with their arms outwards, *qi* flows into the body from the tips of the fingers and toes and through the soles of the feet. In this model there is talk of transport points – points that transport *qi* into the body.

For half of the channels there is no conflict between the two systems. *Qi* flows in the same direction in both systems. It is in the other half of the channels that there is an apparent discrepancy. This therefore raises the issue of whether we are discussing two different types of *qi* or whether *qi* can move in two directions at the same time, in the same way as cars on a road.

Personally, I think that we should separate direction of flow and dynamic from each other when looking at the channels. In the cyclic system, there is talk of *qi direction*, i.e. *qi* flows to and from the body; in the earlier centripetal model, there is talk of *qi dynamic*. The *qi* dynamic changes in the channels between the acupuncture points on the tips of the toes and fingers and the torso.

An analogy for the channel system that unites these two models is a bus route that transports passengers from its end station in the suburbs to the city centre. If the outer *jing*-well point, which is located on the tip of a toe or a finger, is the end station in the suburb, the *he*-sea point will be a bus stop in the city itself. The bus will start its journey from the end station with only a very few passengers. The closer the bus gets to the centre of the city, the more passengers get on the bus. When the bus is travelling in the opposite direction, the passenger dynamic will be the same, even though the direction of movement is the opposite. The further away from the city that you are, the fewer the passengers. This is the same principle as one of the aspects of the five *shu*-transport points. The strength, depth, breadth and volume of *qi* increases the closer the channel is to the elbow or knee, no matter whether the channel is flowing to or from the torso.

A second aspect of the channel dynamic that is described through the *shu*-transport points is that at the *jing*-well and *ying*-spring points there is not that much volume, but on the other hand *qi* is very volatile, dynamic and fast-moving. It is just like a stream, flowing down a hillside. When it reaches the sea, i.e. the *he*-sea points at the elbows and knees, there is a lot more *qi*. At the sea, the river is deeper and broader and more voluminous, but it is also slower and more sluggish. It has lost the rapid dynamic and become calmer but also more forceful. Again, if we only focus on *qi* direction, then this analogy would not make sense for half of the channels. On the other hand, if we think about a piston in a petrol engine, then there is a similar dynamic. The pressure is greatest when the piston is at the top of the stroke, no matter whether it is on the way up or down. The opposite is the case at the bottom of the stroke. The pressure is lowest here, whether the piston is moving upwards or downwards. Instead of pressure, we can perhaps think of *yin/yang* dynamics. At the tips of the fingers and toes, the *qi* polarity of the channel changes. The closer you get to the tip, the more tension there is. *Yin* and *yang* are at their strongest just before they change polarity. Just think of a balloon. The pressure is greatest, i.e. the balloon is most *yang*, just before it bursts and becomes *yin*, i.e. limp.

The five *shu*-transport points are also classified as Five Phase points. *Yin* channel *jing*-well points are always Wood points, and the subsequent *shu*-transport points on the *yin* channels are Fire, Earth, Metal and Water, in that order. *Yang* channel *jing*-well points are classified as Metal, and the subsequent *shu*-transport points on the *yang* channels are Water, Wood, Fire and Earth, in that order. This concept does not clash with the comprehension of either the direction or dynamic in a channel. This classification is mainly used in the treatment of the Five Phases, where the points are used as tonifying or draining points, depending on which imbalances there are between the Five Phases.

Yin channel *shu* points are as follows.

	Jing Wood	*Ying* Fire	*Shu* Earth	*Jing* Metal	*He* Water
Lung	Lu 11	Lu 10	Lu 9	Lu 8	Lu 5
Spleen	Sp 1	Sp 2	Sp 3	Sp 5	Sp 9
Heart	He 9	He 8	He 7	He 4	He 3
Kidney	Kid 1	Kid 2	Kid 3	Kid 7	Kid 10
Pericardium	Pe 9	Pe 8	Pe 7	Pe 5	Pe 3
Liver	Liv 1	Liv 2	Liv 3	Liv 4	Liv 8

Yang channel *shu* points are as follows.

	Jing Wood	*Ying* Fire	*Shu* Earth	*Jing* Metal	*He* Water
Large Intestine	LI 1	LI 2	LI 3	LI 5	LI 11
Stomach	St 45	St 44	St 43	St 41	St 36
Small Intestine	SI 1	SI 2	SI 3	SI 5	SI 8
Urinary Bladder	UB 67	UB 66	UB 65	UB 60	UB 40
San jiao	SJ 1	SJ 2	SJ 3	SJ 6	SJ 10
Gall Bladder	GB 44	GB 43	GB 41	GB 38	GB 34

The five *shu*-transport points and their actions

Jing-well points

Jing means well – a place where water bubbles up to the surface. *Jing*-well points are either the first or the last points on a channel. They will always be the point on a channel that is most distal from the body. Almost all of them are located in the junction of the line drawn along one of the borders of the nail and the base of the nail. Kid 1 and Pe 9 are exceptions, but they are still the most distal point on their respective channels. The *yang* channel *jing*-well points are Metal points, whilst they are Wood points on *yin* channels. *Jing*-well points are the place where the channel is most superficial. *Jing*-well points are located just below the surface of the skin.

One of the explanations of why these points are so dynamic is that it is here that *yin* and *yang* transform into each other. It is the spot where the polarity changes. The *Nanjing* describes these points as having an outward movement of *qi*, which is consistent with water bubbling up from underground. It is also for this reason that it is said that *qi* emanates here. These factors together result in the *qi* being very volatile here and in a state of flux. This is the reason why *jing*-well points have some of the therapeutic actions that they have.

The actions attributed to these acupuncture points are as follows.

- **Drain *shi* conditions and disperse stagnations:** *Jing*-well points are often used to treat acute *shi* conditions, both invasions of exogenous *xie qi* and chronic blockages of channels, such as joint pain. Because of the dynamic that these acupuncture points have, they can be used to disperse stagnations and accumulations, not just of *qi*, but also of Phlegm and *xue*. This means that *jing*-well points can be used in the treatment of severe pain along the pathway of the channel and to disperse physical accumulations. Lu 11, for example, is used to treat mumps. These points can be bled when there are *xue* stagnations, resulting in very painful joints. One of the classic indications that *Nanjing*, Difficulty Sixty-Eight, ascribes to these points is that they can treat fullness below the Heart. Many of these acupuncture points have the common indication that they treat stagnations in the thorax and costal regions. A classic indication of SI 1 is to promote lactation.

- **Expel exogenous *xie qi*, especially Heat:** *Jing*-well points can be used to treat invasions of Wind-Heat. A good example of this is the use of Lu 11 in the treatment of a sore throat due to an invasion of Wind-Heat.

- **Treat problems at the opposite end of the channel:** In common with all distal points, *jing*-well points affect the equivalent area on the opposite end of the channel. In the case of *jing*-well points, this will be the area around the channel's last or first point, depending on the directional flow of the channel. This is reflected in many of these acupuncture points being recommended for the treatment of toothache, problems in the mouth and gums, earache, eye problems, etc., especially when these are due to *shi* conditions.

- **Affect *shen*:** There are two major areas where these acupuncture points are used to affect *shen*. One is fainting and loss of consciousness. All *jing*-well points apart from GB 44, UB 67 and SJ 1 can be used to restore consciousness. The second area where these points are often used is to drain Heat that is agitating *shen*. This is often done by bleeding these points. Pe 9 and He 9 can, for example, be bled when there is insomnia. Several other *jing*-well points also have powerful *shen*-calming effects, in particular Kid 1 and St 45.

- Other situations where these acupuncture points are used are as local points when treating local problems in the immediate area, such as numbness or pain in the fingers and the toes. Some *jing*-well points have very specific indications that are unique to just one or two of these points. Sp 1 and Liv 1 can, for example, be treated with moxa to stop bleeding.

Ying-spring points

Ying means a spring – a place where water trickles out of the ground and starts flowing down the hillside. *Ying*-spring points are the penultimate or second acupuncture point on the channel, dependent on the direction of the channel. *Ying*-spring points are located in the joints of the fingers and toes. The *qi* begins to flow along the channel here, but it is very swirling and fast in its movement, like a mountain brook. It is here that the water begins to rush down the mountainside. The volume of the *qi* channel is increasing, but the channel is very shallow. There is still a lot of dynamic in these points and this is reflected in their areas of usage.

Ying-spring points are used to do the following.

- **Clear Heat:** *Ying*-spring points clear Heat, both *xu* and *shi* Heat. This is the main action that has traditionally been attributed to this category of acupuncture points. Several of the *ying*-spring points are some of the body's most powerful Heat-draining points. Liv 2, St 44, GB 43, He 8 and Pe 8 are all frequently used to drain *shi* Heat in their own organ. Kid 2 and Lu 10 are used to control and clear *xu* Heat. These points do not just drain Heat from the organ level, but they are also used in the same way as *jing*-well points to drain Heat from the opposite end of the channel and they will often be used for conditions of Heat and pain in the head. One of the indications for the use of these acupuncture points that is mentioned in chapter forty-four of *Huang Di Nei Jing – Ling Shu* is skin colour change. This is because Heat rises upwards and causes the skin to become red, either in the whole head or in the area at the opposite end of the channel.

- **Expel exogenous *xie qi* and eliminate internally generated *xie qi*:** These acupuncture points have a powerful dynamic and they can therefore be used to expel exogenous *xie qi* when it has invaded the channel. *Ying*-spring points can also be used to drain and eliminate internally generated *xie qi* such as Wind and Fire and to clear *yin xu* Heat.

Shu-stream points

The word *shu* in *shu*-stream is the same word as used in the overall category of *shu*-transport points, which these points are a sub-category of. It is also the same term that is used in the name of the back-*shu* points. The character *shu* has the same denotation here, i.e. transportation or conveyance. I have, however, chosen not to call these points *shu*-transport points, to avoid confusion with the other point categories. In keeping with other books, I have chosen also to call these points *shu*-stream points. This is because the channel has deepened and widened and the flow is stronger and steadier. The stream is now so deep and steady flowing that objects can float in it and thereby be transported along its course – thus the name *shu*.

This ability to transport objects inwards along the channel is, though, not necessarily beneficial. Exogenous *xie qi* can enter into the channel and be transported deeper into the realm of the body via *shu*-stream points. It is probably for this reason that *wei qi* also gathers in these points. This means that *shu*-stream points can be used to expel exogenous *xie qi*.

Yuan qi also enters the channel at this point in the *yin* channels, as these points are also the *yuan*-source point on the *yin* channels. This means that they are some of the most important points to tonify their associated organ and the body as a whole. This is not the case in *yang* channels.

Shu-stream points are, with the exception of GB 41, the third or third from last acupuncture point on the channel, depending on the channel's direction of flow.

The actions attributed to *shu*-stream points are as follows.

- **Expel exogenous *xie qi*:** These points can be used when Wind and Dampness have invaded the body. In the classical texts, these acupuncture points are recommended in the treatment of *bi* syndromes (painful obstruction of the channel), where invasions of Wind-Damp-Cold have blocked the channel, and there is pain and/or heaviness along the path of the channel, especially in the joints.

- **Intermittent pain:** *Huang Di Nei Jing – Ling Shu,* chapter forty-four, recommends using these acupuncture points when there are chronic conditions characterised by pain that 'comes and goes'.

- **Damp *bi*:** *Nanjing,* Difficulty Sixty-Eight, recommends the use of *shu* points to treat a heavy body and joint pain.

- **Treat *yin* organs:** *Huang Di Nei Jing – Ling Shu* recommends the use of these points to treat *yin* organs. This is relevant for the *yin* channels' *shu*-stream point. This ability probably relates to the fact that these points are simultaneously the *yuan*-source point on the *yin* channels.

Jing-river points

Even though *jing* is spelled in the same way as in *jing*-well point, the Chinese character *jing* is a completely different character and is pronounced differently. This character refers to something that passes through. In English these points are referred to as 'river' points. *Jing*-river points are located in areas where there is more flesh and muscle. The channel is deeper and wider here, resulting in a difference in the channel's dynamic. The flow is calmer and slower, but due to the depth and volume of water it is also more powerful.

Xie qi that has entered the channel can deviate from the channel itself and into the joints, muscles and bones.

Jing-river points are all located between the ankle and knee or between the wrist and elbow.

Jing-river points are used to do the following.

- **Treat respiratory problems, wheezing and coughs:** The *Nanjing* recommends the use of *jing*-river points in the treatment of respiratory problems where there is wheezing, breathing difficulty, coughing and breathlessness. Many *jing*-river points have these indications as a part of their area of action. This probably is related to the fact that these points are the Metal point on the *yin* channels.

- **Expel exogenous *xie qi* from the channel:** These acupuncture points can be used to expel exogenous *xie qi* that has invaded the channel and is starting to affect the joints, bones and tendons. This means that these points can be used in the treatment of *bi* (painful obstruction) syndrome.

- **Treat the voice:** *Huang Di Nei Jing – Ling Shu* states that these points can be used if there are changes in a person's voice. This will often be the case if there is a respiratory problem. Many *jing*-river points also have indications where there are problems with the voice that do not relate to Lung imbalances. For example, LI 5, St 41 and Pe 5 are used to treat a person who is manic and is raving. Pe 5, SJ 6, Kid 7 and He 4 can, on the other hand, be used if a person has difficulty talking for a variety of reasons.

He-sea points

He means to unite or to gather. When rivers flow into the sea, they unite. *He*-sea points are characterised as having a deep, wide and slow movement of *qi*, especially compared with the *jing*-well points. The *qi* is not as volatile and cannot be as easily affected here. Whereas *jing*-well points are ascribed an outward movement, these points are defined by an inward movement of *qi*, like a river flowing into a delta. Because the flow of the channel is slower and steadier, but also more powerful, these points can be used to regulate *qi*, especially in the *fu* organs. *He*-sea points are located in fleshy areas in and around the knees and the elbows.

Something that is unique for *he*-sea points is that, unlike the other *shu*-transport points, there are three extra *he*-sea points on the legs. These are known as the lower *he*-sea points. There is one for each of the three arm *yang* channels. Two of them are located on the Stomach channel – St 37 and St 39, which are the Large Intestine and the Small Intestine's lower *he*-sea points respectively. UB 39 is the lower *he*-sea point of *san jiao*. These lower *he*-sea points are more frequently used than the *he*-sea point on the arm channel in the treatment of imbalances in the associated organ.

He-sea points are mainly used to do the following.

- **Treat diarrhoea and rebellious *qi*:** All *he*-sea and lower *he*-sea points, with the exception of SI 8, treat diarrhoea and/or vomiting. Several *he*-sea points are amongst the most important points used in the treatment of digestive problems in the Stomach or Intestines. *He*-sea points have a regulatory effect on the *qi* of these organs. All *he*-sea points on the legs drain Dampness and Damp-Heat downwards, as does LI 11.

- **Treat problems in the *fu* organs:** *He*-sea points, as we have just seen, regulate *qi* in the Stomach and the Intestines. Their action, however, is not just limited to these three organs. Several *he*-sea points have the ability to regulate *qi* and drain Dampness and Damp-Heat from the Urinary Bladder, Gall Bladder and the Uterus.

- **Treatment of skin ailments:** Several *he*-sea points are regularly used in the treatment of skin problems. Points such as LI 11, Lu 5, Pe 3, He 3, UB 40, Liv 8 and SJ 10 all treat skin problems, especially when these disorders are caused by Heat.

The five *shu*-transport points can also be used in other situations than those described above. These points have traditionally been used to treat according to the seasons and according to the Five Phases.

The five *shu*-transport points and treatment according to the seasons

Both *Huang Di Nei Jing – Ling Shu* and *Huang Di Nei Jing – Su Wen* recommend the use of the five *shu* points for use in seasonal treatments, i.e. using specific *shu*-transport points in different seasons. There is, though, discrepancy between the individual chapters' approach. The use of specific points to treat according to the calendar is similar to the *Tian Gan Di Zhi* or 'Stems and Branches' approach. The focus in this approach is to adapt treatments to the *yin/yang* dynamic of the circadian rhythms, the seasonal rhythms and the sixty-year cycle. Stems and Branches is a fascinating, but also complex, system, based on *yin* and *yang* rhythms, astrology and numerology.

In seasonal treatments, the *jing*-well points are used in winter. In the spring, *ying*-spring points are used, whilst *shu*-stream points are used in summer. *Jing*-river points are used by the late summer and *he*-sea points in the autumn. It can be difficult to base a treatment on this approach, in the same way that it can be difficult to base treatments according to the 'midday/midnight' principle of the horary cycle. There are, however, situations in which it is possible to incorporate or adapt the treatment in relation to these rhythms.

The five *shu* points – transport and treatment in relation to the Five Phases

Each of the five *shu* points are classified in relation to the Five Phases. There is, however, a difference in the sequence between the *yin* and *yang* channels. *Yin* channels have Wood points as their *jing*-well points, whilst *yang* channels have Metal points as theirs. Various acupuncture systems, especially those practised outside of mainland China, base their treatment on the use of points in relation to their Five Phase properties. *Shu*-transport points will be used to tonify and drain *qi* in the various phases and to create a flow of *qi* from one phase to another. Furthermore, each of the phase points are attributed characteristics and qualities that are manifestations of that phase.

This approach is a source of many discussions and disagreements between some acupuncturists. Many TCM-trained acupuncturists consider that this system is too rigid and not always consistent with the physiological and pathological reality, and therefore should not be used literally. It is not only modern TCM practitioners, but also teachers and writers who are more classically orientated, who take this view. Professor Wang Ju Yi, for example, writes in his book *Applied Channel Theory in Chinese Medicine*:

> …theory is dependent on application in the clinic, not the other way around. The points do not conform to five-phase theory; rather five-phase theory represents an attempt to categorize points based on their natural function…they should not be used inflexibly when clinical reality suggests otherwise. (Wang and Robertson 2008, p.484)

As an example he uses He 9 and He 7. In Five Phase theory the Heart's Wood point, He 9, is used to tonify Heart *qi*, and its Earth point, He 7, is used to drain Heart *qi*. In practice, it is more common to use these points oppositely. Another example is Sp 2, which according to Five Phase theory should be one of the most important acupuncture points to nourish the Spleen and the Earth phase. Sp 2 is, however, a Spleen channel point that is rarely used to do this compared with other Spleen and Stomach channel points.

Five Phase treatments are mainly based on *Nanjing*, Difficulty Sixty-Nine. Here it states: 'In case of depletion, fill the respective mother. In case of depletion, drain the respective child.' The mother is the acupuncture point on the channel that is the same phase as the previous phase in the *sheng* cycle. For example, the mother point on the Liver channel is Liv 8. This is because Liv 8 is a Water point and Water is the preceding phase in the *sheng* cycle. By the same logic, it would be appropriate to use the son point Liv 2 when there is a *shi* condition in the Liver. This is because Liv 2 is a Fire point and the Fire Phase succeeds the Wood Phase in the *sheng* in the cycle. The mother point is manipulated with a tonifying needle technique, whereas the son point is manipulated with a draining technique.

Channel	Mother point (tonify)	Son point (drain)
Lung	Lu 9	Lu 5
Large Intestine	LI 11	LI 2
Stomach	St 41	St 45
Spleen	Sp 2	Sp 5
Heart	He 9	He 7
Small Intestine	SI 3	SI 8
Urinary Bladder	UB 67	UB 65
Kidney	Kid 7	Kid 1
Pericardium	Pe 9	Pe 7
San jiao	SJ 3	SJ 10
Gall Bladder	GB 43	GB 38
Liver	Liv 8	Liv 2

The five *shu*-transport points' resonance with certain phases will mean that they also have an influence on the various *xie qi*, which also have a resonance with this phase. This means that these phases or *shu*-transport points can be used to treat precisely this form of *xie qi* when it creates an imbalance in the channel or an organ. GB 34, for example, can be used to treat Dampness and Damp-Heat in the Gall Bladder. This is because GB 34 is an Earth point and Dampness is the *xie qi* that resonates with the Earth Phase.

- Wood points are used to treat Wind.
- Fire points are used to treat Heat or Fire.
- Earth points are used to treat Dampness.
- Metal points are used to treat Dryness.
- Water points are used to treat Cold.

OTHER ACUPUNCTURE POINT CATEGORIES

Many point categories have been created through the years. These can be acupuncture points that one or more writers consider to be points that have an influence on a certain type of *qi* or points that have common characteristics. Other acupuncture point categories are collections of acupuncture points that an author considers to be very effective, a kind of acupuncture point Top Ten.

The acupuncture point categories that I will discuss are:

- the four Sea points
- Gao Wu command points
- Window of Heaven points
- the thirteen ghost points
- Ma Dan Yang twelve Heavenly Star points
- entry/exit points.

The four Sea points

This acupuncture point category is to be found in *Huang Di Nei Jing – Ling Shu*, chapter thirty-three. There are four 'seas' that will have specific symptoms and signs when they are out of balance. The text then lists the acupuncture points that will have an effect on these seas and therefore can be used in the treatment of these imbalances.

Sea	Symptoms and signs in *shi* conditions	Symptoms and signs in *xu* conditions	Acupuncture points
Qi	Distended chest, rapid breathing, red face.	Breathless, the person has no desire to speak.	St 9, Ren 17, Du 15, Du 14
Xue	Feeling of the body growing larger. Discomfort in the body without being able to clarify what it is.	The feeling that the body is shrinking. Vague feeling of illness and unease.	UB 11, St 37, St 39
Nourishment	Distended abdomen.	Hunger, but no desire to eat.	St 30, St 36
Marrow	Lightness of the body, great vigour and strength.	Dizziness, tinnitus, weak legs, blurred vision, desire to lie down and sleep.	Du 20, Du 16

Gao Wu command points

This category originally consisted of four acupuncture points that Gao Wu considered to have powerful influence on certain areas of the body.

These acupuncture points were as follows.

Acupuncture point	The area of the body that the point commands
St 36	Abdominal cavity
LI 4	Face and the mouth
Lu 7	Back of the head
UB 40	Back and lumbar

Two additional points were later added.

Acupuncture point	The area of the body that the point commands or the condition it treats
Pe 6	Thorax
Du 26	Loss of consciousness

Window of Heaven points

These acupuncture points seem to have generated more interest in the West than they traditionally have in China. These ten points are mentioned in *Huang Di Nei Jing – Ling Shu* and have been commented upon by later commentators. They were listed as group acupuncture points, each with their own individual indications, but they are not referred to as a coherent group.

Many Western acupuncturists, especially those who have been trained in 'Worsley style' Five Element acupuncture, view these points as having a powerful influence on a person's *shen* and the person's relationship to the Heavenly *qi*. This is not something that is confirmed by the traditional indications and actions of these acupuncture points, apart from the fact that many of these points have the word *tian* (Heaven) in their names.

Other writers, such as Peter Deadman, believe that *tian* should be seen more as a reference to the fact that the majority of these acupuncture points are located on the neck (Deadman and Al-Khafaji 1998, p.49). The neck is the area between the torso, which is the Earth, and the head, which is Heaven. Most of these acupuncture points' classic indications seem to confirm this view. Window of Heaven points' actions and indications generally relate to the regulation of *qi* between the head and neck. This can be interpreted as having an effect on *shen*, but this will be because they regulate the movement of *qi* to and from the head in the same way that an acupuncture point such as Du 20 does.

The ten Window of Heaven points

- St 9: *Renying*
- LI 18: *Futu*
- SJ 16: *Tianyou*
- UB 10: *Tianzhu*
- Lu 3: *Tianfu*
- Ren 22: *Tiantu*
- SI 16: *Tianchuang*
- SI 17: *Tianrong*
- Du 16: *Fengfu*
- Pe 1: *Tianchi*

Some authors have, through the years, disputed whether SI 17 should in reality be GB 9: *Tianchong*; the logic being that all six *yang* channels would then be represented.

There are five broad areas of treatment that these acupuncture points have in common.

- Regulation of *qi*.
- Problems with the throat and neck.
- Acute disorders.
- Mental-emotional disorders.
- Problems with the head and sensory organs.

Regulation of qi

Window of Heaven point	Can be used to regulate
St 9	Rebellious Lung *qi* – distended feeling in chest, shortness of breath Rebellious Stomach *qi* – vomiting Rebellious Liver *qi* – dizziness, headache, red face
LI 18	Rebellious Lung *qi* – distended feeling in chest, shortness of breath
Lu 3	Rebellious Lung *qi* – distended feeling in chest, shortness of breath, bloody cough
SJ 16	Rebellious Liver *qi* – headache, dizziness
UB 10	Rebellious Liver *qi* – headache, dizziness
Ren 22	Rebellious Lung *qi* – distended feeling in chest, shortness of breath, cough Rebellious Stomach *qi* – vomiting
SI 16	Rebellious Liver *qi* – headache, dizziness
SI 17	Rebellious Lung *qi* – distended feeling in chest, shortness of breath, cough Rebellious Stomach *qi* – vomiting
Du 16	Rebellious Lung *qi* – distended feeling in chest, shortness of breath Rebellious Stomach *qi* – vomiting Rebellious Liver *qi* – dizziness, headaches
Pe 1	Rebellious Lung *qi* – distended feeling in chest, shortness of breath Rebellious Liver *qi* – dizziness, headaches

Problems with the throat and neck

Window of Heaven point	Can be used to treat
St 9	Goitre, swollen lymph nodes, swollen throat, problems swallowing
LI 18	Goitre, swollen lymph nodes, swollen and painful throat, problems swallowing
SJ 16	Goitre, swollen throat
UB 10	Swollen throat
Ren 22	Goitre, swollen lymph nodes, swollen and painful throat, problems swallowing, cold feeling in the throat, neck pain, 'plumstone *qi*', phlegm in the throat
SI 16	Goitre, swollen throat
SI 17	Goitre, swollen or blocked sensation in the throat
Du 16	Swollen or painful throat

Acute disorders

Window of Heaven point	Can be used to treat
St 9	Sudden diarrhoea and vomiting
LI 18	Sudden loss of voice
SJ 16	Sudden deafness
UB 10	Epilepsy, muscle spasms
Ren 22	Asthma
SI 16	Sudden loss of voice after a stroke
Du 16	Sudden loss of voice after a stroke

Mental-emotional disorders

Window of Heaven point	Can be used to treat
SJ 16	Disturbing dreams
UB 10	Mania, hallucinations, epilepsy, seeing ghosts, incessant chattering
Du 16	Mania, sorrow, anxiety, palpitations, desire to commit suicide, sadness
Lu 3	Increased sleep, insomnia, melancholy, sadness, tearfulness, forgetfulness, 'ghost talking'

Problems with the head and sensory organs

Window of Heaven point	Can be used to treat
St 9	Dizziness, headache, red face
Lu 3	Dizziness
SJ 16	Earache, deafness, dizziness, swollen face, visual disturbances, inability to smell, blocked nose and sinuses
UB 10	Eye pain, blurred vision, watery eyes, speech impairment, blocked nose, inability to smell, headache, dizziness
Ren 22	Red head or face, feeling of heat in the head and face, speech impairment
SI 16	Deafness, tinnitus, ear pain
SI 17	Tinnitus, deafness, swollen face
Du 16	Headache, dizziness, speech impediments, blurred vision, nose bleeds

The thirteen ghost points

Sun Si Miao wrote in 652 CE about thirteen acupuncture points that could be used to treat 'ghosts' or *gui* that disturbed a person's *shen*. He recommended them for the treatment of symptoms, similar to the symptoms that are seen in disorders such as bipolar depression (manio-depression), schizophrenia and epilepsy. *Gui* points were to be inserted in a specific order, starting on the left-hand side in men and right-hand side in women.

Acupuncture point	Name	Alternative name
Du 26	*Renzhong*	*Guigong* (Ghost palace)
Du 16	*Fengfu*	*Guizhen* (Ghost pillow)
Du 23	*Shangxiang*	*Guitang* (Ghost hall)
Ren 24	*Chengqiang*	*Guishi* (Ghost market)
Lu 11	*Shaoshang*	*Guixin* (Ghost faith)
LI 11	*Quchi*	*Guitui* (Ghost leg or Ghost minister)
St 6	*Jiache*	*Guichuang* (Ghost bed)
Sp 1	*Yinbai*	*Guilei* (Ghost eye or Ghost pile)
Pe 7	*Daling*	*Guixin* (Ghost heart)
Pe 8	*Laogong*	*Guicu* (Ghost cave)
UB 62	*Shenmai*	*Guilu* (Ghost road)
Extra point	*Haiquan*	*Guifeng* (Ghost seal)
Extra point	*Yumentou* (in women) or *Yinxiafeng* (for men)	*Guicang* (Ghost store or Ghost hidden)

There have historically been differences in which points were included in this category. Some sources have suggested that *guixin* was Lu 9 and not Pe 7, and also that Pe 5 or Pe 8 should be *guilu*. Gao Wu was of the opinion that you should use Du 24, St 17, GB 34 and Liv 2, instead of UB 62, Du 23, LI 11 and *yumentou/yinxiafeng*.

Ma Dan Yang twelve Heavenly Star points

This is a list of the twelve acupuncture points that Ma Dan Yang felt were some of the most effective points – an acupuncture points hit list. Liv 3 was added at a later date, so today the list is as follows.

- St 9
- Lu 7
- LI 4
- LI 11
- St 36
- St 44
- He 5
- UB 40
- UB 57
- UB 60
- GB 34
- GB 39
- Liv 3

Entry/exit points

This point category does not exist in modern TCM texts. The category is, though, used by some Five Phase acupuncturists, especially for those who are inspired by the teachings of J. R. Worsley.

The following acupuncture points will be used when there is a blockage preventing *qi* from flowing from one channel to the next in the twelve-channel *qi* cycle. Entry/ exit points are usually the first or the last acupuncture point on a channel, but this is not always the case. In treatment, the exit point of a channel is used together with the entry point of the subsequent channel in the twelve-channel *qi* cycle.

Entry point	Exit point
Lu 1	Lu 7
LI 4	LI 20
St 1	St 42
Sp 1	Sp 21
He 1	He 9
SI 1	SI 19
UB 1	UB 67
Kid 1	Kid 22
Pe 1	Pe 8
SJ 1	SJ 22
GB 1	GB 41
Liv 1	Liv 14

ACUPUNCTURE POINTS' ACTIONS AND INDICATIONS

INTRODUCTION

In this section I will describe the actions and indications of the various acupuncture points. An action is the properties that an acupuncture point has. An indication is the situations in which this point can be used. The terms used to describe many of the actions attributed to the points can be confusing and incomprehensible to many people who do not have a training in acupuncture or Chinese medicine. This is because many of these terms are direct translations from the Chinese, but also because many of the actions appear to be the same or very similar. There are, however, often significant differences in the actions, even though they sound as if they are identical. For example, expelling Heat and draining Heat are not the same at all. Expelling Heat involves causing a light sweat, so that the exogenous *xie qi* is driven upwards and outwards through the pores. To drain Heat means to drain downwards, so that *xie* Heat is sent downwards and out of the body together with the stools or the urine.

I have summarised many of the actions referred to in the descriptions of the acupuncture points' actions. Most of the actions are obvious and don't need a thorough explanation; others though can seem slightly mysterious or strange.

Activate	Needling LI 4 can, for example, activate *wei qi*, i.e. it creates a movement and circulation of *wei qi*, so *wei qi* is able to carry out its functions. This will in general involve the use of a needle technique that spreads *qi*.
Anchor	Holds something down. For example, treating Kid 4 can help the Kidneys to grasp and anchor the *qi* that the Lung has sent down through the body. It generally requires the use of a tonifying needle technique.
Astringe	Draws together and keeps vital substances such as *jinye* and *jing* inside the body. For example, He 6 holds sweat inside the body, especially when there are night sweats. It generally requires the use of a tonifying needle technique.
Benefit	This action refers to an acupuncture point having a beneficial influence. This will usually be on a sense organ or a specific area of the body. This could be achieved by the acupuncture point expelling *xie qi*, draining Heat or drawing *qi* and *xue* to the area. The technique will depend on the condition being treated.

Brighten	This action is only seen in the context of the eyes. To brighten the eyes means to make the vision clearer and sharper. It generally, but not always, requires the use of a tonifying needle technique.
Calm	*Shen*-calming points are used when *shen* is agitated, such as when there is nervousness or insomnia. Internal Wind conditions, such as dizziness, will also be treated with acupuncture points that calm internal Wind. Once again, both tonifying or draining needle techniques can be applicable, depending on the imbalance.
Clear *xu* Heat	*Shi* Heat must either be expelled through the exterior aspects of the body or drained downwards and out through the stool or the urine. *Xu* Heat on the other hand is cleared. This is done by nourishing *yin* and thereby eliminating the Heat. It generally requires the use of a tonifying needle technique.
Control	Acupuncture points that control can stop sweating or restrain *yang* that rises up to the head. The technique will depend on the underlying condition.
Cool	This action is required when there is *xue* Heat. A draining technique is utilised.
Disperse	Accumulations and severe stagnations need to be dispersed and dissolved. A strong draining and spreading needle technique is relevant here.
Drain	When *xie qi* is in the exterior it must be expelled through the skin. When *xie qi* is in the interior, it must be drained downwards and out of the body, usually through the Intestines or the Urinary Bladder. This will require the use of a draining needle technique.
Expel	When exogenous *xie qi* is still in the exterior, it must be expelled from the exterior aspects of the body. This requires a strong stimulation of the needle to induce perspiration.
Extinguish	This term is used for acupuncture points that can eliminate internally generated Wind, which rises up to the head. This requires a draining needle technique.
Generate fluid	Some acupuncture points enable the body to create more *jinye* or draw *jinye* to a specific area. This requires a tonifying needle technique.
Harmonise	When an acupuncture point harmonises, it creates balance. This is typically necessary when one organ invades another, disturbing its functions. Liv 13, for example, harmonises the Liver and the Spleen when stagnant Liver *qi* invades the Spleen or the Spleen is weak and gets invaded. The technique involved can be a tonifying, draining or even technique, depending on the underlying imbalances.
Heat	Burning of moxa on some acupuncture points will be able to Heat and thereby tonify *yang* when there are *xu* Cold conditions.
Induce labour	These points can be used to start the birth process. This will usually involve a draining technique. These acupuncture points are prohibited during pregnancy.
Lower	Descends *yang qi* or Phlegm downwards.
Move	Used on acupuncture points that move *qi* and *xue* when these are stagnant. This involves a needle technique that is spreading.

Nourish	To nourish is a tonifying quality. *Yin* substances are nourished. *Yin* substances include *yin*, *xue* and *jing*. *Yang* and *qi* will, on the other hand, be tonified, strengthened or warmed. This will once again require a tonifying needle technique.
Open	To open can have multiple definitions. An acupuncture point can open by spreading *qi* in a particular area of the body, such as the chest. This will involve a needle technique that is spreading. To open is also used for acupuncture points that activate and move *qi* in a channel. Finally, to open is used to describe the action of the opening points of the eight extraordinary channels.
Raise	When *yang* is *xu*, it is not able to raise things upwards. Acupuncture points that raise *yang* are stimulated with tonifying techniques that cause *yang* to ascend. These points will usually be stimulated with moxa.
Regulate	To regulate is most commonly used when an acupuncture point moves stagnant *qi* or *xue* or makes *qi* flow in the right direction. Points that regulate are also used when *xie qi* is locked in the *shaoyang* aspect of the body. A spreading technique is generally used.
Rescue *yang*	When *yang* collapses, a person loses consciousness. This is an acute and serious condition. These acupuncture points are therefore used in extreme situations. Moxa is usually a necessity.
Restore consciousness	These acupuncture points will be used when a person is unconscious, either because *yang* has collapsed or because *shen* is blocked by Wind and Phlegm. In *shi* conditions a draining technique or bleeding will be used. When *yang* has collapsed, moxa will be used.
Restrain ascending *yang*	This term refers to the ability of an acupuncture point to control *yang* that is ascending upwards. This requires a draining needle technique.
Send	This action refers to the ability of an acupuncture point to send *qi* in a certain direction. The needle technique is dependent on the underlying imbalance.
Spread	Stagnations of *qi*, *xue* and to some extent Phlegm need to be dispersed. This requires a spreading needle technique.
Stop bleeding	Some acupuncture points have the ability to stop bleeding. The needle technique will depend on the character of the underlying imbalance.
Tonify	General description of techniques that strengthen and increase the quantity and quality of the vital substances or optimise the functions of the organs.
Transform	*Yin* pathogens such as Phlegm and Dampness should be transformed. This may require a tonifying technique in *xu* conditions or a draining technique when it is a *shi* condition.

LUNG CHANNEL ACUPUNCTURE POINTS

Type	Point
Yuan-source	Lu 9
Luo-connecting	Lu 7
Xi-cleft	Lu 6
Mu-collecting	Lu 1
Back-*shu*	UB 13
Jing-well	Lu 11
Ying-spring	Lu 10
Shu-stream	Lu 9
Jing-river	Lu 8
He-sea	Lu 5
Wood	Lu 11
Fire	Lu 10
Earth	Lu 9
Metal	Lu 8
Water	Lu 5
Entry point	Lu 1
Exit point	Lu 7
Five Phase tonifying point	Lu 9
Five Phase draining point	Lu 5

Lung 1 *Zhongfu* (Central Mansion)

- *Mu*-collecting point.
- Meeting point of the Spleen and Lung channels.
- Entry point.
- Starting point of the Lung divergent channel.

Actions

- Sends Lung *qi* downwards and outwards.

- Transforms Phlegm, drains Heat and regulates the water passages.

- Sends Stomach *qi* downwards.

- Opens the channel and moves *qi* and *xue* in the channel and in the local area.

Indications

- **Shortness of breath, dyspnoea, wheezing and shallow breathing:** There are three reasons why Lu 1 has an effect on the functions of the Lung. Lu 1 is the Lung *mu*-collecting point, it is a local point and Lu 1 is an acupuncture point on the Lung channel. This means that Lu 1 can be used to strengthen the Lung in its function of dissipating and descending *qi*. At the same time, Lu 1 transforms Phlegm, Phlegm-Dampness or Phlegm-Heat that have accumulated in the Lung and block the Lung *qi ji*. Lu 1 can, like all local points in the thorax, circulate *qi* in the upper *jiao* when Lung *qi* is blocked by stagnations. Lu 1 can therefore be used in most situations where there is breathing difficulty or where the breathing is affected.

- **Cough:** Lu 1 can be used in the treatment of both chronic and acute coughs. This applies to all types of cough. This is because Lu 1 can regulate rebellious Lung *qi*, descend and dissipate Lung *qi*, transform Phlegm and drain Heat from the Lung.

- **Chest oppression:** In common with other local points in the chest, Lu 1 can circulate *qi* in the thorax. Lu 1 will also regulate the Lung and thereby help the Lung to descend and dissipate *qi*, so that it does not accumulate in the chest. By circulating *qi* in the chest, Lu 1 can also be used for tension in the upper back.

- **Facial oedema:** The Lung spreads *jinye* through the whole body. If the Lung is blocked by exogenous *xie qi*, it can result in oedema in the face. This is the reason why people are often slightly puffy around the eyes when they have a cold.

- **Vomiting, hiccups and abdominal distension:** By sending Lung *qi* downwards, Lu 1 supports the Stomach function of sending *qi* downwards from the middle *jiao*. Furthermore, the Lung channel has its origin in the Stomach. Lu 1 can therefore be used for both Lung *qi* and Stomach *qi* that is rebellious or will not descend.

- **Pain, discomfort and numbness along the course of the channel or in the local area.**

Lung 2 *Yunmen* (Cloud Gate)

Actions

- Regulates Lung *qi*.
- Drains Heat from the Lung.
- Opens the channel and moves *qi* and *xue* in the channel and in the local area.

Indications

Lu 2 is mainly used to treat stagnations of *qi* and *xue* in the local area. It will often be used when there is pain on the front of the shoulder. Lu 2 also has the ability to drain Heat from the Lung and to regulate Lung *qi*. Lu 2 is therefore also applicable in the treatment of coughs, dyspnoea, shallow breathing, shortness of breath and wheezing.

Lung 3 *Tianfu* (Heavenly Mansion)

- Window of Heaven point.

Actions

- Regulates Lung *qi*.
- Drains Heat from the Lung.
- Cools *xue* and stops bleeding.
- Calms *po*.
- Opens the channel and moves *qi* and *xue* in the channel and in the local area.

Indications

- **Shortness of breath, wheezing, dyspnoea, shallow breathing and superficial breathing:** By regulating Lung *qi*, Lu 3 can be used in the treatment of coughs, breathing difficulties, shortness of breath and wheezing.

- **Cough:** Lu 3 can be used to treat coughs, because it regulates Lung *qi*. Lu 3 also drains Heat from the Lung and can therefore be used when the Heat creates Phlegm in the Lung or causes Lung *qi* to become rebellious. Lu 3 also cools *xue* in the Lung and stops bleeding. Lu 3 can therefore be used when Heat agitates *xue* in the blood vessels in the Lung, resulting in the coughing up of blood or blood in the sputum.

- **Nose bleeds:** Lu 3 can be used for spontaneous bleeding in the Lung's sensory organ, the nose. This is because Lu 3 can drain Heat and cool *xue* in the Lung.

- **Somnolence, insomnia, sadness, depression, crying and melancholy:** Lu 3 has the specific action of calming *po*, which is the *shen* aspect of the Lung. This means that Lu 3 can be used in the treatment of mental-emotional problems that relate to a *po* imbalance.

- **Pain, discomfort, numbness and sensory disturbances along the course of the channel and in the local area.**

Lung 4 *Xiabai* (Guarding White)
Actions

- Regulates Lung *qi*.

- Regulates *qi* and *xue* in the thorax.

- Opens the channel and moves *qi* and *xue* in the channel and in the local area.

Indications

Lu 4 is mainly used for stagnations of *qi* and *xue* in the local area. As with all Lung channel points, Lu 4 will have a regulatory effect on the Lung organ. Lu 4 can therefore also be used in the treatment of breathing difficulties, coughs, etc. Lu 4 can also be used to regulate *qi* and *xue* in the chest. This means that Lu 4 can be used to treat the Lung, the Heart and the upper *jiao* in general. Lu 4 is therefore applicable in the treatment of chest oppression, palpitations, pain, etc.

Lung 5 *Chize* (Foot Marsh)

- *He*-sea point.

- Water point.

- Five Phase draining point.

Actions

- Drains Heat from the Lung.

- Regulates Lung *qi*.

- Regulates the water passages.

- Opens the channel and moves *qi* and *xue* in the channel and in the local area.

Indications

- **Shortness of breath, wheezing, shallow breathing and dyspnoea:** As the channel's Water point, Lu 5 will be able to regulate Lung *qi* by draining Heat from the Lung. *Xie* Heat in itself will block the Lung's ability to send *qi* downwards. In addition, Heat, by virtue of its *yang* dynamic, will cause Lung *qi* to rise upwards and become rebellious. The Heat will also lead to the formation of Phlegm, which will further disrupt the Lung *qi* dynamic.

- **Cough:** Heat can both cause Lung *qi* to become rebellious and can create Phlegm in the Lung. By draining Heat from the Lung, Lu 5 can be used to treat coughs. The Heat can also agitate *xue*, causing the blood vessels in the Lung to burst, resulting in the coughing of blood or blood in the sputum.

- **Fever, low-grade fever in the evening and fever on exertion:** Lu 5 can be used to treat both *xu* and *shi* Heat in the Lung.

- **Chest oppression:** By regulating Lung *qi*, Lu 5 will help to spread and send *qi* downwards, so that *qi* does not accumulate in the chest.

- **Vomiting, diarrhoea and abdominal distension:** Lu 5 is a *he*-sea point. *He*-sea points have the common property that they can treat diarrhoea and rebellious *qi*. Furthermore, the Lung channel has its source in the Stomach and passes through the Large Intestine. Lu 5 can therefore be used in the treatment of various digestive problems that involve these organs.

- **Skin disorders:** Bleeding Lu 5 can drain the Heat that is causing skin problems.

- **Oedema of the limbs, blocked urination and frequent urination:** If the Lung is blocked by exogenous *xie qi*, it will interfere with its functions with regards to fluid physiology in two ways: *xie qi* can block the Lung, so that it cannot spread the transformed fluids. This can result in oedema. The blockage will also prevent the Lung from sending impure fluids down to the Urinary Bladder, resulting in a lack of urination. Frequent urination can, on the other hand, be seen when there is Lung *qi xu*. This is because the Lung will not be capable of carrying out its transforming and spreading functions. This can result in an increased amount of fluids, which seep down through the body to the Urinary Bladder. Lu 5, which is the Lung *he*-sea point, is appropriate in both of these situations.

- **Pain, discomfort, numbness and sensory disturbances in the elbow and along the path of the channel:** Lu 5 is an important point in the treatment of pain in the elbow. Lu 5 is also used in the treatment of pain further up the arm when the pain can be related to the Lung channel. Lu 5 can also be used as a 'cross channel' point, when there is pain in the knee on the opposite side of the body.

Lung 6 *Kongzui* (Collection Hole)

- *Xi*-cleft point.

Actions

- Regulates Lung *qi*.
- Stops bleeding.
- Drains Heat from the Lung.
- Expels exogenous *xie qi*.
- Opens the channel and moves *qi* and *xue* in the channel and in the local area.

Indications

- **Cough, wheezing, dyspnoea and shortness of breath:** Like other *xi*-cleft points, Lu 6 is used in the treatment of acute and painful conditions in its corresponding organ and channel. This means that Lu 6 is commonly used to treat acute respiratory problems such as asthma, cough or the consequences of an invasion of exogenous *xie qi* of the Lung.

- **Pain along the path of the channel:** Lu 6 can be used for acute pain along the path of the channel.

- **Bleeding in the Lung, bloody cough, blood in the sputum and nose bleeds:** *Xi*-cleft points on *yin* channels have the additional action that they can stop bleeding. For this reason, Lu 6 can be used in the treatment of nose bleeds, bloody cough and cough with blood in the sputum.

Lung 7 *Lieque* (Broken Sequence)

- *Luo*-connecting point.
- Opening point for *ren mai*.
- Ma Da Yang Heavenly Star point.
- Gao Wu command point.
- Exit point.

Actions

- Regulates Lung *qi*.

- Opens to the exterior and expels Wind.

- Activates *wei qi*.

- Opens the nose.

- Calms Wind.

- Benefits the back of the head and neck.

- Opens and regulates the water passages.

- Opens *ren mai*.

- Opens the channel and moves *qi* and *xue* in the channel and in the local area.

Indications

- **Cough, wheezing, shallow breathing and dyspnoea:** Lu 7 is one of the most important points on the Lung channel, and thereby also the body, to treat respiratory disorders. This is because Lu 7 is the Lung channel's *luo*-connecting point. Lu 7 is especially good at regulating Lung *qi* and thereby helping the Lung to descend and dissipate *qi*. It also has, as we will see below, a huge influence on the spreading of *wei qi*. Lu 7 can be used in all situations in which the ability of the Lung to descend and dissipate *qi* is disrupted. This means that Lu 7 can be used in *xu* and *shi*, external and internal and chronic and acute conditions. It is due to these wide-scoping and powerful actions that Lu 7 is one of the Ma Dan Yang Heavenly Star points.

- **Sneezing, colds, itching in the nose, blocked nose, runny nose, polyps in the nose, poor sense of smell and nose bleeds:** The use of Lu 7 in the treatment of problems in the nose is due to two main factors. The first is that many nasal problems are caused by Lung imbalances, especially when these imbalances lead to the formation of Phlegm and/or rebellious Lung *qi*. The second reason is the relationship that Lu 7 has to the Large Intestine channel. The Large Intestine channel terminates its course at the nose and thereby has a powerful influence on the nose. Lu 7 is a *luo*-connecting point and connects to the Large Intestine channel. Lu 7 is also the place on the Lung channel where a branch separates from the primary channel and connects to LI 1 and is thereby the crossing point between the two channels. It is here that *qi* continues its path from one channel to the next.

- **Fever, aversion to cold, lack of sweating and spontaneous sweating:** Lu 7 has the ability to activate the Lung's function of descending and, not least, dissipating *qi*. This is extremely important with regards to the circulation of *wei qi*. Lu 7 is one of the body's most important acupuncture points to spread and activate *wei qi*. Lu 7 is therefore often used to expel all forms of exogenous *xie qi* that block or disturb the circulation of *wei qi*.

- **Headache, stiffness in the neck and pain in the neck:** Lu 7 is a Gao Wu command point for the back of the head and neck. This is witnessed by the fact that Lu 7 can be used for many disorders that manifest with pain, stiffness or discomfort in this area. The Lung channel does not have a direct connection to the area, but Lu 7 is connected to the Large Intestine channel, which connects to Du 14. Lu 7 also expels exogenous Wind, which is often the cause of problems in the neck and head.

- **Facial paralysis, spasms of facial and neck muscles, tics, loss of consciousness, foaming at the mouth and vomiting:** These disorders can be the result of either exogenous or internally generated Wind. Lu 7 can both expel exogenous Wind and calm internally generated Wind.

- **Retained placenta, retention of a dead foetus and pain in the external genitalia:** The ability of Lu 7 to be used for problems with the retention of the placenta or of a dead foetus can be explained by the fact that Lu 7 can send Lung *qi* downwards. This will support the expulsion from the uterus. Furthermore, Lu 7 is the opening point for *ren mai*, which flows through the *bao*, i.e. the uterus. This relationship to *ren mai* is also the reason why Lu 7 can be used to treat the external genitalia.

- **Blood in the urine, urinary difficulty and painful urination:** The Lung plays an active role in the transformation and transportation of body fluids. A weakening of the Lung's functionality in *xu* conditions and invasions of exogenous *xie qi* can therefore lead to problems with urination. Lu 7 can be used both to treat *xu* and *shi* conditions of the Lung.

- **Poor memory, inappropriate laughter, frequent yawning, sadness and crying:** All *yin* channel *luo*-connecting points have a *shen*-calming effect. Lu 7 can therefore be used to calm *shen*. Lu 7 will be particularly relevant when sadness, sorrow, anxiety and melancholy are a part of the presentation. Lu 7 is especially beneficial in the treatment of sorrow, because it helps the Lung to disperse *qi*, so that the accumulated emotion can be spread and released. Furthermore, by descending *qi* the Lung *qi* creates space so that pure *qi* can come up to the upper *jiao* and thereby also to the Heart. This helps to explain some of the other effects that Lu 7 has on the psyche and memory.

- **Pain, discomfort, stiffness, numbness and sensory disturbances along the pathway of the channel and in the local area:** Lu 7 can be used to treat acute pain along the path of the channel in general and for pain along the pathway of the *luo*-connecting vessel in particular. As a *luo*-connecting point, Lu 7 can also be used to treat pain, discomfort and stiffness in the Large Intestine channel.

Lung 8 *Jingqu* (Channel Gutter)

- *Jing*-river point.
- Metal point.

Actions

- Regulates Lung *qi*.
- Opens the channel and moves *qi* and *xue* in the channel and in the local area.

Indications

Lu 8 is mainly used to treat stagnations of *qi* and *xue* in the local area. As with all Lung channel points, Lu 8 will have a regulatory effect on the Lung organ. This means that Lu 8 can also be used to treat breathing difficulties, coughing, wheezing, etc. By regulating Lung *qi*, Lu 8 can also be used to regulate *qi* and *xue* in the chest and therefore to treat chest oppression and pain in the chest.

Lung 9 *Taiyuan* (Great Abyss)

- *Yuan*-source point.
- *Shu*-stream point.
- Earth point.
- *Hui*-gathering point for the blood vessels.
- Five Phase tonifying point.

Actions

- Regulates Lung *qi*.
- Transforms Phlegm.
- Tonifies Lung *qi*.
- Nourishes Lung *yin*.
- Tonifies *zong qi*.
- Promotes the circulation of *xue* in the vessels and channels.
- Opens the channel and moves *qi* and *xue* in the channel and in the local area.

Indications

- **Cough with sputum, chest oppression, dyspnoea, shortness of breath and shallow breathing or wheezing:** Lu 9 is the Lung *yuan*-source point and thus one of the most important points, together with the Lung back-*shu* point UB 13, to tonify Lung *qi* and nourish Lung *yin*. Lu 9 can be used for all chronic *xu* conditions in the Lung. Lu 9 can also be used in *shi* conditions to transform Phlegm in the Lung, even though its primary focus is on *xu* and interior conditions. This is in contrast to Lu 7, which is more frequently used to treat exterior and *shi* conditions that involve the Lung.

- **Poor circulation:** Lu 9 is the *hui*-gathering point for the blood vessels. This is because Lu 9 can be used to tonify *zong qi*, which is the driving force behind the movement of *xue* through the blood vessels. This means that Lu 9 can be used for problems with poor circulation due to *qi xu*.

- **Pain, discomfort, stiffness, numbness and sensory disturbances in the wrist and along the path of the channel.**

Lung 10 *Yuji* (Fish Border)

- *Ying*-spring point.
- Fire point.

Actions

- Regulates Lung *qi*.
- Drains Heat from the Lung.
- Benefits the throat.
- Harmonises the Stomach and Heart.
- Opens the channel and moves *qi* and *xue* in the channel and in the local area.

Indications

- **Sore throat and dry mouth:** Lu 10 and Lu 11 are the primary acupuncture points on the Lung channel for the treatment of a sore throat. Lu 11 will most often be used at the beginning of an invasion of exogenous Wind-Heat and exclusively in *shi* conditions. Lu 10 on the other hand can be used for both *xu* and *shi* Heat affecting the throat.

- **Cough and rapid and shallow breathing:** Lu 10 is the Fire point of the Lung channel and can be used to treat both *xu* and *shi* Heat conditions affecting the Lung. As with all Lung channel points, Lu 10 can also be used to regulate Lung *qi*, but the most important action of this point is to drain Heat from the Lung and thereby regulate Lung *qi*.

- **Mental restlessness, irritability, anger and mania:** Heat in the Lung can spread to its neighbour organ, the Heart, causing *shen* to become restless and agitated. By draining Heat from the Lung, Lu 10 can ameliorate conditions of mental restlessness, irritability, mania and anger.

- **Pain, discomfort, stiffness, numbness and sensory disturbances in the thumb and along the course of the channel.**

Lung 11 *Shaoshang* (Lesser Shang[6])

- *Jing*-well point.
- Wood point.
- Sun Si Miao ghost point.

Actions

- Expels exogenous Wind.
- Regulates Lung *qi*.
- Benefits the throat.
- Eliminates internal Wind, opens the orifices and restores consciousness.
- Opens the channel and moves *qi* and *xue* in the channel and in the local area.

Indications

- **Sore throat, dry throat, mumps and swollen glands in the throat:** Lu 11 is used primarily in the treatment of sore throats. Lu 11 will most often be used in the initial stages of an invasion of exogenous Wind-Heat and exclusively in *shi* conditions. The ability of Lu 11 to treat acute sore throats is due to two reasons: Lu 11 is a *jing*-well point and also, via the internal pathway of the Lung channel, a distal acupuncture point for the throat.

- **Loss of consciousness:** Like most *jing*-well points, Lu 11 can be used to restore consciousness when internal Wind has swirled up Phlegm and blocked the orifices of the Heart.

- **Mental restlessness, anger, mania, chest oppression or a distended sensation in the chest:** Heat in the Lung can spread to its neighbour organ, the Heart, agitating *shen* so it becomes restless. By draining Heat from the Lung, Lu 11 relieves conditions of mental restlessness, irritability, mania and anger. In addition, *jing*-well points relieve a 'sense of fullness below the Heart'.

- **Pain, discomfort, stiffness, numbness and sensory disturbances in the thumb and along the path of the channel.**

LARGE INTESTINE CHANNEL ACUPUNCTURE POINTS

Type	Point
Yuan-source	LI 4
Luo-connecting	LI 6
Xi-cleft	LI 7
Mu-collecting	St 25
Back-*shu*	UB 25
Jing-well	LI 1
Ying-spring	LI 2
Shu-stream	LI 3
Jing-river	LI 5
He-sea	LI 11
Metal	LI 1
Water	LI 2
Wood	LI 3
Fire	LI 5
Earth	LI 11
Entry point	LI 4
Exit point	LI 20
Five Phase tonifying point	LI 11
Five Phase draining point	LI 2

Large Intestine 1 *Shangyang (Shang[7] Yang)*

- *Jing*-well point.
- Metal point.

Actions

- Expels exogenous Heat.
- Restores consciousness.
- Opens the channel and moves *qi* and *xue* in the channel and in the local area.

Indications

- **Pain in the throat, jaw and teeth:** Conjunctivitis, tinnitus and deafness. LI 1 can expel Wind-Heat that has invaded the body, and it can drain Toxic-Fire. Both conditions can result in pain, inflammation or swellings in the neck, eyes, teeth, gums and ears. These are all areas that the Large Intestine channel connects to. As a distal point and *jing*-well point, LI 1 can alleviate disorders in these areas.

- **Loss of consciousness:** Similar to most *jing*-well points, LI 1 is used to restore consciousness when internal Wind has swirled up Phlegm and blocked the orifices of the Heart.

- **Pain, discomfort, stiffness, numbness and sensory disturbances in the index finger and along the path of the channel, especially shoulder pain.**

Large Intestine 2 *Erjian* (Second Space)

- *Ying*-spring point.
- Water point.
- Five Phase draining point.

Actions

- Drains Heat.
- Expels Wind-Heat.
- Opens the channel and moves *qi* and *xue* in the channel and in the local area.

Indications

- **Pain in the throat, jaw and teeth, conjunctivitis, nose bleeds and blocked nose:** *Ying*-spring points have the common function that they can treat *xu* and *shi* Heat. LI 2 can expel Heat from the *yangming* channel's upper aspects in the face. Heat in the *yangming* channel can be exogenous or can be internally generated.

- **Fever and chills:** LI 2 can expel exogenous Wind and Heat. Invasions of Wind-Heat will interrupt and block *wei qi*, resulting in simultaneous fever and chills.

- **Propensity to fright and somnolence:** Both LI 2 and LI 3 can be used if a person is skittish or has a tendency to somnolence.

- **Pain, discomfort, stiffness or numbness and sensory disturbances in index finger and along the path of the channel, especially shoulder pain.**

Large Intestine 3 *Sanjian* (Third Space)

- *Shu*-stream point.
- Wood point.

Actions

- Expels Wind-Heat.
- Benefits the teeth and throat.
- Regulates the intestines.
- Opens the channel and moves *qi* and *xue* in the channel and in the local area.

Indications

- **Pain in the throat, jaw, teeth and gums, conjunctivitis, sinusitis, nose bleeds, dry nose and blocked nose:** LI 3 can expel Heat from the upper reaches of the *yangming* channel in the face and thus treat Heat disorders in the regions that the channel connects to. LI 3 with LI 4 is an often used combination in the treatment of toothache.

- **Diarrhoea and borborygmi:** The *yang* channels on the arm are characterised by rarely being indicated in the treatment of their corresponding organ. Disorders of the Large Intestine are usually treated with Stomach channel points or with the Large Intestine's back-*shu*, *mu*-collecting or lower *he*-sea points. LI 3 is however one of the few Large Intestine channel points that has specific Large Intestine disorders amongst its indications.

- **Fever and chills:** LI 3 can expel exogenous Wind and Heat. Invasions of Wind-Heat will interrupt and block *wei qi*, resulting in simultaneous fever and chills.

- **Propensity to fright and somnolence:** Both LI 2 and LI 3 can be used if a person is skittish or has a tendency to somnolence.

- **Pain, discomfort, stiffness, numbness and sensory disturbances in the index finger, hand and along the path of the channel, especially shoulder pain.**

Large Intestine 4 *Hegu* (Union Valley)

- *Yuan*-source point.
- Gao Wu command point.
- Ma Dang Yan Heavenly Star point.
- Entry point.

Actions

- Opens to the exterior and expels Wind.
- Activates and regulates *wei qi* and controls sweating.
- Regulates Lung *qi*.
- Stops pain.
- Regulates the face, mouth, nose, eyes, ears, gums and teeth.
- Induces labour.
- Revives *yang*.
- Opens the channel and moves *qi* and *xue* in the channel and in the local area.

Indications

- **Fever, chills, sneezing, headache, lack of or spontaneous perspiration and superficial pulse:** LI 4 is one of the most important acupuncture points of all. LI 4 is especially used to expel exogenous *xie qi* that has invaded the body's external aspects. It can be discussed whether LI 4 is most effective for invasions of Wind-Heat or Wind-Cold. Some authors recommend LI 4 to expel Wind-Cold and SJ 5 to expel Wind-Heat; others the opposite. Both acupuncture points in reality activate *wei qi* and open to the exterior. LI 4 does this by virtue of its relationship to the Lung, whilst SJ 5 is the opening point of *yang wei mai* and thereby controls the body's external aspects. LI 4 can therefore be used for all external invasions of *xie qi*. LI 4 has a close relationship to *wei qi* and thus also the pores. This point will be used to induce a sweat in invasions of Wind-Cold, where Cold has blocked *wei qi* and the pores. LI 4 can, however, also be used together with Kid 7, with a tonifying needle technique, to treat profuse and spontaneous sweating.

- **Stops pain:** LI 4 has a powerful *qi*-moving effect. This is, for example, seen in the much-used point combination LI 4/Liv 3, which moves *qi* and *xue* in the whole body. LI 4 can be used in the treatment of pain in general due to this *qi*-moving ability. It is particularly relevant in the treatment of pain in the face and head. By moving *qi*, LI 4 has a relaxing effect on the muscles and LI 4 is therefore used to relax the body.

- **Headache:** LI 4 can be used in the treatment of several different types of headaches. Headaches due to invasions by exogenous *xie qi* can be relieved when LI 4 activates *wei qi*. LI 4 is used together with Liv 3 to treat headaches due to ascending Liver *yang* and Liver *qi* stagnation. LI 4 can also be used to treat a headache caused by Phlegm.

- **Pain, discomfort, inflammations, bleeding, tenderness, swelling and other disturbances of the throat, nose, eyes, ears, mouth, lips, gums, teeth and face:** Both Ma Dan Yang and Gao Wu classified LI 4 as one of the most important acupuncture points in the body. This is reflected by the effect that LI 4 has on all the sensory organs, the face and the head. The list of disorders that LI 4 is able to treat is almost endless – blocked nose, sneezing, nose bleeds, running nose, dry nose, loss of sense of smell, sinusitis, red eyes, painful eyes, blurred vision, itchy eyes, dry throat, burning sensation in the throat, sore throat, 'plumstone *qi*', swollen glands, mumps, toothache, jaw pain, abscesses, swollen or bleeding gums, facial paralysis, earache, deafness, tinnitus and much more.

- **Induces labour:** LI 4 has the empirical effect of moving *qi* in the uterus and thereby inducing labour. This is the reason that LI 4 is contraindicated in pregnancy. In contrast, LI 4 is used to induce labour, expel the placenta after the birth and as a pain-relieving point during labour. The relationship between LI 4 and the movement of *qi*, and thereby *xue*, in the uterus is the reason that LI 4 can also be used in the treatment of amenorrhoea.

- **Loss of consciousness:** LI 4 can be used to revive a person who has lost consciousness when *yang* has collapsed.

- **Pain, discomfort, stiffness, paralysis or numbness and sensory disturbances in the hand and along the path of the channel:** LI 4 is generally used as a pain-relieving point. As a distal point on the Large Intestine channel, LI 4 will have a strong effect on pain, stiffness, numbness, sensory disturbances, etc. along the path of the channel. LI 4 is an important acupuncture point in the treatment of shoulder and elbow problems, such as frozen shoulder, tennis elbow and other forms of repetitive strain injuries or traumas.

Large Intestine 5 *Yangxi* (*Yang* Cleft)

- *Jing*-river point.
- Fire point.

Actions

- Expels Wind and opens to the exterior.
- Drains *yangming* Heat.
- Calms *shen*.
- Benefits the nose, ears, eyes and throat.
- Opens the channel and moves *qi* and *xue* in the channel and in the local area.

Indications

- **Fever, chills, headache, lack of or spontaneous perspiration and superficial pulse:** Like LI 4, LI 5 can be used to activate *wei qi* and open to the exterior and thereby expel exogenous *xie qi*.

- **Blocked nose, nose bleeds, sneezing, sore eyes, red eyes, sore throat, earache and toothache:** LI 5 can be used both when Wind-Heat has invaded the sense organs and when internally generated Heat has risen up through the *yangming* channel to these areas.

- **Fever:** When exogenous *xie qi* has penetrated to the *yangming* stage, it will create a condition of extreme Heat in the body. This will manifest with a high fever. LI 5, which is the Fire point of the *yangming* arm channel, can drain this Fire.

- **Mania, mental restlessness, insomnia, anxiety and inappropriate laughter:** *Shi* Heat in the *yangming* aspect can ascend and agitate *shen*, resulting in manic behaviour. LI 5 can drain this Fire and thereby calm *shen*.

- **Pain, discomfort, stiffness, paralysis, numbness and sensory disturbances in the wrist and along the path of the channel.**

Large Intestine 6 *Pianli* (Veering Passageway)

- *Luo*-connecting point.

Actions

- Expels Wind-Heat.
- Regulates the water passages.
- Opens the channel and moves *qi* and *xue* in the channel and in the local area.

Indications

- **Fever, chills, headache, lack of or spontaneous perspiration and superficial pulse:** LI 6 activates *wei qi* and opens to the exterior, expelling exogenous *xie qi*.

- **Blocked nose, nose bleeds, sneezing, sinusitis, sore eyes, red eyes, sore throat, earache and toothache:** LI 6 can expel invasions of Wind-Heat in the sense organs, as well as draining internally generated Heat that has ascended via the *yangming* channel to these areas.

- **Oedema and blocked urination:** LI 6 is the *luo*-connecting point and connects to the Lung channel. LI 6 can therefore be used when *xie qi* has disturbed the ability of the Lung to spread fluids throughout the body and to send impure fluids down to the Urinary Bladder. The oedema will be acute and in the upper part of the body, face and arms.

- **Pain, discomfort, stiffness, paralysis, numbness and sensory disturbances on the course of the channel and in the local area.**

Large Intestine 7 *Wenliu* (Warm Flow)

- *Xi*-cleft point.

Actions

- Drains Heat and Fire-Toxins.
- Regulates the Intestines and Stomach.
- Moderates acute conditions.
- Drains *yangming* Heat and calms *shen*.
- Opens the channel and moves *qi* and *xue* in the channel and in the local area.

Indications

- **Sore throats, ulcers and sores in the mouth, inflammation in the skin, abscesses and toothache:** LI 7, which is a *xi*-cleft point, can be used for acute and *shi* conditions along the course of the channel. These will usually be caused by Heat, Fire and Fire-Toxins affecting the *yangming* channel.

- **Fever:** When exogenous *xie qi* penetrates to the *yangming* level, it will create intense Heat in the body. The Heat will result in a state of fever. LI 7, which is a *xi*-cleft point of the *yangming* arm channel, can drain this Fire.

- **Mania, mental restlessness, insomnia, anxiety and inappropriate laughter:** *Yangming shi* Heat can ascend and agitate *shen*, resulting in manic behaviour. LI 7 can drain this Fire and calm *shen*.

- **Borborygmi and abdominal distension:** LI 7 is one of the few *yang* points on the arms that can treat imbalances in its corresponding organ.

- **Pain, discomfort, stiffness, paralysis, numbness and sensory disturbances in the wrist and along the path of the channel.**

Large Intestine 8 *Xialian* (Lower Ridge) and Large Intestine 9 *Shanglian* (Upper Ridge)

Actions

- Harmonise the Intestines.

- Open the channel and move *qi* and *xue* in the channel and in the local area.

Indications

LI 8 and LI 9 can be used to treat problems in the Intestines such as diarrhoea, bloody stools and distension. In practice, LI 8 and LI 9 are, however, not used that often in these situations and are mainly used for pain and discomfort in the arm.

Large Intestine 10 *Shousanli* (Arm Three Mile)

Actions

- Regulates the Intestines and Stomach.

- Tonifies *qi*.

- Opens the channel and moves *qi* and *xue* in the channel and in the local area.

Indications

- **Abdominal pain, diarrhoea and vomiting:** Large Intestine channel points are not used as much as the organ's lower *he*-sea point St 37 and its *mu*-collecting point St 25 to regulate the Intestines. LI 10 can, however, be used to treat *xu* and *shi* conditions in the Large Intestine.

- **Fatigue:** LI 10 is located in the corresponding place on the arm that St 36 is located in on the leg. They also have similar names. Many, but not all, authors therefore recommend the use of LI 10 in the treatment of *qi xu* conditions.

- **Pain, discomfort, stiffness, paralysis, numbness and sensory disturbances in the forearm and along the path of the channel:** LI 10 is an important acupuncture point in the treatment of pain, tenderness and stiffness of the forearm and as an auxiliary point in the treatment of pain in the elbow, shoulder and neck when these conditions are located in the Large Intestine channel.

Large Intestine 11 *Quchi* (Pool at the Crook)

- *He*-sea point.

- Earth point.

- Ma Dang Yan Heavenly Star point.

- Sun Si Miao ghost point.

- Five Phase tonifying point.

Actions

- Drains Heat.

- Cools *xue.*

- Extinguishes Wind and stops itching.

- Drains Dampness and Damp-Heat.

- Regulates the Intestines.

- Opens the channel and moves *qi* and *xue* in the channel and in the local area.

Indications

- **Fever, thirst, profuse sweating and hot skin:** LI 11 is one of the most important acupuncture points to drain *shi* Heat in the body. LI 11 can be used in all Heat conditions, both internally generated Heat and *yangming* stage Heat. LI 11 is usually used to treat Heat in the interior, whereas points such as LI 4 and SJ 5 are used to expel Wind-Heat.

- **Eczema, psoriasis, acne, rosacea, urticaria, dry or red skin, itchy skin or weeping sores:** LI 11 is an important acupuncture point to treat skin disorders. LI 11 can drain Heat and Damp-Heat, cool *xue* and extinguish Wind. This means that LI 11 can be used in the treatment of many different types of skin disorder.

- **Diarrhoea, constipation and blood in the stools:** LI 11 can drain Damp-Heat, which can result in acute and chronic diarrhoea and blood in the stool. LI 11 can also drain *shi* Heat and Fire, which can result in constipation.

- **Sore throat, toothache, abscesses, bleeding gums, nose bleeds, sore throats and ear and eye pain:** LI 11 drains Heat from the *yangming* channel and thus can relieve inflammations and painful conditions in the areas that the channel connects to.

- **Vomiting, acid regurgitation, heartburn, burning pain in the stomach, insatiable hunger, bad breath and increased thirst:** LI 11 can drain Heat and Fire from the Stomach.

- **Mania, mental restlessness, insomnia:** *Shi* Heat in the *yangming* aspect can ascend and agitate *shen*, resulting in manic behaviour. LI 11 can drain *yangming* Heat and thereby calm *shen*.

- **Pain, discomfort, stiffness, paralysis, numbness and sensory disturbances in the elbow and along the path of the channel, particularly where there is swelling and the skin is hot and red.**

Large Intestine 12 *Zhouliao* (Elbow Bone-Hole), Large Intestine 13 *Shouwuli* (Arm Five Mile) and Large Intestine 14 *Binao* (Upper Arm)

LI 14 is a meeting point of the Large Intestine, Small Intestine and Urinary Bladder channels. Some authors also state that *yang qiao mai* meets the Large Intestine channel here.

Actions

- Open the channel and move *qi* and *xue* in the channel and surrounding area.

Indications

LI 12, LI 13 and LI 14 are mainly used to treat pain, stiffness, inflammation and other channel problems in the arm, elbow and shoulder.

Large Intestine 15 *Jianyu* (Shoulder Bone)

- Meeting point of the Large Intestine channel and *yang qiao mai*.

Actions

- Opens the channel and moves *qi* and *xue* in the channel and in the local area.

Indications

- **Shoulder problems:** LI 15 and SJ 14 are two of the most important local points to treat shoulder problems, such as pain and lack of mobility.

Large Intestine 16 *Jugu* (Large Bone)

- Meeting point of the Large Intestine channel and *yang qiao mai*.

Actions

- Opens the channel and moves *qi* and *xue* in the channel and in the local area.

Indications

LI 16 can be used as a local point to treat shoulder problems such as pain and lack of mobility.

Large Intestine 17 *Tianding* (Heavenly Tripod)

Actions

- Opens the channel and moves *qi* and *xue* in the channel and in the local area.

Indications

Local point for treatment of problems that manifest in the throat.

Large Intestine 18 *Futu* (Supports the Prominence)

- Window of Heaven point.

Actions

- Benefits the throat and voice.

- Transforms Phlegm and regulates *qi*.

- Opens the channel and moves *qi* and *xue* in the channel and in the local area.

Indications

Local point for treatment of problems in the throat, such as pain, dryness of the throat, sore throats, itching in the throat, 'plumstone *qi*' (feeling of a lump in the throat, which is not relieved by swallowing), mumps, loss of voice and goitre. Because LI 18 can regulate and transform Phlegm, it can also be used to treat coughs, phlegm in the throat, wheezing or dyspnoea.

Large Intestine 19 *Kouheliao* (Grain Bone-Hole)

Actions

- Expels Wind and opens the nose.

- Opens the channel and moves *qi* and *xue* in the channel and in the local area.

Indications

Local point for the treatment of problems in the nose, such as sneezing, blocked nose, running nose, dry nose, loss of sense of smell and nose bleeds.

Large Intestine 20 *Yingxiang* (Welcome Fragrance)

- Meeting point of the Large Intestine and Stomach channels.

- Exit point.

Actions

- Expels Wind and opens the nose.

- Opens the channel and moves *qi* and *xue* in the channel and in the local area.

Indications

- **Sneezing, blocked nose, running or dry nose, nose bleeds, inability to smell, polyps, sinusitis, blocked sinuses and sores in the nose:** LI 20 is one of the most important acupuncture points for the treatment of problems in the nose.

STOMACH CHANNEL ACUPUNCTURE POINTS

Type	Point
Yuan-source	St 42
Luo-connecting	St 40
Xi-cleft	St 34
Mu-collecting	Ren 12
Back-*shu*	UB 21
Jing-well	St 45
Ying-spring	St 44
Shu-stream	St 43
Jing-river	St 41
He-sea	St 36
Metal	St 45
Water	St 44
Wood	St 43
Fire	St 41
Earth	St 36
Entry point	St 1
Exit point	St 42
Five Phase tonifying point	St 41
Five Phase draining point	St 45

Stomach 1 *Chengqi* (Tear Container)

- Entry point.

- Meeting point of the Stomach channel, *yang qiao mai* and *ren mai*. *Du mai* also meets here, according to some sources.

Actions

- Benefits the eyes and stops lacrimation.

- Expels Wind and Heat.

- Opens the channel and moves *qi* and *xue* in the channel and in the local area.

Indications

- **Conjunctivitis, red, itchy, dry or painful eyes, increased pressure in the eyes, blurred vision, visual disturbances, night-blindness, spontaneous and increased lacrimation, short-sightedness and long-sightedness:** St 1 is an extremely important local point for the treatment of all kinds of eye disorders.

Stomach 2 *Sibai* (Four Whites)
Actions

- Benefits the eyes and stops lacrimation.

- Expels Wind and Heat.

- Opens the channel and moves *qi* and *xue* in the channel and in the local area.

Indications

- **Conjunctivitis, red, itchy, dry or painful eyes, increased pressure in the eyes, blurred vision, floaters, night-blindness, spontaneous and increased lacrimation, short-sightedness, long-sightedness, tics and sinusitis:** St 2 does not have as strong an effect on the eyes as St 1 does, but is sometimes used instead of St 1, as the risk of bruising is significantly less.

Stomach 3 *Juliao* (Large Bone-Hole), Stomach 4 *Dicang* (Earth Granary), Stomach 5 *Daying* (Big Reception), Stomach 6 *Jiache* (Jawbone) and Stomach 7 *Xiaguan* (Below the Joint)

- St 3 is a meeting point of the Stomach channel and *yang qiao mai*.

- St 4 is a meeting point of the Stomach and Large Intestine channels, as well as *ren mai* and *yang qiao mai*.

- St 5 is a meeting point of the Stomach and Gall Bladder channels.

- St 6 is a Sun Si Miao ghost point.

- St 7 is a meeting point of the Stomach and Gall Bladder channels.

Actions

- Expel Wind.

- Open the channel and move *qi* and *xue* in the channel and in the local area.

Indications

The *yangming* channel is rich in *qi* and *xue*. This means that its points are well suited to move *qi* and *xue* in the local area and in the channel. St 3, St 4, St 5, St 6 and St 7 are all important local points in the treatment of imbalances that manifest in the face and the jaw. Their scope is very broad and covers everything from acne and skin diseases to facial paralysis, toothache, tics, pain and discomfort, etc.

Stomach 8 *Touwei* (Head Corner)

- Meeting point of the Stomach and Gall Bladder channels, as well as *yang wei mai*.

Actions

- Benefits the eyes.

- Expels Wind.

- Transforms Phlegm in the head.

- Opens the channel and moves *qi* and *xue* in the channel and in the local area.

Indications

- **Dizziness, headache, heaviness in the head, fuzzy sensation in the head, feeling of being in a bubble, brain fog and difficulty concentrating:** St 8 transforms Phlegm, thereby allowing pure *yang qi* to ascend to the head. St 8 is therefore an important acupuncture point in the treatment of all disorders and symptoms that are caused by Dampness and Phlegm in the head.

- **Eye problems:** St 8 can be used in the treatment of many eye problems, especially tics, lacrimation, pain in the eyes and blurred vision.

Stomach 9 *Renying* (Man's Reception)

- Window of Heaven point.

- Meeting point of the Stomach and Gall Bladder channels.

Actions

- Regulates *qi* and *xue* and controls rebellious *qi*.

- Benefits the throat and neck.

- Opens the channel and moves *qi* and *xue* in the channel and in the local area.

Indications

St 9 is not used as often as its actions justify. This is because it is a difficult place to insert needles and it requires qualified instruction and practice. As with all 'Window of Heaven' points, St 9 lowers rebellious *qi*, which ascends upwards through the neck.

- **Nausea, vomiting, acid regurgitation and hiccups:** St 9 can lower rebellious Stomach *qi*.

- **Asthma, coughs and other respiratory disorders:** St 9 can send rebellious Lung *qi* downwards and therefore be used to treat asthma and coughs.

- **Headaches, dizziness, hypertension and a red face:** St 9 can be used to restrain and sink ascending Liver *yang*.

- **Problems in the local area such as mumps, swollen glands, goitre, sore throat and weak voice.**

Stomach 10 *Shuitu* (Water Prominence) and Stomach 11 *Qishe* (Qi Abode)

Actions

- Benefit the throat and neck.

- Send *qi* downwards.

- Open the channel and move *qi* and *xue* in the channel and in the local area.

Indications

- **Local problems in the throat and neck:** St 10 and St 11 can be used to treat local disorders in the throat and neck. They can also be used in the treatment of respiratory problems, because they can send rebellious Lung *qi* downwards.

Stomach 12 *Quepen* (Empty Vessel)

- Meeting point of the Stomach, Large Intestine, Small Intestine, *san jiao* and Gall Bladder channels, as well as *yin qiao mai*.

Actions

- Sends rebellious *qi* downwards.

- Drains Heat from the throat.

- Opens the channel and moves *qi* and *xue* in the channel and in the local area.

Indications

- **Asthma, cough, chest oppression, hiccups, acid regurgitation, nausea and vomiting:** St 12 can be used to send rebellious Stomach and Lung *qi* downwards. This means that St 12 can be used in the treatment of both respiratory and gastric disorders.

- **Problems in the local area:** St 12 is a local point that can be used to treat shoulder problems.

Stomach 13 *Qihu* (Qi Door), Stomach 14 *Kufang* (Storeroom), Stomach 15 *Mount Wuyi* (Roof) and Stomach 16 *Yingchuan* (Breast Window)

Actions

- Regulate *qi* in the chest.
- Open the channel and move *qi* and *xue* in the channel and in the local area.

Indications

- **Coughs, asthma, chest oppression, heaviness in the chest and shortness of breath:** St 13, St 14, St 15 and St 16 can all be used to regulate *qi* in the chest and the breasts.

Stomach 17 *Ruzhong* (Centre of the Breast)

St 17 is used only as a reference point and is not used therapeutically due to its location on the nipple.

Stomach 18 *Rugen* (Root of the Breast)

Actions

- Benefits the breasts.
- Regulates Stomach *qi*.
- Opens the channel and moves *qi* and *xue* in the channel and in the local area.

Indications

- **Distension or tenderness of the breasts or the nipples, mastitis, lumps or breast abscesses and poor lactation:** St 18 is mainly used in the treatment of problems that relate to the breasts.

- **Chest oppression and heaviness in the chest:** As well as influencing the breasts, St 18 can also be used to regulate *qi* and *xue* in the chest. St 18 can therefore be used in the treatment of respiratory problems.

Stomach 19 *Burong* (Not Contained) and Stomach 20 *Chengman* (Supporting Fullness)

Actions

- Harmonise the middle *jiao* and regulate Lung and Stomach *qi*.

- Open the channel and move *qi* and *xue* in the channel and in the local area.

Indications

- **Coughs, shortness of breath, asthma and dyspnoea:** These two acupuncture points can be used as local points and have a regulatory effect on Lung *qi*.

- **Nausea, vomiting, food stagnation, acid regurgitation, hiccups, abdominal distension and borborygmi:** These two acupuncture points can be used as local points and have a regulatory effect on Stomach *qi*.

Stomach 21 *Liangmen* (Beam Door)

Actions

- Regulates *qi* in the middle *jiao*.

- Harmonises the middle *jiao* and transforms food stagnation.

- Raises Spleen *qi*.

- Opens the channel and moves *qi* and *xue* in the channel and in the local area.

Indications

- **Gastric and abdominal pain, acid regurgitation, hiccups, burping, nausea, vomiting, diarrhoea, burning sensation in the epigastrium and borborygmi:** St 21 can treat digestive problems due to disturbances of the Stomach *qi*, food stagnation or Stomach and Spleen *qi xu*.

Stomach 22 *Guanmen* (Gate Door)
Actions

- Regulates *qi* in the Stomach and the Intestines.
- Opens the channel and moves *qi* and *xue* in the channel and in the local area.

Indications

- **Abdominal distension, abdominal pain, constipation, diarrhoea, flatulence and borborygmi:** St 22 can be used as a local point to treat imbalances of *qi* in the Stomach and the Intestines.

Stomach 23 *Taiyi* (Supreme One) and Stomach 24 *Huaroumen* (Slippery Flesh Door)
Actions

- Harmonise the middle *jiao*.
- Transform Phlegm and calm *shen*.
- Open the channel and move *qi* and *xue* in the channel and in the local area.

Indications

- **Abdominal distension, abdominal pain, constipation, diarrhoea, flatulence and borborygmi:** These two acupuncture points can be used as local points and have a regulatory effect on the Stomach and Intestines. They are particularly relevant when there are psycho-emotional aspects underlying these symptoms.

- **Manic behaviour and mental restlessness:** The points can also be used to drain Phlegm-Heat and thereby calm *shen*.

Stomach 25 *Tianshu* (Heavenly Pivot)

- *Mu*-collecting point of the Large Intestine.

Actions

- Regulates the Intestines.
- Regulates the Stomach and Spleen.

- Drains Dampness and Damp-Heat.

- Opens the channel and moves *qi* and *xue* in the channel and in the local area.

Indications

- **Diarrhoea, blood in the stool, constipation, undigested food in the stool, borborygmi and flatulence:** St 25 is the Large Intestine *mu*-collecting point. St 25 can therefore be used in the treatment of most disorders that manifest in the Intestines. As well as being the Large Intestine *mu*-collecting point, St 25 is also an acupuncture point on the Stomach channel and thereby will also affect the Stomach, which has a great influence on the transformation of food and its transportation down through the Intestines.

- **Vomiting, nausea, gastric and intestinal pain, abdominal oedema and abdominal distension:** St 25 regulates *qi* in the Intestines and Stomach. This will affect the Stomach organ in two ways. First, by being a Stomach channel point, St 25 will affect the Stomach organ itself. Second, St 25 is an acupuncture point that regulates the Intestines so that *qi* flows freely and is not blocked here. This creates space so that Stomach *qi* can descend. This is important, because when there are stagnations in the Intestines that block the Stomach *qi*, and when there is Stomach *qi xu*, the Stomach will be unable to send its *qi* downwards, resulting in the symptoms listed above.

- **Uterine fibroids, lumps and accumulations in the uterus, dysmenorrhoea, irregular menstruations, clotted, dark menstrual blood and red and white vaginal discharge:** As the Chinese name of the point suggests, St 25 is a pivot in the body. St 25 is located on the border between the middle and lower *jiao*. St 25 not only has a huge influence on the regulation of *qi* in the middle *jiao*, it also has a similar action in the lower *jiao*. The *yangming* channel is rich in *qi* and *xue* and is therefore well suited to dispersing stagnations. This means that St 25 can be used to treat more than just digestive problems; St 25 can also be used to treat gynaecological problems caused by a stagnation.

- **Mania and mental restlessness:** Heat in the Stomach and the Intestines can ascend and agitate *shen*. St 25 can drain Heat from these organs and expel it together with the stool.

Stomach 26 *Waling* (Outer Mound)
Actions

- Opens the channel and moves *qi* and *xue* in the channel and in the local area.

Indications

- **Abdominal distension, pain and discomfort in the local area:** St 26 has a regulatory effect on *qi* and *xue* in the lower *jiao*.

- **Dysmenorrhoea:** St 26 can move *qi* and *xue* in the Uterus and thus be used for painful or irregular periods.

Stomach 27 *Daju* (Large Giant)
Actions

- Tonifies the Kidneys and astringes *jing*.

- Regulates *qi* and promotes urination.

- Opens the channel and moves *qi* and *xue* in the channel and in the local area.

Indications

- **Difficult, blocked or painful urination:** Apart from being a local point and a point that can affect the rest of the channel, St 27 mainly influences the Kidneys and the Urinary Bladder. It can be used to promote urination.

- **Premature ejaculation and nocturnal emissions:** St 27 can also astringe *jing*.

Stomach 28 *Shuidao* (Water Path)
Actions

- Regulates *qi* in the lower *jiao*.

- Opens the channel and moves *qi* and *xue* in the channel and in the local area.

Indications

- **Blocked or painful urination, oedema, distension in the lower abdomen, dysmenorrhoea, irregular periods and infertility:** Apart from being a local point and a point that can affect the rest of the channel, St 28 mainly influences the Urinary Bladder and the Uterus. St 28 can be used to treat blocked and painful urination, oedema, distension in the lower abdomen, painful and irregular menstruations, infertility due to cold in the uterus and lumbar pain.

Stomach 29 *Guilai* (Return)

Actions

- Warms the lower *jiao*.

- Opens the channel and moves *qi* and *xue* in the channel and in the local area.

Indications

- **Amenorrhoea, irregular menstruation, fibroids, uterine prolapse, infertility, vaginal discharge and pain and swelling of the vagina:** St 29 creates a circulation of *qi* and *xue* in the internal and external genitalia.

- **Pain in the testicles and penis, testicles that have not descended to the scrotum, premature ejaculation, nocturnal emissions, nocturia and impotence:** St 29 creates a circulation of *qi* and *xue* in the internal and external genitalia.

Stomach 30 *Qichong* (Qi Thoroughfare)

- Meeting point of the Stomach channel and *chong mai*.

Actions

- Regulates *qi* and *xue* in the lower *jiao*.

- Regulates *qi* and *xue* in *chong mai*.

- Opens the channel and moves *qi* and *xue* in the channel and in the local area.

Indications

- **'Running piglet *qi*':** 'Running piglet *qi*' is a sensation that arises when rebellious *qi* ascends uncontrolled up through *chong mai*. It can feel like 'butterflies' in the Stomach and chest, but it can also feel like a panic attack. There are often palpitations, chest oppression, a choking sensation in the throat and an inner turmoil. As well as being an acupuncture point on the Stomach channel, St 30 is also a *chong mai* point. St 30 can therefore be used to anchor rebellious *qi* in *chong mai*.

- **Irregular menstruation, dysmenorrhoea, amenorrhoea, spotting, heavy menstrual bleeding, fibroids, retained placenta and poor lactation:** St 30 is a local point whilst at the same time being a *chong mai* point. *Chong mai* passes through the uterus and at the same time has a powerful influence on the supply and movement of *xue* in the uterus. This means that St 30 is often used in the treatment of gynaecological disorders. *Chong mai* travels up to the breasts and supplies them with *xue*, which is the root of the breast milk. This is why St 30 is used to treat breast problems.

- **Swollen or painful genitals and impotence:** St 30 is both a *chong mai* point and a local point. This means that St 30 can move *qi* in the lower *jiao* and in the internal and external genitalia.

- **Pain, distension, tenderness in the lower abdomen, constipation, blocked or difficult urination and painful urination:** The *yangming* channel is rich in *qi* and *xue* and can therefore have a powerful effect on circulating stagnated *qi* and *xue* in the areas that it passes through.

Stomach 31 *Biguan* (Thigh Gate), Stomach 32 *Futu* (Crouching Rabbit) and Stomach 33 *Yinshi* (*Yin* Market)

- St 31 is the starting point of the Stomach divergent channel.

Actions

- Expel Wind-Dampness.
- Open the channel and move *qi* and *xue* in the channel and in the local area.

Indications

- **Weakness, stiffness, heaviness in the legs, muscle atrophy, numbness or paralysis of the leg:** St 31, St 32 and St 33 all have in common that they can activate the channel in the leg and/or waist, circulate *qi* and expel Wind and Dampness. This makes them useful acupuncture points to treat *bi* syndromes in the legs, i.e. painful blockages of *qi* in the channel.

Stomach 34 *Liangqiu* (Beam Mound)

- *Xi*-cleft point.

Actions

- Regulates rebellious Stomach *qi*.

- Expels Wind-Dampness.

- Opens the channel and moves *qi* and *xue* in the channel and in the local area.

Indications

- **Vomiting, nausea, acid regurgitation and abdominal pain:** As a *xi*-cleft point, St 34 can treat acute conditions in the Stomach organ, especially when there is rebellious Stomach *qi*.

- **Pain along the path of the channel, particularly in the thigh and knee:** St 34 is able to treat acute pain, swelling, stiffness or paralysis in the knee and/or leg.

Stomach 35 *Dubi* (Calf's Nose)

Actions

- Expels Wind-Dampness.

- Opens the channel and moves *qi* and *xue* in the channel and in the local area.

Indications

- **Knee problems:** St 35 is an important acupuncture point for the treatment of all kinds of knee disorders, especially if Dampness and Cold are present.

Stomach 36 *Zusanli* (Leg Three Miles)

- *He*-sea point.

- Earth point.

- Ma Dan Yang Heavenly Star point.

- Gao Wu control point.

Actions

- Tonifies Stomach and Spleen *qi*.

- Nourishes Stomach *yin*.

- Regulates Stomach *qi*.

- Transforms Dampness and Phlegm.

- Nourishes *xue*.

- Tonifies *yuan qi*.

- Drains Stomach Fire and calms *shen*.

- Expels Cold and Damp.

- Rescues *yang* and restores consciousness.

- Opens the channel and moves *qi* and *xue* in the channel and in the local area.

Indications

- **Abdominal pain, nausea, vomiting, hiccups, burping, abdominal distension, vomiting of blood, poor appetite, easily sated, insatiable appetite, gnawing hunger and acid regurgitation:** St 36 is one of the body's most important acupuncture points. It is therefore both a Gao Wu command point and a Ma Dan Yang Heavenly Star point. St 36 has a very wide scope of action. St 36 is used to treat both *xu* and *shi* imbalances in the Stomach and the Spleen, which manifest with digestive symptoms. Typical patterns of imbalance, which can manifest with the above symptoms and which St 36 treats, are Stomach and Spleen *qi xu*, Stomach Fire, Stomach *yin xu*, Dampness, Damp-Heat, food stagnation, invasions of Dampness and Cold in the Stomach and the Intestines, and rebellious Stomach *qi*.

- **Diarrhoea, undigested food in the stool, borborygmi and flatulence:** *He*-sea points can, in general, be used to treat diarrhoea and rebellious *qi*. St 36 has, furthermore, a powerful tonifying effect on both the Stomach and the Spleen. Its capacity is not limited to *xu* forms of diarrhoea and imbalances in the Intestines. St 36 can also be used to expel Cold and Dampness from the Stomach and Intestines and to disperse food stagnation in the Stomach.

- **Fatigue, shortness of breath and feeling run down:** St 36 is an Earth point on an Earth channel and tonifies both Stomach and Spleen *qi*. St 36 can be used in the treatment of all *xu* conditions in these organs. St 36 is one of the most effective *qi*-tonifying acupuncture points. By optimising the production of *qi* in the middle *jiao*, St 36 tonifies *qi* in the whole body.

- **Low immunity, frequent colds and sickness:** The Spleen is the post-heavenly root of *wei qi*. Tonifying St 36 will increase the production of *gu qi* and thereby *wei qi*.

- **Dizziness, palpitations, scanty menstrual bleeding, blurred vision, floaters and dry and pale skin:** Tonifying St 36 will increase the production of *gu qi*, which is the post-heaven root of *xue*.

- **Mania, manic singing, mental restlessness, raving, anger and fear:** Heat in the Stomach can ascend to the Heart and agitate *shen*, whilst Phlegm can block *shen*. By draining Stomach Fire and Phlegm-Fire, St 36 will be able to calm *shen*.

- **Loss of consciousness:** Direct moxa on St 36 can rescue *yang* and restore consciousness.

- **Oedema, heaviness in the arms and legs and lack of urination:** When the Spleen does not transform and transport optimally, Dampness will arise. This can manifest as oedema and heaviness of the limbs, and there will be lack of urine. St 36 is one of the best acupuncture points in the body to tonify the Spleen.

- **Pain along the path of the channel:** St 36 can be used to treat pain in the breasts, mastitis, pain along the tibia, pain in the knee or thigh and paralysis in the legs.

Stomach 37 *Shangjuxu* (Upper Large Emptiness)

- Large Intestine lower *he*-sea point.

Actions

- Regulates the Stomach and Intestines.

- Tonifies Stomach and Spleen *qi*.

- Transforms food stagnation.

- Drains Dampness and Damp-Heat.

- Opens the channel and moves *qi* and *xue* in the channel and in the local area.

Indications

- **Diarrhoea, undigested food in the stool, blood in the stool, borborygmi, flatulence, abdominal distension, constipation and intestinal pain:** St 37 is the lower *he*-sea point of the Large Intestine. *He*-sea points have the common indication of treating diarrhoea and rebellious *qi*. The use of St 37 is recommended for all symptoms that manifest in the Intestines, not only diarrhoea. This is because St 37 will regulate *qi* in the Large Intestine whilst at the same time tonifying Stomach and Spleen *qi*.

- **Shortness of breath, shallow breathing and chest oppression:** St 37 is a distal point for the chest. Furthermore, stagnations in the Large Intestine can disrupt the Lung from sending its *qi* downward.

- **Mania and mental restlessness:** Heat in the Stomach can ascend to the Heart and agitate *shen*. St 37 can calm *shen* by draining Heat from the Stomach and the Large Intestine via the stool.

- **Pain in the shin and weakness or paralysis in the leg:** As a local and a channel point, St 37 can affect the lateral aspect of the tibia and the muscles in this region.

Stomach 38 *Tiakou* (Narrow Opening)

Actions

- Expels Wind-Dampness.

- Benefits the shoulder.

- Opens the channel and moves *qi* and *xue* in the channel and in the local area.

Indications

- **Pain in the lower limb, atrophy of the muscle and swelling, weakness or paralysis of the leg:** As a local channel point, St 38 can affect the lower leg, particularly in *bi* syndrome.

- **Shoulder pain and frozen shoulder:** St 38 is a distal point on the *yangming* channel and is often used for pain and lack of movement in the shoulder when this manifests in the Stomach or Large Intestine channels.

Stomach 39 *Xiajuxu* (Lower Large Emptiness)

- Small Intestine lower *he*-sea point.

Actions

- Moves *qi* in the Small Intestine.

- Regulates the Intestines and drains Damp-Heat and Dampness.

- Opens the channel and moves *qi* and *xue* in the channel and in the local area.

Indications

- **Diarrhoea, undigested food in the stool, blood in the stool, borborygmi, flatulence, abdominal distension and intestinal pain:** *He*-sea points have the common action of being able to treat diarrhoea and rebellious *qi*. St 39 is the lower *he*-sea point of the Small Intestine. This is why St 39 is able to treat not only diarrhoea and rebellious *qi*, but also all imbalances that relate to the Small Intestine organ.

- **Pain in the lower abdomen and pain that radiates down to the testis and to the lumbar region:** These symptoms appear when Cold has invaded the Small Intestine and stagnates *qi*. As the lower *he*-sea point for the Small Intestine, St 39 can regulate *qi* in this organ.

- **Pain along the path of the channel:** St 39 can treat pain in the breasts, mastitis, pain along the tibia, pain in the knee or thigh, paralysis of the legs and atrophy of the muscle in the lower leg and foot.

Stomach 40 *Fenglong* (Abundant Bulge)

- *Luo*-connecting point.

Actions

- Transforms Phlegm and Dampness.

- Opens the chest.

- Drains Stomach Fire and Heat.

- Calms and opens *shen*.

- Opens the channel and moves *qi* and *xue* in the channel and in the local area.

Indications

- **Asthma, cough, dyspnoea, wheezing, sputum in the throat and chest and blocked nose:** St 40 is the primary acupuncture point in the treatment of Phlegm. Phlegm can take on many forms and is involved in many disorders. Phlegm has a tendency to accumulate in the Lung and interfere with its functions. St 40 can be used to treat Phlegm imbalances in the Lung, both because of its ability to transform Phlegm and because it is a distal point that moves *qi* in the chest.

- **Chest oppression, palpitations, heaviness in the chest, difficulty breathing deeply, 'plumstone *qi*' and swelling in the throat:** St 40 is one of the most important acupuncture points to spread *qi* in the chest and the upper *jiao*. St 40 will often be used in combination with Pe 6 and Ren 17 for this purpose.

- **Mental unrest, mania, raving, manic singing and aggression:** St 40 can both transform Phlegm and drain Fire downwards. This means that St 40 can be used to treat mental-emotional imbalances where Phlegm blocks *shen* and Fire agitates *shen*. The combination of these two factors is very typical and is often the root cause of bipolar depression (manio-depression), schizophrenia and similar conditions.

- **Heavy head, headache, dizziness, nausea, fuzzy sensation in the head and difficulty concentrating:** These symptoms are typical of Phlegm-Dampness, which blocks off the orifices of the Heart and blocks *shen*. St 40 can alleviate these symptoms by transforming Phlegm.

- **Heaviness of the body, fatigue and lethargy:** Many people who complain of fatigue and tiredness do not have a *xu* condition but have some form of stagnation, for example Phlegm-Dampness. There can, of course, often be a combination of Spleen *qi xu* and Phlegm-Dampness simultaneously. St 40 can help *qi* circulate freely in the body by transforming Phlegm. This will result in the person feeling lighter and more energetic. Transforming Phlegm and Dampness will also support the Spleen, which is burdened by Dampness.

- **Obesity:** St 40 can be used in the treatment of obesity, because it transforms Phlegm-Dampness that has accumulated in the body.

- **Constipation:** St 40 is an acupuncture point on the Stomach channel and thus an acupuncture point that can tonify the Stomach so it is better able to send its *qi* downwards through the Intestines. At the same time St 40 is an acupuncture point that transforms Phlegm. Some forms of constipation are caused by Phlegm blocking the movement of the stool down through the Intestines.

- **Acid regurgitation and burning pain in the epigastric region:** St 40 can drain Fire and Heat from the Stomach, alleviating pain and regulating the *qi* that has become rebellious due to the Heat.

- **Lipomas, lumps in the breast, ganglions and goitre:** Phlegm can physically accumulate in the tissue and under the skin. St 40 is often involved in the treatment of these accumulations, as it can transform Phlegm.

- **Pain along the path of the channel:** This can be pain in the breasts and chest, pain along the tibia, pain in the knee or thigh, paralysis in the legs and atrophy of the muscle in the lower leg and foot.

Stomach 41 *Jiexi* (Cleft Divide)

- *Jing*-river point.

- Fire point.

- Five Phase tonifying point.

Actions

- Drains Stomach Heat.

- Calms *shen*.

- Opens the channel and moves *qi* and *xue* in the channel and in the local area.

Indications

- **Pain or swelling in the face, frontal headache, dizziness, visual disturbances, red face or reddish rashes and skin diseases in the face:** St 41 is both a Fire point and a distal point on the Stomach channel. This means that St 41 can affect the areas in the head that are traversed by the Stomach channel, especially if there is Heat present.

- **Abdominal distension, constipation, abdominal pain, gnawing hunger and burping:** As the Fire point on the Stomach channel, St 41 can be used to treat Heat conditions in the Stomach. St 41 can be combined with LI 11 in these situations.

- **Mania, mental restlessness, epilepsy and muscle spasms:** Heat in the Stomach and the Intestines can agitate *shen*. St 41 is the Stomach Fire point and therefore can drain Heat from the Stomach, which rises up and agitates *shen* or generates Wind.

- **Fever:** As the Fire point of the Stomach channel, St 41 can be used when exogenous *xie qi* has invaded the body and generated Heat.

- **Pain along the path of the channel:** St 41 can be used to treat pain, swellings, paralysis and other disturbances of *qi* and *xue* in the ankle, foot and the lower leg.

Stomach 42 *Chongyang* (Thoroughfare *Yang*)

- *Yuan*-source point.

- Exit point.

Actions

- Drains Stomach Heat.

- Regulates Stomach *qi*.

- Calms *shen*.

- Tonifies Stomach *qi*.

- Opens the channel and moves *qi* and *xue* in the channel and in the local area.

Indications

- **Pain or swelling in the face, toothache, bleeding gums, red face or reddish rashes and skin diseases in the face:** St 42 is a distal point on the Stomach channel and can therefore be used to treat disorders at the opposite end of the channel. St 42 can affect the areas of the head that are traversed by the Stomach channel, in particular if there is Heat present.

- **Mania, mental restlessness, epilepsy and muscle spasms:** Heat in the Stomach and the Intestines can agitate *shen*. St 42 can drain Heat from the Stomach, which rises up and agitates *shen* or generates Wind.

- **Fatigue, poor appetite, nausea, loose stool and other digestive problems:** Some sources state that St 42, which is a *yuan*-source point, can be used to tonify Stomach and Spleen *qi*.

- **Pain along the path of the channel:** St 42 can be used to treat pain, swelling, paralysis and other disturbances of *qi* and *xue* in the ankle and foot.

Stomach 43 *Xiangu* (Sunken Valley)

- *Shu*-stream point.

- Wood point.

Actions

- Regulates Spleen *qi* and drains oedema.

- Regulates the Stomach and Intestines.

- Opens the channel and moves *qi* and *xue* in the channel and in the local area.

Indications

- **Facial oedema, swelling and pain around the eyes:** St 43 is both a distal point for the face and a Stomach channel point. This means that it has an influence on its partner organ, the Spleen. Both these factors mean that St 43 can be used to treat accumulations of fluid in the face.

- **Abdominal distension, borborygmi, burping and chest oppression:** St 43 can regulate *qi*, both in the areas that the Stomach channel traverses and in the Stomach organ itself. This means that St 43 can be used to treat disturbances of *qi* in the chest, and it can support the Stomach's function of sending *qi* downwards and through the Intestines.

- **Pain along the path of the channel:** St 43 can be used to treat pain, swelling, paralysis and other disturbances of *qi* and *xue* in the foot, leg and face.

Stomach 44 *Neiting* (Inner Courtyard)

- *Ying*-spring point.
- Water point.
- Ma Dan Yang Heavenly Star point.

Actions

- Drains Heat from the Stomach.
- Drains Damp-Heat from the Intestines.
- Calms *shen*.
- Opens the channel and moves *qi* and *xue* in the channel and in the local area.

Indications

- **High fever, profuse sweating, great thirst and rapid heartbeat:** St 44 can be used to drain Heat when exogenous *xie qi* has penetrated down to the *yangming* level. St 44 will often be used together with LI 11 in these situations.

- **Toothache, abscesses, bleeding gums, nose bleeds, sore throats, styes and red and sore eyes:** *Xie* Heat in the Stomach or Stomach channel can ascend to the head, resulting in Heat in the sensory organs that the channel connects to. As a Water point and a distal point, St 44 can drain Heat from the opposite end of the channel.

- **Insatiable hunger, acid regurgitation, burning pain in the epigastric region, bad breath and great thirst:** St 44 is the Stomach channel Water point and can be used to treat *shi* Heat conditions in the Stomach.

- **Diarrhoea, blood in the stool, foul-smelling stool, burning sensation into the rectum and constipation:** St 44 is an effective acupuncture point to drain Damp-Heat from the Large Intestine.

- **Mania and mental unrest:** In common with other Stomach channel points, St 44 can calm *shen* by draining Heat from the body. Fire in the Stomach can rise up to the Heart and agitate *shen*. St 44 and St 45 also have depression as one of their indications. The use of St 44 is recommended when the person 'has a need for silence and cannot cope with the sound of other people's voices'. This can be seen both in depression and when the mind is very agitated, with the person having a need for peace and quiet.

- **Pain along the path of the channel:** St 44 can be used to treat pain, lumps, paralysis and other disturbances of *qi* and *xue* in the ankle and foot.

Stomach 45 *Lidui* (Severe Mouth)

- *Jing*-well point.
- Metal point.
- Five Phase draining point.

Actions

- Drains Heat from the Stomach channel.
- Drains Heat, calms *shen* and restores consciousness.
- Opens the channel and moves *qi* and *xue* in the channel and in the local area.

Indications

- **Toothache, abscesses, bleeding gums, nose bleeds, sore throats, styes, red, sore eyes and dry and cracked lips:** *Xie* Heat in the Stomach or Stomach channel can ascend to the head, resulting in Heat in the sensory organs that the channel connects to. As a distal point on the Stomach channel, St 45 can drain Heat from the opposite end of the channel.

- **Insatiable hunger, acid regurgitation, burning pain in the epigastric region, bad breath and great thirst:** St 45 can be used to drain Stomach Fire. It will often be combined with LI 11.

- **Loss of consciousness:** Similar to most *jing*-well points, St 45 can be used to restore consciousness when internal Wind has swirled up Phlegm and blocked the orifices of the Heart.

- **Mania, mental restlessness, epilepsy and muscle spasms:** Heat in the Stomach and the Intestines can ascend to the Heart and agitate *shen*. Both St 44 and St 45 are in some texts recommended for the treatment of depression.

- **Pain along the path of the channel:** St 45 can be used to treat pain, lumps, paralysis and other disturbances of *qi* and *xue* in the foot and toes, as well as in the face, eyes and mouth.

SPLEEN CHANNEL ACUPUNCTURE POINTS

Type	Point
Yuan-source	Sp 3
Luo-connecting	Sp 4
Xi-cleft	Sp 8
Mu-collecting	Liv 13
Back-*shu*	UB 20
Jing-well	Sp 1
Ying-spring	Sp 2
Shu-stream	Sp 3
Jing-river	Sp 5
He-sea	Sp 9
Wood	Sp 1
Fire	Sp 2
Earth	Sp 3
Metal	Sp 5
Water	Sp 9
Entry point	Sp 1
Exit point	Sp 21
Five Phase tonifying point	Sp 2
Five Phase draining point	Sp 5

Spleen 1 *Yinbai* (Hidden White)

- *Jing*-well point.

- Wood point.

- Sun Si Miao ghost point.

- Entry point.

Actions

- Stops bleeding.

- Regulates the Spleen and the middle *jiao*.

- Calms *shen.*

- Restores consciousness.

- Opens the channel and moves *qi* and *xue* in the channel and in the local area.

Indications

- **Bleeding:** Burning moxa on Sp 1 is an empirical treatment to stop bleeding, especially bleeding from the uterus. Sp 1 shares this characteristic with Liv 1, which is also on the root of the big toenail. Sp 1 can stop all types of bleeding, both bleeding due to *xu* and *shi* conditions and bleeding anywhere in the body. This action can partly be explained by the Spleen's function of holding *xue* in the vessels.

- **Abdominal distension, swollen limbs, diarrhoea, vomiting and poor appetite:** Because Sp 1 is a *jing*-well point, it can be used to regulate Spleen *qi* when it is disturbed by exogenous *xie qi*. Sp 1 can therefore be used to treat the above-mentioned disorders when they are acute and caused by invasions of *xie qi*.

- **Mental unrest, chest oppression, a feeling of unrest in the chest, bipolar depression, insomnia and depression:** There are several reasons that explain the *shen*-calming ability of Sp 1. The internal branch of the Spleen channel terminates in the Heart, and the primary channel terminates in the chest. Sp 1 is therefore a distal point for this region. Furthermore, the Spleen channel connects to the Heart channel in the chest. The *Nanjing* also states that *jing*-well points treat 'fullness below the Heart'.

- **Loss of consciousness:** Similar to most *jing*-well points, Sp 1 can be used to restore consciousness when internal Wind has swirled up Phlegm and blocked the orifices of the Heart.

- **Pain, discomfort, numbness and sensory disturbances in the big toe and along the path of the channel.**

Spleen 2 *Dabu* (Huge Metropolis)

- *Ying*-spring point.

- Fire point.

- Five Phase tonifying point.

Actions

- Drains Dampness and Heat.

- Regulates the Spleen and the middle *jiao*.

- Calms *shen*.

- Opens the channel and moves *qi* and *xue* in the channel and in the local area.

Indications

- **Abdominal distension, diarrhoea, constipation, vomiting, poor appetite, restlessness when hungry and dizziness after eating:** Sp 2 is the Fire point of the Spleen channel. From a Five Phase point of view, Sp 2 is the primary tonifying point on the Spleen channel. In TCM-style acupuncture Sp 2 is viewed as being less important than many other Spleen points in the treatment of Spleen *xu* conditions. Sp 2 is instead seen as being more relevant in the treatment of *shi* Heat conditions and to treat local disorders and channel disorders. This is because Sp 2 is a *ying*-spring point and Fire point and can therefore drain Damp-Heat and Heat, as well as spreading *qi* in the local area.

- **Mental unrest, chest oppression, feeling of unrest in the chest, bipolar depression, insomnia and depression:** There are several factors that explain the *shen*-calming ability of Sp 2. The internal branch of the Spleen channel terminates in the Heart, and the primary channel terminates in the chest. Sp 2 is therefore a distal point for this region. Furthermore, the Spleen channel connects to the Heart channel in the chest. Sp 2 can drain Heat from the channel and from the middle *jiao* – Heat that can rise up and agitate *shen*.

- **Pain, discomfort, swelling, numbness and sensory disturbances in the big toe and along the path of the channel.**

Spleen 3 *Taibai* (Great White)

- *Shu*-stream point.

- *Yuan*-source point.

- Earth point.

Actions

- Tonifies Spleen *qi*.

- Transforms Dampness and Phlegm.

- Regulates Stomach and Spleen *qi*.

- Opens the channel and moves *qi* and *xue* in the channel and in the local area.

Indications

- **Fatigue, weakness in the arms and legs and poor memory:** The Spleen is the root of the post-heaven *qi*, and Sp 3 is the *yuan*-source point on the Spleen channel. This means that Sp 3 is one of the most important acupuncture points that can tonify the Spleen and thus *qi* in general.

- **Abdominal distension, poor appetite, easily sated, nausea, loose stool, borborygmi, flatulence and fatigue after meals:** These symptoms can be signs of Spleen *qi xu* or Dampness blocking the movement of *qi* in the middle *jiao*. Spleen *qi xu* can also lead to the formation of Dampness. The Dampness will be a burden on the Spleen. Tonifying Sp 3 can strengthen the Spleen, so the Spleen is better able to transform Dampness. Sp 3 can also be drained directly to reduce Dampness.

- **Dizziness, poor concentration, heavy headaches, fuzzy feeling in the head, sensation of being in a bubble and heavy arms and legs:** Dampness can block pure *yang qi* so that it cannot ascend to the head. Dampness can also block the orifices of the Heart (the five senses). Sp 3 can transform or drain Dampness as described above.

- **Pain, discomfort, swelling, numbness and sensory disturbances in the foot and along the path of the channel.**

Spleen 4 *Gongsun* (Grandfather Grandson)

- *Luo*-connecting point.

- *Chong mai* opening point.

Actions

- Tonifies Spleen *qi*.

- Regulates the middle *jiao*.

- Transforms and drains Dampness.

- Regulates the Intestines.

- Regulates Stomach and Spleen *qi*.

- Calms *shen*.

- Opens *chong mai*.

- Opens the channel and moves *qi* and *xue* in the channel and in the local area.

Indications

- **Abdominal distension, pain in abdomen, vomiting, diarrhoea, blood in the stool, poor appetite, easily sated, nausea, loose stool, borborygmi and flatulence:** Sp 4 is the *luo*-connecting point of the Spleen channel. The Spleen *luo*-connecting vessel travels from Sp 4 up through the entire intestinal tract and into the Stomach. This means that Sp 4 is able to regulate *qi* in these organs. Sp 4 will also tonify Spleen and Stomach *qi* and transform Dampness. This means that Sp 4 is one of the body's most important acupuncture points to treat disturbance of *qi* in the whole digestive system.

- **Bipolar depression, mental unrest, depression, anxiety and insomnia:** In common with other *yin* channel *luo*-connecting points, Sp 4 can treat mental-emotional imbalances. The Spleen has an influence on the Heart and *shen* in a number of ways. The Spleen is the post-heaven root of *xue*, which nourishes and anchors *shen*. The Spleen also transforms Dampness, which can become Phlegm or Phlegm-Heat, which can either block or agitate *shen*. The Spleen channel also connects to the Heart and the Heart channel.

- **Cardiac pain and chest pain:** Sp 4 is both a channel point and opening point for *chong mai*. Both the Spleen channel and *chong mai* traverse the chest and the Heart. Sp 4 can therefore be used in the treatment of pain here.

- **Irregular menstruation, dysmenorrhoea, amenorrhoea and placental retention:** Sp 4 is the opening point for *chong mai* and can be used to regulate *chong mai*. By so doing, Sp 4 can influence the movement of *xue* in the uterus.

- **Pain, discomfort, swelling, numbness and sensory disturbances in the foot and along the path of the channel.**

Spleen 5 *Shangqiu* (*Shang*[8] Hill)

- *Jing*-river point.

- Metal point.

- Five Phase draining point.

Actions

- Tonifies Spleen *qi*.

- Drains Dampness and Damp-Heat.

- Regulates the Intestines.

- Calms *shen.*

- Benefits sinews and bones.

- Opens the channel and moves *qi* and *xue* in the channel and in the local area.

Indications

- **Fatigue, somnolence, desire to lie down and lethargy:** Sp 5 tonifies Spleen *qi* and thus gives a person more energy. Sp 5 tonifies Spleen *qi* in two ways. Sp 5 can, like all other Spleen channel points, directly tonify Spleen *qi*. Sp 5 can also indirectly tonify Spleen *qi* by draining Dampness.

- **Abdominal distension, diarrhoea, loose stool, borborygmi and flatulence:** Sp 5 can be used in the treatment of digestive system problems by tonifying Spleen *qi* and draining Dampness.

- **Bipolar depression, manic behaviour, mental restlessness, melancholy, excessive worrying, inappropriate laughter and nightmares:** The Spleen has an influence on the Heart and *shen* in several ways. The Spleen is the root of *xue*, which anchors and nourishes *shen*; the Spleen transforms Dampness, which can lead to Phlegm or Phlegm-Heat, thus blocking and/or agitating *shen*; and the Spleen channel connects to the Heart channel in the Heart.

- **Pain, discomfort, swelling, numbness and sensory disturbances in the foot, ankle and along the path of the channel:** There is a feeling of heaviness in the body and pain in the bones (bone *bi*). Sp 5 is used as both a local and a distal point, in the treatment of disturbance of *qi*, along the path of the channel. Sp 5 can also be used to drain Dampness, both in the local area and in the knee.

Spleen 6 *Sanyinjiao* (Three *Yin* Meeting Point)

- Meeting point of the three leg *yin* channels.

Actions

- Tonifies Stomach and Spleen *qi*.

- Drains Dampness and Damp-Heat.

- Calms *shen.*

- Tonifies the Kidneys.

- Regulates the Uterus and menstruation.

- Induces labour.

- Nourishes *xue* and *yin*.

- Cools *xue*.

- Invigorates *xue*.

- Spreads Liver *qi*.

- Harmonises the lower *jiao*.

- Opens the channel and moves *qi* and *xue* in the channel and in the local area.

Indications

- **Tiredness and fatigue, fatigue or weakness of the arms and legs, loose stool, diarrhoea, borborygmi, poor appetite, abdominal pain, abdominal distension and vomiting:** Sp 6 is one of the body's most important or main points to tonify *qi*, *xue* and *yin*. This means that Sp 6 can be used in the treatment of many *xu* conditions in the body. As it is a Spleen channel point, Sp 6 has a particularly strong influence on the digestive system and on a person's appetite. Sp 6 can however also be used to treat *shi* conditions, such as Dampness, Damp-Heat and Liver *qi* stagnation. These *shi* conditions will also be able to disrupt the digestive system.

- **Oedema, heaviness in the arms and legs and heaviness in the body:** Dampness can accumulate in the body tissue and produce a feeling of heaviness. Sp 6 can directly drain Dampness, and Sp 6 can also tonify the Spleen so that it is better able to transform Dampness. A build up of fluids can be caused by *xu* conditions in both the Spleen and Kidneys. Sp 6, which is a channel point on both of these organs' channels, is therefore applicable in both situations.

- **Irregular, scanty or heavy menstruations, amenorrhoea, dysmenorrhoea, spotting, uterine prolapse, vaginal discharge, uterine fibroids, infertility, placental retention, retention of lochia and delayed labour:** Sp 6 is an acupuncture point that can move, cool and nourish *xue*, as well as strengthening the Spleen's ability to hold *xue* and organs in place. This means that Sp 6 is indisputably one of the body's most important acupuncture points in the treatment of gynaecological disorders. The ability of Sp 6 to create movement of *xue* in the uterus and to induce labour means that it is contraindicated in pregnancy.

- **Premature ejaculation, nocturnal emissions, exaggerated libido, impotence, genital pain, blocked urination, painful urination and cloudy urine:** As an acupuncture point on the Kidney channel, Sp 6 influences Kidney *qi* and Kidney *yin*. Sp 6 spreads Liver *qi* and drains Dampness, which can also be a factor in several of these problems.

- **Palpitations, insomnia and being easily startled:** Sp 6 has a *shen*-calming effect. It does this mainly by nourishing *xue* and *yin*, both of which anchor and nourish *shen*.

- **Blurred vision, spots in front of the eyes, night-blindness and dizziness:** Sp 6 can be used for dizziness caused by *qi xu* and *xue xu*. In addition, Sp 6 can also be used to treat visual disturbances resulting from Liver *xue xu*.

- **Muscle cramps in the legs, restless legs and pain in the calf, knee and ankle:** In common with all acupuncture points, Sp 6 can be used for pain, numbness, stiffness, tightness, swelling, etc. in the local area and along the channel. Sp 6 is particularly relevant in the treatment of restless leg syndrome (RLS), where a person has restless legs in the evening and at night. This is because Sp 6 nourishes Liver *yin* and Liver *xue*.

Spleen 7 *Lougu* (Dripping Valley)

Actions

- Tonifies Stomach and Spleen *qi*.

- Drains Dampness and Damp-Heat.

- Opens the channel and moves *qi* and *xue* in the channel and in the local area.

Indications

Sp 7 is mainly used as a local point to treat disorders in the local area and along the channel.

Spleen 8 *Diji* (Earth Pivot)

- *Xi*-cleft point.

Actions

- Regulates *qi* and *xue*.

- Drains Dampness and Damp-Heat.

- Regulates the Uterus and menstruation.

- Stops bleeding.

- Opens the channel and moves *qi* and *xue* in the channel and in the local area.

Indications

- **Dysmenorrhoea, irregular or heavy menstrual bleeding and uterine fibroids:** *Xi*-cleft points are used to treat acute and painful conditions. *Yin* channel *xi*-cleft points also have the characteristic that they have a significant influence on *xue*. This is clearly seen in Sp 8, which is a very important point in the treatment of many forms of menstrual imbalances where there is pain or irregular bleeding.

- **Abdominal distension, pain in abdominal cavity, diarrhoea and poor appetite:** As a *xi*-cleft point, Sp 8 is used to treat acute and painful problems that relate to the Spleen's functionality.

- **Pain, discomfort, swelling, numbness and sensations, tightness of muscles, etc. in the local area and along the channel.**

Spleen 9 *Yinlingquan* (*Yin* Mound Spring)

- *He*-sea point.

- Water point.

Actions

- Regulates Spleen *qi*.

- Drains Dampness and Damp-Heat.

- Opens the water passages.

- Controls the lower *jiao*.

- Opens the channel and moves *qi* and *xue* in the channel and in the local area.

Indications

- **Oedema, swollen legs, diarrhoea, urinary disturbances, vaginal discharge, abdominal distension and poor appetite:** The main action that is ascribed to Sp 9 is the ability to drain Dampness. That is why it is a much-used acupuncture point in the treatment of many different disorders that have in common that they are the result of Dampness or Damp-Heat. Due to its *yin* nature, Dampness has a tendency to accumulate in the lower *jiao*. This means that Dampness and Damp-Heat will often disrupt the functions of the organs that are located in the lower *jiao*. Dampness can also accumulate in the middle *jiao* when the Spleen is weak or when food that has a Damp energy has been consumed. The Dampness will then disrupt the Spleen and Stomach *qi* dynamic (*qi ji*) and in general burden the Spleen.

- **Pain, discomfort, swelling, numbness and sensations, tight muscles, etc. in the local area and along the channel:** Sp 9 will in particular be used when there are disturbances along the course of the channel that are the result of Dampness. This will often manifest with swelling and puffiness. Sp 9, by virtue of its location, is a point that is often used in the treatment of problems on the medial aspect of the knee.

Spleen 10 *Xuehai* (Blood Sea)

Actions

- Invigorates *xue*.

- Cools *xue*.

- Stops bleeding.

- Opens the channel and moves *qi* and *xue* in the channel and in the local area.

Indications

- **Skin diseases, such as eczema, psoriasis, rosacea, urticaria and acne:** Sp 10 is a very important acupuncture point in the treatment of many different types of skin disorders. Sp 10 will be used when there is *xue*-Heat or *xue* stagnation. Sp 10 will usually be combined with UB 17 and LI 11 to drain *xue*-Heat and combined with UB 17, Sp 6 and Liv 3 to invigorate *xue*.

- **Dysmenorrhoea, heavy, irregular menstrual bleeding, spotting and amenorrhoea:** Sp 10 has two major effects in the treatment of menstrual disturbances. Sp 10 can both cool and invigorate *xue*. Some sources state that Sp 10 has a third action that is relevant in both dermatology and gynaecology. They state that Sp 10 can be used to nourish *xue*. Sp 10 can, in the same way as other Spleen acupuncture points, be used to strengthen the Spleen's production of *qi*, which is the post-heaven root of *xue*, and to hold *xue* in the blood vessels. Other authors however are of the opinion that this effect is secondary to the ability of Sp 10 to cool and invigorate *xue*. Their view is that there are other acupuncture points, for example Sp 6, that are better suited to nourish *xue*. On the other hand, Sp 10 is one of the body's most important acupuncture points to drain *xue*-Heat and invigorate stagnant *xue*.

Spleen 11 *Jimen* (Winnowing Door)

- Starting point of the Spleen divergent channel.

Actions

- Regulates Spleen *qi*.

- Drains Dampness and Damp-Heat.

- Opens the channel and moves *qi* and *xue* in the channel and in the local area.

Indications

Sp 11 can be used to treat disorders in the Urinary Bladder and around the genitalia that are the result of Dampness and Damp-Heat. Sp 11 is, however, mainly used as a local point in clinical practice.

Spleen 12 *Chongmen* (Thoroughfare Door) and Spleen 13 *Fushe* (Bowel Abode)

- Both points are the meeting points of the Spleen and Liver channels.

- Sp 12 is also a meeting point of the Spleen channel and *yin wei mai*.

Actions

- Spread *qi* and invigorate *xue*.

- Drain Dampness and Damp-Heat.

- Open the channel and move *qi* and *xue* in the channel and in the local area.

Indications

These two acupuncture points, which are located in the inguinal area, are mainly used to treat local disorders and problems in the Urinary Bladder.

Spleen 14 *Fujie* (Abdominal Knot)
Actions

- Warms and benefits the lower *jiao*.

- Regulates *qi* and controls rebellious *qi*.

- Opens the channel and moves *qi* and *xue* in the channel and in the local area.

Indications

Sp 14 is used mainly to treat local disorders in the lower *jiao*, especially in the Intestines. Sp 14 can also be used to control rebellious *qi* that rises up from the lower *jiao* and disrupts the functions of the Heart and Lung.

Spleen 15 *Daheng* (Large Horizontal)

- Meeting point of the Spleen channel and *yin wei mai*.

Actions

- Regulates *qi* in the Intestines.

- Opens the channel and moves *qi* and *xue* in the channel and in the local area.

Indications

- **Intestinal pain, constipation, diarrhoea and abdominal pain:** Sp 15 is an important local point used to treat all forms of *qi* disturbance in the local area and in particular in the Large Intestine.

Spleen 16 *Fuai* (Abdominal Lament)
Actions

- Regulates *qi* in the Intestines.

- Opens the channel and moves *qi* and *xue* in the channel and in the local area.

Indications

Sp 16 is mainly used as a local point in the treatment of disorders manifesting in the Intestines.

Spleen 17 *Shidou* (Food Hole), Spleen 18 *Tianxi* (Heavenly Cleft), Spleen 19 *Xiongxiang* (Chest Village) and Spleen 20 *Zhourong* (Encircling Glory)

Actions

- Regulate *qi* in the chest and costal area.

- Open the channel and move *qi* and *xue* in the channel and in the local area.

Indications

These acupuncture points are mainly used as local points to treat disorders manifesting in the chest.

Spleen 21 *Dabao* (Large Wrapping)

- Great *luo*-connecting point.

- Exit point.

Actions

- Invigorates *xue* in the *luo*-connecting vessels.

- Benefits the sinews.

- Regulates *qi* in the chest and costal region.

- Opens the channel and moves *qi* and *xue* in the channel and in the local area.

Indications

- **Pain in the whole body:** As the 'great' *luo*-connecting point, Sp 21 is said by some to have the ability to invigorate *xue* in the small *luo*-connecting vessels in the whole body. Others believe that this action is more limited to the costal region.

- **Cough, chest oppression, shortness of breath and dyspnoea:** Sp 21, in common with other channel points, can move *qi* and *xue* both in the local area and along the path of the channel.

HEART CHANNEL ACUPUNCTURE POINTS

Type	Point
Yuan-source	He 7
Luo-connecting	He 5
Xi-cleft	He 6
Mu-collecting	Ren 14
Back-*shu*	UB 15
Jing-well	He 9
Ying-spring	He 8
Shu-stream	He 7
Jing-river	He 4
He-sea	He 3
Wood	He 9
Fire	He 8
Earth	He 7
Metal	He 4
Water	He 3
Entry point	He 1
Exit point	He 9
Five Phase tonifying point	He 9
Five Phase draining point	He 7

Heart 1 *Jiquan* (Highest Spring)

- Entry point.
- Starting point of the Heart divergent channel.

Actions

- Opens the chest.
- Calms *shen.*
- Opens the channel and moves *qi* and *xue* in the channel and in the local area.

Indications

- **Shoulder disorders and axillary and chest pain:** He 1 is mainly used in the treatment of local disorders, such as problems with raising the shoulder, axillary pain and chest oppression.

- **Cardiac pain and irregular heartbeat:** He 1 will also have an influence on the Heart organ and can be used to treat both cardiac pain and an irregular heartbeat and to calm *shen*.

Heart 2 *Qingling* (Blue-Green Spirit)

Actions

- Opens the channel and moves *qi* and *xue* in the channel and in the local area.

Indications

He 2 is used mainly in the treatment of disorders of the upper arm.

Heart 3 *Shaohai* (Lesser Sea)

- *He*-sea point.
- Water point.

Actions

- Drains Heat and transforms Phlegm in the Heart.
- Calms *shen*.
- Opens the channel and moves *qi* and *xue* in the channel and in the local area.

Indications

- **Cardiac pain and chest oppression:** He 3 can move *qi* and *xue* in the Heart.
- **Manic behaviour, mental restlessness and uncontrolled laughter:** He 3 will, as a Water point, drain Heat from the Heart. Heart Fire, especially in combination with Phlegm, has a very disruptive effect on *shen*. He 3 drains Phlegm-Fire from the Heart.
- **Dizziness, red eyes, toothache and ulcers on the tongue and gums:** He 3 will, as a Water point, drain Fire and Heat downwards. Heat and Fire are *yang* in nature and thus tend to ascend to the head.

- **Local pain, numbness, tremors or problems with movement in the elbow and along the path of the channel.**

Heart 4 *Lingdao* (Spirit Path)

- *Jing*-river point.
- Metal point.

Actions

- Calms *shen.*
- Regulates the sinews.
- Opens the channel and moves *qi* and *xue* in the channel and in the local area.

Indications

- **Tremors, spasms and pain in the lower arm:** He 4 is mainly used for the treatment of local disorders along the channel in the forearm, especially if there are tremors and spasms in the lower arm, the wrist or the elbow muscles and tendons.

Heart 5 *Tongli* (Internal Connection)

- *Luo*-connecting point.
- Ma Dan Yang Heavenly Star point.

Actions

- Regulates the Heart.
- Benefits the tongue.
- Calms *shen.*
- Benefits the Urinary Bladder.
- Regulates the Uterus.
- Opens the channel and moves *qi* and *xue* in the channel and in the local area.

Indications

- **Heart palpitations, irregular heartbeat, chest oppression, cardiac pain and pain in the chest:** The Heart *luo*-connecting vessel connects to the Heart and the chest. He 5 can therefore circulate and tonify *qi* and *xue* in the Heart and chest. He 5 is an important acupuncture point used in the regulation of the heartbeat.

- **Pain of the tongue, speech impediments, stuttering, loss of voice and stiffness of the tongue:** The Heart has a close relationship to the tongue, both because the tongue is the sense organ of the Heart and because the Heart *luo*-connecting vessel connects directly to the tongue. He 5, which is the Heart *luo*-connecting point, can therefore be used to treat the majority of problems that manifest in the tongue.

- **Insomnia, anxiety, fear, mental restlessness, sadness and depression:** In common with most Heart channel points, He 5 is an important acupuncture point to calm *shen*.

- **Heavy menstrual bleeding:** The Heart is connected to the Uterus via *bao mai*. One of the functions that the Heart has is to ensure that *bao* (the Uterus) can 'open' when this is relevant in the menstrual cycle. If there is too much Heat in the Heart, the Heat may be transmitted down to the Uterus via *bao mai* and agitate *xue* in the Uterus. This will result in the Uterus opening too much, with heavy menstrual bleeding as a consequence.

- **Incontinence and painful urination:** The Heart is connected to the Urinary Bladder via the Small Intestine channel and via the divergent channel of the Urinary Bladder. This means that emotional imbalances, which create Heat in the Heart, can disrupt the functioning of the Urinary Bladder when Heat is transmitted from the Heart to the Urinary Bladder via the Small Intestine channel or the Urinary Bladder divergent channel. Because He 5 is the *luo*-connecting point, it connects directly to the *taiyang* channel, which consists of the Small Intestine and Urinary Bladder channels.

- **Pain, swelling, numbness and stiffness of the wrist and along the path of the channel.**

Heart 6 *Yinxi* (*Yin* Cleft)

- *Xi*-cleft point.

Actions

- Calms *shen*.

- Nourishes Heart *yin* and clears *yin xu* Heat.

- Controls sweat.

- Regulates Heart *xue.*

- Controls rebellious *qi.*

- Opens the channel and moves *qi* and *xue* in the channel and in the local area.

Indications

- **Night sweats:** Kid 7 and He 6 is a classic acupuncture point combination to treat night sweats that have resulted from Heart and Kidney *yin xu*. Both of these acupuncture points nourish *yin* in their respective organs and both acupuncture points can hold sweat inside the body.

- **Insomnia, mental restlessness and palpitations:** Heart *yin xu* will result in the *shen* lacking nourishment and not being anchored. In addition, the resultant Heat can agitate *shen*. By nourishing Heart *yin*, He 6 can calm *shen*. He 6 is also able to calm the physical aspects of the Heart in *yin xu* conditions; for example, He 6 can be used to treat palpitations.

- **Cardiac and chest pain, and chest oppression:** As a *xi*-cleft point on a *yin* channel, He 6 can invigorate *xue* in the channel and in its associated organ. He 6 can therefore be used to treat stabbing and sharp pain in the chest and cardiac region.

- **Nose bleeds and bloody vomit:** Rebellious *qi* and ascending Heat can cause nose bleeds and bloody vomiting. As a *xi*-cleft point, He 6 can treat acute conditions of rebellious *qi* and uncontrolled bleeding.

- **Pain, swelling, numbness, stiffness of the wrist and disorders along the path of the channel.**

Heart 7 *Shenmen* (*Shen* Door)

- *Shu*-stream point.

- *Yuan*-source point.

- Earth point.

- Five Phase draining point.

Actions

- Calms *shen.*

- Nourishes Heart *yin* and Heart *xue.*

- Fortifies Heart *yang* and Heart *qi.*

- Opens the channel and moves *qi* and *xue* in the channel and in the local area.

Indications

- **Insomnia, mental restlessness, depression, lack of joy, sorrow, sadness, fear, anxiety and poor memory:** He 7 is the *yuan*-source point of the Heart and has therefore a fundamental tonifying effect on Heart *qi*. Furthermore, He 7 is one of the most important acupuncture points to nourish Heart *yin* and Heart *xue*. In particular, its capacity to nourish Heart *xue* and Heart *yin* means that He 7 is used to nourish and anchor *shen*. This is in stark contrast to the properties attributed to He 7 in Five Phase acupuncture, where He 7 is used as a point to drain *qi* from the Fire Phase.

- **Heart palpitations:** Because it can tonify all aspects of the Heart, He 7 can be used to treat disturbances in the physical aspects of the Heart, such as palpitations.

- **Itching:** By calming *shen*, He 7 can have a soothing effect when there is itchy skin.

- **Pain, swelling, numbness, stiffness of the wrist and disorders along the path of the channel.**

Heart 8 *Shaofu* (Lesser Mansion)

- *Ying*-spring point.

- Fire point.

Actions

- Calms *shen.*

- Drains Fire from the Heart and Small Intestine.

- Drains Phlegm-Fire from the Heart.

- Regulates Heart *qi.*

- Opens the channel and moves *qi* and *xue* in the channel and in the local area.

Indications

- **Insomnia, mental restlessness, palpitations, manic behaviour and anxiety:** He 8 is mainly used to treat *shi* Heat conditions, such as Heart Fire and Phlegm-Heat in the Heart, when Heat agitates *shen*. He 8 has a powerful effect on draining Heart Fire. He 8 may, however, also be used to clear *xu* Heat that has arisen in Heart *yin xu* conditions.

- **Painful urination, incontinence, itchy genitalia and genital pain:** He 8 can be used to drain Heat from the Heart that has been transmitted to the Urinary Bladder via the Small Intestine channel.

- **Pain, swelling and numbness or stiffness in the hand or the little finger, as well as along the path of the channel.**

Heart 9 *Shaochong* (Lesser Thoroughfare)

- *Jing*-well point.
- Wood point.
- Five Phase tonifying point.
- Exit point.

Actions

- Drains Heat from the Heart and calms *shen*.
- Extinguishes internal Wind and restores consciousness.
- Drains Fire and benefits the tongue, eyes and throat.
- Opens the channel and moves *qi* and *xue* in the channel and in the local area.

Indications

- **Insomnia, palpitations, mental restlessness, manic behaviour and anxiety:** He 9 has a powerful draining effect on Heat conditions in the Heart. For example, this point is often bled when Heat agitates *shen*, resulting in insomnia.

- **Cardiac pain, pain in the chest and palpitations:** *Jing*-well points have the common indication that they can treat 'fullness below the Heart'. He 9 is also the terminal point on the Heart channel and is, therefore, a distal point that can be used in the treatment of pain, discomfort and disturbance of *qi* and *xue* in the Heart and chest.

- **Loss of consciousness and epilepsy:** Like many *jing*-well points, He 9 is used to restore consciousness when Wind-Phlegm blocks the 'orifices of the Heart'.

- **Pain in the tongue and swollen tongue:** As a distal point, He 9 can treat disruptions of *qi* in the opposite end of the channel. The Heart divergent channel terminates in the throat, and the Heart *luo*-connecting vessel connects to the tongue.

- **Red eyes, pain in the eyes, swelling in the throat and dryness in the throat:** As a distal point, He 9 can treat disruptions of *qi* in the opposite end of the channel. The Heart divergent channel terminates in the throat, and the Heart *luo*-connecting vessel connects to the tongue and the eyes.

- **Pain, swelling, numbness and stiffness in the hand, little finger and along the path of the channel.**

SMALL INTESTINE CHANNEL ACUPUNCTURE POINTS

Type	Point
Yuan-source	SI 4
Luo-connecting	SI 7
Xi-cleft	SI 6
Mu-collecting	Ren 4
Back-*shu*	UB 27
Jing-well	SI 1
Ying-spring	SI 2
Shu-stream	SI 3
Jing-river	SI 5
He-sea	SI 8
Metal	SI 1
Water	SI 2
Wood	SI 3
Fire	SI 5
Earth	SI 8
Entry point	SI 1
Exit point	SI 19
Five Phase tonifying point	SI 3
Five Phase draining point	SI 8

Small Intestine 1 *Shaoze* (Lesser Marsh)

- *Jing*-well point.

- Metal point.

- Entry point.

Actions

- Expels Heat.

- Restores consciousness.

- Benefits the breasts and promotes lactation.

- Opens the channel and moves *qi* and *xue* in the channel and in the local area.

Indications

- **Loss of consciousness:** Similar to most *jing*-well points, SI 1 can be used to restore consciousness when internal Wind has swirled up Phlegm and blocked the orifices of the Heart.

- **Agitation in the chest, a cold sensation and pain or oppression in the chest or in the lateral costal region:** One of the indications that is attributed to *jing*-well points is that they can relieve 'fullness in the area below the Heart'. An internal branch of the Small Intestine channel also traverses the thorax.

- **Febrile diseases, chills, cough, headache and dizziness:** SI 1 can be used to treat symptoms that arise from invasions of exogenous *xie qi*, especially Wind-Heat.

- **Visual disturbances, red eyes, nose bleeds, sore throat, tonsillitis, mouth ulcers and tongue stiffness:** The Small Intestine channel connects to the inner and outer canthus and to the ear. The channel also flows to the throat. As a distal point, SI 1 can be used to treat disorders in the opposite end of the channel. The Small Intestine channel is also connected to the Heart channel, whose *luo*-connecting vessel reaches the tongue. For this reason, SI 1 can also be used when there is a problem with the tongue and in the treatment of mouth ulcers resulting from Heart Fire.

- **Pain or lumps in the breasts, disorders of lactation and breast abscesses:** The primary application area of SI 1 is problems with the breasts, especially when a woman has difficulty breastfeeding due to the breast milk not flowing. SI 1 is often used together with Ren 17 in these situations.

- **Stiffness of the neck and shoulder, neck pain and tension, pain in the arm and the elbow and pain in the little finger:** SI 1 can be used to treat all disturbances of *qi* along the path of the channel. Pain or discomfort in the shoulder and neck region is often the result of a disturbance of the Small Intestine channel.

Small Intestine 2 *Qiangu* (Front Valley)

- *Ying*-spring point.
- Water point.

Actions

- Expels Wind-Heat.
- Benefits the eyes, ears and neck.
- Opens the channel and moves *qi* and *xue* in the channel and in the local area.

Indications

- **Pain or lumps in the neck, mumps, pain in the eyes, red eyes, conjunctivitis, nose bleeds, blocked nose and tinnitus:** *Ying*-spring points have the common characteristic that they can drain *xu* and *shi* Heat. SI 2 can expel Heat from the Small Intestine channel's upper aspect in the face.

- **Fever and chills:** SI 2 can expel exogenous Wind and Heat. Invasions of Wind-Heat will interfere with and block *wei qi*. This can result in simultaneous fever and chills.

- **Stiffness of the neck and shoulder, neck pain and tension, pain in the arm and the elbow and pain in the little finger:** SI 2 can be used to treat all disturbances of *qi* along the path of the channel. Pain or discomfort in the shoulder and neck region is often the result of a disturbance of the Small Intestine channel.

Small Intestine 3 *Houxi* (Rear Cleft)

- *Shu*-stream point.
- Wood point.
- Opening point for *du mai*.
- Five Phase tonifying point.

Actions

- Controls *du mai.*

- Expels exogenous *xie qi* from the *taiyang* level.

- Benefits the neck and the back of the head.

- Calms *shen.*

- Benefits the eyes, nose and ears.

- Opens the channel and moves *qi* and *xue* in the channel and in the local area.

Indications

- **Stiffness, pain or restricted movement in the neck, headache and shoulder pain:** SI 3 is a very important distal point to treat pain, discomfort and inhibited movement in the shoulder, neck and occiput. SI 3 has an effect on this area for three reasons. First, SI 3 is a distal point on the Small Intestine channel, which traverses this area. Second, the Small Intestine channel is also a part of the *taiyang* aspect of the body. *Taiyang* is the exterior aspect that protects the body against invasions of Wind-Cold. When Wind-Cold invades the body, it will often block the circulation of *qi* in *taiyang*, especially in the neck and shoulders and the back of the head. Finally, SI 3 is the opening point for *du mai*, thus having a significant influence on the *yang* aspects of the body, especially the neck and head.

- **Fever and chills, pain or lumps in the neck, mumps, pain in the eyes, red eyes, conjunctivitis, nose bleeds, blocked nose and tinnitus:** As a *shu*-stream point, SI 3 can expel exogenous *xie qi*. As written above, this property is reinforced by the fact that SI 3 is the *shu*-stream point of the *taiyang* channel. This means that SI 3 can be used when there are acute external invasions of *xie qi*. As a distal point, SI 3 will be able to expel and drain *xie qi* from the sensory organs that the *taiyang* channel connects to.

- **Epilepsy and bipolar depression:** SI 3 is the opening point for *du mai*. Two of the indications that relate to *du mai* are epilepsy and symptoms of manio-depression. The treatment of these disorders with SI 3 can be seen in the context of *du mai* connecting to the brain and to the treatment of *yang* pathogens such as internal Wind and Heat.

- **Pain, swelling, numbness or stiffness along the path of the channel:** In addition to the already-mentioned disorders of the occiput, neck, shoulders and sense organs, SI 3 can treat problems in the hand, wrist, elbow and arm.

Small Intestine 4 *Wangu* (Wrist Bone)

- *Yuan*-source point.

Actions

- Drains Damp-Heat.

- Opens the channel and moves *qi* and *xue* in the channel and in the local area.

Indications

- **Stiffness, swelling and pain in the fingers, wrist, elbow, shoulder and neck, headache, tinnitus, jaw pain and lacrimation:** As the *yuan*-source point on a *yang* channel, SI 4 can be used to expel exogenous *xie qi*, which interferes with *qi* along the path of the channel.

- **Jaundice, pain in the costal and hypochondriac region and fever:** SI 4 is an empirical point for treatment of Damp-Heat and Damp-Cold in the Gall Bladder.

Small Intestine 5 *Yanggu* (*Yang* Valley)

- *Jing*-river point.
- Fire point.

Actions

- Drains Heat and reduces swelling.

- Calms *shen*.

- Opens the channel and moves *qi* and *xue* in the channel and in the local area.

Indications

- **Swelling and pain in the neck and jaw, toothache, stiffness of the tongue, visual disturbances, tinnitus, deafness and red and painful eyes:** SI 5 can be used to treat disturbances of *qi* and expel *xie qi* from the channel's upper aspect, which connects to the eyes and ears and traverses the throat and jaw.

- **Manic behaviour:** SI 5 is the Fire point of the Small Intestine channel and can be used to drain Heat and Fire from its partner organ, the Heart.

- **Pain, swelling, numbness and stiffness along the path of the channel.**

Small Intestine 6 *Yanglao* (Supporting the Aged)

- *Xi*-cleft point.

Actions

- Brightens the eyes.

- Relieves acute and painful conditions.

- Opens the channel and moves *qi* and *xue* in the channel and in the local area.

Indications

- **Blurred vision and pain in the eyes:** SI 6 can be used to treat problems with the eyes when these imbalances are caused by Heart or Small Intestine imbalances. This is because the Heart *luo*-connecting channel and the Small Intestine and Heart primary channels all connect to the eyes.

- **Shoulder pain, pain in the upper part of the back around the scapula and lumbar pain:** As a *xi*-cleft point, SI 6 can treat acute and painful conditions along the path of the channel. Both aspects of the *taiyang* channel traverse the upper part of the back, and the Small Intestine channel passes over the shoulder joint. SI 6 can treat acute lumbar pain that is related to the Urinary Bladder channel. This is due to the Small Intestine's *taiyang* relationship to the Urinary Bladder channel.

- **Pain, discomfort, stiffness, paralysis, numbness and sensory disturbances along the path of the channel and in the local area.**

Small Intestine 7 *Wenliu* (Branch to the Correct)

- *Luo*-connecting point.

Actions

- Expels Wind-Heat.

- Calms *shen.*

- Opens the channel and moves *qi* and *xue* in the channel and surrounding area.

Indications

- **Fever and chills, pain and stiffness in the neck and on the back of the head and headache:** As a *taiyang* point, SI 7 can expel exogenous *xie qi* from the exterior aspects of the body. These invasions will often start with fever and chills. When the *taiyang* aspect is invaded by *xie qi*, there will often be a headache and stiffness in the neck and shoulders.

- **Blurred vision and pain in the eyes:** SI 7, which is the Small Intestine channel *luo*-connecting point, can be used to address problems of the eyes when these problems are caused by Heart or Small Intestine imbalances. This is because the Heart *luo*-connecting vessel and the Small Intestine and the Heart primary channels all connect to the eyes.

- **Manic behaviour, mental restlessness, depression, sadness, anxiety and fear:** SI 7 has a *shen*-calming effect, because SI 7 is the Small Intestine *luo*-connecting point. As a *luo*-connecting point, SI 7 can drain Heat from its partner organ, the Heart.

- **Pain, discomfort, stiffness, paralysis or numbness and sensory disturbances in the shoulder and elbow and along the path of the channel:** *Luo*-connecting points are especially useful to expel *xie qi* that blocks the small *luo* network vessels around the large joints.

Small Intestine 8 *Xiaohai* (Small Sea)

- *He*-sea point.
- Earth point.
- Five Phase draining point.

Actions

- Drains Damp-Heat.
- Opens the channel and moves *qi* and *xue* in the channel and in the local area.

Indications

- **Swelling and pain in the neck, jaw, teeth and gums:** As a *he*-sea point, SI 8 can drain *xie qi* from the channel.

- **Pain, discomfort, stiffness, paralysis or numbness and sensory disturbances in the shoulder and elbow and along the pathway of the channel:** As a channel point, SI 8 can be used to address problems in the shoulder and neck. SI 8 can also be used as a local point to treat elbow problems.

Small Intestine 9 *Jianzhen* (True Shoulder), Small Intestine 10 *Naoshu* (Upper Arm Point), Small Intestine 11 *Tianzong* (Heavenly Gathering), Small Intestine 12 *Bingfeng* (Grasping the Wind), Small Intestine 13 *Quyuan* (Curved Wall) and Small Intestine 14 *Jianwaishu* (Outer Shoulder Point)

- SI 10 is a meeting point of the Small Intestine channel, *yang wei mai* and *yang qiao mai*.

- SI 12 is a meeting point of the Small Intestine, Gall Bladder, *san jiao* and Large Intestine channels.

Actions

- Benefit the shoulder and scapula region.

- Open the channel and move *qi* and *xue* in the channel and in the local area.

Indications

- **Local disorders:** What all these acupuncture points have in common is that they are important acupuncture points to disperse stagnated *qi* and *xue* in the local area. They can also expel exogenous *qi* that blocks the channel's *qi* in the local area. These acupuncture points are often sore on palpation when there is shoulder pain. SI 11 can also be used to treat problems in the breasts, such as sores and swellings, as well as poor lactation.

Small Intestine 15 *Jianzhongshu* (Middle Shoulder Point)

Actions

- Regulates Lung *qi*.

- Opens the channel and moves *qi* and *xue* in the channel and in the local area.

Indications

- **Local disorders:** SI 15 is also an important local point to treat problems in the shoulder area. SI 15 can also regulate Lung *qi* and can therefore be used to treat coughs.

Small Intestine 16 *Tianchuang* (Heavenly Window) and Small Intestine 17 *Tianrong* (Heavenly Hood)

- Both acupuncture points are Window of Heaven points.

Actions

- Regulate rebellious *qi*.
- Open the channel and move *qi* and *xue* in the channel and in the local area.

Indications

- **Swellings in the throat, sore throat, goitre, mumps and swollen lymph nodes in the throat, as well as hoarseness and muteness after a cerebral haemorrhage:** Both acupuncture points are Window of Heaven points and thus can be used to regulate *qi* to and from the head and in the throat.

- **Headaches, tinnitus and deafness:** As Window of Heaven points they can regulate the movement of *qi* between the head and the body.

- **Manic behaviour:** SI 16 can also be used to calm *shen* in manic conditions.

Small Intestine 18 *Quanliao* (Cheekbone Hole)

- Meeting point of the Small Intestine and *san jiao* channels.

Actions

- Expels Wind.
- Drains Heat and reduces swelling.
- Opens the channel and moves *qi* and *xue* in the channel and in the local area.

Indications

- **Local disorders:** SI 18 is used as a local point to treat problems in the jaw, teeth, sinuses, mouth and cheek. SI 18 is often used in the treatment of facial paralysis, trigeminal neuralgia and tics.

Small Intestine 19 *Tinggong* (Auditory Palace)

- Meeting point of the Small Intestine, Gall Bladder and *san jiao* channels.
- Exit point.

Actions

- Benefits the ears.
- Opens the channel and moves *qi* and *xue* in the channel and in the local area.

Indications

- **Local disorders:** SI 19 is used in the treatment of all the problems with the ears such as otitis media, deafness, tinnitus and itching in the ears. SI 19 can also be used to calm *shen*.

URINARY BLADDER CHANNEL ACUPUNCTURE POINTS

Type	Point
Yuan-source	UB 64
Luo-connecting	UB 58
Xi-cleft	UB 63
Mu-collecting	Ren 3
Back-*shu*	UB 28
Jing-well	UB 67
Ying-spring	UB 66
Shu-stream	UB 65
Jing-river	UB 60
He-sea	UB 40
Metal	UB 67
Water	UB 66
Wood	UB 65
Fire	UB 60
Earth	UB 40
Entry point	UB 1
Exit point	UB 67
Five Phase tonifying point	UB 67
Five Phase draining point	UB 65

Urinary Bladder 1 *Jingming* (Bright Eyes)

- Meeting point of the Urinary Bladder, Small Intestine, Gall Bladder, *san jiao* and Stomach channels, as well as *yang qiao mai*, *yin qiao mai* and *du mai*.

- Entry point.

Actions

- Benefits the eyes.

- Expels Wind and Heat.

- Opens the channel and moves *qi* and *xue* in the channel and in the local area.

Indications

- **Conjunctivitis, red, itchy, dry or painful eyes, increased pressure in the eye, blurred vision, flickering in front of the eyes, night-blindness, spontaneous lacrimation, short-sightedness and long-sightedness:** UB 1 is a very important local point used to treat all forms of eye problems.

- **Headache:** UB 1 can also be used to treat a headache, especially when the headache is caused by invasions of Cold in the *taiyang* channel.

- **Insomnia:** UB 1 is a meeting point of many channels, but it is particularly its relationship to *yin qiao mai* and *yang qiao mai* that make UB 1 relevant in the treatment of insomnia.

Urinary Bladder 2 *Zanzhu* (Bamboo Gathering)

Actions

- Benefits the eyes and stops lacrimation.
- Expels Wind and Heat.
- Opens the channel and moves *qi* and *xue* in the channel and in the local area.

Indications

- **Conjunctivitis, red, itchy, dry or painful eyes, pressure in or behind the eyes, blurred vision, spots in the visual field, night-blindness, spontaneous lacrimation, short-sightedness, long-sightedness and tics:** UB 2 circulates *qi* and *xue* in the local area.

- **Sinusitis and frontal headaches:** UB 2 is an important acupuncture point in the treatment of sinusitis and can also be used to treat frontal headaches.

- **Haemorrhoids:** Due to the pathway of the Urinary Bladder divergent channel, UB 2 can also be used to treat haemorrhoids.

Urinary Bladder 3 *Meichong* (Eyebrow Thoroughfare), Urinary Bladder 4 *Quchai* (Deviating Bend), Urinary Bladder 5 *Wuchu* (Fifth Place), Urinary Bladder 6 *Chengguang* (Receiving Light) and Urinary Bladder 7 *Tongtian* (Heavenly Connection)

Actions

- Expel Wind, transform Phlegm in the head and relieve pain.

- Benefit and regulate the nose and eyes.

- Open the channel and move *qi* and *xue* in the channel and in the local area.

Indications

- **Local problems:** All of these points can be used as local points in the treatment of headaches, dizziness and a feeling of heaviness in the head. Because of the Urinary Bladder channel's connection to the eyes and upper part of the nose, these points can also be used in the treatment of eye disorders, blocked nose, sneezing and nose bleeds.

Urinary Bladder 8 *Luoque* (Declining Connection)

Actions

- Calms Wind, transforms Phlegm and calms *shen*.

- Benefits the sense organs.

- Opens the channel and moves *qi* and *xue* in the channel and in the local area.

Indications

- **Dizziness, bipolar disorder and epilepsy:** UB 8 can be used in the treatment of Wind and Phlegm that disturbs *qi* in the head.

- **Problems in the eye and nose:** UB 8 circulates *qi* and *xue* in the eyes and nose.

Urinary Bladder 9 *Juzhen* (Jade Pillow)

Actions

- Expels Wind and Cold and relieves pain.

- Benefits the nose and eyes.

- Opens the channel and moves *qi* and *xue* in the channel and in the local area.

Indications

- **Headache and eye and nose problems:** UB 9 can be used to expel invasions of Wind-Cold in the *taiyang* aspect that manifest with a headache. UB 9 can also be used to treat problems in the eye and nose.

Urinary Bladder 10 *Tianzhu* (Heavenly Pillar)

- Window of Heaven point.

Actions

- Expels exogenous Wind and calms internal Wind.

- Opens the orifices.

- Calms *shen*.

- Opens the channel and moves *qi* and *xue* in the channel and in the local area.

Indications

- **Aversion to cold, fever, soreness in the muscles, headache, dizziness, heaviness in the head, stiffness in the neck and muscle spasms:** UB 10 is an important acupuncture point in the treatment of disorders that are caused by both internal and exogenous Wind. This property is shared with GB 20 and Du 16, which are also located in the same region of the neck. UB 10 is particularly important in the treatment of invasions of Wind-Cold, because UB 10 is an acupuncture point on the *taiyang* channel, which protects the body against exogenous Cold.

- **No sense of smell, blocked nose, red and painful eyes, blurred vision and lacrimation:** One of the characteristics of Window of Heaven points is that they can treat problems in the sense organs. The Urinary Bladder channel also connects to the eyes and upper region of the nose.

- **Manic behaviour, incessant talking, epilepsy and upwardly staring eyes:** Many Window of Heaven points have *shen*-calming properties. The Urinary Bladder channel also passes through the brain.

- **Pain in the neck and lumbar:** UB 10 can be used as a local point in the treatment of neck pain and as a distal point to treat lumbar pain.

Urinary Bladder 11 *Dazhu* (Large Shuttle)

- *Hui*-gathering point for bones.

- Meeting point of the Urinary Bladder, Small Intestine, *san jiao* and Gall Bladder channels, as well as *du mai*.

Actions

- Benefits the bones and joints.

- Expels Wind and protects the exterior.

- Regulates Lung *qi*.

- Opens the channel and moves *qi* and *xue* in the channel and in the local area.

Indications

- **Muscular-skeletal disorders, stiffness of the neck and spine, back pain and pain and deformities of the joints:** UB 11 is the *hui*-gathering point for the bones and has traditionally been used in the treatment of bone disorders, including 'bone *bi*', where exogenous *xie qi* has penetrated deep into the joints and become a chronic stagnation, resulting in deformity of the joint.

- **Aversion to cold, sore muscles, lack of sweat, headache and dizziness:** Similar to UB 12 and UB 13, UB 11 is used to expel invasions of Wind-Cold from the *taiyang* stage.

- **Frequent colds and aversion to wind and draughts:** UB 11 can, like UB 12 and UB 13, be used to activate *wei qi* and thus protect the body's exterior aspects.

- **Cough, chest oppression, shortness of breath and shallow breathing:** Like UB 12 and UB 13, UB 11 can be used to regulate Lung *qi*.

Urinary Bladder 12 *Fengmen* (Wind Door)

- Meeting point of the Urinary Bladder channel and *du mai*.

Actions

- Expels exogenous Wind.

- Tonifies *wei qi* and protects the exterior.

- Regulates Lung *qi*.

- Benefits the nose.

- Opens the channel and moves *qi* and *xue* in the channel and in the local area.

Indications

- **Frequent colds and aversion to wind and draughts:** UB 12 has a close relationship to the Lung and can be used to strengthen and activate *wei qi* and thus protect the body's exterior aspect.

- **Aversion to cold, sore muscles, lack of perspiration, sore throat, headache and dizziness:** The three Urinary Bladder channel points at the top of the back can all activate *wei qi* and expel exogenous *xie qi* from the Lung and from the *taiyang* stage.

- **Blocked or running nose, no sense of smell and nose bleeds:** By virtue of its close relationship to the Lung, UB 12 can influence the Lung's sensory organ, the nose. UB 12 can therefore be used to treat disorders that manifest in the nose.

- **Cough, chest oppression, shortness of breath and shallow breathing:** Similar to UB 11 and UB 13, UB 12 can be used to regulate Lung *qi* and thereby treat various types of cough and respiratory problems.

- **Urticaria and pustules on the back:** UB 12 can be used in the treatment of some types of skin disorders on the back. This is because UB 12 is a local point and an acupuncture point that can expel Wind. Furthermore, the skin is an aspect of the Lung, and UB 12 has a close relationship to the Lung.

- **Pain and stiffness in the local area, neck and lumbar region:** As a channel point, UB 12 can be used to treat pain in the local area and along the path of the channel.

Urinary Bladder 13 *Feishu* (Lung *Shu*)

- Lung back-*shu* point.

Actions

- Tonifies Lung *qi* and nourishes Lung *yin*.
- Regulates Lung *qi*.
- Drains Heat from the Lung.
- Transforms Phlegm-Dampness in the Lung.
- Expels Wind.
- Strengthens *wei qi* and protects the exterior.
- Benefits the nose.
- Calms *shen*.
- Opens the channel and moves *qi* and *xue* in the channel and in the local area.

Indications

- **Tiredness, shortness of breath, spontaneous sweating and frequent colds:** UB 13 is the Lung back-*shu* point and thus has a deep, fundamental tonifying effect on the Lung. In these situations, UB 13 is often used together with the Lung *yuan*-source point, Lu 9.

- **Cough, chest oppression, shortness of breath, shallow breathing and dyspnoea:** Lu 13 can be used to treat both *xu* and *shi* conditions that disrupt the functioning of Lung *qi*. This could, for example, be acute invasions of exogenous *xie qi*, accumulation of Phlegm in the Lung, Lung *qi xu* or Lung *yin xu*. Furthermore, UB 13 is used to treat stagnations of *qi* in the u*jiao*.

- **Aversion to cold, sore muscles, sore throat, lack of sweating, headache and dizziness:** As the Lung back-*shu* point, UB 13 activates *wei qi* and expels invasions of *xie qi*.

- **Blocked or running nose, no sense of smell and nose bleeds:** Back-*shu* points can be used to treat disorders that manifest in their *zang* organ's sensory organs.

- **Night sweats, dryness in the throat, blood in the sputum and dry, non-productive cough:** UB 13 is one of the most important acupuncture points, together with Lu 9, to nourish Lung *yin*.

- **Suicidal thoughts and manic behaviour:** UB 13 can calm *shen* by influencing its own *shen* aspect, *po*. This could be appropriate if a person suffers from suicidal thoughts. The same effect is seen in the point Lu 3, which also affects the person's *po*. *Po* is conceived of as being the corporeal spirit. *Po* ceases to exist when the physical body ceases to exist and has a descending *yin* dynamic. This can cause some people to be attracted to death. UB 13 can also calm *shen* by draining Heat from the Lung. Draining Heat from the Lung means that the Heart does not become heated by Heat from the Lung. Heat in the Heart can agitate *shen* and lead to manic behaviour.

- **Epigastric distension, no appetite and vomiting:** There is a close relationship between the Lung and the Stomach. The Lung channel has its origin in the Stomach and both organs send their *qi* downwards. This means that blockages and deficiencies of Lung *qi* can mean that Stomach *qi* is not supported in its downward dynamic. Conversely, a stagnation of *qi* or food in the Stomach can block the descent of Lung *qi*.

- **Pain and stiffness in the local area, neck and lumbar region:** As a channel point, UB 13 can be used to treat pain in the local area and along the path of the channel.

Urinary Bladder 14 *Jueyinshu* (Terminal *Yin Shu*)

- Pericardium back-*shu* point.

Actions

- Regulates Heart *qi*.

- Spreads Liver *qi* and opens the chest.

- Lowers and disperses *qi*.

- Opens the channel and moves *qi* and *xue* in the channel and in the local area.

Indications

- **Cardiac pain and irregular heartbeat:** As the back-*shu* point of the Pericardium, UB 14 can regulate Heart *qi*.

- **Feeling of unrest in the chest and chest oppression:** UB 14 is a local point in the upper *jiao*, whilst simultaneously being the back-*shu* point of the Pericardium, which has a *jueyin* relationship to the Liver. UB 14 can therefore be used to regulate *qi* in the upper *jiao*, especially when it is due to a stagnation of Liver *qi*.

- **Cough, shortness of breath and dyspnoea:** By being able to regulate *qi* in the upper *jiao*, UB 14 has a regulatory effect on Lung *qi*.

- **Back pain:** UB 14 can be used as a local point to treat pain in the upper part of the back.

Urinary Bladder 15 *Xinshu* (Heart *Shu*)

- Heart back-*shu* point.

Actions

- Tonifies Heart *qi* and Heart *yang*.

- Nourishes Heart *yin* and Heart *xue*.

- Regulates Heart *qi* and invigorates Heart *xue*.

- Drains Heat from the Heart.

- Calms *shen*.

- Opens the chest and regulates *qi* in the upper *jiao*.

- Opens the channel and moves *qi* and *xue* in the channel and in the local area.

Indications

- **Cardiac pain, irregular heartbeat and palpitations:** As the back-*shu* point of the Heart, UB 15 can both tonify Heart *qi* and *yang*, nourish Heart *xue* and *yin* and invigorate Heart *xue* and *qi*. This means that UB 15 can be used to treat both *xu* and *shi* conditions that manifest with a disturbance of the Heart *qi*.

- **Sense of agitation in the chest and chest oppression:** Heat in the Heart can agitate *qi* in the chest. Stagnations of *qi* can result in chest oppression. UB 15 can both drain Heat from the Heart and circulate *qi* in the upper *jiao*.

- **Poor memory, insomnia, anxiety, nervousness, manic behaviour, depression, dream-disturbed sleep, dementia and mental confusion:** There are three overall types of *shen* imbalance: *shen* can be undernourished, *shen* can be agitated by Heat and *shen* can be blocked by Phlegm, *xue* stagnation or *qi* stagnation. UB 15 is relevant in all three situations, because UB 15 can tonify and nourish the Heart, drain Heat from the Heart, nourish Heart *yin* and disperse stagnations in the Heart.

- **Cough, shortness of breath and laboured breathing:** By regulating *qi* in the upper *jiao*, UB 15 can have a regulatory effect on Lung *qi*.

- **Back pain:** UB 15 can be used as a local point when there is pain in the upper part of the back.

Urinary Bladder 16 *Dushu* (*Du Shu*)

- *Du mai* back-*shu* point.

Actions

- Regulates *qi* and *xue* in the upper *jiao*.

- Opens the channel and moves *qi* and *xue* in the channel and surrounding area.

Indications

- **Local problems:** UB 16 is mainly used as a local point when there is cardiac pain, gastric pain, borborygmi and abscesses in the breasts or on the back.

Urinary Bladder 17 *Geshu* (Diaphragm *Shu*)

- Diaphragm back-*shu* point.

- *Hui*-gathering point for *xue*.

Actions

- Invigorates *xue*.

- Cools *xue* and stops bleeding.

- Nourishes *xue*.

- Nourishes *yin*.

- Regulates *qi* in the chest and diaphragm.

- Opens the channel and moves *qi* and *xue* in the channel and in the local area.

Indications

- **Pain that is stabbing or sharp in character, dysmenorrhoea, cardiac pain or chest pain, depression and paranoia:** All of these conditions can be caused by *xue* stagnation. UB 17, together with Sp 10, is the main acupuncture point to invigorate *xue* in the whole body.

- **Fever, red skin disorders, bleeding, heavy menstrual bleeding, bloody sputum, blood in the stool, nose bleeds and vomiting of blood:** Heat can agitate *xue* so that there is bleeding. *Xue* Heat can manifest as eczema, rosacea, psoriasis and other skin diseases where the skin is very red. UB 17 and Sp 10 are the two main acupuncture points to drain *xue* Heat.

- **Pale face, fatigue, dizziness, spots in the visual field, palpitations, insomnia, scanty menstrual bleeding or amenorrhoea and poor memory:** UB 17 with direct moxa can nourish *xue*. In these situations, UB 17 will often be used together with the back-*shu* point of the organ, where *xue xu* is manifesting or together with acupuncture points that strengthen the production of *xue* such as St 36, Sp 6, UB 20 or Ren 12.

- **Cough, dyspnoea, hiccups, vomiting, acid regurgitation and food stagnation:** UB 17 can regulate *qi* in the diaphragm and thereby both affect Lung *qi* and Stomach *qi*.

- **Painful *bi* syndrome in the whole body and pain throughout the body:** Persistent blockage of *qi* from exogenous *xie qi* will result in a stagnation of *xue* that will result in pain throughout the whole body.

- **Night sweats, feeling hot at night, burning sensation in the bones and dryness of the throat:** UB 17 and UB 19 are collectively known as 'the four flowers'. The combination of these four acupuncture points can be used to tonify an extreme condition of *yin xu*.

- **Back pain:** UB 17 can be used as a local point to relieve pain in the middle part of the back.

Urinary Bladder 18 *Ganshu* (Liver *Shu*)

- Liver back-*shu* point.

Actions

- Nourishes Liver *xue* and Liver *yin*.

- Spreads Liver *qi*.

- Invigorates Liver *xue*.

- Drains Fire and Damp-Heat from the Liver.

- Benefits the eyes.

- Extinguishes internal Wind and restrains Liver *yang*.

- Opens the channel and moves *qi* and *xue* in the channel and in the local area.

Indications

- **Amenorrhoea, scanty, heavy or irregular menstrual bleeding, dysmenorrhoea, premenstrual breast distension and premenstrual mood-swings:** The Liver has an important influence on the menstrual cycle and menstrual bleeding. This is because the Liver stores *xue*. In addition, the Liver is responsible for the free movement of *qi*, and thereby also of *xue* in the whole body. UB 18 can nourish Liver *xue*, spread Liver *qi* and invigorate Liver *xue*. UB 18 can therefore be used in the treatment of most menstrual disorders.

- **Superficial visual obstruction, blurred vision, red eyes, yellow sclera, pressure or pain in the eye, dry or itchy eyes, lacrimation and night-blindness:** UB 18 can be used in the treatment of many forms of eye disorders. UB 18 can do this because it nourishes Liver *yin* and *xue* when used with a tonifying needle technique, whilst at the same time it can drain Liver Fire and Liver *yang* when used with a draining technique. The eyes are the sense organ of the Liver and Liver *xue*, and Liver *yin* nourish the eyes. Liver Fire and Damp-Heat in the Liver can ascend to the eyes, making the eyes red or yellowish respectively. Ascending Liver *yang* or Liver Fire can result in painful eyes. UB 18 can be used to treat all of these conditions.

- **Irritability, quick temper, mood swings, depression and bipolar depression:** UB 18 can treat mental-emotional imbalances when the underlying pattern of imbalance is Liver *qi* stagnation, Liver *xue xu* or Liver Fire.

- **Hemilateral headache and headache on the top of the head:** Liver imbalances are often a cause of headaches. This is because the Gall Bladder channel, which is the partner channel of the Liver, traverses the side of the head, where many headaches manifest. Furthermore, the Liver channel itself connects up to Du 20. For this reason, Liver imbalances can also give a headache in the region of the vertex.

- **Shoulder and neck tension, muscle spasms, cramps in the muscles and tics:** UB 18 can relieve tension in the muscles and tendons, particularly in the shoulders and neck, by spreading Liver *qi*. Liver *xue xu* and Liver *yin xu* can manifest with cramping and restlessness in the muscles during the night.

- **Dizziness and epilepsy:** UB 18 can be used to calm internal Wind that rises up to the head. In addition, UB 18, by nourishing Liver *xue*, can also be used when there is dizziness arising from Liver *xue xu*.

- **Dream-disturbed sleep:** *Hun* returns to the Liver during the night. If there is Heat in the Liver, *hun* will become agitated and restless. If there is Liver *xue xu*, *hun* will not be anchored. Both situations can manifest with dream-disturbed sleep, and both situations can be treated with UB 18.

- **Tinnitus:** UB 18 can restrain ascending Liver *yang*, which can result in tinnitus.

- **Uterine fibroids, muscle knots and breast lumps:** Physical accumulations are manifestations of Phlegm or *xue* stagnation. UB 18 can help to disperse these accumulations by spreading Liver *qi* and invigorating Liver *xue*.

- **Ulcers or sores around the mouth or genitalia:** UB 18 can be used to drain Damp-Heat from the Liver channel. Damp-Heat in the Liver channel can manifest as red and/or weeping ulcers.

- **Distension or pain in the hypochondriac region, solar plexus or epigastric region, abdominal distension, intestinal pain, lumbar pain, distension of the jaw and pain in the inguinal region:** By moving Liver *qi*, UB 18 can be used in the treatment of pain and muscle tension.

- **Bloody sputum, nose bleeds and vomiting of blood:** Liver Fire can invade the Lung and the Stomach, resulting in bleeding in these organs. UB 18 can drain Fire from the Liver and thereby stop bleeding from these organs.

- **Back pain:** UB 18 can be used as a local point when there is pain in the central area of the back.

Urinary Bladder 19 *Danshu* (Gall Bladder *Shu*)

- Gall Bladder back-*shu* point.

Actions

- Drains Damp-Heat from the Liver and Gall Bladder.

- Regulates the Gall Bladder.

- Tonifies Gall Bladder *qi*.

- Nourishes *yin*.

- Regulates the *shaoyang* aspect.

- Opens the channel and moves *qi* and *xue* in the channel and in the local area.

Indications

- **Jaundice, yellow sclera, bitter taste in the mouth, pain in the region of the physical gall bladder, hypochondriac pain, pain in the costal region, pain in the chest, vomiting and poor appetite:** UB 19 can drain Damp-Heat from the Gall Bladder. UB 19 can therefore be used in the treatment of gallstones, jaundice, cholecystitis and biliary colic.

- **Nervousness, shyness, indecisiveness, reticence, lacking the courage to carry out decisions, palpitations and depression:** As the Gall Bladder back-*shu* point, UB 19 has a powerful tonifying effect on Gall Bladder *qi*. UB 19 can therefore be used to treat psycho-emotional conditions that are a result of Gall Bladder *qi xu*.

- **Fatigue, tiredness, alternating fever and chills, and malaria:** Invasions of *xie qi* can sometimes get stuck in the *shaoyang* aspect of the body. This can result in a state of chronic fatigue, alternating fever and chills, and the person feeling that they have not completely recovered from a bout of illness or that they repeatedly experience relapses of their symptoms. The Gall Bladder is a part of the *shaoyang* aspect and that is why UB 19 can be used to regulate *shaoyang*.

- **Night sweats, feeling hot at night, burning sensation in the bones and dryness in the throat:** UB 17 and UB 19 are collectively known as 'the four flowers'. The combination of these four acupuncture points can be used to treat conditions of *yin xu*.

- **Back pain:** UB 19 can be used as a local point when there is pain in the surrounding area.

Urinary Bladder 20 *Pishu* (Spleen *Shu*)

- Spleen back-*shu* point.

Actions

- Tonifies Spleen *qi* and Spleen *yang*.

- Tonifies Spleen *yang* and holds *xue* inside the blood vessels.

- Transforms Dampness.

- Nourishes *xue*.

- Regulates *qi* in the middle *jiao*.

- Opens the channel and moves *qi* and *xue* in the channel and in the local area.

Indications

- **Fatigue, tiredness, poor appetite, loose stool, watery stool, undigested food in the stool, abdominal distension, nausea, borborygmi, sweet tooth, weak limbs, inability to gain weight and emaciation:** UB 20 is one of the most important acupuncture points in the body to tonify Spleen *qi* and Spleen *yang* and thereby transform food into *qi*. The presence of Dampness and the weakening of Spleen *qi* can result in stagnations of *qi* in the middle *jiao*.

- **Heavy limbs, sticky sensation in the mouth, oedema, increased vaginal discharge and somnolence:** When there is Spleen *qi xu* and Spleen *yang xu*, there will be an ineffective transformation of the food and drink that has been consumed. This can result in Dampness. By tonifying Spleen *qi* and Spleen *yang*, UB 20 can be used in the treatment of symptoms arising from Dampness.

- **Organ prolapse, being easily bruised, menstrual spotting and spontaneous bleeding anywhere in the body:** UB 20 can be used to raise *yang* and strengthen the Spleen's ability to hold *xue* inside the blood vessels.

- **Back pain:** UB 20 can be used as a local point to treat pain in the local area.

Urinary Bladder 21 *Weishu* (Stomach *Shu*)

- Stomach back-*shu* point.

Actions

- Tonifies Stomach *qi* and nourishes Stomach *yin*.

- Regulates Stomach *qi*.

- Regulates *qi* in the middle *jiao*.

- Opens the channel and moves *qi* and *xue* in the channel and in the local area.

Indications

- **Fatigue, poor appetite, emaciation, difficulty gaining weight and weak limbs:** UB 21 can be used to tonify Stomach *qi* and thus improve the Stomach's ability to 'rot and ripen' the food so the Spleen can transform it into *qi*.

- **Pain in the Stomach, vomiting, nausea, acid regurgitation and abdominal distension:** UB 21 can be used to regulate Stomach *qi* and is therefore also able to regulate *qi* in the whole of the middle *jiao*.

- **Back pain:** UB 21 can be used as a local point when there is pain in the local area.

Urinary Bladder 22 *Sanjiaoshu* (*San Jiao Shu*)

- *San jiao* back-*shu* point.

Actions

- Regulates *san jiao*.

- Regulates the water passages and drains Dampness from the lower *jiao*.

- Invigorates *xue* in the lower *jiao*.

- Regulates *shaoyang*.

- Opens the channel and moves *qi* and *xue* in the channel and in the local area.

Indications

- **Oedema, urinary difficulty, cloudy urine, blood in the urine, diarrhoea, borborygmi and abdominal distension:** *San jiao* is responsible for the overall management of the water passages in the whole body. When there are disruptions in this transportation and transformation of fluids, the *yin* nature of water and fluids will result in them seeping down to the lower *jiao*. UB 22 can be used to open the water passages in the lower *jiao* and promote urination so these *yin* fluids can be drained out of the body.

- **Uterine fibroids, lumps, cysts and accumulations in the uterus and the lower abdomen:** UB 22 can disperse stagnations of *xue* in the lower *jiao*.

- **Headache, intermittent fever and chills, bitter taste in the mouth and dizziness:** Exogenous *xie qi* can sometimes get locked in the *shaoyang* level. This can lead to a chronic state of alternating fever and chills, and a person feeling that they have never completely recovered from an illness. *San jiao* is an aspect of *shaoyang* and UB 22 can therefore be used to regulate the *shaoyang* level.

- **Back pain:** UB 22 can be used as a local point when there is pain in the lumbar region.

Urinary Bladder 23 *Shenshu* (Kidney *Shu*)

- Kidney back-*shu* point.

Actions

- Tonifies Kidney *qi* and Kidney *yang*.

- Nourishes Kidney *yin* and Kidney *jing*.

- Strengthens and warms *mingmen*.

- Benefits the Bones and the Marrow.

- Regulates the water passages and promotes urination.

- Benefits and warms the Uterus.

- Strengthens the lumbar region.

- Benefits the eyes and ears.

- Opens the channel and moves *qi* and *xue* in the channel and in the local area.

Indications

- **Impotence, lack of libido, exaggerated libido, infertility, premature ejaculation and nocturnal emissions:** A deficiency of both Kidney *yin* and Kidney *yang* can interfere with a person's sexual function. Heat from Kidney *yin xu* can create an increased desire for sex and the Heat can over-activate the semen, resulting in uncontrolled ejaculation. Kidney *yang xu* leads to a reduction in the libido and men can have problems with their erection. UB 23 can treat both Kidney *yin xu* and Kidney *yang xu*.

- **Oedema, urinary difficulty, cloudy urine, blood in the urine, incontinence, frequent and copious urination and frequent and scanty urination:** Fluid physiology is in general under the influence of Kidney *yang*. The Urinary Bladder is particularly affected by Kidney imbalances. This is because many of the functions that relate to fluid physiology are dependent on Kidney *yang*. Kidney *yang* also actively holds urine inside the Urinary Bladder and expels urine out of the Urinary Bladder upon urination. Kidney *yin xu* can manifest with sparse, dark urine. The Heat generated by Kidney *yin xu* can result in frequent urination. This is due to the *yang* nature of Heat, which will force the urine out of the Urinary Bladder. UB 23 can be used in all these situations, because it strengthens Kidney *qi* and Kidney *yang*, as well as nourishing Kidney *yin*.

- **Watery diarrhoea containing undigested food and borborygmi:** By tonifying Kidney *yang*, UB 23 supports Spleen *yang* in its transformation of food and liquids.

- **Fatigue:** UB 23 is an important acupuncture point in the treatment of tiredness and fatigue, because the Kidneys are the pre-heaven root of *qi*.

- **Dizziness, insomnia and night sweats:** UB 23 can nourish Kidney *yin*. UB 23 is therefore a relevant point in the treatment of *yin xu* disorders, both in the Kidneys and other organs, particularly the Heart.

- **Irregular menstrual cycle, amenorrhoea and whitish or watery vaginal discharge:** The menstrual cycle is dependent on the constant alternation between *yin* and *yang* and there being a sufficient quantity of both. The Kidneys are the root of both *yin* and *yang* in the body. UB 23 can therefore be used in the treatment of many different kinds of gynaecological disorders. In addition, the three extraordinary channels *ren mai*, *du mai* and *chong mai*, which are of great importance for the menstrual cycle, all have their origin in the space between the two Kidneys. This means that UB 23 can be used to influence these channels.

- **Dyspnoea, shortness of breath and asthma:** UB 23 can be used to tonify Kidney *qi*, enabling the Kidneys to grasp the *qi* that has been sent down from the Lung.

- **Tinnitus and deafness:** By nourishing Kidney *yin* and Kidney *jing*, UB 23 can be used to treat tinnitus and deafness when these are a consequence of a *xu* imbalance.

- **Dry eyes, superficial visual obstructions, such as dots in the visual field, and blurred vision:** It is not only Liver *xue* and Liver *yin* that nourish the eyes. By nourishing Kidney *yin*, UB 23 can be used when there are eye problems that are the result of *yin xu*.

- **Weakness, stiffness and tiredness in the lower back and/or the knees, and lumbar pain:** UB 23 can be used as a local point in the treatment of all forms of lumbar problems, including *shi* conditions, such as stagnations of *xue*, Dampness and Cold. UB 23 is of particular relevance in the treatment of lumbar and knee problems that are due to Kidney *xu* conditions.

Urinary Bladder 24 *Qihaishu* (Sea of *Qi Shu*)

Actions

- Strengthens the lumbar region.

- Regulates *qi* and *xue* in the lower *jiao*.

- Opens the channel and moves *qi* and *xue* in the channel and in the local area.

Indications

- **Lumbar pain, haemorrhoids, irregular menstruations, dysmenorrhoea and vaginal discharge:** In spite of its name, UB 24 does not have particularly tonifying qualities. UB 24 is used almost exclusively as a local point to treat disorders in the surrounding area.

Urinary Bladder 25 *Dachangshu* (Large Intestine *Shu*)

- Large Intestine back-*shu* point.

Actions

- Regulates the Intestines.

- Strengthens the lumbar region.

- Opens the channel and moves *qi* and *xue* in the channel and in the local area.

Indications

- **Diarrhoea, constipation, blood in the stool, pus in the stool, undigested food in the stool, borborygmi, abdominal distension, abdominal pain, prolapse of the rectum and haemorrhoids:** UB 25 is the back-*shu* point of the Large Intestine and can therefore be used in the treatment of all disorders that relate to intestinal functioning and stool consistency.

- **Lumbar pain, stiffness, and weakness and fatigue in the lumbar region:** UB 25 is an important local point that can be used in the treatment of all forms of lumbar problems.

Urinary Bladder 26 *Guanyuanshu* (Origin Gate *Shu*)

Actions

- Strengthens the lumbar region.

- Regulates *qi* in the lower *jiao*.

- Opens the channel and moves *qi* and *xue* in the channel and in the local area.

Indications

- **Local problems:** UB 26 is used as a local point in the treatment of lumbar problems, problems with urination, diarrhoea and abdominal constipation, uterine fibroids and lumps and cysts in the lower *jiao*.

Urinary Bladder 27 *Xiaochangshu* (Small Intestine *Shu*)

- Small Intestine back-*shu* point.

Actions

- Supports the Small Intestine function of separating the pure from the impure.

- Regulates the Intestines and Urinary Bladder.

- Drains Dampness and Damp-Heat from the lower *jiao*.

- Opens the channel and moves *qi* and *xue* in the channel and in the local area.

Indications

- **Diarrhoea, constipation, blood in the stool, pus in the stool, undigested food in the stool, borborygmi, abdominal distension, abdominal pain, prolapse of the rectum and haemorrhoids:** UB 27 can be used to influence the Small Intestine's ability to separate the pure and impure. When this function is compromised, Dampness and Damp-Heat can arise. This can manifest with changes in the stool. UB 27 can also be used to circulate *qi* in the Intestine when there is a stagnation.

- **Dark urine, strongly smelling urine, painful or difficult urination and blood in the urine:** The Small Intestine plays a key role in fluid physiology, as well as having a *taiyang* relationship to the Urinary Bladder. This means that UB 27 can be used in the treatment of many different kinds of urinary problems. Furthermore, the Small Intestine has a *biaoli* (external/internal) relationship to the Heart. Heart Fire, which often arises due to emotional imbalances, can drain downwards via the Small Intestine and into the Urinary Bladder, where it can result in painful, frequent and scanty urinations of dark yellow urine that may contain blood.

- **Yellow or white vaginal discharge:** Copious vaginal discharge or changes in the quality of the vaginal discharge are likely to arise when there is Dampness or Damp-Heat seeping down to the lower *jiao*. As a local point and as the Small Intestine back-*shu* point, UB 27 can be used to treat both the cause and manifestation of these imbalances.

- **Pain in the lower abdomen or in the testes:** Stagnations of *qi* in the Small Intestine can cause pain in the lower *jiao* and in the testes. UB 27 can, as the back-*shu* point, regulate *qi* in the Small Intestine.

- **Lumbar pain, stiffness and pain in the sacrum, pain in the buttocks and sciatica:** UB 27 can be used as a local point in the treatment of problems in the surrounding area.

Urinary Bladder 28 *Pangguanshu* (Urinary Bladder *Shu*)

- Urinary Bladder back-*shu* point.

Actions

- Regulates the Urinary Bladder.
- Drains Dampness and Damp-Heat from the lower *jiao*.
- Disperses stagnations and disperses accumulations in the lower *jiao*.
- Regulates the water passages.
- Opens the channel and moves *qi* and *xue* in the channel and in the local area.

Indications

- **Dark urine, strong-smelling urine, painful or difficult urination, incontinence, cloudy urine and blood in the urine:** As the back-*shu* point of the Urinary Bladder, UB 28 can be used in the treatment of most types of urinary problems.

- **Genital itching, genital pain and swelling, and genital ulcers, sores and rashes:** UB 28 can be used to drain Dampness and Damp-Heat out of the body with the urine.

- **Diarrhoea and constipation:** UB 28 can both drain Dampness and move *qi* in the lower *jiao*. UB 28 can therefore be used to influence the stool.

- **Lumps, cysts in the lower *jiao* and uterine fibroids:** UB 28 circulates *qi* and *xue* in the lower *jiao* and can therefore be used to disperse stagnations of *qi*, *xue* and Phlegm in the lower *jiao*.

- **Lumbar pain, stiffness and pain in the sacrum, pain in the buttocks and sciatica:** UB 28 can be used as a local point in the treatment of problems in the surrounding area.

Urinary Bladder 29 *Zhonglushu* (Central Spine *Shu*)

Actions

- Benefits the lumbar region.

- Expels Cold.

- Opens the channel and moves *qi* and *xue* in the channel and in the local area.

Indications

- **Local disorders:** UB 29 is mainly used as a local point in the treatment of problems in the surrounding area. UB 29 can also be used to expel Cold from the lower *jiao*.

Urinary Bladder 30 *Baihuanshu* (White Ring *Shu*)

Actions

- Regulates menstruation.

- Controls the lower orifices.

- Opens the channel and moves *qi* and *xue* in the channel and in the local area.

Indications

- **Local disorders:** UB 30 is mainly used as a local point when there are problems in the sacrum and the buttocks. UB 30 can be used in the treatment of sciatica and lumbar pain. UB 30 also has an influence on the lower orifices and can be used to control vaginal discharge and nocturnal emissions.

Urinary Bladder 31 *Shangliao* (Upper Hole), Urinary Bladder 32 *Ciliao* (Second Hole), Urinary Bladder 33 *Zhongliao* (Centre Hole) and Urinary Bladder 34 *Xiaoliao* (Lower Hole)

Actions

- Regulate *qi* in the lower *jiao* and in the uterus.

- Drain Dampness from the lower *jiao.*

- Tonify Kidney *qi* and control the lower orifices.

- Benefit the stool and urination.

- Open the channel and move *qi* and *xue* in the channel and in the local area.

Indications

- **Dark urine, strongly smelling urine, painful or difficult urination, incontinence, cloudy urine, blood in the urine, diarrhoea, constipation, haemorrhoids and borborygmi:** These acupuncture points have a regulatory influence on the *qi* in the lower *jiao* and at the same time can drain Dampness out of the body.

- **Dysmenorrhoea, irregular menstruations and labour pains:** These acupuncture points have a powerful moving effect on *qi* and *xue* in the uterus. In addition to treating menstrual problems, these acupuncture points can be used to relieve labour pains and to induce labour. It is also for this reason that these points are contraindicated during pregnancy.

- **Infertility:** By tonifying the Kidneys, these acupuncture points can be used in the treatment of infertility.

- **Vaginal discharge:** These acupuncture points can tonify Kidney *qi* and thereby strengthen the Kidneys' ability to control the lower orifices. Furthermore, these points can be used to drain Dampness, which can be the cause of vaginal discharge.

Urinary Bladder 35 *Huiyang* (*Yang* Meeting) and Urinary Bladder 36 *Chengfu* (Hold and Support)

Actions

- Drain Damp-Heat from the lower *jiao.*

- Open the channel and move *qi* and *xue* in the channel and in the local area.

Indications

- **Local disorders:** These acupuncture points are mainly used as local points in the treatment of sacral problems, problems with the coccyx or buttocks, sciatica or pain in the thigh. These two acupuncture points can also be used in the treatment of haemorrhoids.

Urinary Bladder 37 *Yinmen* (Abundance Door) and Urinary Bladder 38 *Fuxi* (Superficial Cleft)

Actions

- Open the channel and move *qi* and *xue* in the channel and in the local area.

Indications

- **Local disorders:** Both of these acupuncture points are mainly used as local points in the treatment of problems along the pathway of the channel.

Urinary Bladder 39 *Weiyang* (Support *Yang*)

- *San jiao* lower *he*-sea point.

Actions

- Regulates *san jiao*.
- Regulates the water passages.
- Opens the channel and moves *qi* and *xue* in the channel and in the local area.

Indications

- **Oedema in the lower half of the body, urinary difficulty, painful urination and constipation:** As the lower *he*-sea point of the *san jiao*, UB 39 can influence fluid physiology, especially in the lower *jiao*.

- **Lumbar weakness, lumbar pain, stiffness in the lumbar region, knee pain, sciatica, haemorrhoids and pain in the foot and ankle:** UB 39 can be used in the treatment of problems in the knee and problems along the path of the channel.

Urinary Bladder 40 *Weizhong* (Centre of the Bend)

- *He*-sea point.
- Earth point.
- Gao Wu command point.
- Ma Dan Yang Heavenly Star point.
- Starting point of the Urinary Bladder divergent channel.

Actions

- Drains Heat and cools *xue*.
- Benefits the lumbar region and knees.
- Expels Summer-Heat.
- Benefits the Urinary Bladder.
- Opens the channel and moves *qi* and *xue* in the channel and in the local area.

Indications

- **Lumbar pain, stiffness and pain in the sacrum, pain in the buttocks, sciatica and weakness of the legs:** UB 40 is an extremely important distal point used in the treatment of all types of problems in the lower back. This is also why UB 40 is one of Ma Dan Yang's Heavenly Star points and Gao Wu's command points. Bleeding UB 40 is recommended in the treatment of acute lumbar pain when it is caused by a stagnation of *xue*. UB 40 can, however, be used for all forms of lumbar problems, whatever the aetiology.

- **Red, itchy skin disorders and nose bleeds:** Bleeding UB 40 can cool *xue*. UB 40 is therefore used in the treatment of skin disorders that are caused by *xue* Heat. In addition, UB 40 is used to treat spontaneous bleeding from the nose caused by *xue* Heat.

- **Fever, vomiting, nausea, diarrhoea and a feeling of heaviness in the body:** UB 40 is one of the few acupuncture points that are specifically recommended for the treatment of invasions of Summer-Heat.

- **Incontinence, urinary difficulty, dark urine and painful urination:** UB 40 is one of the few Urinary Bladder channel points that are specifically recommended to treat problems with urination.

- **Haemorrhoids:** The Urinary Bladder divergent channel separates away from the primary channel at UB 40 and connects to the rectum. UB 40 can, therefore, be used as a distal point in the treatment of haemorrhoids, even though UB 57 is the acupuncture point that is more often used for this purpose.

- **Knee pain:** UB 40 is an important local point in the treatment of knee problems.

Urinary Bladder 41 *Fufen* (Connected Branch)

- Meeting point of the Urinary Bladder and Small Intestine channels.

Actions

- Expels Wind-Cold.
- Opens the channel and moves *qi* and *xue* in the channel and in the local area.

Indications

- **Local disorders:** UB 41 is mainly used as a local point in the treatment of disorders in the surrounding area.

Urinary Bladder 42 *Pohu* (Po Door)

Actions

- Tonifies Lung *qi.*
- Regulates Lung *qi.*
- Calms *po.*
- Opens the channel and moves *qi* and *xue* in the channel and in the local area.

Indications

- **Cough, dyspnoea, shallow breathing, shortness of breath and wheezing:** UB 42, which is located immediately lateral to the Lung back-*shu* point, can be used to tonify and regulate Lung *qi.*

- **Sadness, depression, grief, suicidal thoughts and chest oppression:** The lateral Urinary Bladder channel points on the back are often said to have the ability of having a special effect on the *shen* aspect of the *zang* organ of the back-*shu* point that is medial to their position. UB 42 is recommended, therefore, when there are symptoms and signs that relate to *po*, which is the *shen* aspect of the Lung.

- **Pain and stiffness in the local area, in the neck and in the lumbar region:**
As a channel point, UB 42 can be used to treat pain in the local area and
along the path of the channel.

Urinary Bladder 43 *Gaohuang* (*Gaohuang Shu*)
Actions

- Tonifies and nourishes the Lung, Spleen, Kidneys, Heart and Stomach.

- Nourishes *yin* and clears *xu* Heat.

- Tonifies *yuan qi*.

- Calms *shen*.

- Transforms Phlegm.

- Opens the channel and moves *qi* and *xue* in the channel and in the local area.

Indications

- **Dry or bloody cough, wheezing, fatigue, night sweats, burning sensation
in the bones and weight loss:** UB 43 has traditionally been used in the
treatment of tuberculosis. It is also in this context that the *yin*-tonifying
qualities that are attributed to UB 43 should be seen.

- **Poor memory, palpitations and dizziness:** UB 43 can both nourish Heart
yin and calm *shen*.

- **Nocturnal emissions, premature ejaculation and impotence:** UB 43
can nourish Kidney *yin* and *yuan qi*. UB 43 can therefore be used to treat
problems of the male sexual function.

- **Undigested food in the stool and weak limbs:** Moxa on UB 43 can have
a powerful tonifying effect on *qi* in the body and thus also on Stomach and
Spleen *qi*.

- **Pain and stiffness in the local area, in the neck and in the lumbar region:**
As a channel point, UB 43 can be used to treat pain in the local area and
along the path of the channel.

Urinary Bladder 44 *Shentang* (*Shen* Hall)
Actions

- Calms *shen*.

- Opens the chest.

- Regulates *qi* in the upper *jiao.*

- Opens the channel and moves *qi* and *xue* in the channel and in the local area.

Indications

- **Depression, sadness, desperation, mental restlessness, fear, anxiety, insomnia, poor memory and poor concentration:** The lateral Urinary Bladder channel points on the back are often said to have a special effect on the *shen* aspect of the *zang* organ of the back-*shu* point that is medial to their position. UB 44 is therefore recommended when there are symptoms and signs that relate to an imbalance of the Heart *shen.*

- **Cough, dyspnoea, shallow breathing, breathlessness, wheezing and chest oppression:** UB 44 can be used to regulate *qi* in the upper *jiao*, and UB 44 will therefore also have a regulatory effect on Lung *qi.*

- **Stiffness in the neck and shoulder and pain in the back:** As a channel point, UB 44 can treat problems in the local area and along the course of the channel.

Urinary Bladder 45 *Yixi* (*Yi Xi*[9])
Actions

- Expels Wind-Heat, drains Heat and regulates Lung *qi.*

- Opens the channel and moves *qi* and *xue* in the channel and in the local area.

Indications

- **Local disorders and invasions of Wind-Heat:** UB 45 is mainly used as a local point when there is stiffness, tension or pain in the surrounding area. UB 45 can be used to expel invasions of Wind-Heat and to drain Heat from the Lung whilst regulating Lung *qi.*

Urinary Bladder 46 *Geguan* (Diaphragm Gate)
Actions

- Regulates *qi* in the middle and upper *jiao.*

- Benefits the diaphragm.

- Opens the channel and moves *qi* and *xue* in the channel and in the local area.

Indications

- **Hiccups, burping, sighing, vomiting and tightness of the diaphragm and the back:** UB 46 can be used to regulate *qi* in the diaphragm and the surrounding area.

Urinary Bladder 47 *Hunmen* (*Hun* Door)
Actions

- Calms and anchors the *hun*.

- Spreads Liver *qi* and relaxes the sinews.

- Regulates *qi* in the middle and upper *jiao*.

- Opens the channel and moves *qi* and *xue* in the channel and in the local area.

Indications

- **Depression, sadness, lack of motivation, no goals in life, insomnia and dream-disturbed sleep:** The lateral Urinary Bladder channel points on the back are often said to have a special effect on the *shen* aspect of the *zang* organ of the back-*shu* point that is medial to their position. UB 47 is therefore recommended when there are symptoms and signs that relate to a *hun* imbalance.

- **Abdominal distension, epigastric distension, distension in the solar plexus, irregular bowel movements, diarrhoea, alternating diarrhoea and constipation, nausea, vomiting and borborygmi:** By spreading Liver *qi* in the middle *jiao*, UB 47 can be used in the treatment of digestive problems where Liver *qi* is invading the Spleen and Stomach.

- **Taut tendons and painful joints:** The Liver has a special influence on the sinews and tendons in the body that are nourished by Liver *xue*. At the same time, the Liver ensures the free flow of *qi* in the tendons and joints.

- **Distension or pain in the costal and hypochondriac regions, chest oppression, stiffness in the neck and shoulder and pain in the back:** As a channel point, UB 47 can treat problems in the local area and along the channel.

Urinary Bladder 48 *Yanggang* (*Yang* Headrope)
Actions

- Regulates Gall Bladder *qi* and drains Damp-Heat.

- Regulates *qi* in the middle and upper *jiao*.

- Opens the channel and moves *qi* and *xue* in the channel and in the local area.

Indications

- **Gallstones, jaundice, colitis, dark or cloudy urine, distension, nausea and diarrhoea or irregular stools:** UB 48 is used as a local point in the treatment of pain and tension in the back and costal region. At the same time, UB 48 can be used to regulate *qi* in the Gall Bladder and to drain Damp-Heat from the Gall Bladder.

Urinary Bladder 49 *Yishe* (Yi Abode)
Actions

- Drains Damp-Heat.

- Benefits *yi*.

- Regulates *qi* in the middle *jiao*.

- Opens the channel and moves *qi* and *xue* in the channel and in the local area.

Indications

- **Poor memory, poor concentration, tendency to worry, ponder or think too much and thinking in circles:** The lateral Urinary Bladder channel points on the back are often said to have a special effect on the *shen* aspect of the *zang* organ of the back-*shu* point that is medial to their position. UB 49 is recommended for symptoms and signs that relate to the Spleen's *yi* aspect.

- **Abdominal distension, nausea, diarrhoea, vomiting, yellow sclera, yellow tinge to the skin and dark or cloudy urine:** UB 49 can be used in the treatment of digestive and other problems that are caused by Damp-Heat.

- **Pain in the back or a sore lower back, and tension and rigidity along the channel or in the local area:** UB 49 can be used as a channel point in the treatment of local disorders and when there are disorders along the path of the channel.

Urinary Bladder 50 *Weicang* (Stomach Granary)
Actions

- Regulates *qi* in the middle *jiao*.

- Opens the channel and moves *qi* and *xue* in the channel and in the local area.

Indications

- **Abdominal distension:** UB 50 can be used in the treatment of disorders manifesting in the surrounding area.

Urinary Bladder 51 *Huangmen* (*Huang* Door)
Actions

- Regulates *qi* in the chest.

- Regulates *qi* in the upper *jiao*.

- Opens the channel and moves *qi* and *xue* in the channel and in the local area.

Indications

- **Disorders manifesting in the breasts or chest:** UB 51 is mainly used as a distal point for the breasts and the area behind them. This is reflected in the name, which refers to the same area that the name of UB 43 refers to. UB 51 can also be used when there are disorders manifesting in the local area.

Urinary Bladder 52 *Zhishi* (*Zhi* Chamber)
Actions

- Nourishes Kidney *yin* and Kidney *jing*.

- Benefits urination.

- Benefits *zhi*.

- Strengthens the lumbar region.

- Opens the channel and moves *qi* and *xue* in the channel and in the local area.

Indications

- **Fatigue, dizziness, tinnitus, deafness, nocturnal emissions, impotence and poor memory:** UB 52 has a tonifying effect on the Kidneys in general and on the Kidney *yin* and *jing* aspects in particular. UB 52 is therefore often used in the treatment of symptoms and signs that relate to Kidney *yin xu* and Kidney *jing xu*.

- **Urinary difficulty and dribbling urination:** By nourishing Kidney *yin*, UB 52 will also have a tonifying effect on Kidney *yang* and Kidney *qi*, because these are created from Kidney *yin*.

- **Depression, loss of the will to live and a tendency to be easily discouraged and abandon plans:** The lateral Urinary Bladder channel points on the back are often said to have a special effect on the *shen* aspect of the *zang* organ of the back-*shu* point that is medial to their position. UB 52 is therefore recommended when there are symptoms and signs that relate to the Kidneys' *zhi* aspect.

- **Lumbar problems and sciatica:** UB 52 can be used in the treatment of disorders in the local area and along the path of the channel.

Urinary Bladder 53 *Baohuang* (Bladder *Huang*)
Actions

- Controls the lower *jiao* and opens the water passages.

- Opens the channel and moves *qi* and *xue* in the channel and in the local area.

Indications

- **Distension in the area around the pubic bone, urinary difficulty, retention of urine, borborygmi, constipation, diarrhoea and oedema:** UB 53 can be used to regulate *qi* and the water passages in the lower *jiao* and thereby drain Dampness down and out of the body.

- **Lumbar problems, pain or tenderness in the buttock and sciatica:** UB 53 can treat problems in the local area and along the path of the channel.

Urinary Bladder 54 *Zhibian* (Sequential Limit)
Actions

- Controls the lower *jiao* and opens the water passages.

- Opens the channel and moves *qi* and *xue* in the channel and in the local area.

Indications

- **Urinary problems, retention of urine, haemorrhoids, constipation, diarrhoea, oedema and vaginal discharge:** UB 53 can be used to regulate *qi* and open the water passages in the lower *jiao*, thereby draining Dampness out of the body.

- **Lumbar problems, pain or tenderness in the buttock and sciatica:** UB 54 is an important local point in the treatment of disorders in the surrounding area and in the treatment of sciatica when it is related to the pathway of the Urinary Bladder channel on the back of the leg.

Urinary Bladder 55 *Heyang* (*Yang* Union)

Actions

- Stops bleeding from the uterus and treats pain in the genitalia.

- Opens the channel and moves *qi* and *xue* in the channel and in the local area.

Indications

- **Irregular bleeding from the uterus, vaginal discharge and pain in the genitalia:** UB 55 is mainly used in the treatment of disorders in the local area and as a distal point for disorders in the lumbar region.

Urinary Bladder 56 *Chengjin* (Sinew Support)

Actions

- Controls the lower *jiao* and opens the water passages.

- Opens the channel and moves *qi* and *xue* in the channel and in the local area.

Indications

- **Haemorrhoids, nose bleeds, lumbar pain, dizziness and headache:** UB 56 is used to address problems in the calf muscle and problems along the path of the channel. UB 56 is, however, rarely used in these conditions, since there are other more potent distal points.

Urinary Bladder 57 *Chengshan* (Mountain Support)

- Ma Dan Yang Heavenly Star point.

Actions

- Benefits the rectum.

- Opens the channel and moves *qi* and *xue* in the channel and in the local area.

Indications

- **Haemorrhoids and prolapse of the rectum:** UB 57 is one of the body's most important points for the treatment of haemorrhoids. Urinary Bladder channel points can be used in the treatment of haemorrhoids, because the Urinary Bladder's divergent channel connects to the anus.

- **Muscular pain or spasms in the calf, lumbar problems and sciatica:** UB 57 is an important local point in the treatment of disorders of the calf muscles, such as cramps and pain. Problems in the calf can be both *xu* or *shi* in nature. UB 57 can also be used when there is a problem in the lumbar region, the ankle and along the path of the channel.

Urinary Bladder 58 *Feiyang* (Fly Upwards)

- *Luo*-connecting point.

Actions

- Regulates *qi* upwards and downwards in the body.

- Expels Wind-Cold from the *taiyang* aspect.

- Benefits the rectum.

- Opens the channel and moves *qi* and *xue* in the channel and in the local area.

Indications

- **Headache, dizziness, epilepsy, nose bleeds, blocked nose, neck pain and tension:** As a *luo*-connecting point, UB 58 connects the Kidney and Urinary Bladder channels. The Kidneys are the root of *yin* and *yang* in the body and the Urinary Bladder channel runs from the inner canthus of the eye, up over the head and neck and down the back of the body to the feet. UB 58 is therefore used as a distal point for the head, neck, eyes and nose, and at the same time as an acupuncture point on the Urinary Bladder channel. UB 58 connects the Urinary Bladder channel with the resources stored in the Kidneys, so that Kidney *yin* can control *yang* in the head.

- **Haemorrhoids and rectal prolapse:** Just like UB 57, UB 58 can be used to treat haemorrhoids. Urinary Bladder channel points can be used in the treatment of haemorrhoids, because the Urinary Bladder's divergent channel connects to the anus.

- **Aversion to cold, aching muscles and fever without sweating:** UB 57 can expel Wind-Cold from the *taiyang* aspect of the body.

- **Muscular pain or spasms in the calf, lumbar problems and sciatica:** UB 58 is an important local point in the treatment of disorders of the calf muscles, such as cramps and pain. Problems in the calf can be *xu* or *shi* in nature. UB 58 can also be used when there is a problem in the lumbar region, the ankle and along the path of the channel.

Urinary Bladder 59 *Fuyang* (Instep *Yang*)

- *Xi*-cleft point for *yang qiao mai.*

Actions

- Activates *qi* and disperses stagnations in *yang qiao mai.*
- Opens the channel and moves *qi* and *xue* in the channel and in the local area.

Indications

- **Pain, stiffness, a feeling of heaviness, atrophy or weakness of the muscles on the lateral and posterior aspects of the leg muscles and the back of the legs, sciatica, lumbar problems and pain in the ankle and calf muscle:** UB 59 is a *xi*-cleft point and can therefore be used to treat acute, painful conditions along *yang qiao mai*. UB 59 can also be used as a local and distal point on the Urinary Bladder channel.

Urinary Bladder 60 *Kunlun* (*Kunlun* Mountain)

- *Jing*-river point.
- Fire point.
- Ma Dan Yang Heavenly Star point.

Actions

- Drains Heat and controls ascending *yang.*
- Extinguishes internal Wind.
- Regulates *qi* in the entire Urinary Bladder channel.
- Induces labour.
- Opens the channel and moves *qi* and *xue* in the channel and in the local area.

Indications

- **Headache, dizziness, epilepsy, nose bleeds, blocked nose, neck pain and tension, pain in the eyes and red eyes:** UB 60 is both a Fire point and a distal point on the Urinary Bladder channel. This means that UB 60 can drain Fire, *yang qi* and internal Wind down from the head, the eyes and the nose.

- **Pain and stiffness in the neck, shoulders, lumbar region, sacrum, buttock and legs, sciatica and pain in the ankle:** UB 60 is a very dynamic acupuncture point that can activate *qi* and *xue* in the entire channel. This is seen by the fact that UB 60 is used to treat disorders along the whole course of the channel. It is due to this versatility that UB 60 is classified as a Ma Dan Yang Heavenly Star point.

- **Difficult labour, delayed labour and placental retention:** UB 60 is an empirical point to induce labour. UB 60 is therefore contraindicated during pregnancy.

Urinary Bladder 61 *Pucan* (Subservient Visit)

- Meeting point of the Urinary Bladder channel and *yang qiao mai*.

Actions

- Opens the channel and moves *qi* and *xue* in the channel and in the local area.

Indications

- **Local disorders:** UB 61 is mainly used as a local point when treating problems in the ankle.

- **Disorders manifesting in the head and neck:** UB 61 can also be used as a distal point to treat problems in the head and neck. UB 61 is also said to have *shen*-calming properties.

Urinary Bladder 62 *Shenmai* (Ninth Vessel)

- Opening point for *yang qiao mai*.

- *Yang qiao mai* source point.

- Sun Si Miao ghost point.

Actions

- Calms internal Wind and expels exogenous Wind.

- Calms *shen.*

- Benefits the head and eyes.

- Opens and regulates *yang qiao mai.*

- Opens the channel and moves *qi* and *xue* in the channel and in the local area.

Indications

- **Insomnia, somnolence, difficulty remaining awake and red, painful eyes:** *Yin qiao mai* and *yang qiao mai* meet in the inner canthus of the eye at UB 1. Together they coordinate the opening and closing of the eyes, whilst regulating the balance between *yin* and *yang* in the head. This is why both of these channels' opening points, Kid 6 and UB 62, are used to treat problems with the eyes themselves as well as sleep disturbances. The two opening points will often be used together – one being drained whilst the other is tonified, depending on whether there is too much or too little *yin* or *yang* in the eye.

- **Manic behaviour, mental restlessness and palpitations:** UB 62 has a *shen*-calming effect, as it is the opening point of *yang qiao mai.* It can regulate *yang* in the brain and the head. In addition, the Urinary Bladder primary channel connects to the brain and its divergent channel connects to the Heart.

- **Epilepsy, headache, dizziness, hemiplegia, nose bleeds, tinnitus or upward-staring eyes:** As the opening point of *yang qiao mai*, UB 62 can extinguish internally generated Wind and drain *yang* from the head.

- **Aversion to cold and wind, aching muscles and fever without sweating:** UB 62 is both a *taiyang* channel point and the opening point of *yang qiao mai*. Both qualities mean that UB 62 can expel invasions of Wind-Cold from the body.

- **Imbalances between the right side and the left side of the body, one leg longer than the other, uneven hips, uneven shoulders, weak or tight muscles along the lateral aspect of the leg and unilateral sweating:** *Yang qiao mai* is a part of the body's energetic framework and thus has an impact on the body's physical structure. UB 62 is the opening point for *yang qiao mai* and will often be used together with Kid 6, which is the opening point of *yin qiao mai.* Together they can be used in the treatment of physical differences between one side of the body and the other and to treat differences in the muscle in the leg's medial and lateral aspects.

- **Stiff neck, headache, back pain and pain in the thigh, calf, ankle or foot:** In common with other Urinary Bladder channel points, UB 62 can be used to treat problems in the local area and problems along the path of the channel.

Urinary Bladder 63 *Jinmen* (Metal Door)

- *Xi*-cleft point.
- Meeting point of the Urinary Bladder channel and *yang wei mai*.
- *Yang wei mai* source point.

Actions

- Calms Wind.
- Relieves acute and painful conditions in the channel.
- Opens the channel and moves *qi* and *xue* in the channel and in the local area.

Indications

- **Epilepsy, loss of consciousness, acute pain, acute *shan* disorder and convulsions:** UB 63 is a *xi*-cleft point and can therefore be used in acute and painful conditions along the path of the channel. As with most other *yang* channels' *xi*-cleft points, UB 63 has not traditionally been used to treat its corresponding *fu* organ.

- **Stiff neck, headache, back pain and pain in the legs, ankles or feet:** In common with other Urinary Bladder channel points, UB 63 can be used to treat problems in the local area and problems along the path of the channel.

Urinary Bladder 64 *Jinggu* (Capital Bone)

- *Yuan*-source point.

Actions

- Controls rebellious *qi* that rises up to the head.
- Extinguishes internal Wind.
- Calms *shen*.
- Opens the channel and moves *qi* and *xue* in the channel and in the local area.

Indications

- **Headache, feeling of heaviness in the head, dizziness, epilepsy, red eyes, nose bleeds and shaking of the head:** Just like several of the other Urinary Bladder channel points in the ankle region, UB 64 can be used in the treatment of disorders of the head, especially when these are due to ascending *yang* and internally generated Wind. As a *taiyang* channel point, UB 64 can expel exogenous Wind from the head.

- **Manic behaviour, mental restlessness, palpitations and a tendency to being easily startled:** The Urinary Bladder primary channel connects to the brain and the divergent channel connects to the Heart. UB 64 can therefore have a calming effect on the Heart and mind.

- **Stiff neck, headache, lumbar pain, pain in the legs, pain in the back, ankle problems and pain, and pain in the feet:** Like other Urinary Bladder channel points in the ankle, UB 64 can treat disorders in the local area and at the opposite end of the channel.

Urinary Bladder 65 *Shugu* (Tied Bone)

- *Shu*-stream point.
- Wood point.
- Five Phase draining point.

Actions

- Controls rebellious *qi* that rises up to the head.
- Drains Heat.
- Opens the channel and moves *qi* and *xue* in the channel and surrounding area.

Indications

- **Headache, feeling of heaviness in the head, dizziness, red eyes, nose bleeds and shaking of the head:** Just like several of the other Urinary Bladder channel points in the ankle region, UB 65 can be used in the treatment of disorders of the head, especially when these are due to ascending *yang* and internally generated Wind. As a *taiyang* channel point, UB 64 can expel exogenous Wind from the head.

- **Stiff neck, headache and pain in the back, lumbar region, legs, ankles and feet:** Like other Urinary Bladder channel points, UB 65 can treat disorders in the local area and at the opposite end of the channel.

Urinary Bladder 66 *Zutonggu* (Valley Passage)

- *Ying*-spring point.
- Water point.

Actions

- Controls rebellious *qi* in the head.
- Drains Heat.
- Opens the channel and moves *qi* and *xue* in the channel and in the local area.

Indications

- **Headache, feeling of heaviness in the head, dizziness, red eyes, nose bleeds and shaking of the head:** Like the other Urinary Bladder channel points on the foot, UB 66 can be used as a distal point to drain *yang* and Heat down from the head.
- **Pain, stiffness or swelling of the toes and feet:** UB 66 can be used to treat local disorders.

Urinary Bladder 67 *Zhiyin* (Reaching *Yin*)

- *Jing*-well point.
- Metal point.
- Five Phase tonifying point.
- Exit point.

Actions

- Controls rebellious *qi* that rises up to the head.
- Expels Wind and Heat.
- Opens the channel and moves *qi* and *xue* in the channel and in the local area.

Indications

- **Headache, feeling of heaviness in the head, dizziness, red eyes, nose bleeds and stiffness in the neck:** Most *jing*-well points can be used to restore consciousness, but UB 67 does not possess this quality. However, UB 67 is recommended in the treatment of acute headaches, especially headaches that are caused by internally generated and exogenous Wind. Like other Urinary Bladder points on the foot, UB 67 can be used as a distal point to address problems in the eyes, nose and neck.

- **Malposition of foetus, delayed labour, difficult labour and placental retention:** UB 67 is an empirical point to turn the foetus when it is malpositioned prior to birth. In these situations, UB 67 is heated with moxa during the final month of the pregnancy to create *yang* activity in the Uterus. By creating *yang* activity in the Uterus, UB 67 can also be used to induce labour and expel the placenta after birth.

- **Pain, stiffness or swelling in the toes and feet:** UB 67 can be used to treat local disorders.

KIDNEY CHANNEL ACUPUNCTURE POINTS

Type	Point
Yuan-source	Kid 3
Luo-connecting	Kid 4
Xi-cleft	Kid 5
Mu-collecting	GB 25
Back-*shu*	UB 23
Jing-well	Kid 1
Ying-spring	Kid 2
Shu-stream	Kid 3
Jing-river	Kid 7
He-sea	Kid 10
Wood	Kid 1
Fire	Kid 2
Earth	Kid 3
Metal	Kid 7
Water	Kid 10
Entry point	Kid 1
Exit point	Kid 22
Five Phase tonifying point	Kid 7
Five Phase draining point	Kid 1

Kidney 1 *Yongquan* (Bubbling Spring)

- *Jing*-well point.
- Wood point.
- Five Phase draining point.
- Entry point.

Actions

- Nourishes Kidney *yin* and clears *xu* Heat.

- Harmonises the Kidneys and Heart and thereby calms *shen*.

- Drains *qi* down from the head and controls ascending *yang*.

- Restores consciousness and rescues *yang*.

- Opens the channel and moves *qi* and *xue* in the channel and in the local area.

Indications

- **Loss of consciousness:** Similar to most *jing*-well points, Kid 1 can be used to restore consciousness when internal Wind has swirled up Phlegm and blocked the orifices of the Heart.

- **Insomnia, mental restlessness, manic behaviour and anger:** Kid 1 has a *shen*-calming effect. There are two reasons for this: Kid 1 nourishes Kidney *yin*, which is the root of Heart *yin*, and it is Heart *yin* that nourishes and anchors *shen*. As well as this, Kid 1 is located on the underside of the foot, making it an extremely *yin* acupuncture point that can draw *qi* downwards from the head.

- **Epilepsy, dizziness, headache, a sensation of pressure in the head and tinnitus:** These conditions can arise when there is ascending Liver *yang* or internally generated Wind. Some of these conditions can arise from *yin xu*. Kid 1 can drain *yang* and Wind down from the head, and it can nourish Kidney *yin*, so *yang* is anchored. This means that Kid 1 can be used to treat *xu* and *shi* conditions in the head and in the Kidneys' sense organ, the ear.

- **'Running piglet *qi*':** 'Running piglet *qi*' is a sensation that arises when rebellious *qi* ascends uncontrollably up the course of *chong mai*. It can feel like 'butterflies' in the stomach and there can be palpitations and a sensation of restriction in the chest and throat. If it is more extreme, it can be experienced as a panic attack. The Kidneys have a close relationship to *chong mai*, and Kid 1 can drain the rebellious *qi* downward.

- **Hot flushes, night sweats, dry throat and dry tongue:** The Kidneys are the root of *yin* in the body. Kid 1 can be used to nourish Kidney *yin* and thereby control *xu* Heat.

- **Constipation and urinary difficulty:** By nourishing Kidney *yin*, Kid 1 can be used in the treatment of Kidney *yin xu* conditions where the stool has become dry and hard and where the urine has become very concentrated and scanty. The Kidneys also control the body's lower orifices.

- **Infertility and impotence:** Kid 1 nourishes Kidney *yin* and *jing* and thereby has an influence on sexual function and the ability to reproduce.

- **Pain, discomfort, numbness and sensory disturbances under the foot and along the path of the channel:** Kid 1 is the only acupuncture point on the underside of the foot. Kid 1 can therefore be used to treat numbness and sensory disturbances in the sole of the foot.

Kidney 2 *Rangu* (Burning Valley)

- *Ying*-spring point.

- Fire point.

- *Yin qiao mai* source point.

Actions

- Nourishes Kidney *yin* and clears *xu* Heat.

- Opens the channel and moves *qi* and *xue* in the channel and in the local area.

Indications

- **Night sweats, hot flushes, dryness in the throat, dry tongue and hot or sweaty palms and foot soles:** Kid 2 is a Fire point on the Kidney channel. Kid 2 can both nourish *yin* and clear *xu* Heat arising from Kidney *yin xu*.

- **Anxiety and insomnia:** Kidney *yin* nourishes Heart *yin* and thereby controls Heat in the Heart. Kid 2 is the Kidney channel Fire point and can therefore both nourish *yin* and clear *xu* Heat, which ascends upwards, agitating *shen*.

- **Genital itching, nocturnal emissions, urinary disturbances and *shan*[10] disorders:** Kidney *yin xu* can result in *xu* Heat, which rises up the Kidney channel to the genitalia and the lower *jiao*. As the channel's Fire point, Kid 2 can nourish Kidney *yin* and clear *xu* Heat.

- **Irregular menstruations:** The menstrual cycle is dependent on Kidney *yin*, which is the foundation of the menstrual blood. Kidney *qi* is also used to keep the Uterus 'closed' so that the menstrual blood does not leave the Uterus at the wrong time or in the wrong amounts. *Xu* Heat can agitate *xue* and result in premature menstrual bleeding, heavy bleeding or spotting. Kid 2 can both nourish Kidney *yin* and clear *xu* Heat.

- **Bloody cough, dry cough and dyspnoea:** Kidney *yin* nourishes Lung *yin*. Furthermore, *xu* Heat can itself desiccate the Lung and solidify Phlegm so that Phlegm becomes thick and rubbery. The Heat can agitate *xue* so that there is bleeding in the Lung. Kid 2 can therefore be used as an additional acupuncture point in the treatment of *yin xu* Heat in the Lung.

- **Pain, discomfort, swelling, numbness and sensory disturbances in the foot and along the path of the channel:** As with all acupuncture points, Kid 2 can be used to treat local and distal problems along the path of the channel.

Kidney 3 *Taixi* (Great Ravine)

- *Shu*-stream point.
- *Yuan*-source point.
- Earth point.

Actions

- Tonifies Kidney *yang* and Kidney *qi*.
- Nourishes Kidney *yin* and Kidney *jing*.
- Calms *shen*.
- Strengthens the lumbar region and knees.
- Opens the channel and moves *qi* and *xue* in the channel and in the local area.

Indications

- **Fatigue, tiredness, weakness or fatigue in the lumbar region and/or knees, dizziness, tinnitus and deafness:** Kid 3 tonifies both the Kidney *yin* and *yang* aspects. These are often simultaneously *xu*, especially in middle-aged and older people. Kid 3, which is the Kidney *yuan*-source point, is one of the most tonifying acupuncture points in the body. Kid 3 tonifies and nourishes the pre-heavenly *qi*.

- **Night sweats and hot flushes:** By nourishing Kidney *yin*, Kid 3 can control and clear *xu* Heat.

- **Poor memory and insomnia:** Kidney *jing* nourishes the brain, and Kidney *yin* supports Heart *yin* in its functions of nourishing and anchoring *shen*. Furthermore, the Kidneys are the pre-heavenly root of *qi* and *xue*, which nourish the brain and *shen*. Kid 3 is therefore an important point in the treatment of many *shen* imbalances.

- **Frequent urination, incontinence, urinary difficulty and dribbling urination:** Both Kidney *yang xu* and Kidney *yin xu* can lead to disturbances of the urination. As a *yuan*-source point, Kid 3 will have a fundamental effect on these disorders.

- **Nocturnal emissions, premature ejaculation emissions, lack of libido, impotence and infertility:** Kidney *yin xu* Heat can cause *mingmen* to flare up. The resultant *mingmen* Heat can manifest with an increased libido. Kidney *yin xu* Heat can also force the semen outwards from the *bao*, resulting in premature ejaculation or nocturnal emissions. Kidney *yang xu*, for its part, can manifest with a lack of libido and impotence. Kidney *yang xu* can also be a factor in premature ejaculation and nocturnal emissions, when *yang* is not strong enough to secure the lower orifices and hold the semen in the body. Kidney *yin* and Kidney *jing* are the basis for fertility. As a *yuan*-source point, Kid 3 is one of the most important points to tonify the Kidney.

- **Diarrhoea:** By tonifying Kidney *yang*, Kid 3 is able to treat watery diarrhoea and diarrhoea that contains undigested food. Diarrhoea that is a manifestation of Kidney *yang xu* will often be seen with a person waking up early, sometimes around dawn, with the need to defecate watery stools. The use of moxa on Kid 3 is recommended in the treatment of Kidney *yang xu*.

- **Dyspnoea, cough, shortness of breath and shallow breathing:** By tonifying Kidney *qi*, Kid 3 can help the Kidneys to grasp the *qi* that the Lung has sent down through the body from the upper *jiao*.

- **Irregular, sparse or heavy menstrual bleeding and dysmenorrhoea:** The menstrual cycle is dependent on Kidney *yin*, which is the foundation of menstrual blood. In addition, *xu* Heat can agitate *xue* and result in early bleeding, heavy bleeding or spotting. Kidney *yang* warms the Uterus. Kidney *yang* thereby keeps Cold out of the Uterus, whilst at the same time creating the necessary activity and transformation in the Uterus. Furthermore, Kidney *qi* is used to hold the Uterus closed so that the menstrual blood does not leave the Uterus at the wrong time or in the wrong amounts.

- **Pain, discomfort, swelling, numbness, stiffness and sensory disturbances in the ankle and along the path of the channel:** Kid 3 is an important acupuncture point in the treatment of pain and weakness in the ankle and the Achilles tendon.

Kidney 4 *Dazhong* (Large Cup)

- *Luo*-connecting point.

Actions

- Tonifies Kidney *qi*.

- Harmonises the Kidneys and Lung and anchors Lung *qi*.

- Strengthens *zhi* and calms *shen*.

- Strengthens the lumbar region.

- Benefits urination.

- Opens the channel and moves *qi* and *xue* in the channel and in the local area.

Indications

- **Dyspnoea, cough, shortness of breath, shallow breathing and chest oppression:** Kid 4 is the most important acupuncture point on the Kidney channel to strengthen the ability of the Kidney to grasp the *qi* that the Lung sends down.

- **Depression, a need to keep themselves to themselves and not talk to anyone, fear, anxiety, dementia and manic behaviour:** In common with other *yin* channel *luo*-connecting points, Kid 4 treats mental-emotional imbalances. A special indication that is attributed to Kid 4 is the desire to remain indoors and avoid human contact. The person will often also suffer from anxiety. Manic behaviour can be experienced when Kidney *yin* cannot control Heart Fire.

- **Fatigue, tiredness, somnolence and weakness or fatigue in the lumbar region and/or knees:** Both Kidney *yang xu* and Kidney *jing xu* can manifest with fatigue and exhaustion. Kidney *jing* is the root of the Bones and Bone Marrow. Kidney *yang* fortifies and warms the lumbar region and the knees. Kidney *xu* conditions will often manifest with knee and lumbar problems.

- **Constipation and urinary difficulty:** Kidney *yin xu* can cause the stool to be very dry and hard and the urine to be concentrated and sparse. Kidney *yang xu* can result in frequent urination, copious urination, incontinence, dribbling after urination and a weak flow of urine.

- **Local disorders:** Pain, discomfort, swelling, numbness, stiffness and sensory disturbances in the ankle and along the path of the channel.

Kidney 5 *Shuiquan* (Water Spring)

- *Xi*-cleft point.

Actions

- Regulates the Uterus and menstruation.

- Benefits urination.

- Opens the channel and moves *qi* and *xue* in the channel and in the local area.

Indications

- **Irregular, sparse or heavy menstrual bleeding, spotting and dysmenorrhoea:** The Kidneys have a close relationship to the Uterus and menstrual cycle, due to Kidney *jing* being the foundation of *tian gui* or menstrual blood. The cycle itself is dependent on the constant alternation of *yin* and *yang* throughout the month. This means that most Kidney channel points have an influence on menstrual bleeding. Kid 5 has a specific influence on menstrual bleeding, because Kid 5 is a *xi*-cleft point. *Xi*-cleft points on *yin* channels are used to regulate bleeding disturbances.

- **Urinary difficulty:** *Xi*-cleft points can be used for acute and painful conditions that relate to their organ. Kid 5 is therefore relevant in the treatment of acute and painful urinary disturbances, for example cystitis.

- **Local disorders:** Pain, discomfort, swelling, numbness, stiffness and sensory disturbances in the ankle and along the path of the channel.

Kidney 6 *Zhaohai* (Shining Sea)

- Opening point of *yin qiao mai*.

Actions

- Nourishes Kidney *yin*.

- Calms *shen*.

- Benefits the eyes.

- Benefits the throat.

- Regulates *yin qiao mai*.

- Opens the channel and moves *qi* and *xue* in the channel and in the local area.

Indications

- **Night sweats, hot flushes and hot or sweaty palms and soles of the feet:** Kid 6 nourishes Kidney *yin*, and Kid 6 can thereby clear *xu* Heat. Kid 6 is therefore an acupuncture point that is widely used in the treatment of *yin xu* conditions. It can be combined in these situations with Lu 7, the opening point of *ren mai*.

- **Insomnia, somnolence, difficulty remaining awake, red eyes, sore eyes and superficial visual disturbances:** *Yin qiao mai* and *yang qiao mai* meet in the internal canthus of the eye at UB 1. Together they coordinate the opening and closing of the eyes, whilst at the same time regulating the balance between *yin* and *yang* in the head. This is why both channels' opening points, Kid 6 and UB 62, are used to treat problems with the eyes and especially to treat sleep disturbances. The two opening points will often be used together, one being drained and the other is tonified depending on whether there is too much or too little *yin* or *yang* in the eye. The two points are often combined with UB 1 in the treatment of insomnia.

- **Mental restlessness, anxiety, fear and palpitations:** Kidney *yin xu* can result in *shen* being agitated due to the *xu* Heat ascending up to the Heart. Also, because Heart *yin* is not nourished, it will not be able to nourish and anchor *shen*. *Yin qiao mai* also connects to the Heart and Kidney channels, as well as regulating *yin* in the body. For these reasons Kid 6 is a very important acupuncture point to calm *shen*.

- **Dizziness and epilepsy:** *Yin xu* can in itself result in dizziness, due to the Brain not being nourished. In addition, *yin xu* can result in the generation of Wind and in not being able to control *yang*. Both of these conditions can result in dizziness. Internally generated Wind can trigger epilepsy.

- **Dryness in the throat, swelling in the throat, 'plumstone *qi*' and dry, itchy cough:** Both the Kidney channel and *yin qiao mai* connect to the throat. Kid 6 is a very important distal point in the treatment of throat disorders when there is *yin xu*.

- **Genital itching, nocturnal emissions, involuntary erections, distension above the pubic bone and *shan* disorder:** Kidney *yin xu* can result in *xu* Heat, which rises up along the Kidney channel to the genitalia and the lower *jiao*. Kid 6 is one of the most important *yin*-nourishing points on the Kidney channel.

- **Constipation:** Kid 6 and Sp 6, which are both *yin*-nourishing acupuncture points, are often used together to treat constipation due to *yin xu*.

- **Irregular, sparse or heavy menstrual bleeding and dysmenorrhoea:** The menstrual cycle is dependent on Kidney *yin*, which is the foundation of menstrual blood. In addition, *xu* Heat can agitate *xue* and result in early periods, heavy bleeding or spotting. Kid 6 is an important point to nourish Kidney *yin*.

- **Imbalances between the right-hand and left-hand sides, one leg longer than the other, uneven hips or shoulders, weak, cramping or tense muscles along the medial aspect of the leg, and unilateral sweating:** *Yin qiao mai* is a part of the body's energetic framework and therefore has an influence on the body's physical structure. Kid 6 is the opening point for *yin qiao mai* and will often be used together with UB 62, which is the opening point for *yang qiao mai*. Together they can be used in the treatment of physical differences between one side of the body and the other, and to treat differences in the medial and lateral muscles in the leg.

- **Local disorders:** Pain, discomfort, swelling, numbness, stiffness and sensory disturbances in the ankle and along the path of the channel.

Kidney 7 *Fuliu* (Recover Flow)

- *Jing*-river point.

- Metal point.

- Five Phase tonifying point.

Actions

- Tonifies Kidney *yang* and nourishes Kidney *yin*.

- Regulates the water passages.

- Regulates sweating.

- Strengthens the lumbar region.

- Drains Dampness and Damp-Heat.

- Opens the channel and moves *qi* and *xue* in the channel and in the local area.

Indications

- **Urinary difficulty, incontinence, frequent urination, cloudy urine, blood in the urine, oedema, night sweats, spontaneous sweating, uncontrollable sweating and lack of sweating:** The Kidneys have a fundamental influence on all the processes involved in fluid physiology. Kidney *yang* is involved in many aspects of these processes, with regard to the transformation and transportation of fluids, but also in relation to urination and sweating. Kidney *yang* is used by the Urinary Bladder, both to keep the urine inside the Urinary Bladder and to drive the urine out of the Urinary Bladder when urinating. The Kidneys are also the root of *wei qi*, and thus the Kidneys have a powerful influence on the ability to keep the pores in the skin closed. This means that Kidney channel points in general can be used to influence fluid physiology, urination and sweating. Kid 7 though has a special ability to regulate fluid physiology and to regulate sweating. Kid 7 can be used when there is Kidney *yang xu* manifesting with oedema, frequent and copious urination and spontaneous sweating. Kid 7 can also be utilised when Kidney *yin xu* affects the body fluids. Kid 7 combined with He 6 is a classic combination for controlling night sweats when there is Heart and Kidney *yin xu*. Kid 7 can also be used in the treatment of sparse, very dark urine. Kid 7 can also be used for urinary tract disorders, caused by Damp-Heat. This is because Kid 7 can treat both the cause and the manifestation, as Kid 7 has Damp-Heat draining properties. At the same time Kid 7 can tonify Kidney *yang*, which is often the reason that the Urinary Bladder is invaded by Cold and Dampness, which can be the root cause of Damp-Heat. Dampness can also collect in the lower *jiao*, when fluids have not been transformed optimally.

- **Diarrhoea and borborygmi:** By tonifying Kidney *yang*, Kid 7 can be used to treat watery diarrhoea and diarrhoea that contains undigested remains. Diarrhoea, caused by Kidney *yang xu*, will often manifest very early in the morning, with the person waking up because they need to pass very watery stools. Kid 7 is also said to have Damp-Heat draining properties. This means that Kid 7 can be used in the treatment of haemorrhoids and diarrhoea when there is Damp-Heat and to treat stools containing blood or pus.

- **Lumbar and back problems and weak or cold knees:** Kid 7 is an important acupuncture point to tonify Kidney *yang*, especially when Kid 7 is stimulated with moxa. This means that Kid 7 is particularly good at strengthening the lumbar region and knees.

Kidney 8 *Jiaoxin* (Connecting Faith)

- *Xi*-cleft point of *yin qiao mai*.

Actions

- Regulates the Uterus and stops bleeding.

- Drains Dampness and Heat from the lower *jiao*.

- Opens the channel and moves *qi* and *xue* in the channel and surrounding area.

Indications

- **Irregular, heavy periods, amenorrhoea and spotting:** Kid 8 is recommended for all types of bleeding from the Uterus, both *xu* and *shi* bleeding. The ability of Kid 7 to hold the menstrual blood inside the Uterus should be seen in light of the fact that Kid 8 is the *xi*-cleft point of *yin qiao mai*. As a *xi*-cleft point, Kid 8 has an influence on *xue*. The Kidneys, via *bao luo*, also ensure that the Uterus remains closed when appropriate so that menstrual blood and the foetus remain in the Uterus until the right moment for their release. This is an example of the Kidney function of controlling the lower orifices.

- **Diarrhoea, abdominal distension, urinary problems, genital itching and swollen and painful genitalia:** Kid 8 can drain Damp-Heat from the lower *jiao*.

- **Local disorders:** Pain, discomfort, swelling, numbness and stiffness in the local area and along the channel.

Kidney 9 *Zhubin* (Guest House)

- *Xi*-cleft point of *yin wei mai*.

- *Yin wei mai* source point.

Actions

- Nourishes Kidney *yin*.

- Calms *shen*.

- Opens the channel and moves *qi* and *xue* in the channel and in the local area.

Indications

- **Fear, anxiety, palpitations, manic behaviour and mental restlessness:** Kid 9 is the source point of *yin wei mai*. Kid 9 can therefore be used in the treatment of Heart imbalances, in particular Heart *xue xu* and Heart *yin xu*.

- **Night sweats, hot flushes, dizziness, tinnitus and dry throat:** Kid 9 can be used to nourish Kidney *yin*.

- **Chest oppression and heaviness in the chest:** As the *xi*-cleft point of *yin wei mai*, Kid 9 can be used when there are acute stagnations in the channel. This means that Kid 9 can be used in the treatment of pain and chest oppression in the chest, as well as cardiac pain.

- **Local disorders:** Pain, discomfort, swelling, numbness and stiffness in the local area and along the channel.

Kidney 10 *Yingu* (*Yin* Valley)

- *He*-sea point.

- Water point.

- Starting point of the Kidney divergent channel.

Actions

- Tonifies and nourishes the Kidneys.

- Drains Damp-Heat from the lower *jiao*.

- Opens the channel and moves *qi* and *xue* in the channel and in the local area.

Indications

- **Dark urine, strongly smelling urine, cloudy urine, difficult or painful urination and blood in the urine:** Kid 10 can drain Damp-Heat from the lower *jiao* and the Kidneys' partner organ, the Urinary Bladder.

- **Genital itching, impotence, *shan* disorder, pain or distension in the inguinal area and around the pubic bone, vaginal discharge and uterine bleeding:** Like other *he*-sea points, Kid 10 can drain Damp-Heat from the lower *jiao*, particularly from the urinary system and the genitalia.

- **Lumbar problems, tinnitus, dizziness, night sweats, hot flushes and a dry throat:** By nourishing Kidney *yin*, Kid 10 can be used in the treatment of Kidney *yin xu*.

- **Local disorders:** Pain, discomfort, swelling, numbness and stiffness of the knees and along the channel.

Kidney 11 *Henggu* (Pubic Bone)

- Meeting point of the Kidney channel and *chong mai*.

Actions

- Circulates *qi* and *xue* in the lower *jiao*.

- Drains Dampness and Heat from the lower *jiao*.

- Opens the channel and moves *qi* and *xue* in the channel and in the local area.

Indications

- **Urinary difficulty, dribbling urination, lack of urination, painful urination, blood in the urine, cloudy urine and copious vaginal discharge:** Kid 11 is one of the many Kidney channel points that are a point on the Kidney channel and at the same time a *chong mai* point. This means that these acupuncture points can be used to influence both of these channels and their spheres of influence. Kid 11 is mainly used as a local point when treating Dampness and Damp-Heat in the urinary system and genitalia. Kid 11 can also, by virtue of its relationship to *chong mai*, be used to treat *xue* stagnations in the lower *jiao*.

Kidney 12 *Dahe* (Great Brightness)

- Meeting point of the Kidney channel and *chong mai*.

Actions

- Nourishes the Kidneys and astringes *jing*.

- Opens the channel and moves *qi* and *xue* in the channel and surrounding area.

Indications

- **Watery vaginal discharge, nocturnal emissions and premature ejaculation:** Kid 12 is mainly used as a local point to treat stagnations in the lower *jiao*, especially in the Uterus, and to 'astringe' *jing*. To astringe *jing* means that Kid 12 can be used to hold *jing* in the Kidneys.

- **Infertility and impotence:** Kid 12 can also be used to stimulate Kidney *jing*.

Kidney 13 *Qixue* (Qi Cavern)

- Meeting point of the Kidney channel and *chong mai*.

Actions

- Regulates *qi* and *xue* in the lower *jiao*.
- Regulates the Uterus.
- Opens the channel and moves *qi* and *xue* in the channel and in the local area.

Indications

- **Infertility, dysmenorrhoea, irregular periods and urinary problems:** As an acupuncture point on the Kidney channel and *chong mai*, Kid 13 has a significant influence on the *bao* or Uterus. This is witnessed by Kid 13 being used when there are disruptions of the menstrual cycle and to relieve menstrual pain. Kid 13 can also be used in the treatment of infertility in women. In addition, Kid 13 is used to treat urinary problems and disturbances of *qi* and *xue* in the lower abdomen.

- **'Running piglet' syndrome:** Kid 13, Kid 14 and Kid 15 can all be used to treat 'running piglet' syndrome, where rebellious *qi* rises uncontrolled up *chong mai*, with symptoms such as turmoil in the abdomen and chest, palpitations, mental unrest and a sense of constriction in the throat and chest.

Kidney 14 *Siman* (Four Fullness)

- Meeting point of the Kidney channel and *chong mai*.

Actions

- Moves *qi* and *xue* in the lower *jiao*.

- Regulates the Uterus.

- Opens the water passages in the lower *jiao*.

- Opens the channel and moves *qi* and *xue* in the channel and in the local area.

Indications

- **Infertility, dysmenorrhoea, irregular periods and urinary problems:** Kid 14 is mainly used to move *qi* and *xue* in the lower *jiao*, especially in the Uterus. Kid 14 can therefore be used in the treatment of irregular or painful menstrual bleeding. Kid 14 can also be used when there are intestinal problems, such as distension, constipation and diarrhoea. By regulating the lower *jiao*, Kid 14 can be used in the treatment of copious vaginal discharge.

- **'Running piglet' syndrome:** Kid 13, Kid 14 and Kid 15 can all be used to treat 'running piglet' syndrome, where rebellious *qi* rises uncontrolled up *chong mai*, with symptoms such as turmoil in the abdomen and chest, palpitations, mental unrest and a sense of constriction in the throat and chest.

Kidney 15 *Zhongzhu* (Central Flow), Kidney 16 *Huangshu* (Huang[11] Point), Kidney 17 *Shangqu* (Shang[12] Bend) and Kidney 18 *Shiguan* (Stone Crossing)

- Meeting points of the Kidney channel and *chong mai*.

Actions

- Move *qi* and *xue* in the lower *jiao* and middle *jiao*.
- Regulate the Intestines.
- Open the channel and move *qi* and *xue* in the channel and in the local area.

Indications

- **Abdominal distension, abdominal pain, constipation, diarrhoea and borborygmi:** Kid 15, Kid 16, Kid 17 and Kid 18 are most often used when there are stagnations and other disturbances of *qi* in the Intestines.

Kidney 19 *Yindu* (*Yin* Metropolis), Kidney 20 *Futonggu* (Abdominal Connecting Valley) and Kidney 21 *Youmen* (Dark Door)

- Meeting points of the Kidney channel and *chong mai*.

Actions

- Regulate *qi* in the middle *jiao*.
- Harmonise the Stomach.
- Open the channel and move *qi* and *xue* in the channel and the surrounding area.

Indications

- **Epigastric pain, vomiting, nausea, acid regurgitation, hiccups, constipation and diarrhoea:** Kid 19, Kid 20 and Kid 21 are usually used to regulate *qi* and *xue* in the Stomach and the middle *jiao*.

- **Chest oppression, cough and shortness of breath:** By regulating *qi* in the middle *jiao*, these acupuncture points can be used to create sufficient space so that *qi* can descend from the upper *jiao*.

- **Breast distension and problems with lactation:** Kid 21 can also tonify the Spleen and spread Liver *qi*. By spreading Liver *qi*, Kid 21 can be used in the treatment of breast distension and problems with lactation.

Kidney 22 *Bulang* (Corridor Walk), Kidney 23 *Shenfeng* (*Shen* Seal), Kidney 24 *Lingxu* (Supported Ruins), Kidney 25 *Shencang* (*Shen* Storehouse), Kidney 26 *Yuzhong* (Elegant Centre) and Kidney 27 *Shufu* (*Shu* Mansion)

- Kidney 22 is the channel's exit point.

Actions

- Regulate Lung and Stomach *qi*.

- Regulate *qi* in the upper *jiao* and open the chest.

- Benefit the breasts.

- Open the channel and move *qi* and *xue* in the channel and in the local area.

Indications

- **Chest oppression, respiratory problems, cough, nausea, vomiting, breast distension, cardiac pain and palpitations:** Several of these Kidney channel points have names containing the words *shen* and *ling*. Both words refer to the body's spiritual aspects. This has led 'Worsley-style Five Element' acupuncturists to ascribe these points *shen*-calming qualities. This does not appear to be the case in Japanese acupuncture and modern TCM. Instead these acupuncture points are used as local points to regulate Lung and Stomach *qi*, open the chest and affect the breasts themselves.

PERICARDIUM CHANNEL ACUPUNCTURE POINTS

Type	Point
Yuan-source	Pe 7
Luo-connecting	Pe 6
Xi-cleft	Pe 4
Mu-collecting	Ren 17
Back-*shu*	UB 14
Jing-well	Pe 9
Ying-spring	Pe 8
Shu-stream	Pe 7
Jing-river	Pe 5
He-sea	Pe 3
Wood	Pe 9
Fire	Pe 8
Earth	Pe 7
Metal	Pe 5
Water	Pe 3
Entry point	Pe 1
Exit point	Pe 8
Five Phase tonifying point	Pe 9
Five Phase draining point	Pe 7

Pericardium 1 *Tianchi* (Heavenly Pool)

- Entry point.
- Starting point of the Pericardium divergent channel.
- Meeting point of the Pericardium, Liver, Gall Bladder and *san jiao* channels.
- Window of Heaven point.

Actions

- Opens the chest.

- Transforms Phlegm and regulates *qi* in the upper *jiao*.

- Disperses knots.

- Benefits the breasts.

- Opens the channel and moves *qi* and *xue* in the channel and in the local area.

Indications

- **Cough, chest oppression, chest pain, breast pain, poor lactation, breast abscesses and breast lumps:** Pe 1 is mainly used to treat stagnations in the breasts and the costal region. Pe 1 can also regulate Lung *qi*, and Pe 1 can therefore be used in the treatment of coughs.

Pericardium 2 *Tianquan* (Heavenly Spring)

Actions

- Opens the chest.

- Opens the channel and moves *qi* and *xue* in the channel and in the local area.

Indications

- **Pain and numbness in the upper arm and pain and tension in the chest:** Pe 2 is mainly used in the treatment of local disorders, for example pain in the upper arm. Pe 2 can regulate *qi* and *xue* in the upper *jiao* and can therefore be used in the treatment of pain and distension in the chest.

Pericardium 3 *Quze* (Marsh at the Bend)

- *He*-sea point.

- Water point.

Actions

- Drains Heat and cools *xue*.

- Calms *shen*.

- Invigorates *xue* in the chest.

- Regulates Stomach *qi*.

- Calms internally generated Wind.

- Opens the channel and moves *qi* and *xue* in the channel and in the local area.

Indications

- **Febrile diseases, delirium, red skin rashes, agitation and mental restlessness, thirst, dry tongue, vomiting of blood and bloody cough:** Pe 3 can be used to drain Heat and cool *xue*. Pe 3 is used in particular when exogenous *xie qi* has penetrated down to the *qi*, *ying* or *xue* level of the 'Four level' diagnosis.

- **Skin diseases caused by *xue* Heat or *qi*-level Heat, for example eczema, rosacea and psoriasis:** Pe 3 can drain Heat from the *qi* level, *ying* level and *xue* level. This means that Pe 3 can be used in the treatment of chronic and acute skin diseases where there is *xie* Heat in the body, creating *xue* Heat and *xue* stagnation.

- **Vomiting, nausea, abdominal pain, diarrhoea and constipation:** According to the *Nanjing*, *he*-sea points such as Pe 3 can be used to treat rebellious Stomach *qi* and diarrhoea. Furthermore, the Pericardium channel passes through the Stomach and Intestines. Pe 3 can therefore regulate *qi* in these areas of the body.

- **Palpitations and pain in the chest:** *Xie* Heat can boil *xue* so that it becomes thick and sticky. This will lead to *xue* stagnation. By cooling *xue* Heat, and by invigorating *xue* in the chest, Pe 3 can be used when there are *xue* stagnation conditions in the upper *jiao* caused by *xue* Heat.

- **Tremors and shaking of the hands or head:** Pe 3 cools *xue*, and Pe 3 can therefore be used when Heat has generated internal Wind.

- **Local disorders:** Pain, numbness, tremors or lack of mobility of the elbow and along the path of the channel.

Pericardium 4 *Ximen* (Cleft Door)

- *Xi*-cleft point.

Actions

- Invigorates *xue* and disperses stagnation.

- Cools *xue* and stops bleeding.

- Calms *shen*.

- Opens the channel and moves *qi* and *xue* in the channel and in the local area.

Indications

- **Stabbing, sharp or cramping pain in the chest, cardiac pain and palpitations:** Pe 4 is the *xi*-cleft point on the Pericardium channel. This means that Pe 4 is an important acupuncture point in the treatment of acute and painful conditions along the course of the channel and in the organ. In addition, *yin* channel *xi*-cleft points also have *xue*-invigorating properties. Pe 4 can therefore be used in the treatment of acute cardiac pain and chest pains.

- **Agitation, mental restlessness, depression, melancholy, anxiety and fear:** Pe 4 can affect *shen*, both by invigorating stagnant *xue* and by cooling *xue*. *Xue* stagnation can by itself block the movement of *shen*. The stagnated *xue* can also prevent fresh *xue* from reaching the Heart and nourishing *shen*.

- **Nose bleeds, bloody cough and vomiting of blood:** Pe 4 can stop bleeding, because it is a *xi*-cleft point and Pe 4 can cool *xue*.

Pericardium 5 *Jianshi* (Intermediate Messenger)

- *Jing*-river point.

- Metal point.

Actions

- Calms *shen*.

- Transforms Phlegm, drains Heat and opens the Heart's orifices.

- Regulates Stomach *qi*.

- Regulates the Uterus.

- Opens the channel and moves *qi* and *xue* in the channel and in the local area.

Indications

- **Bipolar depression, manic behaviour, insomnia, anxiety attacks, fear, mental restlessness, sadness, depression, amnesia, epilepsy and 'plumstone *qi*':** Pe 5 can drain Heat from the Heart, as well as transforming and draining Phlegm from the Heart. This means that Pe 5 is one of the most important points in the treatment of Phlegm-Fire in the Heart, where the Heat from Fire agitates *shen* and Phlegm blocks the orifices of the Heart and obscures *shen*. Pe 5 will often be used in combination with St 40 in these situations.

- **Chest oppression, palpitations, cardiac pain and chest pain:** Pe 5 can circulate *qi* and transform Phlegm in the upper *jiao*.

- **Abdominal pain, nausea and vomiting:** The Pericardium channel passes through all three *jiao*. Pericardium channel points can therefore be used to regulate *qi* in the Stomach and the middle *jiao*.

- **Heavy or irregular menstrual bleeding and dark and clotted menstrual blood:** Through its *jueyin* relationship to the Liver, the Pericardium channel can regulate the movement of *xue* in the Uterus. This means that Pe 5 can be used in some gynaecological treatments.

- **Local disorders:** Pain, swelling, numbness and stiffness of the wrist and along the path of the channel.

Pericardium 6 *Neiguan* (Inner Gate)

- *Luo*-connecting point.
- Opening point for *yin wei mai*.

Actions

- Regulates *qi* in the upper and middle *jiao*.
- Regulates Heart *qi*.
- Calms *shen*.
- Drains Heat.
- Spreads Liver *qi*.
- Opens *yin wei mai*.
- Opens the channel and moves *qi* and *xue* in the channel and in the local area.

Indications

- **Pain in the chest, cardiac pain, chest oppression, irregular heartbeat, palpitations, cough and asthma:** Even though Pe 6 was not one of the original four 'command' points recommended by Gao Wu, Pe 6 was later added to the list as the body's most important distal point for the treatment of disorders in the chest and costal region. Pe 6 can be used for all kinds of stagnation and disturbance of *qi* in the chest and costal region. As we will see below, the scope of the point also includes it being a distal point for disorders in the middle *jiao* and abdomen. This means that Pe 6 is one of the body's most utilised acupuncture points.

- **Nausea, vomiting, hiccups, burping and abdominal pain:** The Pericardium channel passes through all three *jiao*. Pericardium channel points can therefore be used to regulate *qi* in the Stomach and the middle *jiao*. Pe 6 has a very strong effect on rebellious *qi* in the Stomach and, together with St 36, is the primary acupuncture point in the treatment of all types of nausea, including morning sickness.

- **Insomnia, mental restlessness, manic behaviour, anxiety, poor memory, sadness and depression:** The Pericardium envelops the Heart and thus has a very close relationship to the Heart and thereby *shen*. Pe 6 can move stagnant *xue* and *qi* in the Heart and can drain Heat from the Heart. This means that Pe 6 is a much-used acupuncture point in the treatment of *shen* disorders.

- **Hypertension, epilepsy and headache:** Pe 6 can drain Heat, which can be the root cause of internally generated Wind. Pe 6 also has a close relationship to Liver *qi*, and Pe 6 can be used to treat stagnations of Liver *qi*.

- **Irregular or painful menstrual bleeding:** Through its relationship to Liver *qi*, Pe 6 can spread Liver *qi* and thereby Liver *xue*. Pe 6 can therefore be used in the treatment of painful and irregular menstrual bleeding.

- **Poor memory or speech impediment following a stroke:** Pe 6 can be used to treat the consequences of a stroke. This is because Pe 6 directly affects *shen* and because Pe 6 can invigorate stagnant *xue* by spreading Liver *qi*.

- **Pain, swelling, numbness and stiffness of the wrist and along the path of the channel:** Pe 6 can be used as a local point to treat problems in the wrist and forearm, including carpal tunnel syndrome.

Pericardium 7 *Daling* (Large Mound)

- *Shu*-stream point.
- *Yuan*-source point.
- Earth point.
- Sun Si Miao ghost point.
- Five Phase draining point.

Actions

- Calms *shen*.

- Drains Heat from the Heart.

- Drains Heat and cools *xue*.

- Opens the chest.

- Regulates Stomach *qi*.

- Opens the channel and moves *qi* and *xue* in the channel and in the local area.

Indications

- **Insomnia, mental restlessness, depression, lack of joy, sadness, fear, anxiety and poor memory:** Pe 7 was originally used instead of He 7 as the *yuan*-source point of the Heart. At this time the Pericardium channel was used to treat the Heart. The two acupuncture points also have many similar actions and indications, but there are, however, also differences between the two points. Although both acupuncture points calm *shen*, Pe 7 is used more to drain Heat that is agitating *shen*. He 7, on the other hand, is used more to nourish Heart *yin* and Heart *xue*, and in this way calm *shen*. Just like He 7, Pe 7 can be used as a draining acupuncture point in 'Five Phase' acupuncture treatments, because it is an Earth point on a Fire channel.

- **Pain in the chest, cardiac pain, chest oppression, irregular heartbeat and palpitations:** The primary effect that Pe 7 has, in relation to a disturbance of *qi* in the upper *jiao*, is that it is a Heat-draining point. Heat in the upper *jiao* can agitate and create an overactivity of *qi* in the Heart and thereby both disrupt and accelerate the rhythm of the heartbeat.

- **Nausea, vomiting, hiccups, burping and abdominal pain:** The Pericardium channel passes through all three *jiao*. This means that Pericardium channel points can be used to regulate *qi* in the Stomach and in the middle *jiao*. Pe 7 is, however, not used as often in the treatment of the problems of the abdominal area as the previous point on the channel, Pe 6.

- **Fever, thirst, red eyes, yellow sclera, eczema, ulcer, boils and urticaria:** Pe 7 can be used to drain Heat and cool *xue*. This means that Pe 7 can be used both in the treatment of febrile illnesses and to treat certain skin disorders.

- **Pain, swelling, numbness and stiffness of the wrist and along the path of the channel:** Pe 7 can be used as a local point to treat problems in the wrist and forearm, including carpal tunnel syndrome.

Pericardium 8 *Laogong* (Palace of Toil)

- *Ying*-spring point.

- Fire point.

- Sun Si Miao ghost point.

- Exit point.

Actions

- Drains Fire from the Heart and calms *shen*.

- Drains Fire from the Pericardium and restores consciousness.

- Regulates Stomach *qi* and drains Heat from the middle *jiao*.

- Opens the channel and moves *qi* and *xue* in the channel and in the local area.

Indications

- **Insomnia, mental restlessness, manic behaviour, fear and uncontrollable anger or laughter:** Pe 8 is mainly used in the treatment of *shi* Heat conditions, such as Heart Fire and Phlegm-Heat in the Heart, where Heat agitates *shen*. Pe 8 has a powerful effect in draining Heart Fire.

- **Loss of consciousness, coma, stroke, epilepsy, febrile conditions and hypertension:** Pe 8 can be used to restore consciousness when Wind-Phlegm obscures and blocks the 'orifices of the Heart'. Pe 8 can be used to drain Heat from the *ying* level when *xie* Heat has penetrated down to this level. In addition, Pe 8 can drain *xue* Heat.

- **Pain in the chest, cardiac pain, chest oppression, irregular heartbeat and palpitations:** By draining Heat from the upper *jiao*, Pe 8 can regulate *qi* and *xue* that has been agitated by the Heat.

- **Vomiting of blood, nose bleeds and haemorrhoids:** Pe 8 can control bleeding resulting from *xue* Heat.

- **Pain, swelling, numbness and stiffness in the palm, little finger or along the path of the channel and skin diseases in the palm of the hand:** Pe 8 can be used as a local point to treat problems in the palm of the hand. Because Pe 8 can drain Heat, it is useful in the treatment of skin diseases, such as eczema in the palm of the hand.

Pericardium 9 *Zhongchong* (Central Thoroughfare)

- *Jing*-well point.
- Wood point.
- Five Phase tonifying point.

Actions

- Drains Heat from the Pericardium and restores consciousness.
- Drains Fire and benefits the tongue.
- Expels Summer-Heat.
- Opens the channel and moves *qi* and *xue* in the channel and in the local area.

Indications

- **High fever, fever with physical and mental restlessness, lethargy, headache, pain or stiffness of the tongue and hypertension:** Because it is a *jing*-well point, Pe 9 has a very dynamic effect when treating acute invasions of *xie qi* that have generated extreme Heat, swirling up Wind and Phlegm to the head.

- **Acute vomiting, diarrhoea and fever:** Pe 9 can expel invasions of Summer-Heat.

- **Pain in the chest, cardiac pain, chest oppression, irregular heartbeat and palpitations:** By draining Heat from the upper *jiao*, Pe 9 can regulate *qi* and *xue* that has been agitated by Heat. Pe 9 is also a *jing*-well point and can therefore be used to treat 'fullness below the Heart', i.e. a distended feeling in the chest.

- **Local disorders:** Pain, swelling, numbness and stiffness in the hand, little finger and along the path of the channel.

SAN JIAO CHANNEL ACUPUNCTURE POINTS

Type	Point
Yuan-source	SJ 4
Luo-connecting	SJ 5
Xi-cleft	SJ 7
Mu-collecting	Ren 5
Back-*shu*	UB 22
Jing-well	SJ 1
Ying-spring	SJ 2
Shu-stream	SJ 3
Jing-river	SJ 6
He-sea	SJ 10
Metal	SJ 1
Water	SJ 2
Wood	SJ 3
Fire	SJ 6
Earth	SJ 10
Entry point	SJ 1
Exit point	SJ 22
Five Phase tonifying point	SJ 3
Five Phase draining point	SJ 10

San jiao 1 *Guanchong* (Thoroughfare Gate)

- *Jing*-well point.
- Metal point.
- Entry point.

Actions

- Expels Heat.
- Benefits the eyes and ears.
- Opens the channel and moves *qi* and *xue* in the channel and in the local area.

Indications

- **Tinnitus, deafness, earache, conjunctivitis, sore eyes, red eyes and jaw pain:** In common with other *jing*-well points, SJ 1 can be used as a distal point to treat disorders in the sensory organs that the channel connects to or the sensory organs that the channel traverses. SJ 1 can in particular be used to expel and drain acute Heat disorders in the eyes and ears.

- **Febrile diseases, chills, stiff tongue, pain in the tongue, thirst, dry mouth, dry lips and bitter taste in the mouth:** SJ 1 can be used when there are symptoms that arise at the beginning of an invasion of *xie qi*, especially Wind-Heat.

- **Shoulder and neck pain, tension, stiffness in the neck and shoulders and pain in the arm, the elbow or the ring finger:** SJ 1 can be used to treat all forms of disturbance of *qi* along the path of the channel. It will in particular be in the shoulder area that there are blockages of the *san jiao* channel's *qi*.

San jiao 2 Yemen (Fluid Door)

- *Ying*-spring point.
- Water point.

Actions

- Expels Heat and benefits the ears.
- Calms *shen*.
- Opens the channel and moves *qi* and *xue* in the channel and in the local area.

Indications

- **Febrile diseases, chills, thirst, dry mouth, dry lips, tinnitus, deafness, earache, conjunctivitis, sore eyes, red eyes and jaw pain:** In common with other *ying*-spring points, SJ 2 can be used to expel Heat. In addition, SJ 2 is used as a distal point in the treatment of disorders of the sensory organs that the channel connects to or that the channel traverses. SJ 2 can in particular be used to expel and drain acute Heat disorders in the eyes and ears.

- **Fear, anxiety, palpitations, confused speech, mania and epilepsy:** Because *san jiao* has a *biaoli* or external/internal relationship to the Pericardium, SJ 2 can drain Heat from the Heart and calm *shen*.

- **Shoulder and neck pain, tension, stiffness in the neck and shoulders and pain in the arm, the elbow or the ring finger:** SJ 2 can be used to treat all forms of *qi* disturbances along the path of the channel. It is often in the shoulder area that there are often blockages of the *san jiao* channel *qi*.

San jiao 3 Zhongxu (Central Island)

- *Shu*-stream point.
- Wood point.
- Five Phase tonifying point.

Actions

- Expels Heat.
- Drains Heat from the head.
- Drains ascending Liver *yang* and Liver Fire.
- Benefits the ears.
- Harmonises *shaoyang*.
- Opens the channel and moves *qi* and *xue* in the channel and in the local area.

Indications

- **Tinnitus, deafness, earache, conjunctivitis, sore eyes and red eyes:** SJ 3 is both a *shu*-stream point and a very important distal point in the treatment of the ears. SJ 3 is used to expel invasions of *xie qi* or to drain *yang* or Fire from the ears. SJ 3 can also be used as a distal point in *xu* conditions that manifest with problems in the ears, such as Kidney *yin xu* tinnitus and deafness. In addition, SJ 3 is a distal point for eye disorders where Wind-Heat has invaded the eyes or internal Heat has ascended to the eyes.

- **Itching all over the body and red face:** SJ 3 can expel *xie qi* that has penetrated the body and started to generate Heat.

- **Headache and dizziness:** SJ 3 is in particular used to treat hemilateral, throbbing headaches and for the treatment of temporal headaches. This is because the *san jiao* channel has a *shaoyang* channel relationship with the Gall Bladder channel. As the Wood point of the *san jiao* channel, SJ 3 has a further resonance with the Liver and can be used to restrain Liver *yang*, Liver Fire and Liver Wind when these ascend up the Gall Bladder channel to the head. This is also the reason that SJ 3 can be used to treat dizziness.

- **Febrile diseases where there is an alternation between periods of fever and periods of chills and malaria:** SJ 3 is one of several *shaoyang* channel points that can be used to expel invasions of *xie qi* that have become locked in the *shaoyang* aspect of the body.

- **Shoulder and neck pain, tension, stiffness in the neck and shoulders, pain in the arm and elbow or pain and stiffness in the hand or fingers:** SJ 3 can be used for all kinds of *qi* disturbances along the path of the channel. It is often in the shoulder area that there are blockages of the *san jiao* channel *qi*.

San jiao 4 Yangchi (Yang Pool)

- *Yuan*-source point.

Actions

- Drains Heat.

- Tonifies *yuan qi*.

- Expels invasions of *xie qi*.

- Opens the channel and moves *qi* and *xue* in the channel and in the local area.

Indications

- **Stiffness, swelling and pain in the fingers, wrist, elbow, shoulder and neck, headache, tinnitus and jaw pain:** As a *yuan*-source point on a *yang* channel, SJ 4 can be used to expel invasions of *xie qi* that disrupt *qi* along the path of the channel.

- **Febrile diseases where there is an alternation between periods of fever and periods of chills, and malaria:** SJ 4 is one of several *shaoyang* channel points that can be used to expel *xie qi* that has become locked in the *shaoyang* aspect.

- **Fatigue and exhaustion:** There is a difference in how this acupuncture point's actions are viewed in Japanese and Chinese acupuncture traditions. The *san jiao* organ has a very close relationship with *yuan qi* and is responsible for the distribution of *yuan qi* from the Kidneys through the whole body. SJ 4 is the *yuan*-source point of the *san jiao* channel and is therefore used in Japanese acupuncture to tonify *yuan qi*. Chinese-based textbooks do not attribute SJ 4 these tonifying properties.

San jiao 5 Waiguan (Outer Gate)

- *Luo*-connecting point.

- Opening point of *yang wei mai*.

Actions

- Expels invasions of *xie qi*.

- Benefits the head and ears.

- Drains Heat.

- Restrains ascending Liver *yang*.

- Opens *yang wei mai*.

- Activates the channel and moves *qi* and *xue* in the channel and surrounding area.

Indications

- **Fever, chills, acute pain in the head and aversion to cold:** SJ 5 is an important acupuncture point to expel invasions of *xie qi*. SJ 5 operates on two levels. First, like a great many *shaoyang* channel points, SJ 5 can be used to expel exogenous *xie qi* that has become locked in the *shaoyang* aspect. Second, SJ 5 can be used to expel invasions of *xie qi* from the *wei qi* level. This means that SJ 5 can be used to treat acute invasions of exogenous *xie qi*.

- **Febrile diseases where there is an alternation between periods of fever and periods of chills, and malaria:** SJ 5 is one of the body's most important acupuncture points to expel *xie qi* that has become locked in the *shaoyang* aspect. Here, SJ 5 will often be used in combination with GB 34 or GB 40.

- **Headache, dizziness and neck pain:** SJ 5 is a very important distal point in the treatment of all the disorders in the head that manifest along the course of the *shaoyang* channel. In addition, SJ 5 restrains ascending Liver *yang*, Liver Fire and Liver Wind. This means that SJ 5 can be used in the treatment of hemilateral, throbbing headaches and temporal headaches. By opening to the exterior, SJ 5 can be used when there is a headache that is caused by an invasion of *xie qi*. Ascending Liver *yang* can also result in stiffness and pain in the neck and shoulders. In addition, SJ 5 can be used in the treatment of dizziness by calming Liver Wind.

- **Tinnitus, deafness, earache, conjunctivitis, sore eyes, red eyes and lacrimation:** SJ 5 can be used as a distal point in the treatment of disorders of the ear and eyes, especially when these are the result of invasions of exogenous *xie qi* or ascending Liver *yang*.

- **Constipation, abdominal pain, chest oppression and distension and pain in the costal region:** The *san jiao* channel passes through all three *jiao*. This means that SJ 5 can drain Heat that is locked in the interior, disrupting the circulation of *qi* and damaging fluids. The Heat will often rise up to the head. SJ 5 can therefore also be used to treat toothache, cracked lips and nose bleeds.

- **Pain, swelling, numbness and stiffness along the path of the channel:** SJ 5 is often used as a distal point to treat pain in the shoulder and neck. SJ 5 can also be used to treat local disorders in the area of the wrist and as a distal point to treat elbow problems, jaw aches and problems in the throat such as mumps, goitre or swollen lymph nodes.

San jiao 6 Zhigao (Branch Gully)

- *Jing*-river point.
- Fire point.

Actions

- Drains Heat from all three *jiao*.
- Regulates *qi* in all three *jiao*.
- Benefits the chest and costal region.
- Moves the stool.
- Opens the channel and moves *qi* and *xue* in the channel and in the local area.

Indications

- **Constipation:** SJ 6 is an extremely important acupuncture point in the treatment of constipation. However, it cannot treat all forms of constipation. SJ 6 is used to circulate *qi* and drain Heat from the Intestines. This means that SJ 6 is most suitable in the treatment of constipation in *shi* conditions.

- **Abdominal pain, distension, pain in the chest, pain in the costal region, cough and vomiting:** By circulating *qi* in all three *jiao*, SJ 6 can be used in the treatment of many different forms of stagnation. SJ 6 will often be combined with GB 34 in these situations.

- **Febrile disorders, muscle tremors, tinnitus, deafness, earache, conjunctivitis, sore eyes, red eyes, swollen throat, sore throat and tonsillitis:** As a Fire point and a *jing*-river point, SJ 6 can drain Heat from the areas that the channel connects to.

- **Local disorders:** Pain, discomfort, stiffness, paralysis, numbness and sensory disturbances along the path of the channel.

San jiao 7 Huizong (Gathering Meeting)

- *Xi*-cleft point.

Actions

- Benefits the ears.

- Opens the channel and moves *qi* and *xue* in the channel and in the local area.

Indications

- **Tinnitus, deafness, earache, conjunctivitis, sore eyes and red eyes:** As a *xi*-cleft point, SJ 7 can be used in the treatment of acute and painful conditions in the areas that the channel connects to.

- **Pain, discomfort, stiffness, paralysis, and numbness and sensory disturbances in the shoulder, elbow and along the path of the channel:** As a *xi*-cleft point, SJ 7 is used to treat acute and painful conditions along the path of the channel.

San jiao 8 Sanyangluo (Three Yang Luo)
Actions

- Opens the channel and moves *qi* and *xue* in the channel and in the local area.

Indications

- **Local and channel disorders:** SJ 8 is mainly used to treat disorders in the local area and along the path of the channel. Apart from pain, numbness and stiffness, the indications will also include sudden loss of voice and deafness.

San jiao 9 Sidu (Four Rivers)

Actions

- Opens the channel and moves *qi* and *xue* in the channel and in the local area.

Indications

- **Pain and stiffness in the lower arm, sudden loss of voice, sore throat, acute tinnitus and toothache:** SJ 9 is mainly used when there are disorders in the local area and along the path of the channel.

San jiao 10 Tianjing (Heavenly Well)

- *He*-sea point.
- Earth point.
- Five Phase draining point.

Actions

- Transforms Phlegm and dissolves accumulations.
- Regulates *qi*.
- Calms *shen*.
- Drains Heat from the *san jiao* channel.
- Opens the channel and moves *qi* and *xue* in the channel and in the local area.

Indications

- **Goitre, swollen lymph nodes in the neck and armpit, productive cough, vomiting of mucus and blood, chest oppression and poor appetite:** According to the *Nanjing*, *he*-sea points can be used to regulate *qi*. SJ 10, because it transforms Phlegm, can also be used to treat coughing and vomiting of Phlegm, as well as dispersing accumulations of Phlegm along the course of the channel.

- **Pain in the chest, abdomen and costal region:** The *san jiao* channel traverses all three *jiao*, as well as being a part of the same great channel as the Gall Bladder channel. SJ 10 can therefore be used to treat pain and distension in the costal region, abdomen and chest.

- **Epilepsy, manic behaviour, anxiety, fear, sadness and palpitations:** SJ 10 can be used to treat mental-emotional disorders caused by Phlegm-Heat. This is because SJ 10 can transform Phlegm, and because *san jiao* has a *yin/yang* relationship to the Pericardium.

- **Pain, discomfort, stiffness, paralysis, and numbness and sensory disturbances in the shoulder, elbow and along the path of the channel:** SJ 10 is mainly used in the treatment of pain in the elbow. Some of the classical texts have said that SJ 10 can treat *bi* (painful blockage of the channel) syndromes in the whole body.

San jiao 11 *Qinglengyuan* (Clear Cold Abyss) and *san jiao* 12 *Xiaoluo* (Dispersing Riverbed)

Actions

- Open the channel and move *qi* and *xue* in the channel and in the local area.

Indications

- **Local disorders:** SJ 11 and SJ 12 are used mainly to treat disorders in the local area and along the path of the channel.

San jiao 13 *Naohui* (Upperarm Gathering)

- According to some authors, SJ 13 is a meeting point of the *san jiao* channel and *yang wei mai*.

Actions

- Regulates *qi* and transforms Phlegm.

- Opens the channel and moves *qi* and *xue* in the channel and in the local area.

Indications

- **Swellings in the throat and axillary region:** In addition to being an acupuncture point that can be used when there are disorders in the local area and along the path of the channel, SJ 13 can be used in the treatment of swollen lymph nodes in the armpit and throat and for the treatment of goitre.

San jiao 14 *Jianliao* (Shoulder Bone-Hole)

Actions

- Expels Wind-Dampness.

- Opens the channel and moves *qi* and *xue* in the channel and surrounding area.

Indications

- **Pain and lack of mobility in the shoulder:** SJ 14 is a very important acupuncture point in the treatment of all kinds of problems in the shoulder joint. SJ 14 will, in these situations, often be combined with LI 15, as well as points in the local area and distal points along the channel.

San jiao 15 *Tianliao* (Heavenly Hole)

- Meeting point of the *san jiao* and Gall Bladder channels and *yang wei mai.*

Actions

- Expels Wind-Dampness.

- Regulates *qi* and opens the chest.

- Opens the channel and moves *qi* and *xue* in the channel and in the local area.

Indications

- **Tension, pain and limited movement in the shoulder, neck and chest:** SJ 15 can be used to treat tension and pain in the area between the shoulder and neck. SJ 15 can also be used to move and descend *qi* in the chest. In this way, SJ 15 can treat chest oppression, turmoil in the chest or heaviness in the chest.

San jiao 16 *Tianyou* (Window of Heaven)

- Window of Heaven point.

Actions

- Regulates *qi* and descends *qi* from the head.

- Benefits the head and the sense organs.

- Opens the channel and moves *qi* and *xue* in the channel and in the local area.

Indications

- **Headache, dizziness and swollen lymph nodes in the throat:** As a Window of Heaven point, SJ 16 can regulate *qi* to and from the head and in the throat.

- **Acute deafness, impaired hearing, blurred vision, lacrimation, running nose and nose bleeds:** SJ 16 is a Window of Heaven point and can therefore be used in the treatment of disorders of the sense organs.

- **Pain or stiffness in the neck:** SJ 16 can be used when there is pain and discomfort in the local area.

San jiao 17 Yifeng (Wind Screen)

- Meeting point of the *san jiao* and Gall Bladder channels.

Actions

- Benefits the ears.

- Expels Wind and Heat.

- Opens the channel and moves *qi* and *xue* in the channel and in the local area.

Indications

- **All disorders of the ear:** SJ 17 is a very important acupuncture point that can be used to treat all kinds of disorders in the ears – disorders that are caused by both *xu* and *shi* conditions. SJ 17 can also be used to treat disorders along the path of the channel and in the surrounding area.

San jiao 18 Qimai (Spasm Vessel), san jiao 19 Luxi (Skull Rest) and san jiao 20 Jiaosun (Minute Angle)

- SJ 20 is the meeting point of the *san jiao*, Gall Bladder and Small Intestine channels.

- SJ 20 is the starting point of the *san jiao* divergent channel.

Actions

- Benefit the ears.
- Open the channel and move *qi* and *xue* in the channel and in the local area.

Indications

- **All disorders of the ear:** These acupuncture points can be used to treat local disorders, including ear problems.

San jiao 21 *Ermen* (Ear Door)

Actions

- Benefits the ears.
- Expels Wind and Heat.
- Opens the channel and moves *qi* and *xue* in the channel and in the local area.

Indications

- **All disorders of the ear and jaw:** SJ 21 is often used in combination with SJ 17, SI 19 and GB 2 as a local point in the treatment of all types of ear symptoms and jaw problems.

San jiao 22 *Erheliao* (Ear Harmony Bone-Hole)

- Meeting point of the *san jiao*, Gall Bladder and Small Intestine channels.
- Exit point.

Actions

- Benefits the ears.
- Opens the channel and moves *qi* and *xue* in the channel and surrounding area.

Indications

- **All disorders of the ear and jaw:** SJ 22 can be used in the treatment of local disorders, such as ear and jaw problems.

San jiao 23 Sizhukong (Silk Bamboo Hole)

Actions

- Benefits the eyes.

- Expels Wind.

- Opens the channel and moves *qi* and *xue* in the channel and in the local area.

Indications

- **Eye disorders and temporal headaches:** SJ 23 can be used as a local point in the treatment of all forms of eye problems. SJ 23 can also be used as a local point to treat headaches.

GALL BLADDER CHANNEL ACUPUNCTURE POINTS

Type	Point
Yuan-source	GB 40
Luo-connecting	GB 37
Xi-cleft	GB 36
Mu-collecting	GB 24
Back-*shu*	UB 19
Jing-well	GB 44
Ying-spring	GB 43
Shu-stream	GB 41
Jing-river	GB 38
He-sea	GB 34
Metal	GB 44
Water	GB 43
Wood	GB 41
Fire	GB 38
Earth	GB 34
Entry point	GB 1
Exit point	GB 41
Five Phase tonifying point	GB 43
Five Phase draining point	GB 38

Gall Bladder 1 *Tongziliao* (Pupil Bone-Hole)

- Entry point.
- Meeting point of the Gall Bladder, *san jiao* and Small Intestine channels.

Actions

- Benefits the eyes.
- Expels Wind and Heat.
- Opens the channel and moves *qi* and *xue* in the channel and in the local area.

Indications

- **Headaches and eye and jaw disorders:** GB 1 is a very important local point used to treat all forms of eye disorders. These could both be problems caused by invasions of *xie qi* or problems caused by ascending Liver *yang* or Liver Fire. GB 1 can also be used as a local point in the treatment of headaches and jaw problems.

Gall Bladder 2 *Tinghui* (Auditory Gathering)

Actions

- Benefits the ears.

- Expels Wind and Heat.

- Opens the channel and moves *qi* and *xue* in the channel and in the local area.

Indications

- **All disorders of the ear and the jaw:** GB 2 is often used in combination with SJ 17, SI 19 and SJ 22 as a local point in the treatment of all types of ear and jaw problems.

Gall Bladder 3 *Shangguan* (Upper Gate)

- Meeting point of the Gall Bladder, *san jiao* and Stomach channels.

Actions

- Benefits the ears.

- Expels Wind and Heat.

- Opens the channel and moves *qi* and *xue* in the channel and in the local area.

Indications

- **All disorders of the ear and jaw:** GB 3 is used as a local point in the treatment of ear and jaw problems.

Gall Bladder 4 *Hanyan* (Jaw Fullness)

- Meeting point of the Gall Bladder, *san jiao* and Stomach channels.

Actions

- Expels exogenous Wind.

- Calms internally generated Wind and ascending Liver *yang*.

- Opens the channel and moves *qi* and *xue* in the channel and in the local area.

Indications

- **Headaches, dizziness, epilepsy, eye disorders and teeth and jaw problems:** GB 4, GB 5, GB 6 and GB 7 are all important local points in the treatment of hemilateral headaches caused by ascending Liver *yang* and Liver Fire. In addition, GB 4 can be used to expel and calm Wind in the treatment of dizziness, ear symptoms, jaw problems, epilepsy, eye disorders and toothache. GB 4 can, of course, also be used as a local point when there are stagnations of *qi* and *xue* in the local area.

Gall Bladder 5 *Xuanlu* (Suspended Cranium) and Gall Bladder 6 *Xuanli* (Suspended Hair)

- Meeting point of the Gall Bladder, *san jiao*, Large Intestine and Stomach channels.

Actions

- Expel exogenous Wind.

- Calm internally generated Wind and ascending Liver *yang*.

- Open the channel and move *qi* and *xue* in the channel and in the local area.

Indications

- **Headaches, dizziness, epilepsy, eye disorders and teeth and jaw problems:** GB 4, GB 5, GB 6 and GB 7 are all important local points in the treatment of hemilateral headaches caused by ascending Liver *yang* and Liver Fire. In addition, GB 5 and GB 6 are used to expel and calm Wind in the treatment of dizziness, ear symptoms, jaw problems, epilepsy, eye disorders and toothache. These two points can, of course, also be used as local points when there are stagnations of *qi* and *xue* in the local area.

Gall Bladder 7 *Qubin* (Temporal Curve)

- Meeting point of the Gall Bladder and Urinary Bladder channels.

Actions

- Expels exogenous Wind.

- Calms internally generated Wind and ascending Liver *yang*.

- Opens the channel and moves *qi* and *xue* in the channel and in the local area.

Indications

- **Headaches, dizziness, epilepsy, eye disorders and teeth and jaw problems:** GB 4, GB 5, GB 6 and GB 7 are all important local points in the treatment of hemilateral headaches caused by ascending Liver *yang* and Liver Fire. In addition, GB 7 is used to expel and calm Wind in the treatment of dizziness, ear symptoms, jaw problems, epilepsy, eye disorders and toothache. GB 7 can, of course, also be used as a local point when there are stagnations of *qi* and *xue* in the local area.

Gall Bladder 8 *Shuaigu* (Leading Valley)

- Meeting point of the Gall Bladder and Urinary Bladder channels.

Actions

- Expels exogenous Wind.

- Calms internally generated Wind and ascending Liver *yang*.

- Harmonises the Stomach and regulates Stomach *qi*.

- Opens the channel and moves *qi* and *xue* in the channel and in the local area.

Indications

- **Headaches:** GB 8 can be used to treat hemilateral headaches caused by ascending Liver *yang*. GB 8 is particularly relevant when Liver *qi* has invaded the Stomach and there is vomiting and nausea along with the migraine. Because of its ability to treat a headache that is accompanied by vomiting and nausea, GB 8 can also be used to treat the effects of intoxication.

Gall Bladder 9 *Tianchong* (Heavenly Thoroughfare)

- Meeting point of the Gall Bladder and Urinary Bladder channels.
- Some authors are of the opinion that GB 9 is a Window of Heaven point.

Actions

- Calms internally generated Wind and ascending Liver *yang*.
- Drains Heat from the Gall Bladder channel.
- Calms *shen*.
- Opens the channel and moves *qi* and *xue* in the channel and in the local area.

Indications

- **Headaches, dizziness, tinnitus and epilepsy:** GB 9 can be used in the treatment of hemilateral headaches caused by ascending Liver *yang* or Liver Fire. In addition, GB 9 is used to expel and calm Wind in the treatment of dizziness, ear symptoms, tinnitus, epilepsy and spasms. GB 9 is also said to have *shen*-calming qualities, especially when Heat agitates *shen*.
- **Swelling in the throat:** Similar to Window of Heaven points, GB 9 can be used in the treatment of goitre. GB 9 can, of course, also be used as a local point to treat stagnations of *qi* and *xue* in the local area.

Gall Bladder 10 *Fubai* (Floating White)

- Meeting point of the Gall Bladder and Urinary Bladder channels.

Actions

- Restrains ascending Liver *yang*.
- Opens the channel and moves *qi* and *xue* in the channel and in the local area.

Indications

- **Headache and neck and shoulder pain and stiffness:** GB 10 can be used to treat hemilateral headaches caused by ascending Liver *yang*. GB 10 is also used when there is stiffness and pain in the neck and shoulder, goitre or a sore throat. In addition, GB 10 is used to treat disorders along the path of the channel, such as shoulder pain and weakness in the legs.

Gall Bladder 11 *Touqiaoyin* (Head *Yin* Openings)

- Meeting point of the Gall Bladder, *san jiao*, Small Intestine and Urinary Bladder channels.

Actions

- Drains ascending Liver *yang* and Liver Fire.
- Benefits the sense organs.
- Opens the channel and moves *qi* and *xue* in the channel and in the local area.

Indications

- **Headache, pain and stiffness:** GB 11 can be used to treat hemilateral headaches caused by ascending Liver *yang* or Liver Fire. GB 11 is particularly relevant when the sensory organs in the head are disturbed by Liver Fire and Liver *yang*. GB 11 can be used when there is pain, stiffness and other disorders caused by disturbances of *qi* in the Gall Bladder channel and in the local area.

Gall Bladder 12 *Wangu* (Completion Bone)

- Meeting point of the Gall Bladder and Urinary Bladder channels.

Actions

- Calms internally generated Wind and ascending Liver *yang*.
- Calms *shen*.
- Opens the channel and moves *qi* and *xue* in the channel and in the local area.

Indications

- **Headache, tinnitus, dizziness, tics and spasms:** GB 12 can be used in the treatment of hemilateral headaches or tinnitus caused by ascending Liver *yang* or Liver Fire. GB 12 is also used to calm Liver Wind that rises up to the head, giving rise to symptoms such as dizziness, epilepsy, spasm, tics and paralysis in the face.

- **Insomnia, mental restlessness and mania:** GB 12 also has a *shen*-calming effect and can be used in the treatment of insomnia, manic behaviour and mental restlessness.

- **Pain, stiffness and limited movement:** GB 12 can be used when there is pain, stiffness and other disorders caused by disturbance of *qi* in the Gall Bladder channel or in the local area.

Gall Bladder 13 *Benshen* (*Shen* Root)

- Meeting point of the Gall Bladder channel and *yang wei mai*.

Actions

- Calms internally generated Wind and ascending Liver *yang*.

- Calms *shen*.

- Transforms Phlegm.

- Raises *jing* up to the head.

- Opens the channel and moves *qi* and *xue* in the channel and in the local area.

Indications

- **Headache and dizziness:** As with most Gall Bladder channel points in the head, GB 13 can be used in the treatment of headaches and dizziness caused by ascending Liver *yang* and Liver Fire.

- **Epilepsy, spasm and hemiplegia:** As with most Gall Bladder channel points in the head, GB 13 can be used in the treatment of symptoms caused by Liver Wind.

- **Manic behaviour, mental restlessness, fear, depression, jealousy and poor memory:** GB 13 is an important acupuncture point in the treatment of *shen* imbalances. GB 13 will mainly be used when these *shen* imbalances are related to Liver imbalances. GB 13 has, however, the special characteristic that it can draw *jing* up to the head to nourish the Brain. GB 13 can therefore also be used to treat *jing xu* conditions that manifest as *shen* disturbances.

- **Pain, numbness and discomfort in the local area and along the path of the channel.**

Gall Bladder 14 *Yangbai* (*Yang* White)

- Meeting point of the Gall Bladder, *san jiao*, Stomach and Large Intestine channels, as well as *yang wei mai*.

Actions

- Restrains ascending Liver *yang* and Liver Fire.

- Expels exogenous Wind.

- Calms internally generated Wind.

- Benefits the eyes.

- Opens the channel and moves *qi* and *xue* in the channel and in the local area.

Indications

- **Headache and dizziness:** As with most Gall Bladder channel points in the head, GB 14 can be used in the treatment of headaches and dizziness caused by ascending Liver *yang* and Liver Fire, as well as internally generated Wind. As a meeting point of the Gall Bladder and Large Intestine channels, GB 14 can also treat headaches that are caused by *yangming* channel imbalances or invasions of *xie qi*.

- **Eye disorders:** GB 14 is an important acupuncture point in the treatment of all forms of eye disorders. This is because GB 14 is both a local point and a point that can drain Liver *yang*, Liver Fire and Liver Wind, as well as expelling exogenous Wind.

- **Pain, numbness and discomfort in the local area and along the path of the channel:** GB 14 is an important local point to treat pain in the forehead, in particular sinusitis.

Gall Bladder 15 *Toulinqi* (Head Tear Supervisor)

- Meeting point of the Gall Bladder and Urinary Bladder channels, as well as *yang wei mai*.

Actions

- Calms internally generated Wind and ascending Liver *yang*.

- Benefits the eyes.

- Calms *shen*.

- Opens the channel and moves *qi* and *xue* in the channel and in the local area.

Indications

- **Headache and dizziness:** As with most Gall Bladder channel points in the head, GB 15 can be used in the treatment of headaches and dizziness caused by ascending Liver *yang*, Liver Fire and Liver Wind.

- **Epilepsy, spasm and hemiplegia:** As with most Gall Bladder channel points in the head, GB 15 can be used in the treatment of symptoms caused by Liver Wind.

- **Eye disorders:** GB 15 can be used in the treatment of all forms of eye disorders. This is because GB 15 is a channel point that connects to the eye, as well as being an acupuncture point that drains Liver *yang*, Liver Fire and Liver Wind.

- **Obsessive thoughts, mood swings, depression and pensiveness:** Giovanni Maciocia (2009, p.270) recommends this acupuncture point to treat obsessive thoughts and mood swings.

- **Pain, numbness and discomfort in the local area and along the path of the channel.**

Gall Bladder 16 *Muchuang* (Eye Window), Gall Bladder 17 *Zhengying* (Correct Nutrition), Gall Bladder 18 *Chengling* (Spirit Support) and Gall Bladder 19 *Naokong* (Brain Hollow)

- Meeting points of the Gall Bladder channel and *yang wei mai*.

Actions

- Expel Wind.

- Benefit the eyes.

- Calm *shen*.

- Open the channel and move *qi* and *xue* in the channel and in the local area.

Indications

- **Headache, dizziness, eye disorders, nasal problems, insomnia, mania and palpitations:** These acupuncture points can be used in the treatment of eye disorders, headache, dizziness and scalp pain. Furthermore, several of these acupuncture points have *shen*-calming properties and can be used to treat depression, anxiety, manic behaviour and palpitations. GB 18 and GB 19 can also be used to treat a blocked nose, running nose and nose bleeds.

Gall Bladder 20 *Fengchi* (Wind Pool)

- Meeting point of the Gall Bladder and *san jiao* channels and *yang qiao mai* and *yang wei mai*.

Actions

- Expels exogenous Wind.

- Calms internally generated Wind and ascending Liver *yang*.

- Benefits the eyes and ears.

- Opens the channel and moves *qi* and *xue* in the channel and in the local area.

Indications

- **Aversion to cold, fever, soreness in the muscles, headache and muscle spasms:** GB 20 is a very important acupuncture point in the treatment of disorders that are caused by internally generated and exogenous Wind. This property is shared with UB 10 and Du 16, which are located in the same area of the neck.

- **Headache, dizziness, hypertension, heaviness in the head and feeling of being inside a bubble:** GB 20 is one of the body's primary points used in the treatment of headache and dizziness. GB 20 can be used to treat internal imbalances such as ascending Liver *yang*, Liver Fire or Liver Wind and Phlegm and in the treatment of exterior imbalances such as invasions of Wind-Cold, Wind-Heat and Wind-Dampness.

- **Epilepsy, spasms and hemiplegia:** As with most Gall Bladder channel points in the head, GB 20 is used to treat symptoms caused by Liver Wind.

- **Eye disorders:** GB 20 can be used in the treatment of all forms of eye disorders. This is because GB 20 is a channel point that connects to the eye, as well as being an acupuncture point that can drain Liver *yang*, Liver Fire and Liver Wind downwards.

- **Tinnitus, deafness and pain in the ear:** GB 20 is an important channel point in the treatment of ear disorders.

- **Blocked nose, running nose and nose bleeds:** GB 20 can be used to treat nasal disorders. These nasal disorders can have arisen because of internal factors or due to invasions of *xie qi*.

- **Pain, stiffness, numbness, tension and discomfort in the neck, shoulders and along the path of the channel:** GB 20 is an important acupuncture point in the treatment of stiffness, pain and tension in the head and neck, especially when this results in headaches. GB 20 will often be combined with GB 21 and GB 34 in these situations.

Gall Bladder 21 *Jianjing* (Shoulder Well)

- Meeting point of the Gall Bladder, Stomach and *san jiao* channels, as well as *yang wei mai*.

Actions

- Regulates *qi* and transforms Phlegm in the upper *jiao*.

- Descends *qi*.

- Benefits the breasts.

- Opens the channel and moves *qi* and *xue* in the channel and in the local area.

Indications

- **Chest oppression, heaviness in the chest, cough, shortness of breath, goitre and swollen lymph nodes:** GB 21 can be used to descend *qi* and to circulate *qi* in the chest. By circulating and regulating *qi* in the upper *jiao*, GB 21 can also transform Phlegm in the Lung, chest and throat.

- **Difficult labour, placental retention and uterine bleeding:** GB 21 has a powerful downward dynamic and can descend *qi* from the upper *jiao*. This means that GB 21 can be used to expel the foetus and the placenta from the body. GB 21 is therefore contraindicated in pregnancy.

- **Chest pain, poor lactation and breast abscesses and lumps:** GB 21 can regulate *qi* and thereby dissolve Phlegm and *qi* stagnations in the breasts.

- **Pain, stiffness, numbness, tension and discomfort in the neck and shoulders and along the path of the channel:** GB 21 is an important acupuncture point to treat stiffness, pain and tension in the head and neck, especially when this results in headaches. GB 21 will often be combined with GB 20 and GB 34 in these situations.

Gall Bladder 22 *Yuanye* (Armpit Abyss)

Actions

- Regulates *qi* and opens the chest.

- Opens the channel and moves *qi* and *xue* in the channel and in the local area.

Indications

- **Local disorders:** GB 22 is used as a local point to treat pain and distension in the local area, as well as to regulate Lung *qi*.

Gall Bladder 23 *Zheyin* (Sinew Flank)

- Meeting point of the Gall Bladder and Urinary Bladder channels.

Actions

- Regulates *qi* and opens the chest.

- Opens the channel and moves *qi* and *xue* in the channel and in the local area.

Indications

- **Local disorders:** GB 23 is used as a local point when there is pain and distension in the local area, as well as to regulate Lung *qi* and Stomach *qi* when there is coughing and vomiting respectively.

Gall Bladder 24 *Riyue* (Sun and Moon)

- *Mu*-collecting point of the Gall Bladder.
- Meeting point of the Gall Bladder and Spleen channels.

Actions

- Benefits the Gall Bladder and spreads Liver *qi*.
- Regulates *qi* in the middle *jiao*.

- Drains Damp-Heat from the Gall Bladder.

- Opens the channel and moves *qi* and *xue* in the channel and in the local area.

Indications

- **Chest oppression and pain in the costal and hypochondriac regions, gallstones, abdominal pain, epigastric pain, abdominal distension, jaundice, nausea, bitter taste in the mouth and constant yawning and sighing:** GB 24 is the *mu*-collecting point of the Gall Bladder, as well as a local point for the lower ribs. This means that GB 24 can be used to drain Damp-Heat from the Liver and Gall Bladder and to spread stagnant *qi* in the area.

- **Vomiting, acid regurgitation, burping and hiccups:** By moving Liver *qi* and by regulating *qi* in the middle *jiao*, GB 24 can harmonise and regulate Stomach *qi*, especially when the Stomach is invaded by Liver *qi*.

Gall Bladder 25 *Jingmen* (Capital Door)

- *Mu*-collecting point for the Kidneys.

Actions

- Tonifies the Kidneys and regulates the water passages.

- Tonifies the Spleen and Intestines.

- Strengthens the lumbar region.

- Opens the channel and moves *qi* and *xue* in the channel and in the local area.

Indications

- **Urinary difficulty, dark urine, oedema, borborygmi, watery diarrhoea, intestinal pain and abdominal distension:** GB 25 is mainly used to strengthen the relationship between Kidney and Spleen *yang* and can be used when these two organs do not carry out their functions in relation to fluid physiology.

- **Lumbar pain and weakness or fatigue in the lumbar region:** As the *mu*-collecting point of the Kidneys and as a local point, GB 25 can strengthen the lower back.

- **Pain, distension and discomfort along the path of the channel:** GB 25 can be used as a distal point in the treatment of pain in the hip, shoulder and ribs.

Gall Bladder 26 *Daimai* (Belt Vessel), Gall Bladder 27 *Wushu* (Fifth Pivot) and Gall Bladder 28 *Weidao* (Linking Path)

- Meeting points of the Gall Bladder channel and *dai mai*.

Actions

- Regulate *dai mai* and drain Dampness and Damp-Heat.

- Regulate the Uterus.

- Open the channel and move *qi* and *xue* in the channel and in the local area.

Indications

- **Copious vaginal discharge and changes in the quality of the vaginal discharge:** The *dai mai* acupuncture points, GB 26, GB 27 and GB 28, have an extensive influence on Dampness and Damp-Heat in the lower *jiao*. GB 26, GB 27 and GB 28 can therefore be used for all kinds of disturbances in relation to natural discharges from the vagina.

- **Irregular menstrual bleeding, dysmenorrhoea, uterine prolapse and infertility:** GB 26, GB 27 and GB 28 can affect the Uterus and its functionality in several ways: as *dai mai* points they can affect *ren mai* and *chong mai*, they can drain Dampness and Damp-Heat from the lower *jiao* and they can regulate Liver *qi*.

- **Pain in the lumbar region, pain in the inguinal area and hernia:** As local points and *dai mai* points, GB 26, GB 27 and GB 28 can treat disturbances and blockages of *qi* in the local area.

Gall Bladder 29 *Juliao* (Sitting Bone-Hollow)

- Meeting point of the Gall Bladder channel and *yang qiao mai*.

Actions

- Expels Wind, Dampness and Cold.

- Opens the channel and moves *qi* and *xue* in the channel and in the local area.

Indications

- **Pain, stiffness, paralysis and muscle weakness:** GB 29 is an important acupuncture point to treat pain and stiffness of the hip, lumbar region, buttock and thigh, as well as paralysis and weakness in the legs. GB 29 can be used in the treatment of sciatica. GB 29 is also a *yang qiao mai* point, so its effects are not limited to the course of the Gall Bladder channel.

Gall Bladder 30 *Huantiao* (Jumping Circle)

- Meeting point of the Gall Bladder and Urinary Bladder channels.
- Ma Dan Yang Heavenly Star point.
- Starting point of the Gall Bladder divergent channel.

Actions

- Expels Wind-Dampness.
- Opens the channel and moves *qi* and *xue* in the channel and in the local area.

Indications

- **Pain and stiffness in the buttock, waist, lumbar region, coccyx and legs, sciatica and weakness or paralysis in the legs:** GB 30 is a very important acupuncture point in the treatment of pain and stiffness in the hip, lumbar region, buttock and thigh, as well as paralysis and weakness in the legs. GB 30 is a meeting point of the Gall Bladder and Urinary Bladder channels and will therefore be able to treat disorders that relate to both channels' pathways.

- **Pain, stiffness and discomfort along the course of the channel:** GB 30 can be used as a distal point to treat pain in the costal region.

- **Urticaria, eczema and genital itching:** GB 30 can expel Wind and Dampness, not only from the channel, but also from the skin. GB 30 can therefore be used in the treatment of dermatological disorders.

Gall Bladder 31 *Fengshi* (Wind Market)

Actions

- Expels Wind and stops itching.
- Opens the channel and moves *qi* and *xue* in the channel and in the local area.

Indications

- **Urticaria, herpes zoster, eczema and other itchy skin conditions:** GB 31 can expel Wind from the skin. GB 31 can therefore be used in the treatment of skin disorders that are characterised by itching. GB 31 will often be used with SJ 6 in these situations if there is also Heat present in the skin.

- **Pain, stiffness, weakness and discomfort along the course of the channel:** GB 31 is an important local and channel point to treat disturbances of *qi* and *xue* in the thigh and along the path of the channel. GB 31 can treat atrophy of the muscle in legs and paralysis in the leg after a stroke.

Gall Bladder 32 *Zhongdu* (Central Ditch)

Actions

- Expels Wind, Dampness and Cold.

- Opens the channel and moves *qi* and *xue* in the channel and in the local area.

Indications

- **Local disorders:** GB 32 is mainly used as a local point to treat pain, stiffness and atrophy of the muscle or paralysis in the thigh.

Gall Bladder 33 *Xiyangguan* (Knee *Yang* Gate)

Actions

- Expels Wind, Dampness and Cold.

- Opens the channel and moves *qi* and *xue* in the channel and in the local area.

Indications

- **Local disorders:** GB 33 is mainly used as a local point to treat pain, stiffness and swelling in the knee, especially when this radiates up the thigh.

Gall Bladder 34 *Yanglingquan* (*Yang* Mound Spring)

- *He*-sea point.

- Earth point.

- *Hui*-gathering point for the sinews.

- Ma Dan Yang Heavenly Star point.

Actions

- Benefits the sinews.

- Spreads Liver *qi*.

- Drains Damp-Heat from the Liver and Gall Bladder.

- Harmonises *shaoyang*.

- Opens the channel and moves *qi* and *xue* in the channel and in the local area.

Indications

- **Tight tendons, stiff tendons, joint pains, weak joints, stiff joints, tense muscles, sore muscles, knee pain, elbow pain and shoulder pain:** GB 34 has an extensive influence on the muscles and the sinews in the whole body, both because it is the *hui*-gathering point for sinews and because it is an important point to spread stagnant Liver *qi*. GB 34 has a specific influence on the knee, elbow and shoulder, because it is a local point, a 'cross-channel' point and a distal point respectively on the *shaoyang* channel.

- **Irritability, mood swings, stress, depression, constant sighing or yawning and constipation:** GB 34 is one of the body's most important acupuncture points to spread Liver *qi*. GB 34 is therefore used in the treatment of all conditions that arise from Liver *qi* stagnation.

- **Fear, anxiety, being easily startled and palpitations:** GB 34 can be used to tonify Gall Bladder *qi* when there is Gall Bladder and Heart *qi xu*.

- **Costal pain and distension and abdominal distension:** GB 34 can be used both as a distal point and an acupuncture point that spreads stagnant Liver *qi* in the treatment of problems in the abdominal area and costal region. GB 34 will often be combined with SJ 6 in these situations.

- **Bitter taste in the mouth, jaundice, heavy feeling in the body, vomiting and gallstones:** These symptoms will typically be seen when there is Damp-Heat in the Gall Bladder. GB 34 is an important point that can drain Damp-Heat from the Liver and Gall Bladder.

- **Alternating fever and chills, spontaneous sweating, malaria and headache:** GB 34 is, together with GB 40, SJ 3 and SJ 5, one of the most effective points to expel *xie qi* from the *shaoyang* aspect.

Gall Bladder 35 *Yangjiao* (*Yang* Intersection)

- *Xi*-cleft point of *yang wei mai*.

Actions

- Regulates Gall Bladder *qi* and calms *shen*.

- Opens the channel and moves *qi* and *xue* in the channel and in the local area.

Indications

- **Local disorders:** GB 35 is mainly used in the treatment of pain, stiffness, cramps, muscle weakness, muscle atrophy and paralysis in the leg.

Gall Bladder 36 *Waiqiu* (Outer Mound)

- *Xi*-cleft point.

Actions

- Spreads Liver *qi* and Gall Bladder *qi*.

- Drains Heat.

- Opens the channel and moves *qi* and *xue* in the channel and in the local area.

Indications

- **Pain and distension in the costal region, pain and spasms along the path of the channel, muscle atrophy and paralysis along the path of the channel, and headaches:** As a *xi*-cleft point, GB 36 can be used in the treatment of acute and painful conditions along the course of the Gall Bladder channel.

Gall Bladder 37 *Guangming* (Bright Light)

- *Luo*-connecting point.

Actions

- Benefits the eyes.

- Drains Heat.

- Expels Wind-Dampness.

- Opens the channel and moves *qi* and *xue* in the channel and in the local area.

Indications

- **Eye pain, night-blindness, short-sightedness, long-sightedness, itchy eyes, red eyes and pressure in the eyes:** As a *luo*-connecting point, GB 37 addresses problems in the Liver's sensory organ. GB 37 is most effective in treating *shi* conditions in the eyes, which are caused by Liver Fire and ascending Liver *yang*.

- **Hemilateral headache:** There are two reasons that GB 37 can be used to treat hemilateral headaches. GB 37 is a distal point on the Gall Bladder channel, whilst at the same time it is a *luo*-connecting point. GB 37 can therefore also drain Liver Fire and Liver *yang* downwards.

- **Grinding of teeth at night and bitter taste in the mouth:** GB 37 can drain Liver Fire downwards.

- **Distension, pain, spasms, muscle atrophy and paralysis along the path of the channel:** Like all channel points, GB 37 can affect the local area and the course of the channel. This effect is reinforced by the fact that GB 37 can expel Wind-Dampness from the channel.

Gall Bladder 38 *Yangfu* (*Yang* Support)

- *Jing*-river point.
- Fire point.
- Five Phase draining point.

Actions

- Drains Liver *yang*.
- Drains Heat.
- Harmonises *shaoyang*.
- Opens the channel and moves *qi* and *xue* in the channel and in the local area.

Indications

- **Hemilateral headache:** GB 38 can be used to treat headaches. As well as being a distal point on the Gall Bladder channel, GB 38 is also a Fire point. GB 38 can therefore be used to drain Liver Fire and Liver *yang* downwards.

- **Distension and pain in the costal region, axillary region and chest, swollen lymph nodes, a bitter taste in the mouth and a feeling of heat**

in the body: GB 38 can drain Heat and disperse stagnations of *qi* along the course of the Gall Bladder channel. These stagnations of *qi* and Heat will often arise from Liver *qi* stagnation.

- **Alternating fever and chills, pain in the costal region, malaria and headache:** As a Fire point on a *shaoyang* channel, GB 38 can be used to expel *xie qi* from the *shaoyang* aspect.

- **Distension, pain, spasms, muscle atrophy and paralysis along the path of the channel:** As with all channel points, GB 38 can affect the local area and the course of the channel.

Gall Bladder 39 *Xuanzhong* (Suspended Bell)

- *Hui*-gathering point for the Marrow.

Actions

- Benefits the sinews and Bones.

- Nourishes the Marrow.

- Drains Liver *yang*.

- Drains Heat from the channel.

- Expels Wind-Dampness.

- Opens the channel and moves *qi* and *xue* in the channel and in the local area.

Indications

- **Stiffness of the neck and chronic *bi* (painful blockage of the channel) syndrome, heaviness in the body, tense, stiff or weak tendons and numbness, pain or stiffness in the joints:** GB 39 is the *hui*-gathering point of the Marrow, which it nourishes and strengthens, as well as nourishing the sinews. GB 39 can also expel Wind-Dampness and thereby can also be used when *xie qi* blocks the channel and the joints.

- **Hemilateral headache, dizziness, nose bleeds and dryness of the nose:** GB 39 can drain Liver Fire and Liver *yang* downwards. The usage of GB 39 in the treatment of nasal disorders is due to the Gall Bladder sinew channel's connection to the side of the nose.

- **Distension and pain in the costal region, axillary region and chest, swollen lymph nodes, a bitter taste in the mouth and a feeling of heat in the body:** GB 39 can drain Heat and disperse stagnations of *qi* along the course of the Gall Bladder channel. These stagnations of *qi* and Heat will often arise from Liver *qi* stagnation.

- **Hip pain, sciatica, spasms and atrophy and paralysis of muscle along the pathway of the channel:** As with all channel points, GB 39 has an effect in the local area and along the course of the channel.

Gall Bladder 40 *Qiuxu* (Mound Ruins)

- *Yuan*-source point.

Actions

- Spreads Liver *qi* and drains Heat from the Gall Bladder.

- Drains Liver and Gall Bladder Damp-Heat.

- Harmonises *shaoyang*.

- Opens the channel and moves *qi* and *xue* in the channel and in the local area.

Indications

- **Hemilateral headache, eye pain, red eyes and eye strain:** GB 40 is both a distal point on the Gall Bladder channel and an acupuncture point that can spread stagnant Liver *qi* and drain Heat downwards. This means that GB 40 can be used in the treatment of headache and eye problems.

- **Distension and pain in the costal region, shoulders and neck, axillary region and chest, and yawning and sighing:** By spreading Liver *qi* and draining Heat, GB 40 can be used to treat stagnations of *qi* and Fire along the path of the Gall Bladder channel.

- **Herpes zoster, gallstones, nausea and vomiting:** GB 40 can both spread Liver *qi* and drain Damp-Heat from the Liver and Gall Bladder.

- **A bitter taste in the mouth, alternating fever and chills, vomiting and nausea, malaria and headache:** As a *yuan*-source point on a *yang* channel, GB 40 can expel *xie qi*. GB 40 is especially used in the treatment of *xie qi*, which is locked in the *shaoyang* aspect. In these situations, GB 40 will often be used in combination with SJ 5 or SJ 3.

- **Hip pain, sciatica, cramping, atrophy and paralysis of muscles along the path of the channel, ankle pain and weak ankle joint:** As with all channel points, GB 40 has an effect in the local area and along the path of the channel.

Gall Bladder 41 *Zulinqi* (Foot Teardrop Supervisor)

- *Shu*-stream point.

- Wood point.

- Opening point for *dai mai.*

- Exit point.

Actions

- Spreads Liver *qi* and drains Heat from the Gall Bladder.

- Drains Liver *yang.*

- Benefits the breasts, chest and ribs.

- Opens *dai mai.*

- Transforms Phlegm and dissolves accumulations.

- Opens the channel and moves *qi* and *xue* in the channel and in the local area.

Indications

- **Headache, dizziness, eye pain, red eyes, eye strain, tinnitus, deafness, earache, teeth grinding, jaw pain and toothache:** GB 41 is both a distal point on the Gall Bladder channel and an acupuncture point that can spread stagnant Liver *qi* and drain Heat. This means that GB 41 can be used in the treatment of headaches and of the sensory organs of the head that the channel connects to.

- **Distension and pain in the costal region, shoulders, neck, axillary region and chest, swollen lymph nodes in the throat and under the arms, repeated yawning and sighing, and shortness of breath:** By spreading Liver *qi* and draining Heat, GB 41 can be used to treat stagnations of *qi* and disperse Phlegm accumulations along the course of the Gall Bladder channel.

- **Breast distension, swollen breasts, breast lumps and breast abscesses:** Liver *qi* stagnation can easily interfere with the flow of *qi* in the breasts and lead to the formation of the Phlegm and *xue* stagnations. GB 41 can therefore be used in the treatment of many forms of breast disorders.

- **Irregular menstrual bleeding, dysmenorrhoea and PMS:** GB 41 is an important acupuncture point to spread stagnant Liver *qi*. This means that GB 41 can be used in the treatment of menstrual problems.

- **Hip pain, sciatica, pain and swelling of the foot, and pain and cramps in the toes:** As with all channel points, GB 41 has an effect in the local area and along the path of the channel.

Gall Bladder 42 *Diwuhui* (Earth Five Gathering)

Actions

- Spreads Liver *qi* and drains Heat from the Gall Bladder.

- Opens the channel and moves *qi* and *xue* in the channel and in the local area.

Indications

- **Headache, eye disorders, chest oppression and disorders in the feet and toes:** In addition to the treatment of local disorders in the feet and toes, GB 42 can be used to treat headaches, eye disorders and chest oppression.

Gall Bladder 43 *Xia Xi* (Squeezed Stream)

- *Ying*-spring point.

- Water point.

- Five Phase tonifying point.

Actions

- Drains Liver *yang* and Liver Fire.

- Drains Heat from the Gall Bladder channel.

- Drains Damp-Heat.

- Opens the channel and moves *qi* and *xue* in the channel and in the local area.

Indications

- **Headache, dizziness, eye pain, red eyes, eye strain, tinnitus, deafness, earache, teeth grinding, jaw pain and toothache:** Liver *yang* and Liver Fire frequently rise up the Gall Bladder channel to the head. GB 43 is a distal point to the head on the Gall Bladder channel, whilst at the same time draining Liver *yang* and Liver Fire.

- **Distension and pain in the ribs and chest and breast abscesses:** Liver *qi* stagnation can interfere with the flow of *qi* in the Liver and Gall Bladder channels. GB 43 can be used when this stagnant *qi* starts to generate Heat in the channel.

- **Red, hot, swollen feet and fungal infections between the toes:** GB 43 can drain Damp-Heat, especially from the skin in the feet.

- **Pain, stiffness, numbness and sensory disturbances or discomfort in the local area or along the path of the channel.**

Gall Bladder 44 *Zuqiaoyin* (Foot *Yin* Orifice)

- *Jing*-well point.

- Metal point.

Actions

- Drains Liver *yang* and Liver Fire.

- Calms *shen*.

- Brightens the eyes.

- Opens the channel and moves *qi* and *xue* in the channel and in the local area.

Indications

- **Headache, dizziness, eye pain, red eyes, visual disturbances, tinnitus, deafness, earache, grinding of teeth, jaw pain and toothache:** GB 44 is the most distal point on the Gall Bladder channel in relation to the head. At the same time, it is a *jing*-well point. This means that GB 44 can be used to treat acute conditions arising due to Liver Fire and Liver *yang* ascending to the head or when invasions of Wind-Heat disturb the eyes, ears or head.

- **Distension and pain in the costal region and chest and shortness of breath:** GB 44 is a *jing*-well point and can therefore be used to treat 'fullness below the Heart', i.e. a distended sensation in the chest and the ribs.

- **Nightmares, disturbed sleep, insomnia, fear and emotional turmoil:** Heat in the Liver can agitate *hun* and *shen*. This can result in nightmares, dream-disturbed sleep and insomnia. GB 44 can drain Liver Fire and thereby calm *hun* and *shen*.

- **Pain, stiffness, numbness and sensory disturbances or discomfort in the arca or along thc path of the channel.**

LIVER CHANNEL
ACUPUNCTURE POINTS

Type	Point
Yuan-source	Liv 3
Luo-connecting	Liv 5
Xi-cleft	Liv 6
Mu-collecting	Liv 14
Back-*shu*	UB 18
Jing-well	Liv 1
Ying-spring	Liv 2
Shu-stream	Liv 3
Jing-river	Liv 4
He-sea	Liv 8
Wood	Liv 1
Fire	Liv 2
Earth	Liv 3
Metal	Liv 4
Water	Liv 8
Entry point	Liv 1
Exit point	Liv 14
Five Phase tonifying point	Liv 8
Five Phase draining point	Liv 2

Liver 1 *Dadun* (Large Mound)

- *Jing*-well point.

- Wood point.

- Entry point.

Actions

- Regulates *qi* and drains Damp-Heat from the lower *jiao*.

- Benefits the genitalia.

- Regulates Liver *qi*.

- Cools *xue* and stops uterine bleeding.

- Restores consciousness and calms *shen*.

- Opens the channel and moves *qi* and *xue* in the channel and in the local area.

Indications

- **Shan disorders (such as hernias, pain and swelling in the abdomen and swelling of the genitalia), constipation, pain or discomfort in the area above the pubis, feeling of heat in the lower abdomen, genital pain and genital swelling:** Liv 1 can be used in the treatment of many different kinds of disorders in the lower *jiao* and around the genitalia. This is because the Liver channel passes through the inguinal area and the external genitalia, as well as having the specific function of spreading Liver *qi* and draining Damp-Heat from the lower *jiao*. *Shan* disorders can arise when there is a *qi* stagnation and Damp-Heat, as well as from invasions of Cold in the Liver channel. All of these conditions can be treated by Liv 1.

- **Urinary difficulty, frequent urination, painful urination, blood in the urine, Liver *qi* stagnation, Liver Damp-Heat and Liver Fire:** Can all be causes of urinary problems. Liv 1 can therefore be used to treat urinary problems. This is because Liv 1 can spread Liver *qi*, drain Liver Fire and drain Liver Damp-Heat.

- **Irregular menstrual bleeding, heavy menstrual bleeding and spotting:** Whereas Sp 1, which is also located on the root of the big toenail, can stop all forms of menstrual bleeding, Liv 1 will only be used to stop menstrual bleeding arising from *xue* Heat. Liv 1 will be stimulated with moxa in these situations.

- **Nose bleeds:** Liv 1 can stop nose bleeds resulting from ascending Liver Fire.

- **Fear, bipolar depression and insomnia:** By draining Fire downwards, Liv 1 has a *shen*-calming effect.

- **Loss of consciousness and epilepsy:** Similar to most *jing*-well points, Liv 1 can be used to restore consciousness when internal Wind has swirled up Phlegm and blocked the orifices of the Heart.

- **Pain, discomfort, numbness and sensory disturbances in the big toe and along the path of the channel.**

Liver 2 *Xingjian* (Moving Between)

- *Ying*-spring point.

- Fire point.

- Five Phase draining point.

Actions

- Drains Liver Fire.

- Spreads Liver *qi*.

- Extinguishes Liver Wind.

- Drains Heat, cools *xue* and stops bleeding.

- Regulates the lower *jiao*.

- Calms *shen*.

- Opens the channel and moves *qi* and *xue* in the channel and in the local area.

Indications

- **Headache, dizziness, hypertension, eye pain, red eyes, pressure behind the eyes, lacrimation, tinnitus and deafness:** Liver *qi* stagnation can easily lead to ascending Liver *yang* and Liver Fire that rises up to the head. Liver Fire and Liver *yang* can generate internal Wind. As a *ying*-spring point and Fire point, Liv 2 can drain Fire downwards. In addition, Liv 2 spreads Liver *qi* and extinguishes Liver Wind.

- **Quick temper, irritability, mood swings, uncontrollable outbursts of anger, anxiety, manic behaviour, insomnia and palpitations:** Liver *qi* stagnation can, by itself, be the cause of the mood swings. Liver *qi* stagnation will often generate Heat and Fire in the Liver. This Heat can manifest as anger, and Heat can also ascend up to the Heart and agitate *shen*. Liv 2 is a very important acupuncture point to spread Liver *qi* and drain Liver Fire. Compared with Liv 3, Liv 2 is better at draining Liver Fire, whereas Liv 3 is better at spreading stagnant Liver *qi*.

- **Dry throat, pain in the throat and bitter taste in the mouth:** The Liver channel traverses the throat. This means that Liv 2 can be used to treat the throat in disorders that arise from ascending Liver Fire.

- **Epilepsy, loss of consciousness, tight tendons, muscle spasms and tics:** Liv 2 drains and extinguishes internally generated Wind.

- **Genital itching, genital swelling, uncontrollable erection, *shan* disorder (e.g. hernia, pain and swelling in the abdomen, swelling of the genitalia), increased vaginal discharge, herpes and genital ulcers:** The Liver channel encircles the external genitalia. Liver Fire and Liver Damp-Heat can collect in the lower *jiao* and in the external genitalia. As a Fire point and a *ying*-spring point, Liv 2 can drain Fire and Damp-Heat from this area.

- **Urinary difficulty, painful urination, blood in the urine, constipation, diarrhoea and abdominal distension:** Liver *qi* stagnation, Liver Fire and Liver Damp-Heat can all disrupt the Urinary Bladder and urination. Liv 2 can therefore be used in the treatment of urinary problems. In addition, Liv 2 is used to treat constipation and diarrhoea, where these are due to Heat and stagnations of *qi* in the Liver.

- **Irregular menstrual bleeding, heavy menstrual bleeding and spotting:** By draining Heat from the Liver, Liv 2 can cool *xue* and thereby stop uterine bleeding.

- **Bloody cough and bloody vomiting:** When Liver Fire invades the Lung and Stomach, it can result in a bloody cough and bloody vomiting. Liv 2, which is a Fire point, can drain Liver Fire.

- **Distension and pain in the costal region and chest and increased sighing or yawning:** Liver *qi* stagnation can result in a stagnation of *qi* in the chest and the costal region. Liv 2 can be used in these situations because it spreads Liver *qi*.

- **Febrile conditions, great thirst, red face and cold hands and feet:** Liv 2 is an important Heat-draining point, but if Liv 2 is to drain the Heat, this Heat must have its root in the Liver. A paradoxical sign of Liver *qi* stagnation Heat is that the person will often have very cold hands and feet. This is because Liver *qi* stagnation results in the Heat accumulating inside the body and not being circulated out to the extremities.

- **Pain, discomfort, swelling, numbness and sensory disturbances in the big toe and along the path of the channel:** As with all channel points, Liv 2 treats local disorders and disorders along the path of the channel.

Liver 3 *Taichong* (Great Thoroughfare)

- *Shu*-stream point.
- *Yuan*-source point.
- Earth point.
- Ma Dan Yang Heavenly Star point.

Actions

- Spreads Liver *qi.*

- Drains Liver Fire.

- Extinguishes Liver Wind.

- Nourishes Liver *xue* and Liver *yin.*

- Regulates menstruation.

- Opens the channel and moves *qi* and *xue* in the channel and in the local area.

Indications

- **Headache, dizziness and hypertension:** Liv 3 is an important acupuncture point to drain Liver *yang* and Liver Wind that rises up to the head. Liv 3 also spreads Liver *qi* and nourishes Liver *yin* and Liver *xue.* Liver *qi* stagnation, Liver *yin xu* and Liver *xue xu* can all be underlying causes of Liver *yang* and Liver Wind rising up to the head.

- **Blurred vision, superficial visual disturbances, dry eyes, eye pain, red eyes, pressure behind the eyes and lacrimation:** Liv 3 is used in the treatment of eye disorders, both as a tonifying and draining acupuncture point, depending on the point combination and needle technique. Liv 3 nourishes the eyes by nourishing Liver *yin* and Liver *xue.* Liv 3 can also be used with a draining needle technique to restrain ascending Liver *yang,* Liver Fire and internally generated Wind when these disturb the eyes.

- **Dysmenorrhoea, irregular menstrual cycle, PMS, breast distension, scanty or heavy menstrual bleeding and amenorrhoea:** The Liver has an important influence on the menstrual cycle and menstrual bleeding. The Liver ensures the free flow of *qi* and *xue* throughout the cycle and is at the same time a reservoir for *xue.* This means that Liv 3 is a very important acupuncture point in the treatment of menstrual problems. Liv 3 also has a very close relationship to *chong mai,* which terminates its lower course in Liv 3. Some people even use Liv 3 as the opening point to activate *chong mai.*

- **Irritability, outbursts of anger, irascibility, quick temper, depression, mood swings, tearfulness, fear, nervousness, insomnia and dream-disturbed sleep:** Liv 3 is a much-used acupuncture point in the treatment of mental-emotional imbalances. Liv 3 can be used to spread stagnant Liver *qi,* often together with LI 4 or Pe 6. Liv 3 can also be used to nourish Liver *xue.* Liver *xue xu* can itself be one of the underlying causes of Liver *qi* stagnation. Liver *xue xu* can also mean that *hun* is not nourished or anchored adequately.

- **Genital pain or swelling and *shan* disorder (such as hernia, pain and swelling in the abdomen and swelling of the genitalia):** The Liver channel encircles the external genitalia. Stagnations of *qi* in the channel and invasions of Dampness or Cold can lead to pain and swelling in or around the genitalia. Liv 3 can be used as a distal point and as a *qi*-moving point.

- **Muscle cramps, tics, muscle spasms and stiff and tight tendons:** Liver *xue xu* can result in muscles and tendons both lacking nourishment and moisture. Liver Wind can manifest as spasms and convulsions in the muscles. Liv 3 can be used to treat both of these conditions with either tonifying or draining needle techniques.

- **Distension and pain in the costal region or chest, increased sighing or yawning, 'plumstone *qi*' (a feeling that there is a lump in the throat, as if something is stuck) and tense muscles in the neck and shoulders:** Stagnation of Liver *qi* can result in a stagnation of *qi* in the chest, ribs, throat, shoulders or neck. Liv 3 can be used to create a free flow of *qi* in all these areas.

- **Nausea, constipation, diarrhoea, alternating constipation and diarrhoea and abdominal distension:** Liv 3 can be used to spread Liver *qi* when it invades the Stomach, the Spleen or the Intestines.

- **Urinary difficulty:** The Urinary Bladder is dependent on a free flow of *qi* to carry out its functions. Liv 3 can be used to treat urinary problems where the underlying cause is a stagnation of Liver *qi*.

- **Epilepsy:** Liv 3 can be used to calm Liver Wind in epilepsy.

- **Tense muscles, pain, discomfort, swelling, numbness and sensory disturbances in the foot and along the course of the channel:** Liv 3 is an important local and distal point in the treatment of disorders along the path of the channel.

Liver 4 *Zhongfeng* (Central Mound)

- *Jing*-river point.
- Metal point.

Actions

- Spreads Liver *qi* and regulates *qi* in the lower *jiao*.
- Drains Heat.
- Opens the channel and moves *qi* and *xue* in the channel and in the local area.

Indications

- **Genital pain or swelling and *shan* disorder (such as hernia, pain and swelling in the abdomen and swelling of the genitalia):** The Liver channel encircles the external genitalia. Stagnations of *qi* in the channel and invasions of Dampness or Cold can lead to pain and swelling in or around the genitalia. Liv 4 can be used both to spread Liver *qi* and drain Dampness and Cold that have invaded the channel.

- **Premature ejaculation and nocturnal emissions:** The Liver has a relationship to *mingmen* and thus to libido and sexual functionality. Heat can agitate the semen, so that it cannot be held back.

- **Urinary difficulty, painful urination and cloudy urine:** Liv 4 can be used to spread stagnant Liver *qi* and to drain Damp-Cold and Damp-Heat from the Urinary Bladder.

- **Pain, discomfort, swelling, numbness and sensory disturbances in the foot and along the path of the channel.**

Liver 5 *Ligou* (Termite Channel)

- *Luo*-connecting point.

Actions

- Spreads Liver *qi*.

- Benefits the genitalia.

- Drains Damp-Heat from the lower *jiao*.

- Opens the channel and moves *qi* and *xue* in the channel and in the local area.

Indications

- **'Plumstone *qi*' (a feeling that there is a lump in the throat, as if something is stuck), depression, mood swings, anxiety, fear, excessive worrying and palpitations:** *Luo*-connecting points on the *yin* channel have in common that they can be used in the treatment of psycho-emotional imbalances. This property is enhanced by the fact that Liv 5 is at the same time an acupuncture point that can spread stagnant Liver *qi*.

- **Genital pain and swelling, genital itching, uncontrollable erection, *shan* disorder (such as hernia, pain and swelling in the abdomen and swelling of the genitalia) and distension in the area above the pubic bone:** The

Liver *luo*-connecting vessel connects to the external genitalia. This means that Liv 5 is a very effective acupuncture point in the treatment of all forms of genital problems. This effect is reinforced by the fact that Liv 5 can drain Dampness and Heat from the area.

- **Urinary difficulty:** The Urinary Bladder is dependent on the free movement of *qi* in order to carry out its functions. Liv 5 can be used to treat urinary problems where the underlying cause is a stagnation of Liver *qi* or accumulation of Damp-Heat in the lower *jiao*.

- **Dysmenorrhoea, irregular menstrual bleeding, PMS and breast distension:** Harmonious menstrual bleeding is dependent on the free flow of *qi* and *xue*. Liv 5 can be used to treat menstrual disorders by creating a free flow of Liver *qi*.

- **Vaginal discharge:** Liv 5 can be used to treat copious vaginal discharge or changes in the quality of the vaginal discharge when this is due to Damp-Heat.

- **Pain, discomfort, swelling, numbness and sensory disturbances in the calf and along the path of the channel:** Liv 5 can be used as a local and distal point to treat problems in the channel itself. Liv 5 will often be used in combination with Sp 6 in the treatment of cramps and unrest in the legs in the evening and at night.

Liver 6 *Zhongdu* (Central Capital)

- *Xi*-cleft point.

Actions

- Spreads Liver *qi*.

- Invigorates *xue*.

- Drains Dampness.

- Opens the channel and moves *qi* and *xue* in the channel and in the local area.

Indications

- **Persistent flow of lochia and uterine bleeding:** *Xi*-cleft points on *yin* channels have the property that they can regulate the movement of *xue*. This can be seen here in that Liv 6 can stop uterine bleeding.

- ***Shan* disorders (such as hernia, pain and swelling in the abdomen and swelling of the genitalia) and tensions in the area above the pubic bone:** As a *xi*-cleft point, Liv 6 can be used to treat acute and painful conditions along the path of the channel.

- **Damp *bi* (painful blockage of the channel) in the lower legs, weak or shrunken calf muscles, pain and numbness or heaviness along the Liver channel in the leg:** Liv 6 is both a local point and an acupuncture point that can expel Damp-Cold from the channel.

Liver 7 *Xiguan* (Knee Gate)

Actions

- Expels Wind-Dampness.

- Benefits the knees and relaxes the sinews.

- Opens the channel and moves *qi* and *xue* in the channel and in the local area.

Indications

- **Local disorders:** Liv 7 is mainly used as a local point in the treatment of knee disorders, especially when Wind-Dampness has invaded the Liver channel around the knee.

Liver 8 *Ququan* (Spring at the Bend)

- *He*-sea point.

- Water point.

- Five Phase tonifying point.

Actions

- Nourishes Liver *xue* and Liver *yin*.

- Drains Damp-Heat from the lower *jiao*.

- Benefits the genitalia.

- Invigorates *xue* in the Uterus.

- Opens the channel and moves *qi* and *xue* in the channel and in the local area.

Indications

- **Genital pain and swelling, genital itching, uncontrollable erection, impotence, *shan* disorders (such as hernia, pain and swelling in the abdomen and swelling of the genitalia) and distension in the area above the pubic bone:** *He*-sea points on the leg are generally good at draining Damp-Heat from the lower *jiao*. This can be seen here in that Liv 8 can drain Damp-Heat from the genitalia and from the lower *jiao*.

- **Urinary difficulties, dark and cloudy urine and diarrhoea:** Liv 8 can, in the same way as the other *yin he*-sea points, drain Damp-Heat from the lower *jiao*.

- **Amenorrhoea, dysmenorrhoea, uterine fibroids and infertility:** Liv 8 is a frequently used acupuncture point in the treatment of gynaecological disorders. Liv 8 can be used to treat both *shi* conditions, such as Damp-Heat and *xue* stagnation, and *xu* conditions, such as Liver *xue xu*.

- **Headache, dizziness, blurred vision and pressure behind the eyes:** By nourishing Liver *xue* and *yin*, Liv 8 can be used to control ascending Liver *yang* and to nourish the eyes and the Brain.

- **Pain, discomfort, swelling, numbness and stiffness in the knee and along the channel:** Liv 8 can be used to treat knee problems that manifest on the medial aspect of the knee.

Liver 9 *Yinbao* (*Yin* Wrapping)

Actions

- Regulates *qi* and *xue* in the lower *jiao*.
- Opens the channel and moves *qi* and *xue* in the channel and in the local area.

Indications

- **Menstrual disorders:** As well as treating local disorders, Liv 9 can be used in the treatment of menstrual disorders due to stagnation of *qi* and *xue* in the Uterus.

Liver 10 *Zuwuli* (Leg Five Mile)

Actions

- Drains Damp-Heat from the lower *jiao*.
- Opens the channel and moves *qi* and *xue* in the channel and in the local area.

Indications

- **Urinary and genital disorders:** Liv 10 can be used as a local point in the treatment of urinary difficulties and painful, swollen or itchy genitalia.

Liver 11 *Yinlian* (*Yin* Corner)
Actions

- Benefits the Uterus.

- Opens the channel and moves *qi* and *xue* in the channel and in the local area.

Indications

- **Local disorders:** In addition to being a local point that can be used in the treatment of disorders in the inguinal area, Liv 11 can be used to nourish and invigorate *xue* in the Uterus.

Liver 12 *Jimai* (Urgent Pulse)
Actions

- Expels Cold from the Liver channel and the lower *jiao*.

- Opens the channel and moves *qi* and *xue* in the channel and in the local area.

Indications

- **Problems in the local area and genitalia:** Liv 12 can be used in the treatment of *shan* disorder (such as hernia, pain and swelling in the abdomen and swelling of the genitalia) and when there is pain in the inguinal area and the genitalia.

Liver 13 *Zhangmen* (Completion Door)

- *Mu*-collecting point of the Spleen.

- *Hui*-gathering point for *zang* organs.

- *Dai mai* source point.

- Meeting point of the Gall Bladder and Liver channels and *dai mai*.

Actions

- Harmonises the Spleen and Liver.

- Regulates *qi* in the lower and middle *jiao*.

- Spreads Liver *qi*.

- Tonifies Spleen *qi*.

- Opens the channel and moves *qi* and *xue* in the channel and in the local area.

Indications

- **Abdominal distension, abdominal pain, lumps and accumulations in the abdominal cavity, diarrhoea, borborygmi, constipation, nausea and vomiting:** Liv 13 is a local point, an acupuncture point on the Liver channel, the *mu*-collecting point of the Spleen and the *hui*-gathering point for all *zang* organs. This means that Liv 13 is well suited to treat disorders that arise from the Liver 'invading' the Spleen. The Liver and the Spleen become imbalanced in relation to each other when there is a powerful Liver *qi* stagnation that blocks off the Spleen or when the Spleen is *qi xu* and allows itself to be invaded by Liver *qi*. Liv 13 can be used to both tonify Spleen *qi* and spread Liver *qi*, depending on the needle technique.

- **Distension in the chest and costal region, increased tendency to yawn or sigh, shortness of breath, irritability, outbursts of anger and irascibility:** By moving Liver *qi*, Liv 13 can be used to spread *qi* in the upper *jiao* and to affect the state of mind.

- **Fatigue, cravings for sweets and weight loss:** As the *mu*-collecting point of the Spleen, Liv 13 can be used to tonify Spleen *qi*.

- **'Running piglet' syndrome:** By spreading Liver *qi*, Liv 13 can be used to treat 'running piglet' syndrome, where rebellious *qi* rises up through *chong mai*, with symptoms such as turmoil in the abdomen and chest, palpitations, nervousness, anxiety and a feeling of constriction in the throat.

- **Pain and discomfort in the lumbar region and waist and along the channel:** Liv 13 is a local point, a point on the Liver channel and the source point of *dai mai*. This means it can be used to treat problems in the lumbar region and the waist, as well as disorders in the local area and along the course of *dai mai*.

Liver 14 *Qimen* (Cycle Door)

- *Mu*-collecting point for the Liver.

- Meeting point of the Spleen and Liver channels, as well as *yin wei mai*.

- Exit point.

Actions

- Harmonises the Stomach and Liver.

- Regulates *qi* and *xue* in the upper and middle *jiao*.

- Spreads Liver *qi*.

- Opens the channel and moves *qi* and *xue* in the channel and in the local area.

Indications

- **Distension in the chest, costal region, solar plexus and hypochondriac region, tendency to yawn or sigh, shortness of breath, cough, breast distension, swelling or lumps in the breasts, and physical accumulations in the breasts, chest and costal region:** Liv 14 is an important point to regulate *qi* and *xue* in the upper *jiao*, especially when imbalances arise from a stagnation of Liver *qi*.

- **Vomiting, nausea, acid regurgitation, burping, abdominal pain, hiccups, abdominal distension and abdominal pain:** Stomach *qi* can be blocked and become rebellious when the Stomach is invaded by Liver *qi*. Liv 14 can be used to spread Liver *qi* and thus harmonise Stomach *qi*.

- **Mood swings, irritability and irascibility:** By spreading Liver *qi*, Liv 14 can be used in the treatment of mental-emotional imbalances due to Liver *qi* stagnation.

- **'Running piglet' syndrome:** By spreading Liver *qi*, Liv 14 can be used to treat 'running piglet' syndrome, where rebellious *qi* rises up through *chong mai*, with symptoms such as turmoil in the abdomen and chest, palpitations, nervousness, anxiety and a feeling of constriction in the throat.

- **Pain and discomfort in the local area and along the channel:** Liv 14 can be used as a channel point to treat problems in the local area and along the path of the channel.

Type	Point
Opening point	Lu 7
Partner opening point	Kid 6
Source point	Ren 1
Luo-connecting point	Ren 15

Ren 1 *Huiyin* (*Yin* Gathering)

- Meeting point of *ren mai*, *du mai* and *chong mai*.
- Source point of *ren mai*, *du mai* and *chong mai*.
- Sun Si Miao ghost point.

Actions

- Nourishes Kidney *yin*.
- Drains Damp-Heat.
- Calms *shen*.
- Restores consciousness.
- Controls the lower *jiao* and *yin* orifices.
- Opens the channel and moves *qi* and *xue* in the channel and in the local area.

Indications

- **Urinary difficulty, constipation, prostate problems, haemorrhoids, herpes, genital pain, genital ulcers, genital itching, damp and sweaty genitalia, swollen genitalia, impotence, rectal prolapse, amenorrhoea or irregular menstrual bleeding and uterine prolapse:** Ren 1 is an important, but not frequently used, acupuncture point for the treatment of all disorders of the genitalia, rectum and *bao* (which includes the Uterus and prostate). Ren 1 can circulate *qi* and *xue* and drain Damp-Heat.

- **Bipolar depression and manic behaviour:** As a Sun Si Miao ghost point, Ren 1 can be used to calm *shen* when a person is behaving as if they are possessed.

- **Loss of consciousness:** Ren 1 can be used when a person is unconscious after they have drowned.

Ren 2 *Qugu* (Curved Bone)

- Meeting point of *ren mai* and the Liver channel.

Actions

- Regulates the lower *jiao*.

- Benefits the Urinary Bladder and regulates urination.

- Tonifies the Kidneys.

- Opens the channel and moves *qi* and *xue* in the channel and in the local area.

Indications

- **Urinary difficulty, dribbling urination, lack of urination, painful urination, blood in the urine and cloudy urine:** Ren 2 is an important local point in the treatment of the Urinary Bladder and can be used for most imbalances in the Urinary Bladder. In addition, Ren 2 is used to tonify Kidney *qi* and thereby urination.

- **Genital itching, genital pain, genital swelling, genital ulcers, constant erection, *shan* disorder (such as hernia, pain and swelling in the abdomen and swelling of the genitalia), copious vaginal discharge and herpes:** Ren 2 is a meeting point of *ren mai* and the Liver channel. Both channels pass through and around the external genitalia. That is why Ren 2 can be used to treat the majority of disorders that manifest in and around the genitalia.

- **Nocturnal emissions, premature ejaculation and vaginal discharge:** Ren 2 can be used to tonify the Kidneys so that they are better able to hold *jing* inside the body. In addition, Ren 2 can drain Damp-Heat, which agitates the semen and can increase the volume and change the quality of the vaginal discharge.

Ren 3 *Zhongji* (Central Pole)

- *Mu*-collecting point of the Urinary Bladder.

- Meeting point of *ren mai* and the Spleen, Kidney and Liver channels.

Actions

- Benefits the Urinary Bladder and regulates urination.

- Drains Dampness and Damp-Heat.

- Controls the lower *jiao*.

- Benefits the Uterus.

- Tonifies the Kidneys.

- Opens the channel and moves *qi* and *xue* in the channel and in the local area.

Indications

- **Urinary difficulty, dribbling urination, lack of urination, painful urination, blood in the urine, cloudy urine, oedema and pain and distension in the lower part of the abdominal cavity:** Ren 3 is the *mu*-collecting point of the Urinary Bladder. Ren 3 can therefore be used to treat most disorders where the Urinary Bladder's functions are disturbed.

- **Genital itching, genital pain, genital swelling, genital ulcers, constant erection, *shan* disorder (such as hernia, pain and swelling in the abdomen and swelling of the genitalia), copious vaginal discharge and herpes:** Ren 3 is a meeting point of *ren mai* and the Liver channel. Both channels pass through and around the external genitalia. Ren 3 can also drain Damp-Heat from the lower *jiao* and therefore Ren 3 can be used in the treatment of disorders that manifest in and around the genitalia.

- **'Running piglet' syndrome:** Ren 3 can be used to treat 'running piglet' syndrome, where rebellious *qi* rises up through *chong mai*, with symptoms such as turmoil in the abdomen and chest, palpitations, nervousness, anxiety and a feeling of constriction in the throat. The use of Ren 3 is relevant when this syndrome occurs in the context of Kidney *yang xu* and invasions of Cold.

- **Nocturnal emissions, premature ejaculation and vaginal discharge:** Ren 3 can be used to tonify the Kidneys so that they are better able to hold *jing* inside the body. In addition, Ren 3 can drain Damp-Heat, which agitates the semen and which can increase the volume and change the quality of the vaginal discharge.

- **Irregular periods, amenorrhoea, heavy periods and uterine fibroids:** By circulating *qi* and *xue* in the lower *jiao*, Ren 3 can be used to treat most menstrual disorders that have arisen from a stagnation. Ren 3 also has some Kidney tonifying properties and can therefore be used in *xu* conditions. This characteristic is, however, overshadowed by acupuncture points such as Ren 4 and Ren 6.

- **Lumbar pain, pain, distension and disorders in the local area and along the course of *ren mai*:** In common with other acupuncture points, Ren 3 can be used in the treatment of problems in the local area and in areas where the channel connects to.

Ren 4 *Guanyuan* (*Yuan* Gate)

- *Mu*-collecting point of the Small Intestine.

- Meeting point of *ren mai*, *chong mai* and the Spleen, Kidney and Liver channels.

Actions

- Tonifies *yuan qi* and *jing*.

- Nourishes *yin* and *xue*.

- Tonifies the Kidneys.

- Tonifies Spleen *qi* and Spleen *yang*.

- Regulates the Small Intestine.

- Benefits the Uterus.

- Benefits the Urinary Bladder and regulates urination.

- Regulates the lower *jiao*.

- Rescues *yang* and restores consciousness.

- Opens the channel and moves *qi* and *xue* in the channel and in the local area.

Indications

- **Fatigue, tiredness, weakness and fatigue in the lumbar region, weak knees, impotence, vaginal discharge, dizziness and tinnitus:** Although Ren 4 is the *mu*-collecting point of the Small Intestine, Ren 4 is one of the most important acupuncture points to tonify Kidney *yang* and to nourish Kidney *yin* and Kidney *jing*. This means that Ren 4 can be used to treat virtually any disorder where the underlying imbalance is a Kidney *xu* condition.

- **Urinary difficulty, frequent urination, dribbling urination, scanty urination, painful urination, blood in the urine, cloudy urine and oedema:** Like most *ren mai* points below the umbilicus, Ren 4 can be used to treat Urinary Bladder imbalances. Ren 4 will mainly be used when disturbances of the Urinary Bladder's functions are the result of Kidney *yang xu* or Kidney *yin xu* Heat.

- **Amenorrhoea or sparse menstrual bleeding and infertility:** Kidney *jing* is the basis for *tian gui* and *xue*. By nourishing Kidney *jing*, Ren 4 can be used to treat *xu* conditions that disrupt menstruation and fertility.

- **Insomnia, fear, anxiety, palpitations, poor memory and nervousness:** *Shen* is nourished and anchored by Heart *yin* and Heart *xue*. Furthermore, *shen* is agitated by *yin xu* Heat. Heart *yin* is nourished by Kidney *yin*. By nourishing Kidney *yin*, Ren 4 can be used to calm and nourish *shen*.

- **Night sweats, hot flushes and a sensation of heat in the evening and at night:** Ren 4 is an important acupuncture point to nourish Kidney *yin* and hence can be used in the treatment of the *yin xu* Heat conditions in the body.

- **Dry cough and dryness of throat and mouth:** By nourishing Kidney *yin*, Ren 4 supports Lung *yin*.

- **Diarrhoea, watery stools containing undigested food remains and faecal incontinence:** As a meeting point of the Spleen and Kidney channels, Ren 4 can directly tonify Spleen *qi* and Spleen *yang*. Ren 4 can indirectly tonify Spleen *yang* by tonifying Kidney *yang*. Kidney *yang* controls the body's *yin* orifices. This is why Ren 4 can be used in the treatment of faecal incontinence, especially in the elderly, who are often Kidney *xu*.

- **Pain and distension in the lower part of the abdominal cavity:** Ren 4 can, in a similar way to other acupuncture points in the area, be used in the treatment of disorders in the local area.

Ren 5 *Shimen* (Stone Door)

- *Mu*-collecting point of *san jiao.*

Actions

- Opens the water passages.

- Regulates *qi* and *xue* in the lower *jiao.*

- Regulates the Uterus.

- Opens the channel and moves *qi* and *xue* in the channel and in the local area.

Indications

- **Urinary difficulty, frequent urination, dribbling urination, scanty urination, painful urination, blood in the urine, cloudy urine and oedema:** Ren 5 is the *mu*-collecting point of *san jiao*. Ren 5 can therefore be used to regulate the transformation and excretion of fluids in the body, especially in the lower *jiao*.

- **Diarrhoea and watery stools containing undigested food remains:** By controlling the transformation and excretion of fluids in the lower *jiao*, Ren 5 can be used in the treatment of diarrhoea, where fluids have not been transformed and excreted as they should have been.

- **Genital itching, pain and swelling of the genitals and *shan* disorder (such as hernia, pain and swelling in the abdomen and swelling of the genitalia):** Ren 5 can be used to spread *qi* and drain Dampness in the lower *jiao*.

- **'Running piglet' syndrome:** Ren 5 is one of several points in the lower *jiao* that can be used to control a condition where rebellious *qi* rises up *chong mai* with symptoms such as turmoil in the abdomen and chest, palpitations, nervousness, anxiety and a feeling of constriction in the throat.

- **Persistent lochia, vaginal discharge, uterine fibroids, ovarian cysts and accumulations in the Uterus:** Ren 5 can regulate the movement of *qi* and *xue* and drain Dampness and Damp-Heat from the Uterus.

- **Exhaustion, fatigue and tiredness:** Like the other *ren mai* points in the region, Ren 5 can be used to tonify *yuan qi*. This effect is, however, overshadowed by acupuncture points such as Ren 4 and Ren 6.

- **Pain and distension in the lower part of the abdominal cavity:** Ren 5 can, in a similar way to other acupuncture points in the area, be used in the treatment of disorders in the local area.

Ren 6 Qihai (Qi Sea)

- *Yuan*-source point of *huang* (membranes).

Actions

- Tonifies *yuan qi*.
- Tonifies *qi* and *yang*.
- Raises *qi*.
- Rescues *yang*.
- Regulates *qi* and *xue* in the lower *jiao*.
- Opens the channel and moves *qi* and *xue* in the channel and in the local area.

Indications

- **Exhaustion, fatigue, extreme weight loss, muscle weakness and weak voice:** Both Ren 4 and Ren 6 have a very fundamental tonifying effect on the body. Both acupuncture points nourish and tonify the Kidneys and the pre-heaven *qi*. Whereas Ren 4 has a close relationship to Kidney *yin* and *jing*, Ren 6 has a similar close relationship to Kidney *yang* and *yuan qi*. Ren 6 can, therefore, especially when used with moxa, be used to treat both chronic and acute disorders resulting from *yang xu* and *qi xu*.

- **Impotence, organ prolapse, sinking and dragging or collapsing sensation in the body:** Ren 6 with moxa tonifies and raises *yang qi* upwards. Ren 6 will often be used in combination with the moxa treatment of Du 20 in these situations.

- **Loss of consciousness:** When there is a loss of consciousness and collapse, moxa can be used on Ren 6 to 'rescue' *yang*.

- **Cold extremities, abdominal cold, extreme chills, diarrhoea, watery stool with undigested remains and copious amounts of clear urine:** Ren 6 is one of the body's most important *yang* tonifying acupuncture points and can be used in the treatment of *yang xu* conditions in all the organs.

- **Frequent urination, incontinence, copious watery vaginal discharge and heavy and prolonged menstrual bleeding:** Ren 6 can be used by all conditions of *qi xu* where *qi* can no longer hold substances in the body.

- *Shan* **disorders (such as hernia, pain and swelling in the abdomen and swelling of the genitalia):** Ren 6 can warm *yang* and thereby expel Cold. At the same time, Ren 6 can disperse stagnations of *qi* and *xue*.

- **Lumps and physical accumulations in the abdominal cavity, abdominal distension, constipation and pain and distension in the lower part of the abdominal cavity:** In addition to being an important acupuncture point to strengthen *qi*, Ren 6 is a very important acupuncture point to spread *qi* in the middle *jiao* and especially the lower *jiao*.

Ren 7 *Yinjiao* (*Yin* Intersection)

- Meeting point of *ren mai*, *chong mai* and the Kidney channel.

Actions

- Regulates the Uterus.

- Drains Dampness from the lower *jiao*.

- Opens the channel and moves *qi* and *xue* in the channel and in the local area.

Indications

- **Irregular or heavy menstrual bleeding, amenorrhoea and uterine fibroids:** By moving *qi* and *xue* in the lower *jiao*, whilst also being an acupuncture point where *ren mai* and *chong mai* meet, Ren 7 can be used to treat menstrual disorders. Ren 7 will mainly be used to treat *qi* and *xue* stagnations and stagnations due to Dampness or Damp-Heat.

- **Genital itching, pain, ulcers and swelling, constant erection, *shan* disorders (such as hernia, pain and swelling in the abdomen and swelling of the genitalia), copious vaginal discharge and herpes:** Ren 7 can disperse stagnations of *qi* and *xue* in the lower *jiao* and it can drain Dampness and Damp-Heat.

- **'Running piglet' syndrome:** Ren 7 is one of several points in the lower *jiao* that can be used to control a condition where rebellious *qi* rises up *chong mai* with symptoms such as turmoil in the abdomen and chest, palpitations, nervousness, anxiety and a feeling of constriction in the throat.

- **Difficulty urinating and defecating, oedema and borborygmi:** Stagnations of *qi* and *xue*, as well as accumulations of Dampness, can disrupt fluid physiology in the lower *jiao*. Ren 7 can drain Dampness in the lower *jiao* and disperse stagnant *qi* and *xue*.

- **Pain, hardness, distension and cold or hot skin in the area under and around the umbilicus:** Ren 7 can be used as a local point to treat disorders in the local area.

Ren 8 *Shenque* (*Shen* Watchtower)

Actions

- Warms *yang* and rescues collapsed *yang*.

- Warms the Intestines and expels Cold.

- Opens the channel and moves *qi* and *xue* in the channel and in the local area.

Indications

- **Loss of consciousness:** Ren 8 with moxa can be used to 'rescue' *yang* when a person has collapsed and is unconscious.

- **Persistent diarrhoea, cramping pain in the intestines and borborygmi:** Ren 8 with moxa can be used to tonify and warm Spleen *yang* and expel Cold from the Intestines.

- **Pain, hardness, distension, oedema or cold in the area around and under the umbilicus:** Moxa treatment of Ren 8 can circulate *qi* in the umbilical region and in the Intestines and expel Cold.

Ren 9 *Shuifen* (Water Separation)

Actions

- Opens the water passages.

- Regulates *qi* in the Intestines.

- Opens the channel and moves *qi* and *xue* in the channel and in the local area.

Indications

- **Oedema:** Ren 9 can be used in the treatment of all kinds of fluid accumulation in the body. Ren 9 is used in particular when there is oedema in the abdominal cavity.

- **Borborygmi and distension or pain in the area around and under the umbilicus:** Ren 9 can be used as a local point when treating the umbilical region and the Small Intestine.

- **Delayed closure of the fontanelle:** Ren 9 is an empirical point that can be used when the fontanelle is not closed.

Ren 10 *Xiawan* (Lower Cavity)

- Meeting point of *ren mai* and the Spleen channel.

Actions

- Regulates Stomach *qi.*

- Dissolves food stagnation.

- Opens the channel and moves *qi* and *xue* in the channel and in the local area.

Indications

- **Abdominal distension, abdominal pain, nausea, vomiting, poor appetite and undigested food in the stool:** Ren 10 can be used to tonify the Stomach's function of sending *qi* down to the Small Intestine. Ren 10 can therefore be used for conditions of the Stomach *qi xu*, when the Stomach is not strong enough to send the food downwards. Ren 10 can also be used for *shi* conditions such as *qi* stagnation or food stagnation in the Stomach.

Ren 11 *Xiawan* (Strengthen the Interior)
Actions

- Regulates Stomach *qi* and *qi* in the middle *jiao.*

- Disperses food stagnation.

- Opens the channel and moves *qi* and *xue* in the channel and in the local area.

Indications

- **Abdominal distension, abdominal pain, nausea, vomiting, poor appetite and undigested food in the stool:** Ren 11 can be used to tonify Stomach *qi* and to regulate *qi* in the middle *jiao*. Ren 11 can therefore also be used to disperse food stagnations in the Stomach.

Ren 12 *Zhongwan* (Central Cavity)

- *Mu*-collecting point of the Stomach.

- *Hui*-gathering point of the *fu* organs.

- Meeting point of *ren mai* and the Stomach, *san jiao* and Small Intestine channels.

Actions

- Regulates Stomach *qi* and controls rebellious *qi*.

- Tonifies Stomach and Spleen *qi*.

- Transforms Dampness and Phlegm.

- Dissolves food stagnation.

- Calms *shen*.

- Opens the channel and moves *qi* and *xue* in the channel and in the local area.

Indications

- **Fatigue, loose stool, poor appetite and weak limbs:** Ren 12 is an important acupuncture point to strengthen the production of post-heaven *qi*. Ren 12 is the *mu*-collecting point of the Stomach, but at the same time Ren 12 is an acupuncture point that tonifies Spleen *qi*. That is why Ren 12 can be used in the treatment of all the disorders that result from Stomach and Spleen *qi xu*.

- **Abdominal distension, abdominal pain, nausea, vomiting, poor appetite, undigested food in the stool, acid regurgitation and hiccups:** Ren 12 can be used to regulate *qi* in the middle *jiao* in both *xu* and *shi* conditions. When the Stomach and Spleen are *qi xu* they will not be able to send *qi* down and up respectively. Stomach Fire can drive *qi* upwards and Liver *qi* stagnation can block the movement of *qi* in the middle *jiao*.

- **Sticky sensation in the mouth, heaviness in the body, heavy headache and foggy sensation in the head:** By strengthening Spleen and Stomach *qi*, Ren 12 can be used to transform Dampness and Phlegm in the whole body and in the head.

- **Constant worrying and churning thoughts:** When Stomach and Spleen *qi* is weakened, a person can find it difficult to think clearly. This can be due to Phlegm obscuring *shen* or because their *yi* is weak. This will result in a person having difficulty focussing their thoughts, and them not being able to reach a conclusion, because their thoughts keep churning round in their head.

Ren 13 *Shangwan* (Upper Cavity)

- Meeting point of *ren mai* and the Stomach and Small Intestine channels.

Actions

- Regulates Stomach *qi* and controls rebellious *qi*.
- Regulates Heart *qi*.
- Opens the channel and moves *qi* and *xue* in the channel and in the local area.

Indications

- **Abdominal distension, abdominal pain, nausea, vomiting, poor appetite, undigested food in the stool, acid regurgitation, hiccups, borborygmi and lumps and physical accumulations in the upper abdomen:** Ren 13 is especially used to regulate rebellious Stomach *qi* that ascends due to *shi* conditions. Ren 13 can also be used to regulate the movement of *qi* and *xue* in the upper region of the abdominal cavity.

- **Cardiac pain or turmoil in the chest and palpitations:** Ren 13 can be used as a local point to treat pain and unrest in the cardiac region.

- **'Running piglet' syndrome:** Ren 13 is one of several *ren mai* points that can be used to treat 'running piglet' syndrome, where rebellious *qi* rises up through *chong mai* with symptoms such as turmoil in the abdomen and chest, palpitations, nervousness, anxiety and a feeling of constriction in the throat.

Ren 14 *Juque* (Great Watchtower)

- *Mu*-collecting point of the Heart.

Actions

- Regulates Heart *qi*.
- Regulates Lung *qi*.
- Controls rebellious Stomach *qi*.
- Transforms Phlegm and calms *shen*.

- Opens the channel and moves *qi* and *xue* in the channel and in the local area.

Indications

- **Cardiac pain or unrest, palpitations, chest oppression, and pain or distension in the upper back:** Ren 14 is the *mu*-collecting point of the Heart and can be used to treat all forms of stagnations in the Heart. These may be stagnations of *qi*, *xue*, Cold or Phlegm. Ren 14 can also be used when the stagnation results from *xu* conditions, such as Heart *yin xu*, Heart *yang xu* or Heart *xue xu*.

- **Bipolar depression, manic behaviour, anger, irascibility, distress, fear, palpitations, insomnia and mental confusion:** As the *mu*-collecting point of the Heart, Ren 14 has a wide range of actions that affect both the physical and *shen* aspects of the Heart. Ren 14 can be used to treat *xu* conditions where *shen* is not nourished and anchored as it should be. Ren 14 can also be used for *shi* conditions where *shen* is blocked and agitated.

- **Cough, shortness of breath and Phlegm in the Lung:** Ren 14 can be used as a local point to regulate Lung *qi* and *zong qi*.

- **Abdominal distension, abdominal pain, nausea, vomiting, poor appetite, undigested food in the stool, acid regurgitation and hiccups:** Ren 14 can be used as a local point to regulate rebellious Stomach *qi*.

Ren 15 *Jiuwei* (Dove Tail)

- *Luo*-connecting point for *ren mai*.

- *Yuan*-source point for *gao* (fatty tissue or the area between the heart and diaphragm).

Actions

- Regulates Heart *qi*.
- Calms *shen*.

- Opens the chest.

- Opens the channel and moves *qi* and *xue* in the channel and in the local area.

Indications

- **Fear, anxiety, palpitations, insomnia, bipolar depression, manic behaviour, mental confusion, obsessive thoughts and constant worrying:** Ren 15 has a powerful *shen*-calming effect. Ren 15 is effective in the treatment of both *xu* and *shi* conditions.

- **Cardiac pain or unrest, palpitations, chest oppression and distension or pain in the upper back:** Ren 15 can regulate *qi* and *xue* in and around the Heart.

- **Cough, shortness of breath and Phlegm in the Lung:** Ren 15 can be used as a local point to regulate Lung *qi* and *zong qi*.

- **Abdominal distension, abdominal pain, nausea, vomiting, poor appetite, undigested food in the stool, acid regurgitation and hiccups:** Ren 15 can be used as a local point to regulate Stomach *qi*.

Ren 16 *Zhongting* (Central Courtyard)

Actions

- Regulates Stomach *qi*.

- Opens the chest.

- Opens the channel and moves *qi* and *xue* in the channel and in the local area.

Indications

Ren 16 is mainly used as a local point to regulate *qi* in the chest and to control rebellious Stomach *qi*. This is why Ren 16 can be used to treat chest oppression in the local area, as well as nausea, vomiting and acid regurgitation.

Ren 17 *Shanzhong* (Centre of the Chest)

- *Mu*-collecting point of the Pericardium.

- *Hui*-gathering point for *qi*.

- Meeting point of *ren mai* and the Spleen, Kidney, Small Intestine and *san jiao* channels.

Actions

- Regulates *qi* and opens the chest.

- Tonifies *zong qi*.

- Benefits the breasts.

- Opens the channel and moves *qi* and *xue* in the channel and in the local area.

Indications

- **Cough, shortness of breath, Phlegm in the Lung, rattling sound in the chest, asthma, chest oppression or heaviness in the chest, cardiac pain and palpitations:** As the *mu* point for the Pericardium and the *hui*-gathering point for *qi*, Ren 17 is an important acupuncture point to spread *qi* in the upper *jiao*. Ren 17 can therefore be used to regulate Lung *qi*, Heart *qi*, *xue* and *zong qi*.

- **Fatigue, weak voice and spontaneous sweating:** As the *hui*-collecting point for *qi*, Ren 17 can be used to tonify *zong qi*.

- **Poor lactation and lumps and abscesses in the breasts:** Ren 17 can be used to disperse *qi* and *xue* in the breasts and to tonify *qi*.

- **Acid regurgitation, hiccups, vomiting and nausea:** Ren 17 can be used as a local point to descend Stomach *qi*.

Ren 18 *Yutang* (Jade Hall), Ren 19 *Zigong* (Purple Palace) and Ren 20 *Huagai* (Flower Canopy)

Actions

- Regulate *qi* and open the chest.

- Open the channel and move *qi* and *xue* in the channel and in the local area.

Indications

- **Chest oppression, breathing difficulties, cough and disorders of the breasts:** Ren 18, Ren 19 and Ren 20 are mainly used as local points to regulate *qi* in the chest.

Ren 21 *Xuanji* (Purple Pivot)

Actions

- Regulates Stomach *qi*.

- Regulates Lung *qi* and opens the chest.

- Benefits the throat.

- Opens the channel and moves *qi* and *xue* in the channel and in the local area.

Indications

- **Cough, asthma, dyspnoea, acid regurgitation and chest oppression:** Ren 21 is mainly used as a local point to descend Lung and Stomach *qi*.

Ren 22 *Tiantu* (Heavenly Protrusion)

- Meeting point of *ren mai* and *yin wei mai*.

- Window of Heaven point.

Actions

- Regulates Lung *qi* and opens the chest.

- Benefits the throat and the voice.

- Opens the channel and moves *qi* and *xue* in the channel and in the local area.

Indications

- **Cough, shortness of breath, Phlegm in the Lung, rattling sounds in the chest, asthma, chest oppression, heaviness in the chest and cardiac pain:** By descending *qi*, Ren 22 can be used in the treatment of conditions resulting from stagnations of *qi* in the chest or rebellious Lung *qi*.

- **Phlegm in the throat, 'plumstone *qi*', tension in the throat, sore throat, dryness in the throat, loss of voice and goitre:** As a Window of Heaven point, Ren 22 can regulate *qi* and transform Phlegm in the throat. Ren 22 can also be used to draw *yin qi* up to the throat.

Ren 23 *Lianquan* (Corner Spring)

- Meeting point of *ren mai* and *yin wei mai*.

Actions

- Descends *qi*.
- Benefits the tongue.
- Opens the channel and moves *qi* and *xue* in the channel and in the local area.

Indications

- **Swelling of the tongue, speech impediments, sudden loss of voice, aphasia after a stroke, pain in the tongue, tongue ulcers, mouth ulcers and dryness in the mouth:** Ren 23 has a very close relationship to the tongue and can be used to treat most disturbances and problems of the tongue.
- **Cough, dyspnoea and vomiting of mucus:** Ren 23 can descend rebellious *qi*.

Ren 24 *Chengjiang* (Saliva Receptacle)

- Meeting point of *ren mai*, *du mai* and the Stomach and Large Intestine channels.
- Sun Si Miao ghost point.

Actions

- Calms internally generated Wind and expels exogenous Wind.
- Opens the channel and moves *qi* and *xue* in the channel and in the local area.

Indications

- **Manic behaviour, epilepsy and disorders manifesting in the mouth, chin and lips:** Ren 24 is mainly used as a local point in the treatment of internal and exogenous Wind conditions that affect the mouth, chin and lips. As a Sun Si Miao ghost point, Ren 24 can be used in the treatment of manic behaviour and epilepsy.

DU MAI ACUPUNCTURE POINTS

Type	Point
Opening point	SI 3
Partner opening point	UB 62
Source point	Ren 1
Luo-connecting point	Du 1

Du 1 *Changqiang* (Long Strength)

- Meeting point of *du mai*, *ren mai* and the Gall Bladder and Kidney channels.
- *Luo*-connecting point.

Actions

- Regulates the lower *jiao* and the body's *yin* orifices.
- Calms *shen*.
- Calms internally generated Wind.
- Opens the channel and moves *qi* and *xue* in the channel and in the local area.

Indications

- **Urinary difficulty, constipation, prostate problems, haemorrhoids, herpes, genital sores, genital itching, sweaty genitalia, swollen or painful genitalia, impotence, premature ejaculation, nocturnal emissions and rectal prolapse:** Du 1 is an important acupuncture point in the treatment of genital and rectal problems and of the stool and urination. This is because it is a local point in the area and because *du mai* traverses the rectum, Kidneys and the genitalia.

- **Bipolar depression, manic behaviour, epilepsy, tetanus and tremors and shakes:** *Du mai* connects to both the Heart and the Brain, both of which are organs with a close relationship to *shen*. Du 1 can be used as a distal point to calm Wind and drain Heat.

- **Pain and stiffness in the coccyx, sacrum, buttock, lumbar region, back and neck:** Du 1 can be used as a local and distal point to treat problems along the channel and in the vicinity of the rectum and coccyx.

Du 2 *Yaoshu* (Lumbar Point)

Actions

- Expels Wind-Dampness and benefits the lumbar region.

- Calms internally generated Wind.

- Opens the channel and moves *qi* and *xue* in the channel and in the local area.

Indications

Du 2 is mainly used in the treatment of disorders in the local area, especially when there is pain that radiates down the legs. Du 2 can be used to treat spasms and convulsions, because it can calm internal Wind.

Du 3 *Yaoyangguan* (Lumbar *Yang* Gate)

Actions

- Strengthens the lumbar region and legs.

- Expels Wind-Dampness.

- Tonifies Kidney *yang*.

- Regulates *qi* in the lower *jiao*.

- Opens the channel and moves *qi* and *xue* in the channel and in the local area.

Indications

Du 3 is mainly used to treat disorders in the lumbar region and pain that radiates down the legs.

Du 4 *Mingmen* (Gate of Life)

Actions

- Tonifies and warms *mingmen*.

- Tonifies *yuan qi*.

- Tonifies Kidney *yang*.

- Nourishes Kidney *jing*.

- Expels Cold.

- Regulates *du mai*.

- Drains Heat.

- Calms internally generated Wind.

- Strengthens the lumbar region and legs.

- Opens the channel and moves *qi* and *xue* in the channel and in the local area.

Indications

- **Aversion to cold, cold lumbar region, cold knees, cold feet, fatigue and spontaneous sweating:** Du 4 tonifies and warms *mingmen*, which is the pre-heavenly source of *yang* Heat.

- **Weakness and fatigue in the lumbar region and knees and pain and stiffness of the lower back:** Du 4 is an important local point to treat lumbar problems. Whilst warming and tonifying *mingmen*, Du 4 will also tonify Kidney *yang* and expel Cold from the area. This means that Du 4 can treat both the root and the manifestation of the problem.

- **Oedema, incontinence, frequent and copious urination and frequent and scanty urination:** Du 4 is considered to be the most important acupuncture point to tonify and warm *mingmen* and thereby Kidney *yang* and *yuan qi*. This means that Du 4 can be used to treat all disturbances of fluid physiology when these are due to *yang xu* conditions.

- **Impotence, lack of libido, premature ejaculation and nocturnal emissions:** By strengthening and warming *mingmen*, *yuan qi* and Kidney *yang*, Du 4 can be used to influence the sexual functions and activate the libido. One of the functions of Kidney *yang* is to withhold the semen until it should be released. Du 4 can also be used for premature or nocturnal emissions, as it will strengthen the Kidneys' controlling of the *yin* orifices.

- **Dizziness, tinnitus, depression, lack of willpower, mental confusion and poor concentration:** Du 4 can strengthen *yuan qi* and *yang* in general. Du 4 can therefore be used to raise *yang qi* up to the head, transform *jing* to *shen* and activate *shen*. Furthermore, Du 4 can be used in *jing xu* conditions, because Du 4 can also nourish Kidney *jing*.

- **Epilepsy, tremors, severe headaches, extreme rigidity and spasm of the muscles and febrile conditions:** Du 4 can be used to extinguish and to calm internal Wind. Du 4 is also attributed Heat-draining characteristics in the classical texts, similar to those that Du 14 has. This reflects the fact that *du mai* is the *yang* governing channel and that *du mai* points can therefore be used to control *yang shi* conditions.

- **Pain and stiffness in the back and neck:** Du 4 can be used to treat *qi* and *xue* stagnations along the path of the channel.

Du 5 *Xuanshu* (Suspended Pivot)

Actions

- Strengthens the lumbar region.

- Regulates *qi* in the lower *jiao*.

- Opens the channel and moves *qi* and *xue* in the channel and in the local area.

Indications

- **Local disorders:** Du 5 is mainly used to treat disorders of the lower back.

Du 6 *Jizhong* (Spine Centre)

Actions

- Tonifies the Spleen.

- Strengthens the lumbar region.

- Opens the channel and moves *qi* and *xue* in the channel and in the local area.

Indications

- **Local disorders:** Du 6 can be used to treat conditions caused by Spleen *qi xu* and disorders in the local area.

Du 7 *Zhongshu* (Central Pivot)

Actions

- Strengthens the spine.

- Benefits the middle *jiao*.

- Opens the channel and moves *qi* and *xue* in the channel and in the local area.

Indications

- **Local disorders:** Du 7 is mainly used to treat disorders in the central area of the spine, as well as disturbances of *qi* in the middle *jiao*, such as abdominal distension.

Du 8 *Jinsuo* (Sinew Contraction)

Actions

- Drains Liver Fire and Liver Wind.

- Calms *shen*.

- Opens the channel and moves *qi* and *xue* in the channel and in the local area.

Indications

- **Epilepsy, muscle tremors, stiffness and cramping in the muscles and stiffness in the back:** Du 8 can be used in a similar way to UB 18 (which this point is located next to) to calm Liver Wind.

- **Manic behaviour and raving:** By draining Liver Fire, Du 8 can calm *shen*.

Du 9 *Zhiyang* (*Yang* Extremity)

Actions

- Drains Damp-Heat.

- Regulates *qi* in the middle *jiao*.

- Opens the chest.

- Opens the channel and moves *qi* and *xue* in the channel and in the local area.

Indications

- **Jaundice, heaviness in the whole body, heaviness in the arms and legs, nausea, vomiting, poor appetite and abdominal distension:** Du 9 can be used to drain Damp-Heat from the middle *jiao*.

- **Cough, shortness of breath, hiccups and chest oppression:** Du 9 can, in the same way as UB 17 (which this point is located next to), be used to regulate *qi* in the chest and in the diaphragm.

- **Pain, stiffness and problems in the central area of the back, as well as along the channel:** Du 9 can, in the same way as other channel points, be used in the treatment of local disorders and disorders along the path of the channel.

Du 10 *Lingtai* (Spirit Tower)

Actions

- Regulates *qi* in the upper *jiao*.

- Drains Fire-Toxins.

- Opens the channel and moves *qi* and *xue* in the channel and in the local area.

Indications

- **Abscesses, folliculitis and respiratory disorders:** Du 10 is mainly used to treat disorders in the upper part of the back, as well as cough and dyspnoea, by regulating *qi* in the upper *jiao*. Du 10 can also be used for the treatment of abscesses and folliculitis, because it can drain Fire-Toxins.

Du 11 *Shendao* (*Shen* Path)

Actions

- Tonifies and nourishes the Heart.

- Tonifies Lung *qi*.

- Calms *shen*.

- Drains Heat.

- Extinguishes internally generated Wind.

- Opens the channel and moves *qi* and *xue* in the channel and in the local area.

Indications

- **Depression, sadness, anxiety, fear, poor memory, palpitations, tendency to be easily startled, insomnia and lack of courage:** Du 11 can be used in the same way as UB 15 (which this point is located next to) to nourish and tonify the Heart and thereby calm *shen*.

- **Epilepsy, muscle tremor and tetanus:** Du 11 can, as is the case with many other *du mai* points, extinguish internally generated Wind.

- **Febrile conditions:** Like many other *du mai* points, Du 11 can drain Heat. This is an example of how *du mai* is the *yang* governing vessel.

- **Shortness of breath, shallow breathing, dyspnoea and cough:** Du 11 can be used to tonify *zong qi* and thereby Lung *qi*.

- **Pain, stiffness and problems in the upper part of the back, as well as along the channel:** Du 11 can, like other channel points, be used in the treatment of local disorders and disorders along the path of the channel.

Du 12 *Shenzhu* (Body Pillar)

Actions

- Drains Heat from the Heart and Lung.

- Tonifies Lung *qi*.

- Calms *shen*.

- Extinguishes internally generated Wind.

- Opens the channel and moves *qi* and *xue* in the channel and in the local area.

Indications

- **Heat and agitation in the chest, dyspnoea, shortness of breath, cough, thirst, headache and fever:** Du 12 can be used to drain Heat that has accumulated in the chest, agitating and disrupting Lung and Heart *qi*.

- **Manic behaviour, uncontrolled anger, urge to kill and raving:** By draining *shi* Heat from the Heart, Du 12 can calm *shen*.

- **Epilepsy, muscle tremor and tetanus:** Du 12 can extinguish internally generated Wind, especially when the Wind has been stirred up by Fire.

- **Fatigue, weak voice, breathlessness and spontaneous sweating:** Du 12 is located adjacent to UB 13 and they share similar properties, including the ability to tonify Lung *qi*.

- **Pain, stiffness and problems in the upper part of the back, as well as disorders along the course of the channel:** Du 12 can, like other channel points, be used in the treatment of local disorders and disorders along the path of the channel.

Du 13 *Taodao* (Joyous Path)

- Meeting point of *du mai* and the Urinary Bladder channel.

Actions

- Drains Heat.

- Regulates *shaoyang*.

- Opens the channel and moves *qi* and *xue* in the channel and in the local area.

Indications

- **Fatigue, alternating feeling of fever and chills, malaria and burning sensation in the bones:** Invasions of *xie qi* can get stuck in the *shaoyang* aspect of the body. This can result in both acute or chronic conditions, characterised by alternating fever and chills, as well as fatigue. Du 13 can expel *xie qi* from the *shaoyang* aspect.

- **Pain, stiffness and problems in the upper part of the back and neck and along the course of the channel:** Du 13 can, like other channel points, be used in the treatment of local disorders and disorders along the path of the channel.

Du 14 *Dazhui* (Large Vertebra)

- Meeting point of *du mai* with all the *yang* channels.

Actions

- Expels Wind and calms internally generated Wind.

- Activates *wei qi*.

- Drains Heat.

- Tonifies *yang*.

- Regulates *shaoyang*.

- Opens the channel and moves *qi* and *xue* in the channel and in the local area.

Indications

- **Aversion to cold, sore muscles, lack of sweating, sore throat and headache:** Du 14 is, together with Du 20, one of the most *yang* points in the body. Du 14 can be used to activate the *yang wei qi* so that *wei qi* can expel invasions of *xie qi* from the body.

- **Frequent colds:** By tonifying *yang* and by activating *wei qi*, Du 14 can be used to treat *wei qi xu*, manifesting with a weak immune system.

- **Febrile conditions, alternating feeling of fever and chills, malaria and burning sensation in the bones:** Du 14 is one of the most important acupuncture points to drain Heat. Du 14 can drain all forms of *shi* Heat. Du 14 can expel exogenous *xie qi* that has invaded the external aspects of the body or got stuck in the *shaoyang* aspect. Du 14 can also drain Heat from the interior aspects of the body.

- **Fatigue, breathlessness and aversion to cold:** As well as draining Heat, Du 14, when treated with moxa, can be used to tonify and warm *yang*.

- **Spontaneous sweating, excessive sweating and night sweats:** Du 14 has a close relationship to *wei qi*. Du 14 can therefore be used to control sweating. Du 14 drains and expels *shi* Heat, so Du 14 can also be used in the treatment of sweating, which occurs when *shi* Heat drives the fluids in the body upwards and outwards.

- **Dizziness, epilepsy, muscle tremor, tetanus and hypertension:** Du 14 can, like many other *du mai* points, be used to extinguish internally generated Wind.

- **Nose bleeds:** *Du mai* connects to the nose. Du 14 can therefore drain Heat from the nose that is agitating *xue*, resulting in bleeding.

- **Pain, stiffness and problems in the neck and the upper part of the back, as well as along the channel:** Du 14 is an important acupuncture point in the treatment of disorders of the neck and along the path of the channel in the upper back.

Du 15 *Yamen* (Mute Door)

- Meeting point of *du mai* and *yang wei mai*.

Actions

- Benefits the tongue and stimulates speech.
- Expels Wind and calms internally generated Wind.
- Benefits the Brain.
- Opens the channel and moves *qi* and *xue* in the channel and in the local area.

Indications

- **Muteness, loss of voice, rigid tongue and flaccid tongue:** Du 15 has a direct influence on the tongue and has traditionally been used for the treatment of muteness.

- **Dizziness, epilepsy, muscle tremor, tetanus and headaches:** Du 15 is one of the many *du mai* points that can be used to calm internally generated Wind.

- **Aversion to cold, sore muscles, lack of sweating, sore throat and headache:** As well as calming internal Wind, Du 15 can also expel invasions of exogenous Wind.

- **Nose bleeds:** *Du mai* connects to the nose. Du 15 can therefore drain Heat from the nose that is agitating *xue*, resulting in bleeding.

- **Poor memory, poor concentration and emptiness in the head:** Du 15 can lift clear *yang qi* up to the head and brain.

- **Pain, stiffness and problems of the neck and the upper part of the back and along the course of the channel:** Du 15 can be used as a local point in the treatment of disorders of the neck and as a distal point to treat problems along the path of the channel.

Du 16 *Fengfu* (Wind Mansion)

- Meeting point of *du mai* and *yang wei mai*.
- Window of Heaven point.
- Sun Si Miao ghost point.

Actions

- Expels Wind and calms internally generated Wind.
- Nourishes the Marrow and the Brain.
- Calms *shen*.
- Opens the channel and moves *qi* and *xue* in the channel and in the local area.

Indications

- **Dizziness and vertigo:** Du 16 is a very important acupuncture point in the treatment of vertigo and dizziness. Du 16 can calm internal Wind and drain

Phlegm down from the head. Du 16 can also be used to nourish the Brain in *jing xu* conditions.

- **Headache:** Du 16 can be used in the treatment of most kinds of headaches, both acute and chronic, *xu* and *shi*. Du 16 can drain *yang qi* and Phlegm down from the head. Du 16 can also expel invasions of exogenous Wind and nourish the Brain.

- **Epilepsy, muscle tremors, tetanus, hemiplegia, upwardly staring eyes and hypertension:** Du 16 is one of the most important acupuncture points to calm internally generated Wind, especially when this affects the head.

- **Aversion to cold, sore muscles, sore throat, headache and 'wind *bi*' (migratory pain in the body):** As well as calming internally generated Wind, Du 16 can also expel invasions of exogenous Wind.

- **Nose bleeds:** *Du mai* connects to the nose. Du 16 can therefore drain Heat from the nose that is agitating *xue*, resulting in bleeding.

- **Manic behaviour, raving, fear, palpitations, depression and suicidal thoughts:** Du 16 can be used to calm *shen*. Some Daoist traditions believe that *shen* has its residence in the Brain. *Du mai* connects to both the Heart and the Brain.

- **Pain, stiffness and problems at the back of the neck, the upper part of the back and along the channel:** Du 16 can be used as a local point in the treatment of disorders of the neck and head, as well as a distal point to treat problems along the path of the channel.

Du 17 *Naohu* (Brain Door) and Du 18 *Qiangjian* (Unyielding Space)

- Du 17 is a meeting point of *du mai* and the Urinary Bladder channel.

Actions

- Calm internally generated Wind.

- Calm *shen*.

- Open the channel and move *qi* and *xue* in the channel and in the local area.

Indications

- **Dizziness, vertigo, epilepsy, tetanus, hemiplegia and headache:** Du 17 and Du 18 are mainly used to calm internal Wind.

- **Manic behaviour, mental restlessness and eye disorders:** These two acupuncture points can also be used in the treatment of eye disorders and to calm *shen*.

Du 19 *Houding* (Behind the Vertex)

Actions

- Calms internally generated Wind.
- Calms *shen*.
- Opens the channel and moves *qi* and *xue* in the channel and in the local area.

Indications

- **Mania, mental agitation, anxiety and insomnia:** Du 19 is a powerful *shen*-calming point.
- **Dizziness, vertigo, epilepsy, tetanus, hemiplegia and headache:** Du 19 calms internally generated Wind.

Du 20 *Baihui* (One Hundred Gathering)

- Meeting point of *du mai* and the Urinary Bladder, Gall Bladder, *san jiao* and Liver channels.

Actions

- Calms internally generated Wind and ascending *yang*.
- Raises *yang*.
- Nourishes the Brain and the sense organs.
- Rescues *yang*.
- Calms *shen*.
- Opens the channel and moves *qi* and *xue* in the channel and in the local area.

Indications

- **Headache:** Du 20 can be used in the treatment of many types of headaches. Du 20 can raise *qi* and *xue* to the head when there are *xu* conditions. In *shi* headaches, Du 20 can send *qi* and Phlegm down from the head. Du 20 is particularly recommended for Liver imbalance headaches, because the Liver internal channel terminates in Du 20.

- **Dizziness, vertigo, hemiplegia, tetanus, epilepsy and tinnitus:** Du 20 is an important acupuncture point in the treatment of internal Wind conditions. Du 20 can both calm Wind and send the ascendant *qi* down from the head.

- **Tinnitus, pressure behind the eyes and blindness:** Du 20 has an influence on most of the sense organs. Du 20 can be used to lift *qi* and thus also *yin* nourishment up to the head. When using a draining technique, Du 20 can send rebellious *yang qi*, Phlegm and Wind downwards.

- **Blocked nose, running nose, nose bleeds and poor sense of smell:** *Du mai* connects to the nose. This means that Du 20 can be used to treat disorders that manifest in the nose.

- **Organ prolapse, haemorrhoids and low blood pressure:** By lifting *yang qi* upwards, Du 20 can be used for all kinds of prolapse and when *qi* is sinking in the body. Moxa is especially appropriate in these situations. Du 20 is particularly suitable in the treatment of some types of haemorrhoids, because Du 20 can lift *yang qi* upwards and at the same time Du 20 is a distal point for the anus.

- **Depression, manic behaviour, sadness, fear, anxiety, palpitations, poor memory and poor concentration:** By descending *yang qi* from the head, Du 20 has a powerful calming influence on *shen* and the Brain. In some old acupuncture and Daoist texts, *shen* was conceived as having its residence in the Brain. A branch of *du mai* connects to the Brain from Du 20. This means that Du 20 can also be used to nourish and stimulate the Brain by using a tonifying needle technique or moxa to raise activating *yang qi* up to the head.

- **Loss of consciousness:** By lifting *yang qi* up to the head, Du 20 can be used to resuscitate people who are unconscious.

Du 21 *Qianding* (In Front of the Vertex) and Du 22 *Xinhui* (Fontanel Gathering)

Actions

- Calm internally generated Wind and ascending *yang*.

- Benefit the head.

- Open the channel and move *qi* and *xue* in the channel and in the local area.

Indications

- **Dizziness, vertigo headache, epilepsy and hemiplegia:** Du 21 and Du 22 can be used to calm internal Wind.

- **Nasal disorders:** Du 22 can be used as a distal point for the treatment of nasal disorders.

Du 23 *Shangxing* (Upper Star)

- Sun Si Miao ghost point.

Actions

- Benefits the nose and eyes.
- Calms *shen*.
- Benefits the head.
- Calms internally generated Wind.
- Opens the channel and moves *qi* and *xue* in the channel and in the local area.

Indications

- **Blocked nose, running nose, nasal polyps, sneezing, nose bleeds and poor sense of smell:** *Du mai* connects directly to the nose, and Du 23 is a very important acupuncture point in the treatment of all types of nasal disorders.

- **Superficial visual disturbances, blurred vision and short-sightedness:** Du 23 can be used in the treatment of eye disorders. This is due to Du 23 being in the vicinity of the eyes and because the path of the channel on the front of the face connects to the eyes.

- **Bipolar depression:** Du 23 and Du 24 have similar characteristics, but whilst Du 23 is mainly used to treat nasal disorders, Du 24 is more used in the treatment of *shen* imbalances.

- **Swollen and red face and throbbing headache:** Du 23 has facial swelling as a traditional indication. By calming internally generated Wind, Du 23 can be used in the treatment of migraines.

Du 24 *Shenting* (*Shen* Courtyard)

- Meeting point of *du mai* and the Urinary Bladder and Stomach channels.

Actions

- Calms *shen.*

- Benefits the nose and eyes.

- Benefits the Brain.

- Calms internally generated Wind.

- Opens the channel and moves *qi* and *xue* in the channel and in the local area.

Indications

- **Bipolar depression, depression, insomnia, lethargy, the person climbs up to high places and sings and the person removes their clothes and runs around naked:** Du 23 and Du 24 have similar characteristics, but whereas Du 23 is mainly used to treat nasal disorders, Du 24 is more used in the treatment of *shen* imbalances. Du 24 has a powerful *shen*-calming effect and is used in particular when Phlegm-Heat agitates and blocks *shen.*

- **Blocked nose, running nose, nasal polyps, sneezing, nose bleeds, lack of smell, flickering on the eye, blurred vision and short-sightedness:** Du 24 is less used than the previous point on the channel, Du 23, in the treatment of nasal and visual disorders. Du 24 can though be used in the treatment of many disorders in the sensory organs.

- **Vertigo, dizziness, headache, upwardly staring eyes, epilepsy and tinnitus:** Du 24 can, like many other *du mai* points, be used to send internally generated Wind down from the head.

Du 25 *Suliao* (White Bone-Hole)
Actions

- Benefits the nose.

- Opens the channel and moves *qi* and *xue* in the channel and in the local area.

Indications

- **Nasal disorders:** Du 25 can be used as a local point in the treatment of all forms of nasal disorders, such as blocked nose, running nose, nasal polyps, sneezing, nose bleeds and having no sense of smell.

Du 26 *Renzhong* (Central Man)

- Meeting point of *du mai* and the Large Intestine and Stomach channels.
- Sun Si Miao ghost point.

Actions

- Restores consciousness.
- Calms *shen*.
- Benefits the nose and face.
- Benefits the spine and lumbar region.
- Calms internally generated Wind and expels exogenous Wind.
- Opens the channel and moves *qi* and *xue* in the channel and in the local area.

Indications

- **Loss of consciousness:** Du 26 is an important acupuncture point to resuscitate people who have suddenly collapsed and are unconscious. Its ability to revive people is the reason why Du 26 was later added to Gao Wu's original group of four command points.

- **Blocked nose, running nose, nasal polyps, sneezing, nose bleeds, no sense of smell, visual disturbances, blurred vision and short-sightedness:** As a local point, Du 26 has a strong effect on the nose. It can also be used for visual problems due to the pathway of *du mai*.

- **Epilepsy, muscle tremor, tetanus, facial paralysis, hypertension and headaches:** Du 26 can be used to calm internally generated Wind and to expel exogenous Wind from the face and head.

- **Bipolar depression, depression and inappropriate laughter:** As with many other *du mai* points in the head, Du 26 has a powerful *shen*-calming effect and can be used to treat *shi* patterns when *shen* is blocked or agitated.

- **Lumbar pain and stiffness:** Du 26 can be used as a distal point to treat acute blockages of *du mai* in the lower back.

Du 27 *Duiduan* (Oral Extremity)

Actions

- Drains Heat, promotes the formation of fluids and benefits the mouth.

- Calms *shen*.

- Opens the channel and moves *qi* and *xue* in the channel and in the local area.

Indications

- **Local disorders:** Du 27 is mainly used as a local point to treat oral disorders and problems in and around the lips. Du 27 can, however, like many *du mai* points in the head, be used to calm *shen*.

Du 28 *Yinjiao* (Gum Intersection)

- Meeting point of *du mai*, *ren mai* and the Stomach channel.

Actions

- Drains Heat and benefits the gums.

- Benefits the nose and eyes.

- Opens the channel and moves *qi* and *xue* in the channel and in the local area.

Indications

- **Local disorders:** Du 28 is mainly used as a local point in the treatment of the gums. Du 28 can, however, also be used to treat nose and eye disorders.

EXTRA POINTS

Extra points are acupuncture points that are not regular channel points. Some of them are located on the path of the channel but nevertheless are not classified as being channel points. There are myriad extra points. I have only included a limited number of them here. Something that can be confusing is that different books have used different numbering systems to classify these points. I have chosen to follow Claudia Focks's (2008) example of using the WHO's classification of extra points (World Health Organization 1991). The numbering and the lettering of these points is at times different from the classification system used by Peter Deadman and Mazin Al-Khafaji (1998) in *A Manual of Acupuncture*. When there is a conflict between these two classification systems, I have written Deadman and Al-Khafaji's classification in italics under the point's name and the WHO classification.

Ex-HN 1 *Sishencong* (Four Alert *Shen*)
Actions

- Calms *shen.*

- Calms internally generated Wind.

- Benefits the eyes and ears.

Indications

- **Hemiplegia, epilepsy, dizziness, headache and eye disorders:** Like Du 20, *sishencong* can calm internally generated Wind and send *yang qi* downwards.

- **Insomnia, manic behaviour and poor memory:** Like Du 20, *sishencong* has a powerful *shen*-calming effect and these four extra points will often be used together with Du 20.

Ex-HN 3 *Yintang* (Hall of Impressions)
Actions

- Calms *shen.*

- Calms internally generated Wind.

- Benefits the nose.

Indications

- **Insomnia, anxiety, fear, manic behaviour and poor memory:** *Yintang* is one of the body's most important *shen*-calming points. *Yintang* can be used to treat both *xu* and *shi* conditions.

- **Epilepsy, dizziness, vertigo, tremors, headache, hypertension and eye disorders:** Although *yintang* is not classified as a *du mai* point, *yintang* is located on the pathway of *du mai*. *Yintang* also shares many characteristics with *du mai* points. This can be seen, for example, by *yintang* being used to calm *yang* and internal Wind that have risen up to the head.

- **Blocked nose, running nose, nasal polyps, sneezing, nose bleeds, no sense of smell, visual disturbances, blurred vision and short-sightedness:** *Yintang* can be used as a local point in the treatment of nasal and visual disorders.

Ex-HN 4 *Yuyao* (Fish Waist)
Deadman M-HN-6.

Actions

- Benefits the eyes.
- Calms Liver *yang*.

Indications

- **Red eyes, tics, itchy eyes, blurred vision, dry eyes, visual disturbances and drooping eyelids:** *Yuyao* can be used in the treatment of both *xu* and *shi* conditions that manifest with eye disorders.

- **Pressure behind the eyes, headache, dizziness and vertigo:** *Yuyao* can be used to treat Liver *yang* rising upwards and creating imbalances in the local area.

Ex-HN 5 *Taiyang* (Great Yang)
Deadman M-HN-9.

Actions

- Expels Wind and Heat.

- Calms Liver *yang*.

- Benefits the eyes.

Indications

- **Red eyes, tics, itchy eyes, blurred vision, dry eyes, visual disturbances and drooping eyelids:** *Taiyang* can be used in the treatment of both *xu* and *shi* conditions that manifest as eye problems.

- **Pressure behind the eyes, headache, dizziness and vertigo:** *Taiyang* can be used to restrain Liver *yang* from rising up and creating imbalances in the local area.

Ex-HN 6 *Erjian* (Ear Tip)
Deadman M-HN-10.

Actions

- Drains Heat and reduces swelling.

- Benefits the ears and eyes.

Indications

- **Febrile conditions, red and swollen eyes, red and painful throat and headache:** *Erjian* has a powerful Heat-draining effect, especially when bled.

Ex-HN 7 *Qiuhou* (Behind the Ball)
Deadman M-HN-8.

Actions

- Benefits the eyes.

Indications

- **All forms of eye disorders:** *Qiuhou* is a very important local point in the treatment of all forms of eye disorders.

Ex-HN 8 *Bitong* (Clear Nose)
Deadman M-HN-14.

Actions

- Benefits the nose.

Indications

- **Blocked nose, running nose, nasal polyps, sneezing, nose bleeds, poor sense of smell, blocked sinuses and sinusitis:** *Bitong* is an important local point used in the treatment of problems of the nose and sinuses.

Ex-HN *Anmian* (Peaceful Sleep)
Deadman M-HN-54.

Actions

- Calms *shen.*
- Calms the Liver.

Indications

- **Insomnia, mental restlessness, restless desperation and palpitations:** *Anmian* has characteristics very similar to GB 12, which it is located next to. *Anmian*, however, has a stronger effect on insomnia.

- **Vertigo, dizziness, headache, tinnitus, epilepsy and hypertension:** In line with GB 12, *anmian* can be used to calm Liver *yang* and Liver Wind.

Ex-B-1 *Dingchuan* (Calm Breathlessness)
Deadman M-BW-1.

Actions

- Regulates Lung *qi.*
- Moves *qi* and *xue* in the local area.

Indications

- **Shortness of breath, asthma, wheezing, dyspnoea and cough:** *Dingchuan* is an important acupuncture point in the treatment of acute asthma attacks.

- **Pain, stiffness or discomfort in the neck and the upper part of the back.**

Ex-B-2 *Huatuojiaji* (*Huatuojiaji* Points)
Deadman M-BW-35.

Actions

- Regulate *qi* in the internal organs.

- Spread *qi* and *xue* in the local area.

Indications

These extra points treat disorders in the organs that are located on the same level as the point itself. *Huatuojiaji* points can also be used in the treatment of back pain and disorders in the surrounding area.

Ex-B-3 *Weiwanxiashu* (Stomach Controller Lower *Shu*)
Deadman M-BW-12.

Actions

- Drains Heat and generates fluids.

- Moves *qi* and *xue* in the local area.

Indications

- **Chronic thirst and fever, dry mouth, vomiting and abdominal pain:** *Weiwanxiashu* has traditionally been used in the treatment of diabetes.

- **Pain, stiffness or discomfort in the neck and the upper part of the back.**

Ex-B-7 *Yaoyan* (Lumbar Eyes)
Deadman M-BW-24.

Actions

- Tonifies the Kidneys.

- Moves *qi* and *xue* in the local area.

Indications

- **Lumbar pain, soreness in lumbar region and cold lumbar region.**

Ex-B-8 *Shiqizhuixia* (Under the Seventeenth Vertebra)
Deadman M-BW-25.

Actions

- Tonifies the Kidneys.

- Moves *qi* and *xue* in the local area.

Indications

- **Lumbar pain, soreness in lumbar region and cold lumbar region.**

Ex-CA-1 *Zigong* (Child Palace)
Deadman M-CA-18.

Actions

- Tonifies and raises *qi*.

- Regulates menstruation.

- Moves *qi* and *xue* in the local area.

Indications

- **Uterine prolapse, infertility and irregular menstrual bleeding:** *Zigong* is an important acupuncture point in the treatment of gynaecological disorders.

Ex-CA *Qimen* (Qi Door)

Actions

- Regulates menstruation.
- Moves *qi* and *xue* in the local area.

Indications

- **Infertility and heavy menstrual bleeding:** *Qimen* is an important local point in the treatment of gynaecological disorders.

Ex-CA *Sanjiaojiu* (Triangle Moxa)

Deadman M-CA-23.

Actions

- Regulates *qi* in the intestines.

Indications

- **Diarrhoea:** These three points can be treated with moxa to stop diarrhoea.

Ex-CA *Tituo* (Lift and Support)

Deadman M-CA-4.

Actions

- Raises and regulates *qi*.

Indications

- **Uterine prolapse, dysmenorrhoea and abdominal pain.**

Ex-CA *Zhixie* (Stop Diarrhoea)

Actions

- Regulates *qi* in the intestines.

Indications

- **Diarrhoea.**

Ex-UE 1 *Zhoujian* (Elbow Tip)
Deadman M-UE-46.

Actions

- Transforms Phlegm.

Indications

- **Swollen lymph nodes in the throat and axillary and abscesses:** *Zhoujian* is used exclusively with moxa.

Ex-UE 2 *Erbai* (Two Whites)
Deadman M-UE-29.

Actions

- Raises *qi* in the rectum.

Indications

- **Haemorrhoids and rectal prolapse.**

Ex-UE 7 *Yaotongxue/Yaotongdian* (Lumbar Pain Points)
Deadman M-UE-19.

Actions

- Disperses stagnant *qi* and *xue* in the lower back.

Indications

- **Acute lumbar pain and stiffness of the back.**

Ex-UE 8 *Luozhen/Wailaogong/Xianqiang* (Stiff Neck)
Deadman M-UE-24.

Actions

- Disperses stagnant *qi* and *xue* in the neck.

Indications

- **Acute pain and stiffness in the neck.**

Ex-UE 9 *Baxie* (Eight Pathogens)
Deadman M-UE-22.

Actions

- Circulates *qi* and drains Heat from the fingers.
- Expels Wind-Dampness.

Indications

- **Numbness, swelling and pain in the fingers.**

Ex-UE 10 *Sifeng* (Four Creases)
Deadman M-UE-9.

Actions

- Tonifies the Spleen and disperses accumulations.

Indications

- **Malnutrition, indigestion, fatigue, intestinal pain, constipation, abdominal distension, diarrhoea and colic:** These extra points are especially used to treat digestive problems in small children, where there is an accumulation of food in the intestine.

Ex-UE 11 *Shixuan* (Ten Diffusions)
Deadman M-UE-1.

Actions

- Expels Wind and Heat.
- Expels Summer-Heat.
- Restores consciousness.
- Extinguishes internal Wind.

Indications

- **Loss of consciousness, epilepsy, spasm and hemiplegia:** These extra points can be used when internal Wind and Phlegm have blocked the orifices of the Heart.

- **Febrile diseases, mania, vomiting and diarrhoea:** *Shixuan* can expel Summer-Heat.

Ex-UE *Jianqian/Jianneiling* (Front Shoulder/Inner Shoulder Ridge)
Deadman M-UE-48.

Actions

- Disperses stagnant *qi* and *xue* in the shoulder joint.
- Expels Wind and Cold.

Indications

- **All forms of shoulder disorders.**

Ex-LE 2 *Heding* (Crane Summit)
Deadman M-LE-27.

Actions

- Moves *qi* and *xue* and benefits the knee.

Indications

- **Knee disorders.**

Ex-LE 3 *Baichongwo* (One Hundred Insect Burrow)
Deadman M-LE-34.

Actions

- Cools *xue*.

- Expels Wind and drains Dampness.

Indications

- **Itchy skin disorders, urticaria and ulcers in the lower part of the body.**

Ex-LE 4 *Neixiyan* (Inner Knee Eye)
Deadman M-LE-16.

Actions

- Expels Wind-Dampness.

- Moves *qi* and *xue*.

- Benefits the knee.

Indications

- **Knee disorders.**

Ex-LE 5 *Xiyan* (Knee Eye)

Deadman M-LE-16.

- The point is the same as St 35.

Actions

- Expels Wind-Dampness.
- Moves *qi* and *xue*.
- Benefits the knee.

Indications

- **Knee disorders.**

Ex-LE 6 *Dannang/Dannangxue/ Dannangdian* (Gall Bladder Point)

Deadman M-LE-23.

Actions

- Drains Damp-Heat from the Gall Bladder.

Indications

- **Jaundice, cholecystitis, gallstones and pain in the costal and hypochondriac regions.**

Ex-LE 7 *Lanwei/Lanweixue* (Appendix Point)

Deadman M-LE-13.

Actions

- Moves *qi* and *xue* in the Intestines.
- Drains Fire-Toxins from the Intestines.

Indications

- **Appendicitis.**

Ex-LE 10 *Bafeng* (Eight Winds)
Deadman M-LE-13.

Actions

- Expels Wind-Dampness.
- Moves *qi* and *xue*.

Indications

- **Pain, stiffness, swelling and cramping in the toes.**

NEEDLE TECHNIQUES

When composing an acupuncture treatment, acupuncture points are selected according to their actions and indications, as well as their channel relation. It is not just the point itself that is of importance; the technique used to stimulate the point is of equal importance.

There are many different techniques and theories of how the needles should be stimulated. These techniques have been developed through acupuncture's long history. Some of the techniques are more useful and effective than others. Some needle techniques are difficult and require time and patience, while others can be painful for the patient. The last two factors in particular may mean that these needle techniques are not used that often in clinical practice.

The following is a summary of my own experience, the information I have gathered by examining relevant books and articles, courses I have participated in and the direct instruction I have received through the years. This is far from comprehensive, and you will often meet other practitioners and read other textbooks that have different explanations and different approaches. My own view is that if a needle technique works for a practitioner then this is the correct technique for that therapist. In the words of Deng Xiaoping: 'It does not matter what colour a cat is, as long as it catches mice.'

The four stages of a needle technique

A needle technique can be divided into four separate stages.

The four stages are:

- insertion of the needle through the skin

- achievement of *de qi*[13]

- affecting the person's *qi*

- removal of the needle.

There are a host of variations in how the various stages can be performed. But utilising a needle technique and being able to influence both your own and the patient's *qi* requires undivided attention and mental presence. This is well described in *Huang Di Nei Jing – Su Wen*, chapter fifty-four: 'The acupuncturist must be prepared and careful, as if he was standing on the edge of an abyss. He must hold the needle, as if it were a tiger, firmly grasped and in control. He must have a tranquil mind, only focussing on what he is doing.' When you stand on the edge of an abyss or when you have the arms around a tiger, your attention will be 100 per cent focussed. This is how it should also be when you are holding a needle. *Nanjing*, Difficulty

Seventy-Eight, states, 'The one who knows the needles relies on the left hand. The one who does not know the needles relies on the right hand.' This means that the focus should be as much in the fingers that are not holding the needle as in the fingers that are. The fingers of the hand that is not holding the needle are used to perceive the reaction in the skin and to influence the flow of *qi* to and from the needle. The fingers of this hand are also used to sense the skin when locating the point.

Insertion of the needle

The most important factor in this stage is that the needle punctures the skin in exactly the place where the acupuncture point is located. The needle should also penetrate the skin as rapidly as possible for the sake of the patient. The quicker and smoother the needle penetrates the outer layer of the skin, the less pain will be felt by the patient.

The initial insertion must also take into account the factors of depth and direction.

Obtaining *de qi*

De qi is the *qi* response that is elicited by the needle. *De qi* can be something that is perceived by the patient or it can be something that the therapist can feel through their fingertips. *De qi* indicates that *qi* has arrived in the acupuncture point or that *qi* is activated in the channel and in the body. The classical texts have a lot to say about how important it is to achieve *de qi*. The following three quotes are taken from *Huang Di Nei Jing – Ling Shu*.

- 'The acupuncturist must obtain *de qi*. If *qi* has arrived, fastidiously hold it and do not lose it.'

- 'For acupuncture to be successful, the *qi* must arrive. Acupuncture's effects come about like the clouds blown away by the wind.'

- 'If *qi* does not arrive after the insertion, there must be used as many manipulation methods as needed to achieve it.'

There are differing opinions of what *de qi* is and how it is perceived or measured. I was originally taught in TCM[14] acupuncture that *de qi* is the subjective sensation that a patient feels when the therapist has stimulated the needle. I was taught to manipulate the needle until the patient said that they could feel one of the sensations described lower down. These sensations are not the same sensation as pain, which can sometimes be experienced whilst being needled. When using this approach to needling, it is important to make the patient aware of the difference between actual pain and *de qi* sensations.

Japanese acupuncture generally does not view these palpable reactions in the patient as being necessary – they can in fact even be undesirable. The same sections of the classical texts where *de qi* is discussed are interpreted differently. *De qi*, which signifies the arrival of *qi*, is interpreted as not necessarily being something that the patient subjectively experiences. Instead, *de qi* is something that the therapist objectively observes or perceives. *De qi* will be registered through changes in the radial pulse, changes that can be felt on palpation of the abdomen, an altered sensation in how the needle itself feels or palpable changes in the area around the needle or along the channel.

In the following sections, I will describe *de qi* from the more modern TCM approach, as practised in China today. This does not mean, however, that I disagree with the Japanese approach; on the contrary. In my own practice, I use my own subjective perception of *de qi* as a guide when needling patients. My own experience is that many patients, for various reasons, do not necessarily perceive *de qi* when being needled, as the sensations can be extremely subtle. I previously often had the experience in the clinic that I could clearly perceive *de qi* in the needle or in the skin around the needle, but the patient did not report anything. This meant that I then repeatedly manipulated the needle, changing the direction and depth until they reported a sensation. In reality this resulted in the acupuncture point being drained by my attempts to elicit *de qi* when it was already present. I think many patients do not feel *de qi*, not only because the sensation is much more subtle than they are aware of, but also because imbalances such as *qi xu* and stagnations of *xue* and Phlegm can mean that they cannot feel these sensations in their body as clearly.

De qi is obtained by inserting the needle into an acupuncture point to the correct depth. *De qi* is experienced differently from acupuncture point to acupuncture point and from person to person, but the therapist is rarely in doubt that *de qi* has been obtained. *De qi* can feel as if the needle itself becomes taut. It is as if the tissue around the needle grasps the needle or as if the needle is sucked in. *De qi* occurs when the body's *zheng qi* gathers around the needle.

If there is *xie qi* present in the exterior, it can feel as if the tissue tightly grasps the needle, making it more difficult to rotate. It is important to distinguish between *de qi* and the sensation there will be in the needle if muscle fibres have got wrapped around the needle when it is turned. This is something that is especially important when using poor quality needles, which often have a rougher surface, as it can be very painful for the patient.

There is also a difference between *de qi* and the pain that can be caused by the stimulation of a nerve receptor in the skin or in a hair follicle. It is important to make the patient aware of this difference. Pain is not the same as *de qi*. Pain will be experienced as either a stinging, burning, sharp, stabbing or shooting pain. If pain is experienced, the needle should immediately be removed and the skin massaged. The needle can then be reinserted immediately next to the original place.

How *de qi* is perceived

The following needle sensations are all possible. Sometimes *de qi* is only experienced in the acupuncture point itself or its immediate vicinity. At other times, *de qi* sensations can be transmitted up or down the channel or to a specific area of the body. It is often desirable to get the sensation to transmit, as many practitioners believe that it makes the treatment more effective or even is a prerequisite of a successful outcome. This transmission is called 'propagated needle sensation' (PNS) in English and *hao zhen* in Chinese. I will go more into detail about the transmission of *qi* later in this section.

Ma (numbness)

Apart from numbness and an anaesthetised sensation at the site of insertion, buzzing, tingling and electrical sensations are also included in this category of needle sensations. It is useful if these sensations transmit up or down the channel itself.

Ma is viewed as being beneficial when there are *shi* conditions, stagnations and *bi* (painful obstruction) and *wei* (atrophy) syndromes.

Ma should be distinguished from *chu dian* (electric shock), which can occur when hitting a nerve. An electric sensation is a legitimate *de qi* sensation, and the needle does not need to be removed, but it should not be further stimulated, due to the risk of damage to the nerve. I personally usually retreat the needle a fraction upwards upon eliciting an electric sensation.

Zhang (distension)

Zhang is the sensation that is experienced upon being vaccinated or stuck with a hypodermic needle. The area around the site of the needle feels very tight and tense.

This feeling is considered to be beneficial in *shi* conditions and when there is pain.

Suan (aching or soreness)

This soreness feels like lactic acid in the muscles or the sensation there is after being stung by a wasp. *Suan* is more often experienced after the deep insertion of needles. The sensation can also be transmitted along the channel. This sensation is beneficial in *xu* conditions.

Zhong (heaviness)

The area around the needle or the arm or leg feels very heavy.

Kun (tiredness)

The area around the needle or the arm or leg feels very relaxed.

Re (Heat)

Here there is a sensation of warmth in the local area or further up or down the channel. *Re* is considered to be beneficial when there is *yang xu* and *shi* Cold.

Liang (Cold)

Here there is a cold sensation in the immediate area around the needle or further up or down the channel. *Liang* is considered to be beneficial when there is *shi* Heat or *xu* Heat.

Itching

De qi can sometimes be experienced as an itching around the needle or in the skin in the area. My own interpretation of this is that it witnesses the arrival of *wei qi*. Itching in the skin is due to the release of histamine. Histamine is a part of the body's immune response, which *wei qi* can be interpreted as being an aspect of.

Sometimes *de qi* is experienced straight away; at other times it requires effort on the part of the therapist to draw *qi* to the area. The following methods can be utilised to attract *qi* to the needle.

- Hold the handle of the needle between your fingers for a few minutes. This technique is called 'Waiting for *qi*'.

- Lift the needle up slightly or insert it slightly deeper.

- Lift the needle up to just below the surface of the skin and then move it down again in a slightly different direction.

- Tap the skin around the needle with the tip of your finger or with a fingernail.

- Press the skin down around the needle.

- Scrape the handle of the needle.

- Rotate the needle backwards and forwards one hundred and eighty degrees.

- Massage the channel on both sides of the acupuncture point.

- Gently tap the needle with your finger.

- Lift and push the needle up and down quickly, but with small movements.

- Reinsert the needle in a new location. It may be that the acupuncture point was incorrectly localised.

Something that is a common experience for many patients is that they do not experience the initial acupuncture treatments as being painful or unpleasant, but treatments subsequently start to become more painful or unpleasant. What they are actually experiencing is that *de qi* is getting stronger for each treatment. I consider this to be a positive sign. It will either be because their *qi* is getting stronger or there are less stagnations. This is because *de qi* is less palpable if the patient is *qi xu* or if there are stagnations blocking the movement of *qi*.

Techniques to affect *qi*

There are, in general, two overall groups of needle techniques that are used to affect *qi*. The difference between these two main groups is whether the techniques are tonifying or whether they are draining or spreading. Tonifying techniques are used to treat *xu* conditions. Draining or spreading techniques are used in the treatment of *shi* conditions.

Tonifying needle techniques are called *bu fa* and draining or spreading needle techniques are called *xie fa*. A third category is even needle techniques. Even needle techniques are called *ping bu ping xie*, which means 'neither tonifying nor draining' or 'both tonifying and draining'. Even needle techniques are used when you do not wish specifically to tonify or drain the point. An even needle technique is used therefore when you use a needle technique and there is equal focus on both draining and tonifying in the technique itself or when you simply achieve *de qi* and then leave the needle in place without further stimulation.

My personal view is that many needle techniques are methods to focus the therapist's 'intention' or *yi*. This is the reason that some needle techniques appear to be contradictory or that there can be differences from one book to the next with regards to the various techniques, for example which direction the needle should be rotated to tonify or drain *qi*.

In *tai ji quan* you learn as a novice that it is *qi* that initiates the body's movements – that it is *qi* that causes the muscles to move. With experience and instruction you later learn that it is 'intention' or *yi* that leads *qi*. The *yi* is projected and this makes *qi* move. It is with this understanding of *yi* in mind that I have interpreted the various needle techniques. Needle techniques are methods to focus and apply *yi* in treatment. By using my *yi*, I can focus my *qi* and thereby affect the client's *qi*. This means that while I practise a needle technique, I have a very clear focus in my head of what I'm doing with the needle and what I want to achieve with this movement of the needle. It is not without reason that the following quotation from *Huang Di Nei Jing* states, 'The acupuncturist must be prepared and careful, as if he was standing on the edge of an abyss. He must hold the needle, as if it were a tiger, firmly grasped and in control. He must have a tranquil mind, only focussing on what he is doing.' When you are standing on the edge of an abyss and holding onto a tiger, you are very much aware of your every move.

In practice, before you stimulate the needle, you should clearly visualise the difference between active and passive movements and be very aware of what you want to achieve with each movement.

Most techniques are constructed around the elements described below. The individual techniques can be used separately or, as we will see later, they can be combined to create more complex techniques.

Xu ji (fast-slow)

In this technique, there is a rapid insertion of the needle and a slow withdrawal, or a slow insertion and a rapid withdrawal. In other words, the downward and the upward movement of the needle is performed at two different speeds. This difference in the speed of the needle upwards and downwards can be used in two ways. It can be that the speed of insertion into, and withdrawal of the needle from, the skin and the tissue underneath is rapid or slow. It may also be that you repeatedly lift the needle upwards and push the needle down again within the tissue below the skin at different speeds after the needle is inserted and *de qi* has been obtained.

- Rapid downward movements and slow upward movements draw *xie qi* up to the surface and is thus a draining needle technique.

- Slow downward movements and rapid upward movements press *yang qi* down to the interior from the surface and is thus a tonifying needle technique.

Ti cha (lift press)

This needle technique may sound as if it is the same technique as the previous one, but it is actually quite different. In this needle technique it is not the speed of the movement but the relative strength of the movements up and down that is crucial. In order to tonify *qi*, you should press with force in the downward movement and lift without force in the upward movement. Conversely, to pull the needle upwards with force and push the needle down without force is a draining technique.

Personally I interpret lifting and pressing with and without force as being more a mental intention or a way of focussing my *qi* than it is a purely physical action. It is as if my grip on the needle is firmer or more focussed when the motion is with force and that I am mentally pulling the *qi* up from the acupuncture point or sending *qi* down into the acupuncture point when I practise the technique. In this way I can easily combine this technique with the previous one.

Jin tui (forward and reverse)

Acupuncture points can be conceived of as having three levels: *tian* (Heaven), *ren* (Man) and *di* (Earth). *Tian* is the most superficial level of an acupuncture point, whilst *di* is the deepest level.

When utilising this technique you can insert the needle in three distinct, separate stages: Heaven, Man and Earth; and then withdraw the needle to the surface in one movement. This is called three forward and one back. This is a tonifying technique.

To drain the point, the needle is inserted to the deepest level in one movement and then withdrawn to the surface again in three distinct and separate movements through the three levels. This is called one forward and three back.

Yin sui (direction of the needle)

In this technique the direction of the needle is altered after the achievement of *de qi*. The direction of the needle will be either opposite to or in the same direction as the normal directional flow of *qi* in the channel. When the needle is pointing in the same direction as *qi* flows in the channel, it is a tonifying technique. When the needle is pointing in the opposite direction to the *qi* flow in the channel, it is a draining technique.

Nian zhuan (rotation of the needle)

In several books it is stated that rotating the needle between forty-five and ninety degrees in a clockwise direction will tonify *qi*. To drain *qi*, the needle should be rotated in an anti-clockwise direction between one hundred and eighty and three hundred and sixty degrees. Some of the texts also write that the directions should be reversed in men and women. In addition, some texts also recommend reversing these directions for men and women again, depending on whether it is morning or afternoon. Unfortunately, there are also texts where something similar is written, but with the opposite instructions. This makes things, to say the least, slightly confusing.

Something that creates further confusion is that some of the books recommend practising these rotation techniques for two to three minutes. It is difficult to rotate a needle in the one direction for two minutes without rotating more than ninety degrees in total, if you are, for example, practising a tonifying technique. It will therefore be necessary to rotate the needle back again in the opposite direction. This then means that the needle is rotating in the wrong direction. My interpretation of this technique is, therefore, that this is again a difference in focus and intention, i.e. *yi*, rather than a difference in physical movement.

When I want to tonify an acupuncture point, I slowly and carefully rotate the needle in a clockwise direction forty-five to ninety degrees and I have my focus in my fingertips while I turn the needle clockwise. I then release my grip slightly on the handle of the needle, whilst still maintaining contact, and it is as if the needle returns to its original position almost by itself. In the anti-clockwise movement of the needle, I have no focus in my fingertips. In this way, I can repeatedly rotate the needle forty-five to ninety degrees in the same direction and let it return almost by itself to zero. I do this for one to two minutes. The movements will be slow and gentle. Whilst turning the needle clockwise, my *qi* flows outwards into the needle, but it doesn't whilst the needle is returning again.

To practise a draining needle technique, I needle more rapidly and with greater physical force. The movement is one hundred and eighty to three hundred and sixty degrees anti-clockwise. Now the focus and force in the fingertips is present in the anti-clockwise movement. When the needle returns in the clockwise direction, it again almost returns by itself with the minimum of force and focus in my fingers. I repeat this action for two to three minutes. The movement of the needle is faster and more powerful than in the tonifying technique. I personally do not alter the directions of rotation with regard to gender or the time of day.

When practising needle techniques where the needle has repeatedly been rotated, it is important to be aware of how the needle feels when it is being withdrawn upwards. The needle should be able to be easily pulled upwards without resistance. Muscle fibres can sometimes wrap themselves around the needle during repeated rotations. This will cause pain and result in difficulty withdrawing the needle. This can typically be experienced when using low-cost needles, which often have a rougher surface, or if the needle has been rotated too many times in one direction.

Hu xi (breathing)

When utilising breathing in needle techniques, it is the client's respiration that is being referred to. In order to tonify *qi*, the needle should be inserted on an exhalation and lifted upwards or withdrawn on an inhalation. To drain *qi*, the opposite applies. Here the needle is inserted on an inhalation and withdrawn or lifted on an exhalation.

Personally I use the first part of this technique most. Many clients are nervous and afraid of needles. Breathing out whilst I insert the needle enables the client to let go and relax more. This makes the insertion less painful. It is difficult to tense the muscles while breathing out.

Kai he (opening or closing the hole)

Every time a needle penetrates the skin and is removed again, *qi* escapes from the body. This is one of the reasons why some people feel tired after an acupuncture treatment, especially when many needles have been inserted in the treatment. By closing the hole after the withdrawal of the needle and pressing downwards with the finger on a piece of cotton wool, *qi* is closed inside the body. This is recommended if you want to tonify *qi*. If there is *xie qi* present and you want to expel it from the body, you can consciously make the hole where the needle is larger, whilst slowly withdrawing the needle upwards. The slow withdrawal of the needle will draw *xie qi* upwards and, by making the hole larger, *xie qi* can leave the body.

In practice, I often press and hold a piece of cotton wool on the point after withdrawing the needle, even though I have utilised a draining needle technique. This is to stop any bleeding that may occur if I have punctured a blood vessel. I will, however, in invasions of exogenous *xie qi*, almost always make the hole larger and not close it on withdrawing the needle.

Liu Zhen (retaining the needle)

There are different views as to how long the needles should remain in the body or whether they should be retained at all after achieving *de qi* and manipulating the needle with a needle technique.

Huang Di Nei Jing – Ling Shu states in chapter one: 'After *qi* has arrived, there is no further need to retain the needle in the patient's body, because the purpose of the manipulation has been achieved'; and in chapter three: 'The good doctor removes the needle, as soon as *qi* has arrived.' There are therefore some acupuncturists who do not leave the needles in place in the body. Other practitioners believe that needles should be left in the body for about twenty-nine minutes, as this is the time it takes for one circulation of *ying qi* in the channel system. In China I was taught that in *xu* conditions I should let the needles remain in place for fifteen to twenty minutes, whilst in *shi* conditions the needles should be retained for twenty to forty minutes.

A valid argument for letting the client lie with the needles for twenty minutes is that it is often one of the only times during the course of the week that they really let go and sink down into an almost meditative state. All things being equal, this is beneficial for their *yin*. It also means that even though the greatest effect of the needles was achieved upon insertion and the initial manipulation, the effect will have a chance to stabilise and take root before they start rushing around and disrupting the *qi* again.

In the treatment of small children, it is common practice not to let the needles remain in place.

Jui liu (nine-six)

This technique combines the lifting and pressing with the rotating clockwise and anti-clockwise techniques. Nine is a *yang* number and is tonifying. Six is a *yin* number and is draining. When draining or tonifying, the needles are therefore repeatedly lifted and pressed or rotated six or nine times or in multiples of these numbers, e.g. twelve/eighteen/twenty-four, etc., or eighteen/twenty-seven/thirty-six, etc. In addition to the numerological energy that these numbers have, these techniques will have a focussing effect on your own mind whilst you count.

Insertion in the right-hand and left-hand sides in men and women

Some acupuncturists start the treatment by inserting the first needle in the left-hand side of the body in men and on the right-hand side in women.

Time of day

There is a view that treatments should be adapted to utilise the *yang* dynamic that there is in the morning and the *yin* dynamic that there is in the afternoon and evening. This entails reversing the techniques described above, dependent on the time of day – whether it is before or after noon.

The thickness of the needle

Thicker needles are more draining than thinner needles. This is probably because they create a stronger disturbance of *qi* in the channel and thereby also a stronger needle sensation.

The above techniques can be combined with each other or used independently of each other. The more specialised and complex needle techniques described next often combine several of the above methods in a single technique. Such techniques will typically only be used on one or two acupuncture points during a treatment. The same applies to transmitting *qi*, as described later in the advanced needle techniques section. It will not usually be used on all the acupuncture points during treatment.

ADVANCED NEEDLE TECHNIQUES

Shao shan huo (setting fire to the mountain)

This method is very warming and tonifying and is recommended for *yang xu* conditions.

After obtaining *de qi* in the acupuncture point, lift the needle up a few millimetres to the 'Heaven' level and then either lift and press the needle up and down one or two millimetres using a tonifying technique or rotate the needle ninety degrees nine times in order to tonify *qi*. Afterwards press the needle down with force or intention to the 'Man' level and repeat the above procedure. The needle is then pushed further down to the 'Earth' level and the procedure repeated. The needle is then withdrawn upwards, without force, to the 'Heaven' level and the whole procedure is repeated from the beginning. The whole procedure can be repeated several times. The client should experience a warm or burning sensation in the area around the needle. When the needle is withdrawn from the body, it is turned gently clockwise until it is free and is pulled up to just below the surface of the skin. The needle is left in place for a few seconds before it is withdrawn completely and the hole is quickly closed.

Tou tian liang (coolness through penetrating Heaven)

This method is the opposite of the above method. After the achievement of *de qi* the needle should be inserted down to the 'Earth' level, where six draining, lifting and pressing movements are performed or the needle is rotated one hundred and eighty degrees backwards and forwards six times. The needle is withdrawn with force up to the 'Man' level, where there are again performed six draining manipulations of the needle. The needle is then lifted further up with force and intention to the 'Heaven' level and a further six draining manipulations of the needle are performed. The needle can then be completely withdrawn or the whole procedure can be repeated all over again from the 'Earth' level. When the needle is withdrawn completely from the body, the exit hole is enlarged by rotating the needle on the way up and the hole is not closed afterwards.

This technique is very cooling and is used for *shi* Heat conditions.

Coolness-creating needle technique

This method drains *shi* Heat and is used, for example, in Hot *bi* syndromes.

After *de qi* is achieved the needle is lifted one or two millimetres. The tip of the needle is directed towards the area where the Heat is concentrated. The needle is lifted and pressed several times. The needle is then rotated anti-clockwise a few times and held until a cold sensation is felt. A tingling sensation at the tip of the needle should be felt. Sometimes this tingling sensation can be felt in the body as well. If there is no tingling sensation, the procedure should be repeated a second time. When the needle is removed, shake and twist the needle to make the hole larger and then quickly withdraw the needle. The exit hole is not closed.

Transmission of *qi*

Transmission of *qi* is called *hao zhen* in Chinese. The purpose of these needle techniques is to transmit *qi* to the place where you are trying to achieve a therapeutic effect. An example could be that you want to affect the Urinary Bladder and you have inserted a needle in Ren 3 or UB 28. You could then carry out one of the following techniques in order to get *qi* to move from the acupuncture point to the Urinary Bladder. The client should be able to experience the *qi* arriving in the bladder or at least feel the *qi* moving in that direction.

Ti cha (lift press)

Lift (*ti*) the needle up to the skin and press (*cha*) the needle down to the depth of the acupuncture point. Continue until the patient feels *qi* moving in the direction of, or to, the desired location.

Cuo nian (rotation)

The needle is either rotated one hundred and eighty degrees strongly or gently forty-five degrees, depending on whether you are tonifying or draining the point. The needle is only rotated in one direction. The needle must be turned slowly and carefully so that the muscle fibres do not get caught up on it. Continue until the patient feels *qi* moving in the direction of, or to, the desired location.

Pan yao (circle and swing)

After obtaining *de qi*, insert the needle down to the 'Earth' level or to the depth of the acupuncture point, and then lift the needle up to the 'Man' or 'Heaven' level. The needle is then rotated in large circles at an angle of forty-five degrees to the skin. The needle can also be swung vertically back and forth from side to side through an angle of ninety degrees. This is a draining technique. As a general rule, three times is enough to get *qi* to move towards the desired area.

Guan bi (to block)

The left thumb and index finger press on the opposite side of the acupuncture point to the direction *qi* should be sent. It is important that you do not press too hard, otherwise it can block *qi* or even result in *qi* flowing in the wrong direction.

Cang gui tan xue (the green turtle looking for the point)

This is a tonifying technique to move *qi*. When you have achieved *de qi*, the left-hand index finger should be pressed gently on the skin on the opposite side of the needle in relation to the direction in which you would like *qi* to move. The needle is lifted and pressed two millimetres, while moving the needle back and forth in a vertical plane along the channel, i.e. the needle travels in vertical circles.

Cang long yao wei (the green dragon wags its tail)

This technique is also tonifying and makes the *qi* move. There is no rotation, lifting or pressing. After *de qi* has been achieved, the left-hand index finger presses gently on the skin on the opposite side of the needle in relation to the direction in which you would like *qi* to move. The handle of the needle is drawn from side to side across the channel.

Bai hu yao tou (the white tiger shakes its head)

This is a draining technique that simultaneously moves *qi*. When you have achieved *de qi*, the left index finger is pressed gently on the skin on the opposite side of the needle in relation to the direction you would like to have *qi* move. Lift and press, rotate and shake the needle whilst the patient exhales, or rotate the needle and move the handle of the needle from side to side in large movements whilst the patient exhales.

Zi wu dao jiu (pestle and mortar)

This is a very stimulating needle technique that activates channel *qi*. After *de qi* has been obtained, the needle is swiftly pressed inwards to the full depth and then gently withdrawn to below the surface of the skin and rotated nine times anti-clockwise. The needle is then gently pressed slowly inwards to the full depth and swiftly withdrawn to the surface and rotated six times in a clockwise direction.

Feng fan zhang chi (phoenix rises and spreads its wings)

This technique creates a movement of *qi* in the channel. After the needle is inserted to the correct depth, the needle is rotated until resistance is felt and is then suddenly released. This causes a slight tremor in the needle.

Needle techniques for the treatment of *bi* syndromes

The following needle techniques can be used in the treatment of *bi* syndromes, i.e. when there is pain in the channel and especially at the joints. These techniques are summarised from the book *Bi Syndromes* by L. Vangermeersch and Sun Pei-Lin (1994, pp.157–161).

Bao ci – mainly used to treat Wind bi

Insert a needle into an *a-shi* point.[15] The needle is then stimulated with an even or reducing needle technique. The needle is left in situ for a few minutes. In the meantime, a new *a-shi* point is located. When the needle is removed from the first point, a new needle is inserted into the next *a-shi* point and the procedure is repeated.

Hui ci – mainly used to treat sinew or muscle bi and Liver or Spleen organ bi

The needle is inserted vertically into an *a-shi* point. The needle is then lifted and thrust several times. The needle is then angled forty-five degrees and lifted and thrust in four different directions (north, south, east and west).

This technique relaxes muscle spasms and cramping.

Qi ci – used to treat Cold bi pain localised in a small, deep and precise location

A single needle is inserted vertically in the painful spot. Two new needles are then inserted close to the first needle at a slightly oblique angle so that the tips of these two needles point towards each other. Moxa can be used on the needles.

Yang ci – used to treat Cold bi, which is more superficial and covers a larger area of skin or muscle

A needle is inserted vertically down into the middle of the painful area. Four additional needles are inserted superficially at a very oblique angle, so that all four needles point towards the first needle in the middle.

Duan ci – used to treat bone bi

A single needle is inserted into the acupuncture point that is closest to the area of pain or a needle is inserted in the middle of the painful area. After *de qi* has been obtained, the needle is inserted deeper – so deep that the tip gently touches the surface of the bone below. The needle is very carefully rotated forwards and backwards and forwards, up and down. A fine needle technique is required in order to avoid injuring the bone and periosteum.

Fu ci – used to treat sinew, muscle and Cold bi when there are muscle spasms, numbness and muscle atrophy

Two needles are inserted superficially at an angle and away from the middle of the relevant muscle.

He gu ci – used in the treatment of painful muscle bi, which is caused by Cold, Dampness and Wind, especially if there are cramps and spasms

Three needles are used in this technique. The first needle is inserted into the most painful area of the affected muscle. The needle is lifted up and down, both vertically and diagonally. The other two needles are inserted at an angle, parallel with the tendons at both ends of the muscle where they attach to bone. The needles are then lightly stimulated.

COMBINING ACUPUNCTURE POINTS IN A TREATMENT

When it comes to choosing which acupuncture points to use in a treatment, there are many factors that should be taken into account. Reading the descriptions of the individual acupuncture points and analysing their actions and indications can be confusing. When should you choose the one and not the other? What is the difference between them?

First, a treatment must be based on a diagnosis and not just the treatment of a single symptom. Second, there needs to be a treatment strategy.

In Chinese medicine there are two different ways to diagnose and treat disorders. The two methods should not be seen as two separate alternatives. They are combined together in the same treatment. The two ways to diagnose are called: *bian bing lun zhi*, which means 'differentiation of symptoms in relation to disease name', and *bian zheng lun zhi*, which means 'differentiation of symptoms in relation to pattern of imbalance'. *Bian bing lun zhi* is similar to the Western medicine approach, i.e. diagnosing and treating a specific disease or disorder. It is important to remember that you still have to think of this pathological process in a Chinese medicine context. This means that the disorder must be comprehended via the pathomechanisms that underlie it. We need to think about *qi*, *xue*, Phlegm, *zangfu*, etc., not lymphocytes, antibodies, hormone receptors, etc., even though the *bian bing* name is the same as a Western disease category. Dizziness, for example, is a *bian bing lun zhi* diagnosis in Chinese medicine and is called *xuan yun*. Even though dizziness is a disease category in both Chinese and Western medicine, the understanding of why and how dizziness arises is very different. In both Chinese and Western medicine there are various causes and sub-categories of dizziness. The pathomechanisms cannot though be directly translated from one system to the other. In Western medicine dizziness could, for example, be diagnosed as arising when a virus creates an inflammation on the balance nerve. If we just translated this directly into Chinese medicine, we may think that we need to expel an invasion of *xie qi* or drain Fire-Poisons. This, though, is rarely the case in these situations. Dizziness in Chinese medicine can be the result of many factors, such as internal Wind, *xue xu*, Phlegm, etc. Although the disease names and the root causes may sound similar, the treatment focus is often markedly different.

Bian zheng lun zhi is the diagnosis categories that are presented in TCM textbooks. It is the classification of symptoms and signs into the various patterns of imbalance, such as Liver *qi* stagnation, invasion of Wind-Damp, *shaoyin*-stage Cold, etc. As stated, Chinese medicine diagnosis is not a choice of either *bian bing lun zhi* or *bian zheng lun zhi*. If the treatment is to be effective, we must in reality use both differentiations. As always, it helps with an example. GB 20 and the extra point *taiyang* are both effective points used to treat headaches (*bian bing lun zhi* diagnosis – *toutong* or head pain), because these acupuncture points can disperse stagnations of *qi* and *xue*, and they can drain *xie qi* down from the head. GB 20 and *taiyang* are not, though, relevant in the treatment of nausea, which is also a *bian bing lun zhi* diagnosis (*e xin*). This is because they are both points whose primary effect is up in the head. If the headache is due to Phlegm (*bian zheng lun zhi* diagnosis), St 40 and Sp 3 would be obvious additions to the choice of *taiyang* and GB 20. This is because St 40 and Sp 3 can transform Phlegm, which in this example is the cause of the headache. If the cause of the headache was instead an invasion of Wind-Cold (*bian zheng lun zhi* diagnosis), St 40 and Sp 3 would not be relevant, as they do not 'open to the exterior' and expel exogenous *xie qi*. St 40 and Sp 3 can, though, be used to treat nausea (*bian bing lun zhi* diagnosis) if the underlying cause is Phlegm (*bian zheng lun zhi* diagnosis). In this example they would be combined with Ren 12 and Pe 6, which are effective points used to descend Stomach *qi*. Ren 12 and Pe 6 are not suitable, though, in draining Phlegm from the head.

It is also the reason that it is said in Chinese medicine that 'one disorder has many different causes; one cause can result in many different disorders'.

In Chinese medicine there is a straight line between the symptoms or disorder and the choice of acupuncture points. But this straight line has several stages. It is important that we consciously involve all the stages and do not jump directly from the symptom, for example headache, directly to the choice of acupuncture points. Every time you treat a client, you have to formulate a diagnosis and a treatment strategy.

The symptoms and the signs[16] are used as the foundation of the diagnosis. As we have just seen, there are various diagnostic models. These diagnostic models are stencils that can be placed on top of the symptoms in order to be able to see their relationship or pattern. It is only when you have a diagnosis that you can formulate a treatment strategy. The treatment strategy is 100 per cent dependent on the diagnosis. This does not mean that you have to treat the entire diagnosis. It does, though, mean that if you do not treat some aspects of the diagnosis, this must be a conscious choice. You may decide not to treat all the imbalances that are manifesting if a patient has multiple different imbalances. For example, if a patient is manifesting Spleen *qi xu*, Dampness and *xue xu*, we could decide not to treat Dampness or *xue xu*, but to focus singularly on treating Spleen *qi xu*, because this is the root of *xue xu* and Dampness.

The treatment strategy is usually the reverse of the diagnosis. If the diagnosis is Spleen *qi xu*, the treatment strategy will be to tonify Spleen *qi*; if the diagnosis is an invasion of Wind-Cold, the treatment strategy will be to expel Wind-Cold. The moment you have a treatment strategy, you can select acupuncture points that are relevant for this strategy. If the treatment strategy is to tonify Spleen *qi*, for example, you will then select acupuncture points and needle techniques that tonify Spleen *qi* such as St 36, Ren 12, Sp 3 and UB 20 manipulated with a tonifying needle technique. If the treatment strategy is to expel Wind-Cold, then points such as UB 10, UB 12, SI 3 and UB 62 can be stimulated with a draining needle technique.

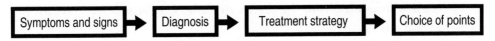

Figure 5.1 Selecting acupuncture points in a treatment

When it comes to selecting acupuncture points for a treatment, there are several characteristics of each acupuncture point that need to be taken into account.

- **Actions:** An acupuncture point can be selected based on its actions. This is particularly relevant when treating the pattern of imbalance, i.e. *bian zheng lun zhi*. If the diagnosis is Dampness, Sp 9 can, for example, be selected, because it is an acupuncture point that drains Dampness.

- **Indications:** Acupuncture points can be selected according to their indications. This approach is relevant in *bian bing lun zhi* or treatment of the disorder itself. Sp 1, for example, can be selected when there is continuous and heavy menstrual bleeding. This is because Sp 1 stops uterine bleeding.

- **Channel relations:** The selection here will be based on which channel the disorder is manifesting itself in. It is important to take into account a channel's internal and external pathways, as well as the course of the *luo*-connecting vessels, divergent channels, sinew channels, etc. It is also important to take into account the channel's *yin/yang* partner channel and hand/foot channel relationships.

- **Point category:** There are many different acupuncture point categories, and each of these categories has specific characteristics that may mean that these point types are relevant in a certain treatment. For example, in a Five Phase treatment, points will be selected based on their Five Phase relationships. In a *zangfu* diagnosis, the choice could fall upon the organ's *mu*-collecting point or its back-*shu* point.

- ***Qi* dynamic:** Some acupuncture points can affect *qi* in certain directions, for example they can raise or descend *qi*. GB 21 is used, for example, to descend *qi* from the upper *jiao*.

- **Empirical effect:** Some acupuncture points have empirical effects that are not necessarily related to the point's relations and dynamics. For example, the extra point *erbai* can be used to treat haemorrhoids.

- **The horary system:** An acupuncture point can be selected according to the relative *qi* dynamic that is in a particular channel at a given time during the day.

- **Stems and branches:** 'Stems and branches' (*tiangan dizhi*) takes account of the relationship between an acupuncture point and not only the time of day, but also the time of year, according to a sixty-year cycle. The acupuncture point will resonate with the precise dynamic that there is between *yin* and *yang* at any given time.

- **Palpation of the points:** When an acupuncture point or a channel is in imbalance, the channel's points or the channel itself will change in nature. This will be felt when palpating along the channel and when palpating the individual points on the channel. Changes can also manifest in an organ's *mu*-collecting or back-*shu* points. There may be changes in the consistency of the tissue, or the skin can feel hot, cold, dry, rough or damp. The acupuncture point or the channel can feel distended or flaccid, or there can be tenderness or pain on palpation. There can also be visible signs, such as colour changes in the skin. If there are changes in an acupuncture point or along the channel then it may be appropriate to treat this acupuncture point or channel. It is not uncommon to be in a situation where there is a choice between several relevant acupuncture points, all of which have similar actions and indications. Palpating the various points and their channels is an effective method to determine which of these points to select.

Whilst taking into account an acupuncture point's actions and indications, it must be remembered that there is a significant difference between selecting a handful of random acupuncture points, all of which have the appropriate actions and indications, and formulating a balanced treatment. It is here that acupuncture becomes an art. The purpose of all treatments is to create harmony in the body. This means that the combination of acupuncture points must be as balanced and harmonious as possible. In practice, this means that the choice of acupuncture points and their location on the body should be harmonious. The treatment should not become a source of imbalance. This means that we must think about: how many needles are to be used; where on the body these points are located; whether they are *yin* or *yang* acupuncture points; on which channel they are located; what other actions the points have; in which direction they send *qi*; which point category they belong to; and much more.

There may well be situations in which we deliberately choose to compose an unbalanced treatment. This will be because, by consciously making such an imbalanced treatment, you will be able to rectify an imbalance and thereby create harmony.

Below are some of the general guidelines that ought to be followed when selecting acupuncture points for a treatment.

Number of points

There can be a great difference from one therapist to the next with regard to how many acupuncture points they usually choose to use in a treatment. There can be valid arguments for using both many and few points in a treatment. I personally try not to use more than six to eight different acupuncture points in a treatment and I usually use fewer needles than this number. As a general rule, I needle the points bilaterally, so the total number of needles does not exceed sixteen needles all together, preferably fewer. It is, however, important not to stick dogmatically to a specific rule about the number of needles. Different situations require different approaches. When there are local stagnations of *qi* and *xue*, such as joint pain due to *bi* syndrome or trauma, then I will quite happily use several needles in the local area to disperse the stagnation. It is a good idea, though, to have a rule of thumb, otherwise you can quickly use too many needles.

The argument behind using a greater number of needles is that the clients we meet in the clinic often have a complex array of many different imbalances. These patterns will often be mutually generating, i.e. imbalances that in themselves generate other imbalances, which in turn are the root cause of other imbalances, or two imbalances that directly generate each other. An example of the latter is Spleen *qi xu* and Dampness. When there is Spleen *qi xu*, Dampness will often arise as a consequence. The presence of Dampness can directly impede the functioning of the Spleen, resulting in Spleen *qi xu*. The presence of multiple patterns of imbalance can become like a Gordian knot. For this reason, some therapists feel that it is important to treat all the imbalances simultaneously, or at least as many as possible, otherwise the untreated patterns will regenerate the treated patterns. This will require the use of many different acupuncture points.

Other practitioners are of the view that as few needles as possible should be utilised. There can be various reasons for this point of view. First, *qi* escapes from the body each time a needle is inserted and withdrawn again. This means that using too many needles will weaken the body's *zheng qi*. It can also be argued that the use of fewer needles has a stronger dynamic effect than using many needles. Each needle sends a signal through the body. If you are sending many signals at the same time, the individual signals will be more blurred and unclear. The body can in this way be compared to a small child. If you say to the child that they must go down to the corner shop and buy a bag of potatoes, the child will easily be able to complete the task. On the other hand, if you say to the child that they should go down to the corner shop and buy potatoes, bread, a newspaper, some butter, jam and a packet of tea, and on the way out take the rubbish out to the bin, post a letter and pop in to see the neighbour to give them back the book you borrowed, then there is a greater chance that not all the items on the itinerary will be carried out with success.

Some acupuncturists even have the concept of 'the golden needle'. They believe that if you diagnose accurately enough, and at the same time have an in-depth understanding of the individual acupuncture point's dynamic, then you will be able to treat the client with a single needle. This also requires that your *qi* and *yi* are very focussed and clear. It is, unfortunately, a level that I am nowhere near achieving. Nevertheless, I agree with the Israeli acupuncturist and lecturer Yair Maimon's view that each additional needle you insert is an expression of doubt in your diagnosis; that you are trying to cover as many bases as possible, due to uncertainty, and that this disperses your focus. Yair Maimon has also constructed a table of the number of needles used in a treatment and the level that you are dealing with. This table is reproduced below.

Diagnosis level	Number of acupuncture points used in the treatment
Shen diagnosis, i.e. the imbalance, and thereby treatment, is related to the person's *shen*	1–3
Five Element/Five Phase diagnosis	3–5
Eight Principle and *zangfu* diagnosis	4–9
Channel-level treatments, treatment of pain in joints and muscles	6–30

Treating *ben* and *biao* (root cause and manifestation)

All symptoms have their root in an imbalance. Chinese medicine therefore distinguishes between *ben* or 'root' and the *biao* or 'branch'. Another term could simply be cause and symptom. When a person has a headache, the headache is the *biao* or manifestation of an underlying imbalance. The cause or *ben* could be anything from Kidney *yin xu* to a local stagnation of *qi* and *xue* in the head. There are times when it is appropriate to treat only the symptoms, for example if a person has an acute and severe headache. In this situation we would probably choose to use only acupuncture points that will relieve the headache itself. More often, though, it will be advisable also to treat the underlying cause of the symptoms. Sometimes we choose to ignore the symptoms themselves and only treat the root cause. This could be because there are many different symptoms that all have a common root or that the symptom is not manifest at the moment of treatment. In the previous example of a person suffering from severe headaches, we might treat the underlying cause when they do not have the headache.

Another example that illustrates the various approaches is a patient seeking treatment because they have a weak immune system and are constantly falling ill. If this patient arrives in the clinic and has flu-like symptoms, we would treat these symptoms, which are *biao* or a manifestation. The treatment would focus on expelling Wind-Heat and/or draining *qi*-level Heat. It would not be appropriate to tonify their *wei qi* at this moment in time, even though *wei qi xu* is the *ben* or root cause of their repetitive respiratory illnesses. On the other hand, we could tonify their *wei qi* the moment they no longer have an acute infection. If we did not do this and only treated the respiratory infection each time they are ill, their immune system would never become strong.

Something that is also important to keep in mind is why the patient has sought treatment. If we only focus on treating the root causes of their disorder and do not relieve the symptoms, there is a danger that the patient will stop coming for treatment before a result has been achieved, because the client does not think that they are gaining any effect from the treatments. We should at least inform the client of our strategy if we choose to work only with the *ben* aspect.

With most of the patients who suffer from chronic diseases, we will usually treat both *ben* and *biao* in the same treatment. We will, however, usually focus more on the one aspect than the other, depending on the patient's condition on that day or our overall strategy.

Something that makes treatment more complex and three-dimensional is that *ben* and *biao* are in some ways similar to the principles of *yin* and *yang*. They are relative to each other and they can constantly be further divided into new aspects. A headache, for example, can be a manifestation of ascending Liver Fire. Liver Fire is therefore *ben* and the headache *biao*. Liver Fire can itself be caused by Liver *qi* stagnation. This means that even though Liver Fire is the cause of the headache, Liver Fire itself is a consequence of Liver *qi* stagnation. Therefore, Liver *qi* stagnation is *ben* in relation to Liver Fire, which is *biao*. Liver *qi* stagnation can itself be a consequence of Liver *xue xu*. Now Liver *qi* stagnation is *biao* and Liver *xue xu* the genuine *ben*. It is like peeling an onion. Each layer often has a layer below it. In fact, the real *ben* of most disorders are the aetiological factors that create the imbalances. That is why it is important to get clients to make changes in their diet and lifestyle if we are really going to create permanent improvements in their condition, otherwise their problems will probably just come back again after some time.

In addition, it is important to remember that the same *biao* can have multiple *ben* and vice versa. For example, a person suffering from tinnitus will probably be manifesting both Kidney *yin xu* and ascending Liver *yang* at the same time. Conversely, Kidney *yin xu* and ascending Liver *yang* can be the cause or the root of many other disparate symptoms and signs, in addition to tinnitus.

When you have made the diagnosis, it can be tempting to start working on all the various imbalances that you can see and forget the actual reason that client has sought treatment. We might think that the disorder that the client wants treating is a banality and that the many other symptoms and signs that are manifestations of their underlying imbalances are more relevant and requiring of treatment. The patient may, for example, want treatment for the pain that they have in their elbow because they have been playing tennis. Even if you immediately become aware of a multitude of other symptoms and signs that are a manifestation of Kidney *yin xu*, Phlegm, Liver *qi* stagnation, ascending Liver *yang*, Spleen *qi xu* and *xue xu*, it is important to remember that they want relief from the pain in their elbow. Again, we can inform the client of our thoughts and observations, especially as they may not be aware that we can treat these things or that there is a common thread in their various symptoms and signs. In the end, though, we must treat the disorder that the client wants treatment for.

To strengthen or drain

The basic premise in Chinese medicine is that *shi* conditions should be drained before tonifying *xu* conditions. Once again, this is a truth with modifications. First, there is a difference between acupuncture and Chinese herbal medicine. In Chinese herbal medicine, it is vital that you do not use nourishing herbs when there is exogenous *xie qi* present. This is because nourishing herbs will also nourish *xie qi* and it would be similar to fertilising a garden full of weeds before you have removed the weeds. Even though your carrots would grow stronger, the weeds would also increase in size. Furthermore, the nourishing herbs can aggravate stagnations, because they often do not move *qi* whilst tonifying it. Needles work in a different way than herbs, especially with regards to tonification and movement. Needles always create a movement of *qi*. In fact, this is also one of the reasons why some people try to limit the amount of needles used in a treatment.

Something else that is relevant to this discussion is that patients in China often receive more frequent acupuncture treatments – daily or every other day – whereas in the West the tendency is to treat once a week or every fortnight. This means that there is not the same possibility to divide treatments and strategies. A third important and determining factor is that the patients we typically see in our clinics have a complex mixture of multiple *xu* and *shi* conditions at the same time. We rarely see pure *shi* conditions. By only draining *qi*, you may weaken a person who is already weak to start with. In practice, this means that I will usually both tonify and drain the patient in the same treatment, unless there is an extreme or acute *shi* condition, such as ascending Liver Fire, Wind or an invasion of exogenous *xie qi*. In these acute or pure *shi* conditions, I will only use draining acupuncture points and draining needle techniques. In chronic conditions where there is a mixture of *xu* and *shi* conditions, I will more probably tonify and drain in the same treatment. However, I will usually have more focus on the one aspect in relation to the other. When *shi* conditions are mixed with *xu* conditions, I will usually start a course of treatments by draining the *shi* conditions whilst tonifying the *xu* aspects. There will most often be a clear focus on draining the *shi* aspect at the beginning of the course of treatments. As the condition improves during the treatment course, the focus in the individual treatments will shift to being more tonifying and less draining. It is, however, extremely important constantly to assess each time the relative balance between *zheng qi* (anti-pathogen or 'correct' *qi*) and *xie qi* (pathogen or 'evil' *qi*) and between *xu* and *shi* conditions. The more *xu* a person is, the more we must tonify their *qi*; and the less *xu* they are, the more we can drain them.

Pure *xu* conditions must, of course, be treated by using tonifying points and needle techniques.

Up and down

As far as is possible, acupuncture points should be utilised in both the upper and the lower part of the body in the same treatment. This will often happen by itself. When it comes to draining Damp-Heat, for example, LI 11 on the elbow is often combined with either Sp 9 below the knee or St 44 on the foot. Thus we have an acupuncture point in the upper part of the body and one in the lower part. There are, however, situations where we deliberately want to a have an unbalanced treatment. Examples of this would be only using moxa on Du 20 to raise *qi* up in the body or by using Kid 1 alone to drain *qi* downwards from the head.

At the same time as selecting acupuncture points in the upper and lower parts of the body, we also need to take into account the dynamic that some acupuncture points have. Some acupuncture points, especially in combination with certain directions of insertion or needling techniques, can send *qi* either upwards or downwards. An acupuncture point such as GB 21, for example, has a clear downward dynamic, whereas an acupuncture point such as Du 20 can be used both to lift *qi* upwards or send *qi* downwards from the head.

Right-hand and left-hand sides

One should preferably treat acupuncture points on both sides of the body. As written earlier, I will almost always treat points bilaterally, i.e. I use a particular acupuncture point on both sides of the body at the same time. This means that I automatically treat the right and left sides of the body. However, there are situations where I will use acupuncture points unilaterally. This could, for example, be in the treatment of joint problems and channel disorders. In these situations, I will often select acupuncture points in the local area and distal points along the affected channel. In these situations, it will also be appropriate to use a few acupuncture points on the opposite side of the body and possibly also in the legs if the problem is in the arm or vice versa. This is, in fact, not particularly difficult to achieve in practice. You can use *luo*-connecting points, you can use 'cross-channel'[17] points and you can use acupuncture points that have specific characteristics that may be relevant. For example, if a person has pain in their left elbow around LI 10 and LI 11, you can, in addition to local and distal points in the left arm Large Intestine channel, use Lu 7, which is the *luo*-connecting point on the right arm. You can also use St 35 and St 36 in the right leg as 'cross-channel' points. You could also use GB 34 in both legs, as this is a *hui*-gathering point for sinews and tendons.

Front and back

Ideally, we should select acupuncture points on both the front and back sides of the body. In practice, this means that when you, for example, needle back-*shu* points, you should preferably also stimulate the acupuncture points of the arms and legs or get that person to lay on their back afterwards and treat a couple of points on the front of the body. Alternatively, you can alternate between treating acupuncture points on the front and on the back in the course of a treatment series, instead of in each individual treatment.

Yin and *yang*

In a balanced treatment there will be a balance in the number of the *yin* and *yang* acupuncture points. However, it will usually be appropriate to make a 'lopsided' distribution of acupuncture points deliberately. In general, though, it is best to include some points of the opposite polarity to create a balance in the treatment. This will often not be something that you have to think consciously about, as there will often be an inbuilt balance in the points chosen. This could be, for example, by using points on the partner channel. For example, when treating a headache that is caused by ascending Liver *yang*, GB 20 and GB 43, which treat the *biao* aspect, will typically be combined with points such as Liv 2 to drain Liver *yang* or the use of St 36 together with Sp 6 to tonify Spleen *qi*. It is also usually very easy to find other acupuncture points that have relevant actions and that have the opposite polarity in relation to the acupuncture points you have chosen. You could, for example, use St 44 and LI 11 to treat Stomach Fire together with Ren 13, or if there is Kidney *yang xu*, you could combine Kid 3 with Du 4.

Channel relationships

When I select acupuncture points, I try as far as possible to limit not only the number of acupuncture points I use, but also the number of channels activated.

In practice, I try to use acupuncture points within the same channel pairs, for example the Stomach and Spleen channels, and within the same great channel or hand/foot channel system, for example the Stomach and Large Intestine, both of which are *yangming* channels. In this situation it would be appropriate to combine relevant Stomach and Large Intestine points with Spleen and Lung points – the Spleen and Lung channels being both *yin* partner channels to the Stomach and Large Intestine channels and at the same time both being a part of the *taiyin* channel. In this way, I have only used two channel systems.

In the clinic, it can be difficult to be as stringent as this, but again it is good to have some guidelines that you try to maintain so that you do not simply take a bunch of random acupuncture points whose actions match the diagnosis. By using a little thought, you can often find suitable acupuncture points within a limited amount of channels.

Channel relationships are vital when treating channel disorders. In these treatments we must use acupuncture points on the affected channel and possibly on its partner channel and/or great (hand/foot) channel. For example, if there are problems along the course of the Large Intestine channel in the arm, we may well use local and distal Large Intestine points along the channel, whilst at the same time needling the *luo*-connecting point on the Large Intestine's partner channel, Lu 7, and possibly also some points on the Stomach channel, with which the Large Intestine shares a *yangming* relationship. This could typically be 'cross-channel' points if there are obstructions and stagnations in the Large Intestine along the channel.

Local, adjacent and distal points

When it comes to treating local disorders, it is most appropriate to use both acupuncture points on the relevant channel in the local area, along with so-called distal points. Distal points are acupuncture points that are located on the same channel but at a distance from the local area. The further towards the one end of a channel a disorder is, the more towards the opposite end of the channel you must choose a distal point. For example, if there is an eye disorder that relates to the Stomach channel, you would choose a Stomach channel point on the foot, because these points are at the opposite end of the channel. In the same way, you choose an acupuncture point further up the Stomach channel on the leg to treat a disorder further down the channel, for example in the chest. An example of this is the use of St 40 to treat stagnations of *qi* and Phlegm in the chest.

You can also use distal points on a channel's hand/foot or great channel partner in the treatment of disorders at the opposite end of its channel. For example, when there is toothache, which is manifesting on the course of the Stomach channel, which is the *yangming* foot channel, you can use LI 4 to treat it because LI 4 is a distal point on the *yangming* hand channel. It is also possible to use St 38 in the treatment of shoulder problems, such as a frozen shoulder, because the shoulder joint is on the pathway of the Large Intestine channel.

Due to the dynamic of *qi* in the channels, acupuncture points distal to the knees and the elbows are more dynamic and potent than acupuncture points further in towards the body. It is therefore the case that these acupuncture points are the most commonly used points in acupuncture.

A second treatment approach, which relates to the use of local and distal points, is the 'chain and lock' approach. When there is a long distance between a local point and a distal point, you can add an acupuncture point on the same channel that has a powerful effect and that is located between the two acupuncture points being treated. For example, if a person has shoulder pain, and you have chosen LI 15 as a local point and LI 4 as a distal point, you can add LI 10. This will amplify the effect of the other two acupuncture points. This is because LI 10 is an acupuncture point that has a strong effect on the *qi* in its own channel. On the other hand, we might select LI 11 if the shoulder joint was red and feels warm on palpation, because LI 11, in addition to being an acupuncture point midway between LI 4 and LI 11, is also an acupuncture point that can drain Heat from the channel.

In addition to local and distal points, 'adjacent' points will often be selected. Adjacent points, as their name suggests, are acupuncture points in the local area. These could be acupuncture points just before and just after the acupuncture point on the same channel where there is pain or a disorder. They could also be acupuncture points on a separate channel in the local area. For example, if there is pain in the shoulder that relates to LI 15, in addition to using LI 4 as a distal point and LI 15 as a local point, we could also use LI 14 and/or LI 16 because they are channel points adjacent to the shoulder joint, or we could use SJ 14 because it is also located on the acromion, adjacent to LI 15.

Cross channel

In pain, especially acute pain in a joint or along the course of a channel, you can select acupuncture points according to the 'cross-channel' approach. This very effective method was developed by Dr Zhou Yu Yan. 'Cross-channel' treatments can also be used if there is a problem that is difficult to treat locally, e.g. an acute sprain. The technique can also be used to treat more chronic diseases. In 'cross-channel' treatment, a disorder is treated by selecting points on the opposite side and in the corresponding area of the opposite limb. If the problem is in the leg, the corresponding area of the opposite arm is selected and vice versa. This means that if there is pain in the medial aspect of the right elbow, the medial aspect of the left knee is needled. In this system, the fingers on one side correspond to their toes in the opposite side, the ankles to the wrists, the elbows to knees, the hips to shoulders and vice versa.

'Cross-channel' points are selected according to the following principles.

- Acupuncture points are selected from a *yin* channel if the disorder is on the medial side and from the *yang* channel if the disorder is on the lateral side.

- Acupuncture points on the right-hand side of the body treat disorders on the left-hand side and vice versa.

- Acupuncture points are selected according to their great channel relationships. For example, if the problem is the *yangming* channel at LI 10 on the right-hand side, you will insert a needle in St 36 on the left-hand side. If a disorder is located in the *taiyin* channel at Sp 5 on the left-hand side, you will needle Lu 9 on the right-hand side, etc.

- A second method is to palpate the equivalent area on the opposite limb on the opposite side, and find the most sensitive point that corresponds to the place where the pain is in the limb. Again – left knee, right elbow; right big toe, left thumb, etc. This area is then palpated with a thin, blunt object in order to find the most sensitive and painful spot. This spot is then investigated with the tip of a needle, the needle is inserted into the most sensitive spot and the needle is strongly stimulated. A needle can subsequently be inserted into the site of the disorder.

Order of insertion and removal of the needles

When the decision has been made with regards to which points are to be utilised in the treatment, you must then determine in which order the needles are to be inserted. Once again, there are some general guidelines that ideally should be followed. There are, however, situations where needles are deliberately inserted into the body in a different order to achieve a specific therapeutic effect.

Generally, insertion of needles starts from the top of the head and goes downwards. Also, acupuncture points on the torso are inserted before points on the arms and legs. Points on the back are inserted before points on the front of the body. Because insertion is from the top downwards, points are inserted on the arms prior to points on the legs. Needles are also withdrawn in this manner, with needles removed from the head first, then the torso, and after that the arms and then the legs. This is to prevent *qi* from rising uncontrolled up to the head.

There are many situations where this principle is deviated from. For example, the opening points of the extraordinary channel are inserted first, before other acupuncture points, even though these opening points are located on the hands and feet. There are also therapeutic situations where other considerations weigh more heavily than the normal order of insertion. This could be when there is too much *qi* in the head, as in a migraine headache, or when a person is very agitated. In these situations, it is common to start treatment by stimulating relevant points on the feet with a draining needle technique to drain *qi* downwards from the head.

In acute channel disorders, it is normal to start the treatment by utilising a draining technique on a distal point on the hand or foot to disperse the stagnation in the channel before needling points further up the channel – in the head, for example.

Another situation in which I do not start the treatment with needles in the head is with new clients who are nervous. This is for psychological reasons. New clients are sometimes nervous of being needled. This nervousness can be accentuated if the first needle to be inserted is in the head or face. It can therefore be better to start with a couple of more 'innocent' points on the torso or limbs, before inserting a needle in the face. Also, I often save points such as Pe 6 for last when treating new clients. This is again for psychological reasons. Points like Pe 6 can sometimes give a very powerful and unpleasant electric shock sensation. If they experience this sensation in the first points that are needled, they will be nervous and tense whilst the remaining needles are inserted. This will also prejudice their experience. If the first needle was unpleasant and painful, they are more likely to interpret the subsequent needles in this light. If, on the other hand, the first eight needles were relatively painless and it was only the last or the penultimate needle that elicited an electric shock, then they will view this more as an anomaly than the norm.

There are also some acupuncturists whose approach is to start the needling on the right-hand side in women and on the left-hand side in men.

Part 6

CAUSES OF DISORDER

CAUSES OF DISORDER

There is a completely different understanding of how physical and mental disorders arise in Chinese medicine than there is in Western medicine. In Chinese medicine there is less focus on the actual disorder and more focus on the underlying disruptions of the body's qi[1] that the disease or disorder is a manifestation of.

When the body is diseased, it will be because there is one or more imbalances of the body's qi. These imbalances are called patterns of imbalance. This is because they are collections of symptoms and signs that the body is manifesting when there is an imbalance in a particular organ, channel, aspect of the body or one or more of the vital substances. Each pattern of imbalance will have its own specific symptoms and signs, and each pattern of imbalance will require its own unique treatment. It is also a characteristic of Chinese medicine that the focus is on treating the individual who is suffering from a disease, rather than treating the disease itself. This certainly does not mean that the disease is not taken into account in the treatment, but it means that as well as treating the symptoms of the disease, the focus of the treatment is also to address and try to rectify the imbalances that have caused the disease to occur.

One disease can be caused by many different imbalances. Whilst at the same time, a single pattern of imbalance can manifest in several different and, from a Western medical perspective, ostensibly unrelated disorders.

Imbalances do not arise by themselves. Imbalances arise because the body has been affected in a negative way. These negative influences that cause imbalances in the body are called aetiological factors.

Diagnosis in Chinese medicine will often move in two directions. When you know what patterns of imbalance a person is manifesting, you will have an idea of the aetiological factors that could be the reason that the imbalance has developed. Similarly, if you know what aetiological factors the person has been exposed to, you can have an idea of possible patterns of imbalances that could develop as a result of these effects. It is important to note though that an aetiological factor in itself is not sufficient to create an imbalance. It depends on the strength and the length of exposure to the influence and the imbalances that the person already has, as well as how their fundamental constitution is. That which creates an imbalance and subsequent disease in one person will not necessarily have any effect on the next person. This means, for example, that we cannot diagnose Liver qi stagnation in a person, just because they have a stressful job and problems in their domestic relationships. You can first diagnose a pattern of imbalance, when there are symptoms and signs that are manifestations of this imbalance. Aetiological factors are not imbalances in themselves, but they can be the cause of them.

It is important to be able to identify the aetiology behind imbalances, both because this will assist the diagnosis, but more importantly because it can also be used as an aspect of the treatment. If you can identify the cause of an imbalance, you can then try to get the person to make changes in their behaviour, diet, lifestyle, etc., so that the imbalance does not deteriorate or reoccur.

Chinese medicine defines three categories of aetiological factors that can result in imbalances and thereby disorders and disease in the body. The first category is the external factors. These are the six forms of climatic *qi* or *liuyin*. These climatic influences surround the body all the time and are a natural part of the environment. We are in fact dependent on these forms of *qi*. Under certain circumstances, however, they may become causes of diseases. This will depend on their intensity and strength, the length of exposure to them and the strength of the body's *wei qi*, which protects the body against invasions of climatic *qi*. When these climatic influences become a form of pathological *qi*, they are called the exogenous *xie qi* or exogenous 'perverse/evil' *qi*. In English they are often called external pathogens.

The second group of aetiological factors are the so-called seven internal causes. These are the emotions or mental-emotional influences that can create imbalances of the body's *qi*. Emotions are neither negative nor positive in themselves. They are in reality nothing more than movements of *qi*. They only become a source of imbalance when they are either very strong, repetitive or constant. Furthermore, if the body is already imbalanced, it will require much less to bring it further out of balance.

The final category of aetiological factors is termed the 'neither internal nor external factors', the 'both internal and external factors' or more simply in English the 'miscellaneous factors'. This category includes all the other possible causes of imbalance, but most importantly factors such as diet, lifestyle and exercise. It is especially within this group of factors that there is the greatest potential for a patient to make positive changes in their lives. It is often in relation to this group of factors that lifestyle and dietary advice is given to the patient.

Aetiological factors	
Exogenous causes	Cold Dampness Heat Dryness Summer-Heat Wind
Internal causes	Anger Sorrow Joy Worry Fear Shock Oppression/anguish
Miscellaneous causes	Constitution Diet Sexual activity Overwork Lack of rest Exercise and physical activity Trauma Burns Incorrect treatment Incorrect medication Parasites Poisoning, including: insect bites, snakebite

THE EXTERNAL
AETIOLOGICAL FACTORS

Like most medical systems, Chinese medicine has a shamanistic past. Initially it was believed that disease arose because the body was invaded by evil spirits. These spirits could, for example, be the person's ancestors who were dissatisfied with their behaviour or rootless spirits that were in the local surroundings. Treatment at that time was based on either expelling the evil spirit from the body or trying to appease the disgruntled ancestor. These evil spirits that caused disease were termed *xie qi*. *Xie* means evil or perverse. These spirits were a perverse or evil form of *qi*, because they were *qi* that only had a negative and disruptive effect on the body. This is in contrast to the body's own *qi*, which is exclusively harmonious, possessing only positive properties. That is why *xie qi* can also be translated as 'pathological *qi*', 'pathogenic *qi*' or simply 'pathogen'. This is because it is a form of *qi* that can result in disease.

Many of the places where *xie qi* was predominant and gathered in were dark, damp or cold – places people instinctively felt were unpleasant. It was observed that people more often fell ill or developed disorders when they stayed in such places. Similar observations could also be made in other places where the climate was more extreme. During the course of time the perception started to change. Evil spirits were less seen as the cause of illness and instead the climate itself was viewed as being the culprit. The relationship between an individual and the world surrounding them became more apparent. The perception changed increasingly to being that people became ill not because they dwelt in cold, dark, damp places, where evil spirits resided, but they became ill because these places were damp and cold – it was the damp and cold that was the *xie qi*.

As analytical observers, Chinese scientists, scholars and doctors saw that people became ill after being exposed to extreme or prolonged climatic influences, and they saw how the condition of a person's own *qi* also played an important role. It was observed how certain climatic conditions, such as cold, dampness, heat, etc., had specific, individual characteristics. The various forms of climatic *qi* affected the physical world in specific and thus predictable ways. For example, if there is an extreme or prolonged period of cold weather, water will freeze. Cold temperatures will also cause things to contract. This is due to the *yin* nature of cold. *Yang* heat, on the other hand, has a very drying quality and injures moisture. It was observed that when people were exposed to prolonged or extreme climatic influences, their bodies reacted in a similar way to the world outside the body when it is exposed to this particular climatic influence. When the body was exposed to cold weather, it was observed that *qi* stagnated in the same way that water does when it freezes.

The designation *xie* was not discarded though, because it was still an appropriate term. The idea is the same – that the body is invaded by a form of *qi* and that this *qi* has negative characteristics and a pathological influence on the body's own *qi*. Whereas before it was an evil spirit that had invaded the body, the conception now was that it was a form of negative climatic *qi* that had invaded the body. This is very typical of Chinese medicine and its way of thinking. An old theory is not rejected, but is instead assimilated into the new understanding of how the body works.

Through the analysis of exogenous *xie qi* and its consequences, six forms of climatic *qi* that can have a pathological effect on the body were defined. There was also observed a resonance between the various climatic influences and specific channels and internal organs – that a certain type of climatic *qi* will be more likely to influence a certain channel or organ than another.

The six forms of exogenous *xie qi* are the following: Wind, Dampness, Cold, Heat, Summer-Heat and Dryness. Each of these six forms of climatic *xie qi* have their own specific *qi* dynamic. *Qi* dynamic is the directional movement that the *qi* has and the way that it affects other forms of *qi*. This *qi* dynamic is a reflection of its relative *yin* or *yang* nature. For example, Heat is a *yang* form of *qi*. Heat's *yang* quality can be seen in that it is a form of *qi* that ascends, it is very drying and Heat creates over-activity in the organs and the vital substances it is in contact with, i.e. it agitates. These *qi* dynamics are of great importance in relation to how the various *xie qi* affect *qi* in the body and what reactions they create.

By understanding the dynamics of the various forms of exogenous *xie qi*, you can recognise their presence in the body. This recognition will be based on the symptoms and signs that the dynamics of each of these forms of *xie qi* produces.

This has meant that an invasion of *xie qi* is defined on the basis of its origin, i.e. how it has arisen. For example, you can be invaded by Damp-Cold if you get cold and soaked after being drenched by the rain in winter. *Xie qi* is, however, also defined just as much by how it manifests, i.e. how it affects the body's *qi*. If something affects the body in the same way as, for example, Cold does, it will be defined as being Cold *xie qi*, even though the person has not been exposed to climatic cold. In general, there is no discrepancy between the way that symptoms and signs manifest themselves and the climatic influences that a person has been exposed to. However, there are circumstances in which there is no climatic influence, yet the person still manifests symptoms and signs of an external invasion of *xie qi*. Allergic rhinitis is a classic example of this. This is because all pathogens, like climatic *qi*, have specific *qi* dynamics. This is of great importance when treating people who have been infected with bacteria, viruses and other 'invisible' forms of infection, and when people react negatively to food additives, chemicals and allergens. If exposure to a particular virus makes the body temperature rise, the eyes red, the thirst increase and the pulse beat faster, then this virus is defined and treated as Heat *xie qi*. This is because these physiological reactions are the reactions that occur when Heat is present in the body. Conversely, if a person feels very cold and has cramping intestinal and gastric pain and watery diarrhoea, this physiological reaction will instead be defined as being a Cold reaction. This will therefore indicate the presence of *xie* Cold in the body, even though the person has not been exposed to cold.

Invasions of *xie qi* are characterised by being both aetiological factors and independent patterns of imbalances. This means that when we diagnosis, say, 'Dampness', there is an understanding that the cause of the imbalance is that the person has been exposed to some form of *qi*, which is Damp in nature, but also that the person manifests specific symptoms and signs that are characteristic of the presence of Dampness. There is, in reality, no distinction between aetiology and manifestation with regard to exogenous *xie qi*. They are one and the same. This stands in contrast to other aetiological factors, such as anger for example, which is one of the seven internal or emotional causes of illness. Anger can be a cause of imbalances, such as Liver Fire, that manifest with specific symptoms and signs, but anger itself is not a pattern of imbalance with specific symptoms and signs.

Something that is also important to remember is that when exogenous *xie qi* invades the body, it can change character and become something else. It is, for example, very typical for invasions of Cold to transform into Heat patterns when the Cold has penetrated into the body.

As stated, each of the six exogenous forms of *xie qi* have their own unique symptoms and signs, which are manifestations of their specific *qi* dynamic. There are, however, some symptoms and signs that will be seen in all invasions of exogenous *xie qi*. This is because exogenous *xie qi* will have a disruptive effect on the body's *wei qi*. When *xie qi* invades the exterior, there will often be an aversion to cold and chills, even if it is an invasion of exogenous *xie* Heat. This is because exogenous *xie qi* blocks *wei qi* so that it no longer can warm the skin. There can also be a slight fever or febrile sensation, even if it is a Cold pathogen. This is because the conflict between *xie qi* and *wei qi* and the subsequent stagnation will generate Heat. The febrile sensation may not be particularly pronounced and may well not be measurable with a thermometer. In Chinese medicine, fever is defined by the patient's own subjective sensation of warmth or if the therapist can observe signs of Heat, such as a red colour in the face or the skin feeling warm on palpation. An important diagnostic sign in invasions of exogenous *xie qi* is that chills and febrile sensations manifest simultaneously. In invasions of exogenous *xie qi*, the pulse will usually be superficial.

The six forms of exogenous *xie qi*

- Cold
- Dryness
- Summer-Heat
- Dampness
- Heat
- Wind

The six forms in detail

Cold

Cold is extremely *yin* in nature. This means that Cold can easily injure *yang*.

Cold is referred to as 'the prevailing *qi* of winter'. This is because cold is the dominant climate at this time of year. This does not mean that Cold cannot or will not invade the body at other times of the year, but that Cold is most prevalent in winter.

Cold's *yin* nature can be seen in its *qi* dynamic, which is contracting. Its contracting nature means that Cold creates stagnations and blocks the movement of *yang*. This is seen in the world around us, where cold freezes water and stops it from moving. Cold does the same in the body. Cold will stagnate *qi*, *jinye* and *xue*, because it blocks their free movement. There is an aphorism in Chinese medicine: 'Where there is stagnation, there is pain; where there is free movement, there is no pain' (*bu tong ze tong, tong ze bu tong*). This means that pain is a key symptom signifying the presence of Cold. The character of pain in Cold is typically cramping or biting in nature. Other typical symptoms are stiffness and a pronounced aversion to cold.

Exogenous *xie* Cold will often invade the body through the skin, where it will disrupt the circulation and the activities of the body's *wei qi*. This means that the symptoms and the signs of an invasion of Cold will be most apparent in the body's external aspects. There can be situations where exogenous *xie* Cold manifests with symptoms and signs in the interior of the body. This will typically be when there is an invasion of Cold in the Stomach and Intestines, the Urinary Bladder or the Uterus, all of which are *fu* organs. An invasion of Cold in the interior is due to either climatic cold penetrating through the skin to the channels or the consumption of food, liquids or medicines that have a Cold nature.

Cold can block the movement and activity of *yang* and thereby prevent it from transforming and transporting fluids. This can result in clear, watery exudations from the nose, vagina or respiratory passages. Diarrhoea caused by Cold will also be watery.

Each of the six climatic *qi* has a resonance with specific organs and channels in the body. Cold has a resonance with the *taiyang* channel. *Taiyang* is the most exterior channel, and it is in these channels that the initial reactions to an attack of Cold manifests according to 'Six Stage' theory.

Dryness

Dryness 'is the prevailing *qi* in autumn'. Whilst it is quite logical that Cold is defined as being the prevailing *qi* in winter, it seems less logical in north-western Europe that Dryness should be the prevailing *qi* in the autumn. Autumnal weather in Britain is often very damp. The reason that Dryness has been ascribed this definition is that in autumn many parts of China are extremely dry, because the prevailing wind is from the West in the autumn. The Gobi Desert is located in West China and this means that the air is extremely dry. Furthermore, autumn is the season of the Metal Phase and the Gobi Desert is located in the West of China, which is the compass direction of the Metal Phase. Dryness is extremely injurious for the Lung, which is the Metal Phase organ. In addition, dryness has a resonance with the *yangming* aspect, which the Metal organs and channels are a part of. Constipation and dry stools are a classic symptom of Dryness in the body.

The British Isles have a damp climate, because of their geographical location. This means that external Dryness has not traditionally been a problem here. Invasions of Dryness can, however, be observed in people who live and work in buildings that have a very dry indoor climate, such as buildings made of concrete.

Dryness is defined as being *yang*. This is because the dominant negative effect Dryness has is that it injures moistness and dries out fluids, i.e. Dryness injures *yin*. The most typical manifestations of an invasion of Dryness are dry mucous membranes, dry throat, dry eyes, dry mouth, dry nose, dry stool and sparse urinations.

Summer-Heat

This pathogen is *yang* in nature. It is 'the prevailing *qi* of summer', but the major difference to the other forms of climatic *qi* is that Summer-Heat is the only form of *xie qi* that is exclusively associated with a specific season. The other forms of exogenous *xie qi* can invade the body all year round, but Summer-Heat invasions are solely seen in the summer. Furthermore, all of the other five forms of climatic *qi* can manifest with equivalent internal imbalances in the body. For example, signs of Cold manifest in a *yang xu* condition or Heat signs manifest in a *yin xu* condition. This is not the case with Summer-Heat. Summer-Heat is exclusively an exogenous form of *xie qi*.

Summer-Heat has an upward and outward dynamic. Most of the signs of Summer-Heat are almost identical to Heat signs. This is because Summer-Heat is a Heat pathogen. Summer-Heat will also injure *yin*. Typical symptoms and signs of an invasion of Summer-Heat are high fever, profound thirst, excessive sweating, red face, headache, rapid, shallow breathing, mental restlessness and agitation. Summer-Heat will result in the heartbeat increasing and therefore a rapid pulse.

Summer-Heat resonates with the *shaoyang* aspect.

Dampness

Dampness is *yin* in nature. It has a descending dynamic and will always seep downwards. This means that Dampness has a tendency to affect the lower parts of the body – the Urinary Bladder, Intestines, Uterus, genitalia and legs.

Dampness is heavy and obstructive. Dampness blocks and slows the movement of *qi*, *xue* and *jinye*. The Spleen, which abhors Dampness, is easily weakened and disrupted by it. Dampness will often disrupt both the Spleen and Stomach *qi ji* and it will be a burden on the Spleen's *yang* aspect. This results in the Spleen failing to carry out its functions optimally, including the transformation of the food and liquids consumed and the Spleen's ability to separate the pure from the impure.

As well as blocking the Spleen's *qi ji* and weakening the Spleen, Dampness has in general a negative influence on the *taiyin* aspect. Many Lung disorders are exacerbated when the climate is damp.

Typical symptoms and signs of Dampness could be poor appetite, nausea, heaviness in the body, especially the limbs, fatigue, cloudy and turbid exudations from the body, loose stools, a greasy tongue coating and a sticky taste in the mouth.

Heat

Heat is *yang* in nature. Heat has an ascending dynamic and it will usually affect the head and the organs in the upper *jiao*. Heat accelerates processes in the body and agitates bodily substances. Heat injures *yin* and dries out *xue* and *jinye*. By agitating *xue*, Heat can result in spontaneous bleeding. Heat can also agitate *shen*. This can lead to anything from a slight unrest and nervousness to outright mania, depending on its strength. An agitated and restless *shen* can often manifest with insomnia.

Heat has a resonance with the *shaoyin* aspect. Heat has an especially damaging effect on both Kidney *yin* and the Heart in general, as well as on the communication between Water and Fire.

Typical symptoms and signs that indicate the presence of Heat can be febrile sensations, thirst, a bitter taste in the mouth, mental restlessness, constipation, red skin, warm or hot skin, bleeding, dark, yellow urine, rapid pulse and a red tongue.

Wind

Wind is a very *yang* form of *xie qi*. Wind is the 'prevailing *qi* in spring'. Invasions of Wind are far from limited to this season, but both wind and spring have a powerful resonance with the Wood Phase and its dynamic, young *yang* energy. Wind's *yang* nature is seen in its mobility and speed. Wind has an expansive and thereby spreading dynamic. Just imagine a pile of leaves that is lying in a heap on the ground. Heat, dampness, cold, etc. will only result in the leaves drying out, becoming heavy and soggy or freezing into a solid mass, but a gust of wind will spread them in all directions and set them in motion. This ability of Wind to spread things apart enables it to penetrate through *wei qi*, whilst at the same time drawing other forms of *xie qi* into the body. This is the reason it is said that Wind is the spearhead that conveys other forms of *xie qi* into the body. This is very important for *yin* forms of *xie qi*, such as Cold, for example. Cold has a contracting nature. Cold therefore results in the pores in the skin contracting and closing, thereby blocking its entry. Wind can spread open the pores and thereby lead Cold in through the skin and into the body. This is similar to a draughty cabin in winter. If the temperature is sub-zero outside, but it is completely windless, it is possible to warm the cabin with a small stove. If, on the other hand, the wind is blowing outside, it is difficult to keep the cabin warm even though the temperature is ten degrees centigrade. This is because the wind will drive the cold into the cabin through the cracks in the walls.

Wind's *yang* nature means that it has a tendency to affect the head and the upper part of the body. Wind's dynamic nature also means that the symptoms and the signs can have a tendency to move from place to place and to be variable in character. Wind's *yang* nature also manifests in its symptoms and signs having a sudden onset.

Wind has a resonance with the *jueyin* aspect. This is reflected by people's eyes watering when it is windy. Both the eyes and tears relate to the Liver through the Five Phases, as does Wind. Internally generated Wind can arise as a consequence of Liver imbalances.

Typical Wind symptoms and signs are symptoms that have a sudden onset, symptoms that move from place to place or symptoms that quickly change character. Wind symptoms are more typical in the upper part of the body and the head. Itching, muscle spasms, tics and tremors are also classic Wind symptoms.

Xie qi	*Yin/yang* nature	Season	Channel	*Qi* dynamic
Cold	*Yin*	Winter	*Taiyang*	Contracting, centripetal
Dryness	*Yang*	Autumn	*Yangming*	
Summer-Heat	*Yang*	Summer	*Shaoyang*	
Dampness	*Yin*		*Taiyin*	Descending
Heat	*Yang*		*Shaoyin*	Ascending
Wind	*Yang*	Spring	*Jueyin*	Outward, spreading, centrifugal

Wei qi is the first level of defence in the body. It protects the body against invasions of exogenous *xie qi*. The sum of the body's anti-pathogenic *qi* is called *zheng qi*.

An invasion of the body by exogenous *xie qi* will be due to one or more of the following factors.

- ***Zheng qi* is weak or weakened:** If *zheng qi*, including *wei qi*, is *xu*, the body will more easily be invaded. This is because the body will not able to protect and defend itself. This will mean that *xie qi* does not need either to be as strong or have affected the body for that long. A weak or weakened *zheng qi* is typically seen in infants, older people, people who are physically run down and people who have been ill. To illustrate this, one could imagine that an old lady and a young man have to go out from their house to the corner shop, which is four hundred metres away. It is freezing cold and both of them are only wearing a thin coat. It is much more likely that this trip to the shop will result in the old lady catching a cold than it will the young man. Her *wei qi* is not strong enough to withstand the onslaught of the Wind and Cold. It is very typical for some people to catch every bug that is going around, whilst others rarely fall ill. This is usually a reflection of the relative strengths of their *wei qi*.

- ***Xie qi* is very strong:** If the body is subjected to a very strong influence of *xie qi*, it will have difficulty keeping it out, even though the *wei qi* is strong. If we return to the young man from the previous analogy, walking down to the shops in a thin jacket in winter will most probably not result in him catching a cold or becoming ill. This is because his *wei qi* is strong. However, it is highly likely that he will catch a cold or fall ill if he falls through the ice and into the freezing cold water below. Even if there is no difference in the length of time he is exposed to the cold, there is a difference in the intensity of the cold he is exposed to. This is also seen in some virulent diseases, where the majority of the population including even strong, healthy individuals fall ill when exposed to the disease.

- **Prolonged exposure of *xie qi*:** A prolonged exposure to a certain form of *xie qi* will wear down the body's defences. If we again imagine the same young man, he will not become sick from walking down to the shops in freezing weather in a thin jacket, but if he had to walk around for two hours in freezing weather with only a thin jacket on, it is more likely that he would become ill afterwards. This time it is not the strength of the cold that is crucial but that he has been subjected to a prolonged exposure to it. Imbalances that arise as a consequence of prolonged exposure to a certain *xie qi* are, for example, seen in people who live or work in an environment that is characterised by a particular climate, for example living or working in a place that is cold and damp.

- **Sudden exposure to *xie qi*:** Illnesses can suddenly occur when seasons change or when the weather is atypical for the season. This could, for example, be sudden cold weather in summer or a mild spell of weather in winter. It is as if *wei qi* does not have time to adjust to this atypical, climatic influence. It is as if *wei qi* has prepared itself to protect the body against something that is, for example, *yin*, and all of a sudden there is something that is *yang*. We often see people catch a cold when there is a period of mild weather in winter or during a cold and wet period in summer. This is also the reason that many people get sore throats and colds from air-conditioning, especially in hot climates. The pores of the skin are wide open due to the heat and then they come into a building that is quite cold and the air-conditioning also creates a draught (Wind). In addition, many people fall ill in the transition from summer to autumn and from winter to spring – the classic spring cold.

- **Presence of imbalances in the body:** A person is more likely to be affected adversely by a specific form of *xie qi* if they already have a similar imbalance. A person with *yang xu* will more quickly be invaded by Cold than a person with *shi* Heat. Also, a person with Spleen imbalances is quicker to be affected by Dampness than a person with *yin xu*.

Internally generated *xie qi*

All six forms of *xie qi* can be exogenous, but only five of them can also be internally generated. Summer-Heat is the only form of *xie qi* that is exclusively exogenous. Whereas exogenous *xie qi* can invade the body when it comes into contact with climatic influences, bacteria, viruses, allergens, etc., internally generated *xie qi* arises when there are internal imbalances in the body, especially *zangfu* organ imbalances. It is important to remember that *xie qi* is defined by its origin, but also by how it manifests. This means that when an internal imbalance manifests with a person having a red face, being excessively thirsty, being mentally restless and having a fast pulse and red tongue, then this imbalance will be defined as Heat. The Heat here though has been internally generated, i.e. it is Heat that has arisen due to internal conditions and not because the person has been in contact with exogenous *xie qi*. As can be seen in this example, internally generated *xie qi* is in many ways similar to exogenous *xie qi*. It is very important to note, however, that internally generated *xie qi* is not classified as an aetiological factor in itself. This is because internally generated *xie qi* is not the original source of the imbalance. The original source of internally generated Heat could, for example, be diet, which is one of the 'miscellaneous aetiological factors', or the Heat could be due to Liver *qi* stagnation that has been caused by frustration and repressed emotions, i.e. the original source of Heat could be emotional or one of the internal aetiological factors. The Heat can also be caused by the exogenous Cold that has penetrated into the body and transformed into Heat and injured the body's *yin* aspects. Exogenous *xie qi* is, though, a root cause. Exogenous *xie qi* has not been caused by anything else and is therefore defined as being an aetiological factor.

As well as there being a difference in their aetiology, the symptoms and the signs of internally generated *xie qi* and exogenous *xie qi* are different in quality, intensity and duration. Exogenous *xie qi* tends to be acute and the symptoms more pronounced. The symptoms and signs of internally generated *xie qi* will more often be chronic and less intense. Exogenous *xie qi* will usually manifest with symptoms and signs relating to the exterior aspects of the body – *wei qi*, skin, muscles, joints and channels. There will probably be an aversion to cold and a slight febrile sensation. Internally generated *xie qi* can affect specific organs and vital substances or it can be systemic. There are, however, also situations where exogenous *xie qi* can manifest in the interior of the body. This will either be because exogenous *xie qi* has penetrated deeper into the body or because there has been a direct invasion of exogenous *xie qi* into the interior.

As previously stated, only five of the six forms of exogenous *xie qi* are generated in the interior. Furthermore, in addition to internal Heat, Cold, Wind, Dampness and Dryness, there are other forms of internally generated *xie qi* that do not exist as exogenous *xie qi*. These are Phlegm, *xue* stagnation and food stagnation, which are also classified as forms of *xie qi*. As stated above, it is important to remember that even though these internally generated forms of *xie qi* can result in disorders and imbalances, they are not defined as aetiological factors. This is because they themselves have resulted from one or more of the internal, external or miscellaneous aetiological factors.

Below is a superficial review of the different forms of internally generated *xie qi*. It is important to remember that the various forms of *xie qi* can combine with each other and in themselves be independent forms of *xie qi*, for example Damp-Heat, Damp-Cold, Phlegm-Dampness, Phlegm-Wind, Phlegm-Heat, Phlegm-Cold, etc. These combined forms of *xie qi* will have characteristics of both of the *xie qi*.

Cold

Internal Cold occurs either when there is a direct invasion of Cold into one of the internal organs or when there is a *yang xu* condition in the body. The first is defined as being a *shi* or excess condition, whilst *yang xu* Cold, as the name suggests, is a *xu* or deficient condition. Internal *shi* Cold is usually of short duration. This is because the Cold will either transform into Heat or injure *yang* and become a *yang xu* Cold. The organs that are usually invaded by Cold are the Stomach, the Intestines and the Uterus. The invasion will either be due to climatic cold invading directly through the skin or channels, or it will be due to the consumption of food, liquids or medicine that have a cold energy or temperature.

Yang xu Cold is characterised by being a Cold condition that has arisen not because the body has been invaded by Cold, but because it is not able to generate warmth. The symptoms and the signs will in many ways be similar to those seen in exogenous Cold, but there will also be differences. First, the symptoms and the signs are generally much milder in *yang xu* Cold. They will also be chronic and will have developed over a longer period of time. An important differentiation between exogenous Cold and *yang xu* Cold is that when there is exogenous Cold, the person will freeze and they will have difficulty keeping warm, even though they put on extra clothes or bedding. In a *yang xu* condition the person feels cold, but if they put on extra clothes or get under the duvet, they will feel warm enough. This is because when exogenous Cold invades the body, it blocks the circulation of the warming *yang qi*. This means that even though there is enough warmth in the body, it does not get circulated around the body. When the body is *yang xu* there is not enough heat in the body, but if the body is insulated and the warmth that is there is prevented from leaving the body, the person will not feel cold.

The pulse will be slow, weak and deep in a *yang xu* condition, but it will be tight and slow when there is *shi* Cold.

Dryness

Internal Dryness arises when *yin* substances in the body, such as *yin* and *xue*, are weakened. Once again, the symptoms and the signs will be chronic and less intense than in an invasion of exogenous Dryness. Typical manifestations of internal Dryness are dry mucous membranes, dry throat, dry eyes, dry mouth, dry nose, dry stool and scanty urinations.

Dampness

Internally generated Dampness is a very common condition. Dampness can arise when the Spleen is weakened and is not strong enough to transform the food and liquids that have been consumed. Dampness can also occur when food and beverages that produce Dampness are consumed. Examples of such foods are dairy products, wheat and sweet substances, as well as certain medicines. There will often be a combination of both causes. Also, the more Dampness that there is present in the body, the more it will burden the Spleen, which abhors Dampness and prefers dryness. This, unfortunately, is often the case with internally generated *xie qi*. Internally generated *xie qi* is often the source of its own production. It quickly becomes a vicious circle. Typical symptoms and signs of Dampness are fatigue, heaviness in the body, nausea and poor appetite, loose stool, sticky sensation in the mouth, cloudy urine, greasy tongue coating and a slippery pulse.

Heat

Internally generated Heat can be both *xu* and *shi* in nature. Internally generated *shi* Heat arises: when there are stagnations of *qi*, *xue* or Phlegm; when exogenous *xie qi* transforms and turns into Heat; when there is a condition of Heat in one or more of the *zangfu* organs; and through the consumption of Hot substances such as food, beverages and medicine. *Xu* Heat can arise when there is too little *yin*, i.e. *yin xu*. This condition results in Heat not being controlled. There are both similarities and differences in the symptoms and signs of *xu* and *shi* Heat. There is also a significant difference in the way these two conditions are treated. *Shi* Heat is drained or expelled from the body by stimulating relevant points with a draining needle technique. *Yin xu* is treated by utilising a tonifying needle technique on acupuncture points that nourish *yin*.

Internally generated *shi* Heat, which is also called full Heat or excess Heat, is characterised by the following symptoms and signs: red face, thirst with a desire for cold drinks, preference for cold foods, constipation, dark urine, mental restlessness or agitation, a red tongue with a yellow coating and a strong, fast pulse. *Yin xu* Heat, also known as empty Heat or deficiency Heat, manifests with symptoms and signs such as night sweats, insomnia, feeling hot in the evening and especially at night, red cheeks, dry mouth and throat, a red tongue without coating and a weak and fast pulse.

Wind

Internally generated Wind can arise from Liver imbalances. These imbalances are generally due to either an excess of Heat in the Liver, Liver *xue xu* or Liver *yin xu*. Internally generated Wind will manifest with symptoms and signs such as itching, dizziness, tics, muscle spasms, tremors or numbness.

There are also three other forms of internally generated *xie qi*: Phlegm, *xue* stagnation and food stagnation. These three have no equivalent external form of *xie qi*. Like the other internal forms of *xie qi*, they are the result of internal imbalances in the body or the consumption of inappropriate foods, liquids and medicine. This again means that even though they cause imbalance and disorder in the body, they are not themselves aetiological factors. This is because they are not the root cause but a consequence of other aetiological factors.

Phlegm

Phlegm is fluids that have congealed, coagulated or thickened. Because these body fluids have changed their form or structure, they have none of the nourishing or moistening qualities that *jinye* has. They have thus gone from being an aspect of *zheng qi* to becoming a form of *xie qi*.

Phlegm can be both substantial, i.e. it can be seen visibly, or insubstantial, i.e. the Phlegm is not visible to the naked eye. Substantial Phlegm can be observed as sputum and mucus in the respiratory passages, stool or menstrual blood. Non-substantial Phlegm can be observed or palpated below the surface of the skin as nodules, ganglion cysts, deformations of bones and cartilage, uterine fibroids, lumps and other physical accumulations in the tissues such as gallstones and kidney stones. Non-substantial Phlegm also manifests as a sensation of heaviness in the body and the head, numbness, fatigue, mental confusion, depression, dizziness, nausea and chest oppression. The pulse can be slippery or wiry. The tongue can be swollen and have a greasy coating.

Xue stagnation

Xue should flow freely and unhindered throughout the body. *Xue* can stagnate for a variety of reasons. *Xue* and *qi* have an extremely close relationship, with *xue* being dependent on *qi* for its movement. This means that *qi* stagnation can directly result in *xue* stagnation. *Qi xu* can also be a cause of *xue* stagnation when *qi* lacks the strength to circulate and spread *xue*. The movement of *xue* can also be blocked by Phlegm and by physical traumas, including surgery. Heat can 'coagulate' *xue*, so that it becomes sticky and clots. Cold can freeze and congeal *xue*.

Just as Phlegm and Dampness have none of the moistening or lubricating qualities that *jinye* has, *xue* stagnation has none of the moistening and nourishing qualities that physiological *xue* has. In fact, stagnant *xue* blocks and thereby prevents fresh, nutritious *xue* from circulating to or through an area.

Xue stagnation can manifest with a characteristic pain that is stabbing, sharp or piercing in character. The pain will be fixed and localised to a specific site. There can be physical accumulations, lumps or hard knots in the muscle or tissue, dry, flaking skin, purple lips, varicose veins and visible purple blood vessels in the skin. The complexion in the face can be dark. Menstrual blood will often be dark and clotted and there can be dysmenorrhoea. The tongue can be dark and purplish or have purple spots. The sub-lingual vein can be dark and swollen. The pulse can be choppy or confined.

Food stagnation

Food stagnation arises when food physically and energetically accumulates in the middle *jiao*. Food stagnation occurs when too much food is consumed at one time, food is eaten too often or too late in the evening or when inappropriate food is eaten, i.e. food that is difficult to transform. Food stagnation can also arise when the Spleen and Stomach are too weak to be able to perform their respective functions.

Food stagnation generally has two consequences that can lead to further imbalances and complications. Food stagnation can block the *qi ji* (*qi* dynamic) of the middle *jiao* and it can create Heat. By physically and energetically blocking *qi* in the middle *jiao*, food stagnation will disrupt and burden the Stomach and Spleen's *qi ji*. This can lead to Stomach and Spleen *qi xu*, rebellious Stomach *qi*, Dampness, Damp-Heat and Phlegm. In addition, a blockage of *qi* in the middle *jiao* can disrupt the communication of *qi* between the lower and upper *jiao* and between the Kidneys and the Heart. Food stagnation can also disrupt Liver *qi* in its spreading function.

When food stagnates in the Stomach, it will manifest with a turgid and distended sensation in the epigastric region. Food stagnation creates Heat. At the same time, it blocks the Stomach *qi* from descending. Both of these factors can cause the Stomach *qi* to rebel. This can manifest as burping, heartburn and acid regurgitation a while after eating. The belching will usually taste of the food that has been consumed and sometimes will also be accompanied by a small amount of semi-digested food. The disruption of the Stomach and the Spleen *qi ji* can result in nausea or poor appetite. When the food is stagnant, it will not be transformed properly and will instead have a tendency to rot and ferment. The combination of untransformed food and Heat can also result in the stool being loose and sticky. The stool can also smell rotten like sewage. Food stagnation can cause constipation by stagnating *qi* in the Stomach and the Intestines.

Food stagnation can manifest on the tongue with a thick, greasy coating in the middle of the tongue. The pulse will often be wiry and slippery in the middle or *guan* positions.

THE INTERNAL
AETIOLOGICAL FACTORS

The internal causes of imbalances are emotions that have a negative effect on the body's physiology. Emotions are a natural aspect of our lives and thereby not a source of imbalance. When we are in balance, the emotions will be an appropriate response to a particular situation. In fact, the lack of a particular emotion in these situations would be a sign of imbalance, as would the constant or excessive manifestation of an emotion or emotions that are inappropriate to a given situation. Emotions are movements of *qi* that resonate with specific organs. The emotions only become causes of imbalance and disease when they are extremely powerful or enduring or when an organ is already out of balance and has difficulty integrating the emotion. Furthermore, because emotions are movements of *qi*, they can also lead to imbalances when they are not expressed.

The emotions are fundamentally different from the exogenous climatic influences. The emotions differ from the six climatic *xie qi* in that the emotions are causes of imbalance and at the same time also a manifestation of an imbalance in the body. Excessive worry and speculation can, for example, weaken the Spleen and lead to Spleen *qi xu*. Spleen *qi xu* will, however, also manifest with a person having a tendency to worry excessively and to have a mind where the thoughts are constantly churning. It will often turn into a vicious circle in which the emotional cause and the emotional reaction reinforce one another and where the cause and manifestation are identical.

Historically, the number of emotions classified as having a direct impact on the human physiology has varied. Different texts have described five, six or seven different emotions as being aetiological factors. There has also not only been a variance in the number of these emotions, but also differences in which emotions are defined as being aetiological factors. Furthermore, there is a difference in the effects that were ascribed to these emotions and to which organs they affected. There have in fact been variations within the same text. For example, *Huang Di Nei Jing – Su Wen*, chapter five, discussed five emotions and their relationship to the five *zang*. In a later chapter there is a discussion of six emotions and the negative effects these will have. This is probably because *Huang Di Nei Jing*, like the Old Testament, is not a coherent book written by a single person but is a collection of texts from a specific period.

The model of pathogenesis that most people utilise today was formulated by Chen Yan in the twelfth century, in his book *Sanyin Jiyi Bingzheng Fanglun*. In this book the causes of diseases are divided up into the three broad categories that we know today. Chen Yan classifies seven emotions as being the internal causes of disease. This ostensibly appears to be a somewhat simplified view of the human psyche. All emotions will, of course, affect the body. These seven emotions should be conceived as being similar to the primary colours: there are only three primary colours, yet the combination of these three colours in various proportions can produce the myriad of colours in the world around us. The seven emotions are similarly the individual components of all the various emotions that a person can experience.

The seven emotions are considered to be significant causes of imbalance in the *zangfu* organs. This is because the seven emotions directly affect the *zangfu* organs. When invasions of *xie qi* penetrate into the body, they must first pass through the exterior aspects of the body before they can disrupt the interior of the body and the *zangfu*. Exogenous *xie qi* will often be expelled before it injures the *qi* of the *zangfu* organs. The seven emotions though will have a direct effect on the *qi* of the *zang* organs in particular. This is because emotions are movements of *qi* that resonate with specific organs' *qi*. This means that repeated or prolonged exposures to certain emotions will create an imbalance in the body's *qi*. Furthermore, the various emotions have their own *qi* dynamic. They can affect *qi* in certain directions. This will influence the various *qi* dynamics inside the body and thus influence the body's physiology.

In addition to the various emotions affecting certain *zang* organs, all emotions will affect the Heart as well as the organs that they resonate with or are an expression of. This is because the Heart is the residence of *shen*, which makes us aware of our emotions. Anger, for example, causes Liver *qi* to ascend and in this way affects the Liver *zang* organ, but it is *shen* and the Heart that make us aware of the fact that we are angry. If it wasn't for *shen*, the various emotions would just be movements of *qi* in the body that we were not aware of. That is why the Heart will always be affected by all of the emotions.

The seven internal aetiological factors

- anger
- worry, speculation and overthinking
- fear
- joy
- sorrow, sadness and melancholy
- shock, fright and terror
- oppression, anguish, obsession and restraint

The seven factors in detail

Anger (nu)

Anger is *nu* in Chinese and primarily affects the Liver. Anger and the Liver resonate with each other, because they both have a dynamic *yang qi*, that is characteristic of the Wood phase. Anger causes Liver *qi* to rise upwards. This is apparent in many of the disorders that anger can precipitate, such as migraines, tinnitus and vertigo.

Anger that is not expressed will stagnate Liver *qi*. Excessive and uncontrolled anger can generate Liver Fire.

Frustration and irritation are also aspects of anger. They are especially relevant as causes of Liver *qi* stagnation. This is because they are characterised by a lack of movement or by something being held back. Unexpressed emotions in general will stagnate Liver *qi*. This is because the Liver is responsible for the free flow of *qi* in the body. Each time *qi* (which emotions also are) is hindered in its movement, it will have a negative effect on the Liver. This is even more apparent in emotions such as irritation and frustration, as anger is a very *yang* emotion.

It must be remembered that no emotion is, in itself, positive or negative. They should only be appropriate to the situation. Anger, which has a *yang* dynamic, can, for example, bring about change. There are many times where anger is justified and necessary, for example when you are confronted with injustice or when someone has transgressed your boundaries of what you think is acceptable. A lack of anger in these situations is just as much a pathological sign as a person who is constantly angry and short tempered.

It is very common to experience people who have difficulty manifesting their anger and who find it difficult to say no and set boundaries. They often find themselves in situations where they are not satisfied and are frustrated. This may be caused by a stagnation of Liver *qi*, resulting in a tendency to internalise their feelings of anger and frustration. This in itself then compounds the frustration that the situation had created. Irritation, frustration and pent-up anger thus become both the cause of Liver *qi* stagnation and its manifestation. People with *xu* conditions in the Liver can also have difficulty manifesting their anger, even when it is actually justified. That is because there is not enough strength in the Liver to project the anger.

The Heart is also affected by anger; the Heart is affected by all prolonged and extreme emotional conditions. The Heart can also be affected when stagnations of Liver *qi* caused by anger result in a stagnation of Heart *qi*. Furthermore, Heat, which often arises from the stagnation of Liver *qi*, can rise up to the Heart and agitate *shen*.

Worry, speculation and overthinking (si)

Si can be translated as worry, speculation or to think too much. *Si* weakens the Spleen and 'knots' *qi*. The knotting of *qi* will disturb the Spleen's *qi ji* or dynamic. It will burden Spleen *qi*. Worry and speculation also have a similar negative effect on Lung *qi*.

To think about things and to speculate are not in themselves negative. They are necessary when we have to deal with things. We should not take ill-considered decisions. They are only negative when speculation gets out of hand and prevents a person from being able to make decisions because they are always thinking in circles and reappraising the situation. As written in the introduction, an imbalance in a *zang* organ will often result in a person manifesting precisely the emotion that has a damaging effect on the organ that is in imbalance. This is very typical of people who are manifesting Spleen imbalances such as Spleen *qi xu* and Dampness. These people tend to overthink and worry a lot.

As with all emotions, the Heart is affected directly not only by the emotion itself, but also when the Lung and the Spleen are disrupted in their functioning. Disturbances of the Lung and the Spleen can lead to *qi xu* and *xue xu* conditions, resulting in the Heart not being adequately nourished.

The stagnated and weakened Lung *qi* will also not be able to support the Liver and supply the strength to move the Liver *qi*. This means that Liver *qi* stagnation can also arise from worry and speculation.

Fear (kong)

Kong includes anxiety and fear. Anxiety and fear mainly have a negative effect on the Kidneys and the Heart, interfering with their communication and cooperation. Anxiety and fear cause *qi* to descend. This is seen clearly when people, especially children, are scared and urinate or even defecate in their pants. This is because fear will weaken Kidney *qi*, so the Kidneys fail to perform their function of controlling the *yin* orifices. At the same time, the downward movement of *qi* that fear creates will send urine and faeces downwards and increase the pressure against these orifices.

By sending *qi* downwards, anxiety and fear interfere with communication between the Kidneys and the Heart. This is the reason that anxiety and fear also manifest with symptoms and signs of Heart imbalances, such as palpitations, mental unrest, insomnia and spontaneous sweating.

Anxiety and fear can also be an aetiological factor when a person lives in a constant state of fear or when they have experienced a sudden and extreme fear. Children are especially vulnerable to all emotional influences, but in particular fear and anxiety, because their organ *qi* is not yet stable. They are therefore easily influenced by the emotions that they are experiencing. Extreme events and prolonged exposure of certain emotions can therefore influence them for the rest of their lives, both on the psychological level and manifesting as physical disorders.

Fear is not only negative; caution is also an aspect of fear. Fear is that which holds us back in perilous situations. A lack of fear can often have disastrous consequences.

Joy (xi and le)

There are two Chinese characters that are used to describe the emotion that resonates with the Heart – *xi* and *le*. *Xi* can be translated as to be excited, euphoric, ecstatic or elated. *Le* is more joy, satisfaction or pleasure. *Xi* is the feelings a child may have when they are excitedly looking forward to their birthday party. *Le* is more the feeling the mother of the child has when looking at her child, who is looking forward to their party.

It sounds improbable that joy and happiness can be an aetiological factor in imbalances, but this can be the case when there is uncontrolled or excessive elation, as there is in *xi*. Joy as an aetiological factor is often seen when there has been a misuse of stimulants, excessive partying, too much sex or stimulation of the senses in general. Excessive happiness spreads the *qi* of the Heart and *shen*. This will weaken Heart *qi* and *jing*, which is the root of *shen*. To be excited or even manic is very exhausting. It results in the Heart *qi* becoming dull.

Le is mainly a source of imbalance in the Heart when it is not present, i.e. when there is a lack of joy. Heart *qi* and *shen* are nourished by joy. Therefore, a person who has Heart *qi xu* will benefit from consciously focussing or meditating on something that makes them happy or on something that they find beautiful for at least five minutes every day to nourish their *shen*.

Sorrow, sadness and melancholy (bei)

Bei can be interpreted as sadness, melancholy or grief.

Grief and melancholy affect the Lung and the Heart. *Bei* binds and hampers *qi* in the upper *jiao*. The stagnated *zong qi* can end up generating Heat, which injures Lung and Heart *yin*, and *bei* can weaken the Lung *qi* by disturbing its *qi* mechanism. That is why it is said that *bei* consumes and dissolves *qi*.

Bei can also affect the Spleen if the person dwells on and speculates about their grief.

Sadness by definition also includes a lack of joy. Sadness will therefore have a debilitating effect on Heart *qi*.

When we mourn something we have lost, a vital part of the process is to let go and release. This resonates with the Metal Phase and its organs. The Lung and the Large Intestine release from the body things that are no longer needed (carbon dioxide and the stool). This creates the necessary space in the body for something new and nourishing (oxygen and food). If we do not let go of things on the emotional level, we will not be capable of allowing something new in. This is one of the reasons that many societies have traditionally allocated periods of time to grieve in. By providing this space for grief, it is easier to let go of its ties.

In most books, the five emotions discussed above are related to the Five Phases and their associated *zang* organs. As can be seen above, this in fact is not a purely one-to-one relationship, but each emotion can have an effect on more than one organ. Furthermore, most books also discuss two or more emotions in addition to these five emotions as being possible causes of disease. These two emotions are shock and oppression. In a way, these two emotions are amplifications of some of the other emotions, but they also have their own *qi* dynamics. Some books place these two emotions together with fear and sorrow when the emotions are classified according to the Five Phases.

Shock, fright and terror (jing)

Jing, or shock, fear or terror, might sound as if it is the same emotion as anxiety and fear, but it is a more violent emotion and it is often more abrupt in its arrival. Also, whereas fear (*kong*) causes *qi* to descend, shock or fright (*jing*) makes *qi* become chaotic in its movements. It spreads *qi*. This means that when a person is exposed to shock or a fright, their *qi* will move chaotically in all directions simultaneously. This can easily be felt if you get a sudden shock. This can result in the body being physically moved by the chaotic *qi*. We can literally jump up from the seat. The chaotic movement of *qi* can also cause a person simultaneously to sweat (outward movement of *qi*), urinate or defecate (downward movement of *qi*) and jump up (upward movement of *qi*). This chaotic movement of *qi* will especially dissipate Heart *qi*. The shock can be so powerful that Heart *qi* has difficulty congregating again. This is seen, for example, in post-traumatic stress syndrome, where the person has been exposed to a very violent experience.

Powerful shocks also draw on a person's reserves when their Kidney *jing* is instantly transformed into *qi* and *shen*. It enables them to act quickly and deal with the situation, but it will also weaken their Kidney *jing*. Extreme sports, etc., where people deliberately seek an adrenaline kick, are therefore not a good idea, because these activities consume Kidney *jing*.

Oppression, anguish, obsession and restraint (you)

You is difficult to translate and has been translated differently into English by various authors. To make the confusion worse, *you* is also translated to the same words in English that are attributed to *bei* and *si* by some authors. For example, Giovanni Maciocia (2009, p.611) translates *you* as worry. I have chosen to follow Father Claude Larre and Elisabeth Rochat de la Vallee's interpretation (1996, pp.145–149). They believe that *you* includes a pronounced aspect of oppression, not necessarily that there is a suppression of a particular emotion, but more that the emotion is so overwhelming and powerful that it is in itself oppressive. *You* intensifies the effect of several of the emotions. Other translations of *you* could be obsessiveness or anguish. Obsession is something that is worse than worry and speculation. A person who overthinks and worries tends to have churning thoughts, but in obsessiveness the person cannot rid themselves of these thoughts, which then overshadow everything.

The dynamic of *you* restricts the free movement of *yang qi* in the organ. This will particularly affect the Spleen, Lung and Heart, but it is something that can affect all organs. This will have an amplifying effect on the other six emotions.

As written in the introduction to this section, the seven emotions can be interpreted as being 'primary' emotions, which all other emotions contain varying proportions of in the same way as all colours are created from the three primary colours. What is important when trying to identify the emotional aspects of a disorder's aetiology is to try to understand how other emotions relate to the seven emotions and what *qi* dynamics this emotion therefore will have.

Some of the most typical emotions that many of the clients who we meet are affected by are guilt, shame, desire, envy, contempt, anger and hatred, as well as mental-emotional conditions such as stress. I will not discuss these emotions and how they affect *qi*, which organs they relate to, etc., as this would only be my own subjective assessment. The enduring strength of Chinese medicine theories is that they are a consensus of knowledge that has been accumulated over a period of several hundred years by thousands of practitioners. Instead, I will recommend that the reader assesses each emotion individually that a patient describes and decide what primary emotions they think it consists of. This is especially important, as there can be a significant difference in the interpretations of the same words that different people use to describe their emotional state. Let us take guilt as an example. Guilt can comprise of many different emotional elements. There can be aspects of speculation and worry when the person constantly speculates over certain words they have spoken or over their actions. There may be aspects of anger towards themselves, because they cannot undo something that has been done. There can be a frustration over not being able to act so that they can make things right again. There may be sorrow in their guilt, because they deeply regret their words or actions. There may be lack of joy or there may be fear and anxiety, as they may be scared that what they have done may become public knowledge, with consequences for their reputation or career. This one emotion or state of mind – guilt – can comprise all these emotions and more, in varying amounts. Guilt though will mean something different from person to person and from situation to situation. This means that we cannot unequivocally say which organs these emotions will affect or what their *qi* dynamic is.

THE MISCELLANEOUS
AETIOLOGICAL FACTORS

This category of aetiological factors was originally called 'neither internal nor external' causes of disease. This category includes all the aetiological factors that are neither climatic nor emotional. This means that this category is very broad and encompassing. Some of the most important causes of disease are to be found in this category. These are the factors that relate to diet and lifestyle. This is because these two areas are often involved in the generation of many patterns of imbalance, and also because it is in these areas that patients themselves can make changes that will have a positive impact on their lives. This means that things like diet and motion can go from being aetiological factors to being part of the treatment.

The miscellaneous aetiological factors

- constitution
- diet
- sexual activity
- overexertion
- lack of rest
- exercise and physical activity
- physical trauma
- incorrect treatment
- incorrect medication
- parasites, poisoning, insect bites and snakebites

Constitution

The constitution that a person is born with will have a determining influence on how their health is throughout their life. It is a person's starting point in life. Most people are lucky and are born with a strong, healthy constitution. Unfortunately, there are others whose constitution is not as strong. This can manifest as congenital disorders and illnesses, developmental problems or simply having a tendency to become ill easily. A person's constitution is determined by the state of their *jing*. *Jing* is what bone, cartilage, teeth, hair, semen, ova, etc. are created from, and also what will determine the development through the seven- and eight-year cycles of women and men. *Jing* is the pre-heavenly root of *qi*, and the entire production of the vital substances is dependent on it. A person with a weak *jing* will therefore tend to develop *xu* conditions in general and will easily be negatively affected by *xie qi*.

There are three things that will have an impact on the state of a person's *jing*.

- The condition of the parents' *jing* at conception.

- The mother's health during pregnancy.

- Lifestyle after birth.

The condition of the parents' jing at conception

The pre-heavenly *jing* that a person is born with is created by the merging of the parents' *jing* at the moment of conception. If one or both of the parents' *jing* was weak at this time, it will result in the pre-heavenly *jing* being weak.

The following factors can result in the parents' *jing* being weak.

- The parents themselves were *jing xu*, i.e. their own *jing* was weak.

- The parents were too old. The older we get, the greater the reduction in the quantity and quality of the *jing*.

- The parents were in poor health at the point of conception.

- The parents were affected by alcohol or drugs at the moment of conception.

The mother's health during pregnancy

The mother's health during pregnancy will have a great impact on the pre-heavenly *jing*, because it is from the mother that the foetus receives nourishment.

The following factors may have importance for pre-heavenly *jing* during pregnancy.

- The mother is sick and her health is poor.

- The mother is overstrained, works too hard or is stressed.

- The mother is affected by substances such as drugs, tobacco or alcohol.

Lifestyle after birth

Even if a person is born with a weak *jing*, they can optimise the *jing* they have through diet, *qi gong*, breathing exercises, meditation and sexual practices and by ensuring that they do not strain their *jing* more than necessary. Conversely, even if a person is born with strong *jing*, it can be weakened through poor lifestyle, which taxes *jing*.

Jing diminishes through the years, because *jing* is at the root of the post-heavenly *qi* and because it is lost through ejaculations and ovulation.

Jing is weakened by:

- using more *qi* than is produced on a daily basis

- not getting enough rest, especially when the body has been strained, for example by overwork or illness

- stress

- ejaculations and ovulations

- births

- drugs.

A weak *jing* can manifest with weak bones, weak teeth, thin hair or baldness, causing fertility problems. Weak *jing* will also be apparent in a person's medical history. *Jing xu* can also be seen in a tongue that is sunken at the rear and a pulse that is weak in the rear (*chi*) positions and in the deepest level.

Diet

Diet is an extremely important factor in the development of patterns of imbalance. Diet can be the primary cause, as well as being a contributing factor that exacerbates already existing tendencies. Diet can have an impact in several ways – through the amount of food that is consumed, how the food is consumed and the food's energetic qualities. The modern world has also added further complicating and aggravating factors in the form of food additives and the chemicals used in the production of food.

The amount of food

The amount of the food eaten is an aetiological factor if too much or too little food is consumed.

Too much food can be a burden on the Stomach and Spleen *qi* and can lead to accumulation of Phlegm and Dampness in the body, as well as food stagnation.

Too little food is usually more of a problem in some developing countries, where poverty can result in people not eating enough. In the first instance, too little food will lead to *qi xu* and *xue xu*. In the longer term, the lack of nutrition can lead to *yin xu* and *jing xu*. In the developed world there are not the same levels of poor nutrition due to poverty as there are in the developing world. There are, however, groups in the population who do not eat enough, as well as people on a low income. This is especially the case with people who suffer from eating disorders and people who follow strict dietary regimes. Furthermore, there are many people who, even though they eat large quantities of food, eat food that contains very little nutrition.

The way the food is consumed

It is not only the quantity of food that is of importance, but how the food is consumed is also significant.

Eating too quickly and not chewing the food enough will create food stagnation and strain the Stomach and Spleen *qi*. Constant consumption of food all day long will also strain the Stomach and Spleen *qi*. The optimal way of eating is to consume regular, small meals, rather than constantly snacking or consuming only one or two large meals. Constantly eating snacks, etc. will mean that the Stomach is never emptied, which weakens both the Stomach and Spleen *qi*. Consuming large amounts of food in one meal is not good either. It will result in the food stagnating and the Spleen will have difficulty transforming it. Eating late in the evening can also lead to food stagnation, as the food is not transformed whilst a person is sleeping.

Not chewing the food enough will mean that the food is not sufficiently broken down. Chewing breaks down the physical structure of the food, making it easier for the Spleen to transform it.

Eating whilst working, watching television, reading or using the computer is very common. On the other hand, it is not something that is to be recommended. It will have two negative consequences. First, having the mental focus somewhere other than on the food itself will mean there is less Spleen *qi* to digest the food, as the Spleen *qi* will also be used to digest information. Second, if the body is misaligned because the person is not sitting upright with a straight back whilst eating, this will impede the downward movement of *qi* from the Stomach.

Incorrect and inappropriate food

The individual foods in themselves are not intrinsically negative. They are only a source of imbalance when their energetic dynamic is detrimental for the person who eats them and when the dynamic does not correspond to the seasonal and the external climatic environment. This means that food that is beneficial for one person or is beneficial to eat, for example, in the summer or in a warm climate may well have a negative effect on another person or, in the example above, when eaten in the winter or if the climate is cold and damp. It is also important that the variety of food consumed is broad and comprehensive, so that all the organs are nourished, whilst also nourishing and tonifying *qi*, *xue*, *jinye*, *yin* and *yang*.

Both the energetic qualities that the food has and its temperature and consistency determine whether a foodstuff will have a positive or negative impact on a person's physiology. Foodstuffs have inherent energetic dynamics. All foodstuffs have an energetic temperature that is independent of its physical temperature. Food that has a Hot energy can create or aggravate Heat conditions and injure *yin*. Similarly, food with a cold energetic dynamic can injure *yang* and can create Cold in the Stomach and the Intestines. The physical temperature is also important. Food that is physically cold and has not been prepared will be a burden on Spleen *yang* and, to some extent, Kidney *yang*. Boiling, steaming, frying and baking food will make it energetically warmer and it will therefore be easier for the Spleen to transform the food, because its structure is already in the process of being broken down. This means that the consumption of raw vegetables, salad, fruit, etc. can weaken Spleen *qi* and Spleen *yang*.

All foodstuffs have specific flavours that determine their physiological effects in the body and which organs they affect. Foodstuffs can therefore have both positive or negative influences, depending on the imbalances a given person has.

Many foodstuffs, however, have qualities that mean it is generally best not to consume too much of them. This is especially important if a person is Spleen *qi xu* or Spleen *yang xu* or if there is Dampness, Damp-Heat, Phlegm or Stomach Fire. This is because the Spleen and Stomach, unlike the other organs, are affected every time a person eats. Foods that typically place a burden on the Spleen and create Dampness and Phlegm are dairy products, sweets, soft drinks, wheat, bananas, nuts and too many raw vegetables. Food and liquids that have a hot energy will aggravate Stomach Fire.

Alcohol and coffee are not foodstuffs, but they are substances that many people consume regularly, and unfortunately both often create and exacerbate imbalances in the body. Alcohol is generally Hot and produces Dampness. Some forms of alcohol are hotter than others and some are more Damp-producing than others. Red wine, for example, is hotter than white wine, and whisky has a very hot energy, whilst beer has a tendency to create a lot of Dampness. All things being equal, this will mean that regular or excessive consumption of alcohol can create Damp-Heat, Phlegm and Fire.

Coffee is very stimulating and affects the Heart directly. At the same time coffee releases Kidney *yang*. This means that coffee places a great strain on Kidney and Heart *yin* and to some extent Kidney *jing*.

In the books *The Art of Diagnosis with Chinese Medicine* (Ching 2009)[2] and *Acupuncture and the Treatment of Disease* (Ching 2005) there is a more in-depth analysis of the individual foods and their energetic characteristics and how these impact on our physiology and pathology.

Additives and chemicals

A lot of the food that people consume has been exposed to chemicals in the manufacturing process as artificial fertilisers and pesticides during the cultivation of vegetables, in the feed of livestock or as medicine or growth promoters, etc. in the production of meat. Furthermore, there is a widespread use of preservatives, dyes, flavouring agents, etc. in the production of the final products. These substances will inevitably have an impact on people's physiology and imbalances. How it affects the body will depend on the individual substance. By looking at the recorded adverse reactions and the symptoms these substances can provoke, you can get an idea of how they affect the body from the perspective of Chinese medicine.

Sexual activity

Chinese medical texts have always placed great emphasis on sexual activity, both as an aetiological factor and in the recommendations given in connection with treating various patterns of imbalance. This in part reflects the influence Daoism has had on Chinese medicine, where the need to protect and nourish the *jing* is a prerequisite for achieving a higher level of consciousness. It is, however, also because it has been observed that the loss of *jing* by having too much sex has a damaging effect on both the Kidneys and the production of the vital substances.

Men lose *jing* each time they have an ejaculation. This means that frequent ejaculations will weaken Kidney *jing*. There is not the same problem for women. Some authors though are of the opinion that women also lose *jing* when orgasming.

How much and how often men should ejaculate without this being a burden on their *jing* is dependent on their age and general health, as well as the season. The older a man is and the poorer his health, the less he should ejaculate. The recommendations vary slightly from book to book.

Giovanni Maciocia (2005) quotes from *The Classic of the Simple Girl*,[3] that when a male is 15 years old he can ejaculate twice a day, if he is in good health, and daily, if his health is weak. As he ages the frequency of how often he should have sex decreases. When he is 30 years old and is in good health, he can still have sex on a daily basis, but only every second day if his health is poor. By the time he is 50, the frequency is down to every fifth day in good health and every ten if his health is poor.

Generally, men should avoid sex when they are ill or physically exhausted. This is because sex will further weaken their *qi*.

Men can reduce the negative consequences of losing *jing* through ejaculation by cultivating Daoist or tantric sexual practices, where an orgasm is achieved without the release of semen. Using techniques to prevent ejaculation, however, can in itself also become a source of imbalance. If the techniques are incorrect it can lead to *qi* stagnations in the lower *jiao*.

Viagra and other medicines that are used to treat impotence are not recommended in Chinese medicine. First, many men are impotent because of Kidney *xu* conditions, especially Kidney *yang xu*. Being enabled to have sex means these men will expend more *jing* and *yang* from the Kidneys. In addition, Viagra's warming and *yang* energy can create and exacerbate conditions of *shi* Heat, ascending *yang* or Wind and it will injure *yin*.

Jing is also weakened through sexual arousal. This is because *mingmen* flares up during sexual arousal and this will in itself consume *jing*, though not to the same degree as ejaculation.

Too little sex can also be a cause of imbalance. Achieving orgasms is a very good way of moving stagnant *qi*. Unfortunately, Liver *qi* stagnation is often a contributory factor that prevents some women from achieving an orgasm and some men from having an erection. The stagnation of Liver *qi* will be further worsened if this in itself then becomes a source of frustration for them.

Sex during menstruation is not recommended in Chinese medicine. This is because the upward movement of *qi* that results when *mingmen* is activated by sexual arousal, as well as the upwards energetic and physical movement of the male genitals, opposes the natural downward movement of menstrual blood from the Uterus. This can be a contributing factor to *xue* stagnations in the Uterus.

Sex at an early age can damage *chong mai* and *ren mai* in girls.

Overexertion

Overexertion is a broad concept and could in reality also include excessive sexual activity, because overexertion is all the situations where a person overuses the resources that they have in their body. Overexertion is when more *qi* is expended than the body is able to produce at that time. This means that overexertion is both different from person to person and different from time to time. When we are very young or when we are old, the body is more easily overtaxed. There is a much better production of *qi* when a person is between the ages of 18 and 30 than there is before or after. This means that it will require more to overstrain a person in this age group than a person who is younger or older. There are, however, differences dependent on many factors other than age. If a person has just been ill, is undernourished, hasn't slept, etc., then there will be less *qi* present to enable the body to perform its functions.

The body can be strained by both physical and mental activities. Some activities are of course more burdensome than others. The more tiring an activity is, the more *qi*-consuming it is. Something that is of great importance is the balance between activity and rest. The more physically and mentally active a person is, the more rest they should have. There should, as always, be a balance between *yin* (rest) and *yang* (activity). Unfortunately, there are a great many people who get too little rest. This is because they are active in both their working hours and leisure time. Activities in leisure time can be physical, such as sport, fitness and physical training, but also watching television, sitting in front of the computer or playing games on a smartphone are also burdensome and cannot be classified as resting and relaxing. Television, and especially computers and smartphones, are mentally stimulating. They activate *shen* and thereby consume *qi* and *yin*.

Overexertion of the body will weaken *qi*, *xue* and *yang* in the short term. This is because it is *qi*, *xue* and *yang* that are immediately consumed by physical and mental activity. If the person continues to consume more *qi* and *yang* than they are able to produce through the food they consume and the air they breathe, they will begin to draw on their *yin* and, in the end, their *jing*. This is unfortunately often the case when people 'burn out' and collapse with stress. It is relatively easy for a person who is *yang xu* or *qi xu* due to overwork to recover their strength. In fact, a good holiday will often be enough. When people are *yin xu* and *jing xu* though, it is a lot more difficult and it will take a very long time. This is also the reason why many people who have burnt out due to stress, even though they feel rejuvenated after they have taken leave from work and relaxed for a month or two, experience that their stress symptoms and fatigue return almost immediately on returning to work. Stress is unfortunately on the increase in modern societies due to some of the above-mentioned factors.

Certain physical activities can be onerous on specific organs or areas of the body – for example, lifting heavy objects weakens the Kidneys; sitting burdens the Spleen.

Constant, repetitive movements can both stagnate and weaken *qi* and *xue* in a certain part of the body. This is seen in repetitive strain injuries such as tennis elbow, computer arm, etc.

Lack of rest

As stated in the previous section, there must be a balance between rest and activity. The more active and *yang* a person is, the more rest and *yin* there should also be. This means that it is important to really relax sometimes and to completely gear down. This is something that acupuncture is really good at doing. A very beneficial aspect of acupuncture treatments is that the client is forced to lie down in an extremely relaxed state for half an hour.

It is also important that people get sufficient sleep and that they sleep at the right times. It is beneficial in relation to the Chinese horary clock that people go to sleep before 11 pm. This is because *xue* returns to the Liver, where it is stored whilst we rest and sleep. Furthermore, the night is the *yin* period, where it is natural to be passively resting and *yin*. Unfortunately, due to the invention of electric lighting, it is now possible to reverse day and night. Previously it was natural and normal to be *yang* active during the day and *yin* passive during the night. This can now be reversed, so that we can be both physically and mentally active at night. This puts a strain on our *yin* and consumes our *yang*. It is unfortunately a necessity for the functioning of society that some people have to work at night. This will, though, be a burden on their *yin*.

Exercise and physical activity

Exercise and physical activity can become sources of imbalances when there is too much and too little of them. Physical activity is necessary to support the circulation of *qi*. People who lead a sedentary lifestyle and who do not get enough physical movement can often have a tendency to have stagnations of *qi*, *xue* and Phlegm. Of course, how much exercise they need varies from one person to the next depending on, amongst other things, how good their *qi* circulation is to start with. It is not only people who are very sedentary who need physical activity. People with stagnations of *qi*, in particular Liver *qi*, as well as Phlegm and *xue* stagnations, will find that their symptoms are often worse when they are physically inactive. The more people tend towards being stagnated, the more physical activity they need. This need for activity however has to be weighed up against the detrimental effects that too much exercise can have. As we have just seen in the section on overexertion, excessive physical activity can weaken the body's *qi*, *xue* and *yang*. Some people 'self-medicate' their Liver *qi* stagnation by excessive training, running, swimming, sport, fitness or similar physical activities. They need the physical exercise to feel good. If they don't train, they immediately start to feel tired, lethargic, irritable and physically and emotionally tense. The problem is though that the excessive training does not treat the underlying problem – *qi* stagnation – just the manifestations of it. In fact, patterns such as Liver *qi* stagnation often get worse in the long term because of it. This is because excessive training can weaken Liver *xue*, so the Liver becomes more rigid and thereby creates more Liver *qi* stagnation, and a vicious circle arises.

Poor posture, sitting hunched forwards with a curved back and sitting with a twisted body or in awkward positions can lead to stagnations of *qi*.

Physical trauma

Physical injuries usually result in stagnations of *qi*, *xue* and *jinye* in the local area, so the area is sore, painful and often swollen. The stagnation of *qi*, *xue* and *jinye* can also generate Heat in the area. This will result in the area being red and feeling warm on palpation. The stagnation of *qi* and *xue* may not always be a local problem. It can also block the channel so there are disturbances further along the path of the channel.

Even if the injury is old, there will often still be stagnations of *qi*, *xue* and Phlegm in the area. In addition, there will also be a poorer circulation of *wei qi* in the area. This will result in the area being more susceptible to invasions of exogenous *xie qi*, which will in turn lead to additional stagnations in the area.

Operations are also included in the category of physical trauma. This is because each time an incision is made into the body, it will stagnate *qi* and *xue*. Scar tissue in fact bears many of the characteristics of stagnated *xue*.

Burns, frostbite and other physical damage to tissues are also a part of this category.

Emotional traumas are classified as being amongst the internal aetiological factors.

Incorrect treatment

This category has traditionally included the imbalances that will have arisen from the use of herbal medicine. These imbalances will arise because either the medicine had a decidedly negative effect on the patient or, even if a prescription acted as intended, there was an adverse reaction. This is one of the major differences between Chinese herbal medicine and Western conventional medicine. In Western pharmaceutical medicine side effects are accepted, and sometimes even expected, as an unfortunate consequence of the treatment. In Chinese medicine, the premise is that if the patient does not get better or if there are side effects, then there are three possibilities: the diagnosis is incorrect; the diagnosis is correct, but the recipe or the dosage of the herbs is incorrect; or there are other imbalances that have not been diagnosed, which are relevant to the treatment.

Acupuncture is more forgiving and it is much more difficult to create problems from an incorrect treatment. Incorrect acupuncture will usually just be ineffective or make the client feel fatigued for a couple of days. The only real form of incorrect treatment with acupuncture is physical damage to organs, blood vessels or nerves caused by the physical structure of the needle.

Some people are of the opinion that moxa can exacerbate conditions of Heat in the body.

Incorrect medication

This is in fact a sub-category of incorrect treatment. I have, however, chosen to discuss incorrect medications as a separate category. This is because many of the patients who we see are medicated with both pharmaceutical medicine and various types of food supplements. Unfortunately, it is beyond the scope of this book to review the various categories of medicine and the various forms of food supplements with regard to the negative consequences they may have. Medicine is by its very nature something that will have a physiological effect on the body. That is why people use it. As I have written above, diagnosis, medication and dosage must match each other, but as I also wrote, adverse reactions are an accepted necessity in many Western pharmaceutical drugs. In order to gain an understanding of the energetic properties of a medicine, and thus be able to gauge how it affects the body when seen from a Chinese medical perspective, you can look at the symptoms that the drug treats and what symptoms it creates as a side effect. Both things will say something about the energetic properties of the substance. Something else you can do with individual clients is to look at their symptom history and see what changes, both for the better and for the worse, there have been whilst taking the medication.

Food supplements such as vitamins and minerals also have energetic characteristics. These will again have an influence on the body's physiology. As with pharmaceutical medicine, we can analyse the beneficial and negative effects that these substances have to gain an idea of their *qi* dynamics.

A second area of incorrect medication is the use and misuse of illicit substances, such as cannabis, cocaine, amphetamine, heroin, LSD, ecstasy, designer drugs, etc. Each of these substances will again have different energetic characteristics, which it will be possible to deduce from the desired effect and the side effects they may have. Many of the illicit substances that people take have an effect on Heart *qi* and *shen*. They will often have an opening, but also a dissipative effect on *shen* and Heart *qi*. Long-term usage will often weaken Heart *qi* and *shen*, whilst at the same time draining *jing* and Kidney *qi*, which is the root of *shen*.

Alcohol is spicy and Hot in its energy; it creates Stomach and Liver Fire, as well as Damp-Heat and Phlegm.

Coffee is spicy, warming and spreading. Coffee weakens Kidney *yin* and Kidney *yang*, whilst over-activating Heart *yang*.

Tobacco is spicy, Warm and drying. Smoking tobacco will therefore injure Lung *yin* and create Phlegm-Heat and Toxic-Heat in the Lung.

Parasites, poisoning, insect bites and snakebites

This category includes the damage that insects and snakes can cause, as well as parasites and the ingestion of poison. It is again beyond the scope of this book to review the energetics of the various types of insect bites, snakebites, poisons, etc. When you know a person has been exposed to any of the above, you can observe which symptoms and signs it has resulted in and from these deduce its energetic qualities.

NOTES

Acknowledgements

1. This is in fact a requoting of Bernard of Chartres, who lived in the twelfth century. Bernard of Chartres wrote: '…we [the Moderns] are like dwarves perched on the shoulders of giants [the Ancients], and thus we are able to see more and farther than the latter. And this is not at all because of the acuteness of our sight or the stature of our body, but because we are carried aloft and elevated by the magnitude of the giants' (Troyan 2004).
2. Burnet rose.

Part 1

1. It might be appropriate to quote Chairman Mao here. When asked about the influence and consequences that the French Revolution had had on the history and development of China, he said, 'It is too early to comment on.'
2. I consistently use the translation 'Five Phases' instead of Five Elements, which is often used to translate the term '*wu xing*'. This is because *xing* in Chinese has the meaning of transformation, movement and something that is changing and not static. Element is a more Western concept that comes from Greek philosophy and medicine.
3. This is not a negative nothingness, but a nothingness that precedes and embraces everything. It is beyond form. It is something that is hard to fathom, because our minds are rooted in dualistic thinking – that something either is or is not.
4. *Dao De Jing* (*Tao Te Ching*) is accredited to Lao Zi.
5. The *Yangming* channel being an exception.
6. There are several types of *qi*. Some of them are mentioned here, but they will be discussed in detail in the chapter on *qi*. *Ying qi* or 'nutritious' *qi* is *yin* compared with *wei qi* or 'defensive' *qi*. This is because *ying qi* nourishes, which is a *yin* quality, and *ying qi* flows in the channels together with *xue*. *Wei qi* on the other hand protects, which is a *yang* quality, and *wei qi* flows just below the skin, which is more exterior than the channels. Both *ying qi* and *wei qi* are *yang* compared with, for example, *gu qi* or 'food' *qi* because *gu qi* is coarse and unprocessed, i.e. is potential, whereas *ying qi* and *wei qi* are a manifestation of this potential.
7. Remember that although *xue* is *yin* compared with *qi*, it is *yang* in relation to food, drink, etc., because it is active and is a manifestation of the potential that the diet contains.
8. A Chinese medicine diagnosis is based on the symptoms and signs that are manifesting. Symptoms are changes in bodily functions, such as diarrhoea, constipation, vomiting and so on. Signs are changes that will not be defined as a symptom of Western medicine. A sign could, for example, be that a person talks rapidly or that they have red cheekbones and their skin feels warm.
9. The various forms of pathological *qi* and the names of organs are both capitalised, to distinguish them from the general definition of the word. In this example, Heat, with a capital H, is a pathological condition that manifests with certain characteristics.
10. *Xu* can be translated as lack of emptiness, deficiency, non-presence, a vacuum.
11. It is important to remember that this and the following examples are included to illustrate the difference between *xu* and *shi* conditions. There will most often be other signs and symptoms not described here; furthermore the symptoms and signs listed here will not be seen every time.
12. *Shi* translates as full, excess, surplus.

13. Daoists had long observed phenomena such as that if you had two string instruments standing in the same room and they were tuned to the same tone, you would be able to hear the same tone emitting from the one instrument when the equivalent tone was struck on the other instrument.

14. Heaven in Chinese cosmology is not heaven as in the Judaic-Christian understanding, but more the universe above us.

15. This understanding of the phases could sometimes be taken quite literally. When Emperor Qin Shihuangdi came to power and founded the Qin dynasty, he understood himself as being a Water or Black Emperor, because he conquered the Zhou dynasty, which understood itself as ruling through the power and principles of Fire. Everything in the realm now had to be arranged in accordance with the principles of Water. For example, it was not enough that all the flags and uniforms had to be black – anything of any importance should be six in number (which is the number of the Water Phase) or six units long. The judicial system was constructed with harsh penalties and strict discipline, in relation to Qin's interpretation of the Water Phase.

16. Japanese and Vietnamese acupuncture, on the other hand, are much more centred around a Five Phase approach to treatment, where specific points on channels are related to specific elements/phases and are thereby used to create a balance between the various phases. There are also English-language schools that define themselves as being Five Element acupuncture schools. Again, their treatments are based on a Five Phase diagnostic approach and subsequent therapeutic use of the points according to their Five Phase dynamics.

17. Either late summer or no season, because Earth is in the centre. Some sources are of the opinion that the Earth Phase is the transitory period between all the seasons.

18. There is variance in the animals listed in different books. I have used as my source two of the oldest references that are to be found in *Huang Di Nei Jing – Su Wen* and *Huainanzi*, but even here there is a difference in the animals in the Wood and Metal Phases.

19. The Lung is singular in Chinese medicine. The Kidneys are the only organ that is plural.

20. The numbers one to five are called *sheng* numbers and the numbers five to nine are called *cheng*. *Sheng* means to create, whilst *cheng* means to take the form or to be complete. Earth is both five and ten.

21. Translation due to be published by Singing Dragon in 2017 as *The Art of Diagnosis in Chinese Medicine.*

Part 2

1. This is confirmed by Western research. Studies have shown that a unit of alcohol a day is enough to reduce your chance of a successful IVF treatment by a fifth. It is interesting that this applies to both men and women. See, for example, Klonoff-Cohen, Lam-Kruglick and Gonzalez (2003).

2. The eight extraordinary vessels will be discussed later in the section on channels (page 224).

3. In addition to the twelve internal organs, there are six so-called extraordinary organs – Uterus, Gall Bladder, Blood Vessels, Bones, Bone Marrow and Brain.

4. Interestingly adrenaline, which is produced by adrenal glands that are located on the kidneys in Western medicine physiology, has many features in common with *mingmen*.

5. *San jiao* is an organ that has function but not form. *San jiao* will be described in the chapter on *zangfu* organs.

6. One translation of *jiao* is cavity. The body is divided into three cavities – *san jiao*. The lower *jiao* is the area between the navel and groin area.

7. The upper *jiao* is the area between the diaphragm and the neck.

8. The *yin/yang* relationship between *wei qi* and *ying qi* can also be seen in the origin of their characters and names in Chinese. *Wei* means 'defensive', and this can be interpreted as the troops that protect the realm. *Ying* can be translated as 'camp', and in the character there is an aspect of a camp fire. *Ying* will be seen as the supply troops who feed, nourish and care for the troops.

9. I have throughout the book capitalised the first letter when referring to the various forms of *xie qi*, as is also the case with the internal organs and physiological substances. This is done to differentiate the term from the Western concept of the term.

10. Zhang Jing-Yue writes in *Lei Jing* (*Systemic Classification of Nei Jing*) (1624): '*Jin* and *ye* are the same, but they have a *yin* and *yang* differentiation: *Jin* is the pure aspect of *ye* while *ye* is the murky aspect of *Jin*. *Jin* can become sweat and move in and out of the exterior tissues, therefore it is *yang*. *Ye* flows into the bones and nourishes the Brain and Bone Marrow, therefore it is *yin*.'

11. There is a divergence in some books in relation to whether it is the pure or impure part of body fluids that is sent from the Small Intestine to the Urinary Bladder. Giovanni Maciocia writes that it is the pure part that is sent down to the Urinary Bladder. In the first edition of *The Foundations of Chinese Medicine* (1989) he is not completely consistent in this description. Several other sources, in particular Steve Clavey (2003), describe the process, as I have done above, where the impure fluids are sent down to the Urinary Bladder and the pure fluids are sent upwards through the body. To me this seems a more logical explanation. First, pure fluids are consistently sent upwards and impure fluids downwards. Second, there is no mixing of pure and impure fluids in the Urinary Bladder in this model.

12. TCM stands for Traditional Chinese Medicine. TCM is not in fact 'traditional', but a mongrel, created by need in post-revolutionary China. China was faced with an acute lack of medical care after the liberation and the Maoists were therefore forced to use the resources at their disposal. Chinese medicine had been seen as being superstitious, backward and unscientific. It was not only the Maoists who had this point of view; Chinese medicine had already been as good as banned by the previous Kuomingtang regime, which had closed all public and private schools that taught Classical Chinese Medicine, with the exception of three institutions. Western medicine was seen by the Kuomintang government as being modern, scientific and superior.

13. Some Daoist traditions developed various sexual techniques in which the man held back his semen when orgasming. The semen is created from *jing*. Every time a man ejaculates, he loses some of his *jing*. By losing *jing*, the material basis for *shen* is also lost. By holding the semen back, the man is thus able to send *jing* up to the Heart to be transformed to *shen* and thereby to consciousness.

Part 3

1. It is popularly believed that in the past in China there was little knowledge of the body's internal anatomy, because the body was considered sacred and therefore surgery and dissection were not permitted. Unfortunately, this is a myth. The Chinese had, amongst other things, a barbaric form of execution, where the organs were removed one by one, whilst the prisoner was still alive. This took place over an extended period of time. It required an extremely good anatomical knowledge and surgical skills in order to be able to carry out this death penalty. It was general practice for doctors to observe these executions, and in this way they would have learnt about the body's internal structure. The battlefield was another place where doctors would gain an in-depth knowledge of what the inside of the body consisted of. In addition, the internal anatomy of other mammals would be apparent when these animals were slaughtered for food. That the Chinese chose to treat the body with other techniques than surgery and that they developed an energetic physiological model is due to other reasons.

2. Historically, there were originally only five *zang* organs. The Pericardium was originally not regarded as a separate organ from the Heart. Later texts assign the Pericardium its own individual place amongst the *zang* organs, but it has limited importance in the diagnosis of patterns of imbalance. The Pericardium channel, however, has always had as much importance as the other channels.

3. The body's physiology is characterised by mutual relationships. All production of post-heaven *qi* is dependent on *jing* and *yuan qi*, but these are at the same time nourished by the surplus from the post-heaven *qi*, after they have carried out their functions in the body.

4. An interesting observation is that humans are the only animal that has to cook its food. One explanation is that when we walked on all fours, like other animals, *mingmen*'s position enabled its transformative power to convert the ingested food in the Stomach to *qi*. As we evolved and began walking upright on

two legs, the fire from *mingmen* began to travel up *du mai* and transformed *jing* to *shen* or to warm the brain, depending on your interpretation. This means that we now have a higher and more developed consciousness but are no longer able to live on a diet of raw food.

5. The Lung has traditionally been referred to in the singular in Chinese medicine, as the two lungs have traditionally been conceived as being the same organ. This is because an organ is more defined by its function than its form. Traditionally, there has been no difference between the two lungs' functions and therefore they have been conceived as being the same organ. This is in contrast to the Kidneys. The left and right Kidney were originally conceived as being two separate organs – first as the Kidney and *mingmen* and later as Kidney *yin* and Kidney *yang*. In modern texts they are conceived as being the same organ, but also in the plural, rather than the singular, which is the case for all the other organs.

6. *Xie* Heat can damage *yin* in the throat and make the voice hoarse; Phlegm can make the voice gravelly or slurred. The Heart controls the tongue and thereby a person's ability to express themselves. For example, when we are nervous we stutter. This shows that the Heart has lost control of the voice. The Liver ensures that *qi* flows freely and without hindrance. If there is Liver *qi* stagnation, the voice can be hard, trimmed and staccato. It can sound like machine gun fire.

7. Traditionally there was no specific distinction between the channels and the blood vessels. In *Huang Di Nei Jing* both names are used to describe the paths of *qi* and *xue* in the body.

8. In sexual stimulation, *hun* is more stimulated by images, pictures and fantasies. *Po* is stimulated through physical touch and stimulation.

9. *Huang Di Nei Jing – Ling Shu*, chapter 8: *Bing jing er chu ru zhe wei zhi po* (*Po* is that which follows the *jing* in its exiting and entering). This indicates that *jing* and *po* have a similar relationship to the *hun* and *shen*, which follow each other in their 'exiting and entering' – *Sui shen wang lai zhe wei zhe wei zhi hun* (that which faithfully follows *shen* in its coming and going indicates *hun*).

10. Some say that *po* enters and exits the body through UB 42 *Pohu* and *hun* via UB 47 *Hunmen*.

11. One of the strategies recommended in the book *The Art of War* (c. 512 BCE) to overcome an enemy whose armies are larger and more powerful than your own is to make the enemy general angry. By making him angry, it will cloud his vision and his actions will be ill considered.

12. *Taiyi Jinhua Zongzhi*, chapter 2: '*Hun* resides in the eyes during the day and resides in the Liver at night. When *hun* is in the eyes, it sees. When *hun* resides in the Liver, it dreams. Dreams are the *hun*'s meanderings through the nine Heavens and nine Earths.' Tang Zhong Hai's view: 'When *hun* travels to the eyes, they can see.'

13. *Huang Di Nei Jing – Ling Shu*, chapter 8: *Sui shen wang lai zhe wei zhe wei zhi hun* (That which faithfully follows the *shen* coming and going indicates *hun*).

14. In Chinese medicine there has traditionally been no clear distinction between the channel and the blood vessels.

15. The Chinese character for the Heart is different to the other organs. Whereas the other *zang* organs have a radical for flesh in their characters, the Heart does not. This indicates the Heart is different from the other *zang* organs – that it is not physical.

16. *Huang Di Nei Jing – Ling Shu*, chapter 8: *Bing jing er chu ru zhe wei zhi po* (*Po* is that which follows *jing* in its exiting and entering); *Sui shen wang lai zhe wei zhe wei zhi hun* (That which faithfully follows *shen* in its entering and exiting indicates *hun*).

17. For a fuller discussion and explanation see Larre and Rochat de la Vallee (1992).

18. Professor Wang Ju Yi believes that the difference between the Heart and the Pericardium can perhaps be understood as the Pericardium controlling the more mechanical and muscular aspects of the Heart's beating and functionality, whereas the Heart is seen more in the electrical control of the heartbeat.

19. There is a very good article on this subject by Qu Lifang and Mary Garvey (2001) in the *Journal of Chinese Medicine*.

Part 4

1. In an older understanding of the *qi* dynamic in the body, *qi* travels centripetally in the channels and not as a circuit, i.e. *qi* flows from the fingers and toes in towards the centre. Man was considered to be the link between Heaven and Earth, and *qi* entered into the body through the tips of the fingers and toes, flowing inwards to the centre of the body. This is one of the explanations of why the dynamic of the so-called *shu*-transport points is sometimes the opposite of the dynamic of the channel's direction. This will be discussed later in the chapter on *shu*-transport points (page 398).

2. The different location of *yangming* and *shaoyang* is due to the fact that 'Diagnosis according to the six stages' is an analysis that charts a pathological development in the body. It is not a physiological model, such as the one that is being reproduced here. When there is an invasion of *xie qi*, the Stomach and the Large Intestine organs are relatively more superficial and thereby more exposed and vulnerable. The Stomach and the Large Intestine are both in direct contact with the exterior, whereas *shaoyang*'s organs are not. This means that exogenous *xie qi* can much more easily penetrate *yangming*. On the other hand, it is also easier for the body to rid itself of exogenous *xie qi* from *yangming*. The passage from *shaoyang* to the exterior is more limited. This means that exogenous *xie qi* has greater difficulty penetrating here, but also that the body has greater difficulty expelling *xie qi* from here. This is also one of the reasons why *xie qi* can have a tendency to get stuck here. Finally, there is a difference in the relationship between *zheng qi* and *xie qi*, which determines the classification of the stages. *Xie qi* penetrates deeper into the body when it is more powerful than the body's *zheng qi* or when the body is weakened. In *taiyang* and *yangming*, *zheng qi* is still strong and this results in powerful and at times violent reactions in the body. When *xie qi* penetrates *shaoyang*, it is because the body's *zheng qi* is weakened and there will not be the same response.

3. *Cun* is an individual anatomical measurement. There is a specific number of *cun* between different anatomical reference points. There are, for example, sixteen *cun* on the lateral side of the tibia from the middle of the malleolus to the lower edge of the patella. One *cun* is approximately the width of a person's thumb joint.

4. Bob Flaws and Honora Wolfe amongst others.

5. For example, Alex Tiberi.

6. The diagnostic model 'Diagnosis according to the six stages' is described in Ching (2009).

Part 5

1. *Huang Di Nei Jing – Ling Shu*, chapter 29, used a different word, *jie*. *Jie* can be translated as notches on a piece of bamboo, a chapter, a rhythm or a holiday. That is, changes in the basic movement, a change in tone or a break in time. It is where something stops. It provides a potential to stop and alter the current form. *Huang Di Nei Jing – Ling Shu*, chapter 1, states that these *jie* are where *shen qi* moves and comes and goes. They are not the same as the skin, muscles, bones and connective tissue. They are something different and greater than this. They can also be understood as the space in the skin, muscles, bones and connective tissue. Acupuncture can thus create activity in this space in the tissue.

2. *Xue* (acupuncture point) is not the same word as *xue* (Blood). It is pronounced differently and has a completely different character.

3. For a deeper analysis of the word *xue* in Chinese and what an acupuncture point is, the reader is referred to an article by Wilcox (2006) in the *Journal of Chinese Medicine* and *Applied Channel Theory in Chinese Medicine* by Wang and Robertson (2008).

4. Modern medicine textbooks in China often use a different term – *xue wei*. *Xue* is still the same term as described in the main text, but *wei* replaces the word *shu*. *Wei* is a fixed point or place.

5. Claudia Focks quotes Solinas *et al.*, who are of the opinion that the Urinary Bladder *luo*-connecting vessel ascends up the back, over the head and to the nose (Focks 2008, p.248).

6. *Shang* is the fifth tone of the Chinese musical scale. *Shang* is also the tone that resonates with the Metal Phase.

7. *Shang* is the fifth tone of the Chinese musical scale. *Shang* is also the tone that resonates with the Metal Phase.

8. *Shang* is the fifth tone of the Chinese musical scale. *Shang* is also the tone that resonates with the Metal Phase.

9. Both *yi* and *xi* are spontaneous sounds a person can express when being palpated.

10. *Shan* can have three definitions. First, it can be an organ or tissue that protrudes forward or prolapses, e.g. a hernia in Western medicine. Second, it can be an extreme abdominal pain, with simultaneous urinary difficulty or constipation. Finally, it may be a disorder that relates to the external genitalia.

11. *Huang* is the area just below the diaphragm.

12. *Shang* is the fifth tone of the Chinese musical scale.

13. *De qi* is the *qi* reaction that the patient's body has to the presence of the needle.

14. TCM or Traditional Chinese Medicine is a modern version of acupuncture created in the second half of the twentieth century. It is based on classical Chinese acupuncture but is also heavily influenced by modern, Western medicine. TCM is the acupuncture style practised in the majority of mainland China today.

15. *A-shi* points are points that have spontaneously arisen. They are places where *qi* and *xue* have stagnated. *A-shi* points can be located both on a channel or in the surrounding tissue. *A-shi* is the sound that the client expresses when the point is pressed.

16. Signs are things that are not actual symptoms, but signify a change in the body's physiology. This could be the quality of the pulse, the colour of the tongue, the posture, the sound of a person's voice, etc.

17. In 'cross-channel' theory, acupuncture points are selected on the opposite side and in the opposite limb according to where the pain is. These acupuncture points must be located either in a similar area, e.g. if the pain is in the lateral side of the right ankle you will select an equivalent point on the lateral side of the left wrist, or the cross-channel point should be located on the equivalent spot on the same great channel, e.g. St 36 on the left side to treat the area corresponding to LI 10 on the right side, because they are both *yangming* channel points.

Part 6

1. *Qi* in this context is the sum of the body's vital substances and organ systems. It is not *qi* as a specific vital substance.

2. Due to be published by Singing Dragon in 2017 as *The Art of Diagnosis in Chinese Medicine*.

3. Maciocia, G. (2005) *The Foundations of Chinese Medicine, Second Edition.* Edinburgh: Churchill Livingstone, p.274.

REFERENCES

Ching, N. (2005) *Akupunktur og Sygdomsbehandling.* Copenhagen: Klitroseforlaget.

Ching, N. (2009) *Kunsten at Diagnosticere.* Copenhagen: Klitroseforlaget.

Clavey, P. (2003) *Fluid Physiology and Pathology in Traditional Chinese Medicine.* Edinburgh: Churchill Livingstone.

Deadman, P. and Al-Khafaji, M. (1998) *A Manual of Acupuncture.* Hove: Journal of Chinese Medicine Publications.

Focks, C. (2008) *Atlas of Acupuncture.* Edinburgh: Churchill Livingstone.

Hicks, A., Hicks, J. and Mole, P. (2004) *Five Element Constitutional Acupuncture.* Edinburgh: Churchill Livingstone.

Klonoff-Cohen, H., Lam-Kruglick, P. and Gonzalez, C. (2003) 'Effects of maternal and paternal alcohol consumption on the success rates of in vitro fertilization and gamete intrafallopian transfer.' *Fertility and Sterility 79.*

Larre, C. and Rochat de la Vallee, E. (1992) *The Heart Master and Triple Heater.* Cambridge: Monkey Press.

Larre, C. and Rochat de la Vallee, E. (1996) *The Seven Emotions.* Cambridge: Monkey Press.

Larre, C. and Rochat de la Vallee, E. (2003) *The Extraordinary Fu.* London: Monkey Press.

Lifang, Q. and Garvey, M. (2001) 'The location and function of the San Jiao.' *Journal of Chinese Medicine 65.*

Maciocia, G. (1989) *The Foundations of Chinese Medicine.* Edinburgh: Churchill Livingstone.

Maciocia, G. (2005) *The Foundations of Chinese Medicine (second edition).* Edinburgh: Churchill Livingstone.

Maciocia, G. (2006) *The Channels of Acupuncture.* Edinburgh: Churchill Livingstone.

Maciocia, G. (2009) *The Psyche in Chinese Medicine.* Edinburgh: Churchill Livingstone.

Montakab, H. (2014) *Acupuncture Point and Channel Energetics.* München: Keiner.

Rochat de la Vallee, E. (2009) *Wu Xing.* Cambridge: Monkey Press.

Rose, K. and Huan, Z. H. (2001) *A Brief History of Qi.* Brookline: Paradigm.

Troyan, S. D. (2004) *Medieval Rhetoric: A Casebook.* London: Routledge.

Vangermeersch, L. and Sun, P. L. (1994) *Bi Syndromes.* Brussels: SATAS.

Wang, J. Y. and Robertson, J. (2008) *Applied Channel Theory in Chinese Medicine.* Seattle: Eastland Press.

Wilcox, L. (2006) 'What is an acu-moxa point?' *Journal of Chinese Medicine 80.*

World Health Organization (1991) *A Proposed Standard International Acupuncture Nomenclature: Report of a WHO Scientific Group.* Geneva: World Health Organization. Available at http://apps.who.int/medicinedocs/en/d/Jh2947e/4.5.html, accessed on 6 April 2016.

Worsley, J. R. (1990) *Traditional Acupuncture: Volume II – Traditional Diagnosis.* Leamington Spa: The Traditional College of Acupuncture.

The following Chinese classical texts have been quoted from in this book:

Dao De Jing

Huainanzi

Huang Di Nei Jing – Ling Shu

Huang Di Nei Jing – Su Wen

Nanjing

Qi Jing Ba Mai Kao

Sanyin Jiyi Bingzheng Fanglun

Shang Han Lun

Taiyi Jinhua Zongzhi

Xue Zheng Lun

FURTHER READING

Aureroche, B., Gervais, G., Auteroche, M., Navailh, P. and Toui-Kan, E. (1983) *Acupuncture and Moxibustion*. Edinburgh: Churchill Livingstone.

Beinfeld, H. and Korngold, E. (1991) *Between Heaven and Earth*. New York: Ballantine Books.

Bromley, M., Freeman, D., Hext, A. and Hill, S. (Trans.) (2010) *Jing Shen*. London: Monkey Press.

Ching, N. (2005) *Akupunktur og Sygdomsbehandling*. Copenhagen: Klitroseforlaget.

Ching, N. (2009) *Kunsten at Diagnosticere*. Copenhagen: Klitroseforlaget.

Clavey, P. (2003) *Fluid Physiology and Pathology in Traditional Chinese Medicine*. Edinburgh: Churchill Livingstone.

Deadman, P. (2001) 'Needle technique.' *Journal of Chinese Medicine 14*.

Deadman, P. (2001) 'Needle technique.' *Journal of Chinese Medicine 15*.

Deadman, P. and Al-Khafaji, M. (1998) *A Manual of Acupuncture*. Hove: Journal of Chinese Medicine Publications.

Dechar, L. (2006) *Five Spirits*. New York: Lantern Books.

Ellis, A., Wiseman, N. and Boss, K. (1989) *Grasping the Wind*. Brookline: Paradigm.

Feit, R. and Zmeiwski, P. (1989) *Acumoxa Therapy: Vols 1 and 2*. Brookline: Paradigm.

Feng, G. F. and English, J. (Trans.) (1973) *Tao Te Ching*. London: Wildwood House.

Focks, C. (2008) *Atlas of Acupuncture*. Edinburgh: Churchill Livingstone.

Golding, R. (2008) *The Complete Stems and Branches*. Edinburgh: Churchill Livingstone.

Hicks, A., Hicks, J. and Mole, P. (2004) *Five Element Constitutional Acupuncture*. Edinburgh: Churchill Livingstone.

Johns, R. (1996) *The Art of Acupuncture Techniques*. Berkeley: North Atlantic Books.

Kaptchuk, T. (1983) *Chinese Medicine: The Web That Has No Weaver*. London: Rider.

Larre, C. (1994) *The Way of Heaven*. Cambridge: Monkey Press.

Larre, C. and Rochat de la Vallee, E. (1989) *The Kidneys*. Cambridge: Monkey Press.

Larre, C. and Rochat de la Vallee, E. (1989) *The Lung*. Cambridge: Monkey Press.

Larre, C. and Rochat de la Vallee, E. (1990) *The Spleen and Stomach*. Cambridge: Monkey Press.

Larre, C. and Rochat de la Vallee, E. (1991) *The Heart*. Cambridge: Monkey Press.

Larre, C. and Rochat de la Vallee, E. (1992) *The Heart Master and Triple Heater*. Cambridge: Monkey Press.

Larre, C. and Rochat de la Vallee, E. (1994) *The Liver*. Cambridge: Monkey Press.

Larre, C. and Rochat de la Vallee, E. (1995) *Rooted in Spirit*. Barrytown: Station Hill.

Larre, C. and Rochat de la Vallee, E. (1996) *The Seven Emotions*. Cambridge: Monkey Press.

Larre, C. and Rochat de la Vallee, E. (1997) *The Extraordinary Meridians*. Cambridge: Monkey Press.

Larre, C. and Rochat de la Vallee, E. (1999) *The Essence, Spirit, Blood and Qi*. Cambridge: Monkey Press.

Larre, C. and Rochat de la Vallee, E. (2003) *The Extraordinary Fu*. Cambridge: Monkey Press.

Larre, C. and Rochat de la Vallee, E. (2003) *The Secret Treatise of the Spiritual Orchard*. Cambridge: Monkey Press.

Lifang, Q. and Garvey, M. (2001) 'The location and function of the San Jiao.' *Journal of Chinese Medicine 65*.

Maciocia, G. (2005) *The Foundations of Chinese Medicine (second edition)*. Edinburgh: Churchill Livingstone.

Maciocia, G. (2006) *The Channels of Acupuncture*. Edinburgh: Churchill Livingstone.

Maciocia, G. (2009) *The Psyche in Chinese Medicine*. Edinburgh: Churchill Livingstone.

Major, J., Queen, S., Mejer, A. S., Roth, H. D., Puett, M. and Murray, J. (Trans.) (2010) *The Huainanzi*. Columbia: Columbia University Press.

Maoshing, N. (1995) *The Yellow Emperor's Classic of Medicine*. Boston: Shambhala.

Montakab, H. (2014) *Acupuncture Point and Channel Energetics*. München: Keiner.

Rochat de la Vallee, E. (2006) *A Study of Qi*. Cambridge: Monkey Press.

Rochat de la Vallee, E. (2006) *Yin and Yang*. Cambridge: Monkey Press.

Rochat de la Vallee, E. (2007) *Essential Woman*. Cambridge: Monkey Press.

Rochat de la Vallee, E. (2009) *Wu Xing*. Cambridge: Monkey Press.

Rose, K. and Zhang, Y. H. (2001) *A Brief History of Qi*. Brookline: Paradigm.

Unschuld, P. (1986) *Nan-Ching – The Classic of Difficult Issues*. Berkeley: University of California Press.

Unschuld, P. and Tessenow, H. (2011) *Huang Di Nei Jing – Su Wen*. Berkeley: University of California Press.

Vangermeersch, L. and Sun, P. L. (1994) *Bi Syndromes*. Brussels: SATAS.

Wang, J. Y. and Robertson, J. (2008) *Applied Channel Theory in Chinese Medicine*. Seattle: Eastland Press.

Wilcox, L. (2006) 'What is an acu-moxa point?' *Journal of Chinese Medicine 80*.

Worsley, J. R. (1990) *Traditional Acupuncture: Volume II – Traditional Diagnosis*. Leamington Spa: The Traditional College of Acupuncture.

Wu, J. N. (2002) *Ling Shu or The Spiritual Pivot*. Honolulu: University of Hawaii Press.

Yi Jing Yi Dazhuan.

GLOSSARY

A-shi **points**	Spots on the body that are sore on palpation or are reactive.
Back-*shu* **points**	Back transport points. Category of acupuncture points, all of which are located on the Urinary Bladder channel. These acupuncture points can transport *qi* directly to their same-name internal organ.
Bao	Envelope, wrapping. The Uterus; the place where the semen is stored; the space between the Kidneys.
Bao luo	The channel that connects the Kidneys and the Uterus.
Bao mai	The channel that connects the Heart and the Uterus.
Bei	Sorrow, sadness, melancholy.
Ben	Root or cause.
Bi	Painful blockage of channel *qi*.
Biao	Branch or manifestation.
Cou li	The space between the skin and muscles; spaces in the tissue.
Cun	Chinese body measurement unit.
Da qi	'Big' *qi* or air *qi*.
Fu	Hollow organ.
Gao	Fatty tissues.
Gu qi	Food or basis *qi*. *Gu qi* is an antecedent and the foundation of *xue* and *zong qi*.
Huang	Membranes.
*Hui-***gathering points**	*Hui* can be translated as 'meeting', 'collecting' or 'gathering'. It is a place where certain energies gather or meet.
Hun	The ethereal spirit. The *shen* aspect of the Liver.
Jiao	Space or burner. There are three *jiao* – *san jiao*. Some people define the three *jiao* as being the organs that are located in that part of the body. Others define the three *jiao* as being the cavity around these organs. A third definition is that *san jiao* is all the spaces in the body, i.e. that *san jiao* can be defined as being the following: the space between the organs; the spaces between connective tissue and the skin; and the spaces in the tissue itself and between the individual cells.
Jin	Thin, light body fluids.
Jin	Tendons.
Jing	Essence or the innate *qi* inherited from the parents. The form of *qi* in the body which is the most *yin*.
Jing	Shock, fright, terror.
Jing luo	Channels and collaterals.
Jinye	Body fluids.
Jueyin	Terminal *yin*. Liver and Pericardium.
Kong	Fear.
Le	Joy.
*Luo-***connecting points**	*Luo*-connecting points, are the place on a channel where the *luo*-connecting vessel branches away from the primary channel.
Mingmen	Gate of fire. The source of all *yang qi* in the body.

Mu-collecting points	Category of acupuncture points that are almost exclusively located on the front of the body. A *mu*-collecting point is the place where an organ's *qi* collects.
Nu	Anger.
Po	Corporeal spirit. *Shen* aspect of the Lung.
Qi	*Qi* is often translated as energy or bio-energy, but it is a very narrow definition of something that is very encompassing and vast. *Qi* is the fundamental substance or energetic matter of the universe. At the same time, *qi* is the energy or the potential that creates all the movement and all change in the universe. In the body *qi* is the sum of all the vital substances and of all physiological activity in the body. At the same time, there are specific forms of *qi* in the body that are further differentiated from each other.
Qi ji	*Qi* mechanism, *qi* dynamic.
Rou	Muscle, meat, flesh.
Shan	*Shan* can have three definitions. It can be an organ or tissue that protrudes or has sunk from its position, for example a hernia in Western medicine. It can be extreme abdominal pain when there is concurrent urinary difficulty or constipation. Finally, it may be disorders that relate to the external genitalia.
Shaoyang	Lesser *yang*. *San jiao* and Gall Bladder.
Shaoyin	Lesser *yin*. Heart and Kidneys.
Shen	*Shen* encompasses concepts such as mind, awareness, consciousness, vitality, spirit. *Shen* is the sum of all the five organs' *shen* aspects, whilst at the same time being the specific *shen* aspect of the Heart. *Shen* is the form of *qi* in the body that is most *yang*.
Shi	Full, excess or surplus.
Shu-transport points	Category of five points on each channel. The five *shu*-transport points are *jing*-well, *ying*-spring, *shu*-stream, *jing*-river and *he*-sea.
Si	Worry, speculation, pensiveness.
Taiyang	Greater *yang*. Urinary Bladder and Small Intestine.
Taiyin	Greater *yin*. Spleen and Lung.
TCM	Traditional Chinese Medicine.
Tian gui	Heavenly or celestial water. Menstrual blood; semen. Created when *jing* is transformed by Heart Fire.
Wei qi	Defensive or protective *qi*. The aspect of *zhen qi* that flows under the skin. *Wei qi* moistens and warms the skin, whilst protecting the body against invasions of *xie qi*.
Wu xing	Five Phases, Five Movements or Five Elements.
Xi	Happiness, joy, ecstasy.
Xi-cleft points	Category of acupuncture points. *Xi*-cleft points are the place where *qi* gathers before plunging deeper into the channel.
Xie qi	Evil, perverse or pathogenic *qi*. It is a pathological form of *qi*.
Xu	Emptiness, vacuum, a lack of. Often translated as deficiency.
Xue	Blood. *Xue* is a more physical form of *qi*. *Xue* is more than just blood in Western physiology. *Xue* nourishes and moisturises the body. *Xue* also nourishes and anchors *shen*.
Yang	One of the two opposing, but at the same time complementary, forces in the universe.
Yangming	*Yang* brightness. Stomach and Large Intestine.
Ye	The denser and more turbid aspect of the body fluids.
Yi	*Shen* aspect of the Spleen. *Yi* can be defined as our mental faculties, as our intellectual focus and as intention.
Yin	One of the two opposing, but at the same time complementary, forces in the universe.

Ying qi	Nourishing *qi*. Nourishes both *zangfu* organs and the whole body. *Ying qi* flows together with *xue* in the channels.
You	Oppression, anguish, restraint.
Yuan qi	Original *qi*. *Yuan qi* is *jing* that has been transformed into *qi*.
Yuan-source **points**	*Yuan* source points are the place on a channel where *yuan qi* enters the channel and the place where *yuan qi* can be accessed.
Yun hua	Transportation and transformation.
Zang	Solid organ.
Zangfu	Internal organs.
Zhen qi	True *qi*, formed when *zong qi* is transformed by *yuan qi*. *Zhen qi* has a *yin* and a *yang* aspect, which are *wei qi* and *ying qi* respectively.
Zheng qi	Correct, upright or healthy *qi*. *Zheng qi* is the sum of the body's anti-pathogenic *qi*. The term is normally only us ed as a contrast to *xie qi*.
Zhi	*Shen* aspect of the Kidneys. Determination, willpower.
Zong qi	Basis, ancestral, inherited or gathering *qi*. *Zong qi* is generated when air inhaled by the Lung is combined with *gu qi*.

Index